Textbook of
VETERINARY
PHYSIOLOGY

Textbook of
VETERINARY PHYSIOLOGY

JAMES G. CUNNINGHAM, DVM, PhD

Associate Professor
Departments of Physiology and of Small Animal Clinical Sciences
College of Veterinary Medicine
Michigan State University
East Lansing, Michigan

W. B. SAUNDERS COMPANY
Harcourt Brace Jovanovich, Inc.

Philadelphia   London   Toronto   Montreal   Sydney   Tokyo

W. B. SAUNDERS COMPANY
Harcourt Brace Jovanovich, Inc.

The Curtis Center
Independence Square West
Philadelphia, PA 19106

Library of Congress Cataloging-in-Publication Data

Textbook of veterinary physiology / editor, James G.
Cunningham.

   p.   cm.

Includes bibliographical references.

ISBN 0–7216–2306–9

1. Veterinary physiology.   I. Cunningham, James G.
   SF768.T49 1992   636.089'2—dc20   91–11374

Editor: Linda Mills
Developmental Editor: Lawrence J. McGrew
Designer: Terri Siegel
Production Manager: Ken Neimeister
Manuscript Editor: Pam Wight
Illustrator: Batvin Kramer
Mechanical Illustrator: Megan Costello
Illustration Specialist: Cecilia Roberts
Indexer: Kathy Garcia

TEXTBOOK OF VETERINARY PHYSIOLOGY   ISBN 0–7216–2306–9

Printed in the United States of America.

Last digit is the print number: 9   8   7   6   5   4   3   2   1

CONTRIBUTORS

JAMES G. CUNNINGHAM, DVM, PhD

Associate Professor, Departments of Physiology and of Small Animal Clinical Sciences, College of Veterinary Medicine, Michigan State University, East Lansing, Michigan
NEUROPHYSIOLOGY (Chapters 2–16)

STEVEN HEIDEMANN, PhD

Professor, Departments of Physiology and of Microbiology and Public Health, Michigan State University, East Lansing, Michigan
THE CELL (Chapter 1)

THOMAS HERDT, DVM

Associate Professor, Department of Large Animal Clinical Sciences, College of Veterinary Medicine, Michigan State University, East Lansing, Michigan
GASTROINTESTINAL PHYSIOLOGY/METABOLISM (Chapters 26–31)

N. EDWARD ROBINSON, BVetMed, MRCVS, PhD

Professor, Department of Physiology, Matilda R. Wilson Professor, Department of Large Animal Clinical Sciences, College of Veterinary Medicine, Michigan State University, East Lansing, Michigan
RESPIRATORY FUNCTION (Chapters 43–48)
HOMEOSTASIS (Chapters 49–51)

GEORGE H. STABENFELDT, DVM, PhD

Professor, Department of Reproduction, School of Veterinary Medicine, University of California, Davis, Davis, California
ENDOCRINOLOGY (Chapters 32 and 33)
REPRODUCTION/LACTATION (Chapters 34–38)

ROBERT B. STEPHENSON, PhD

Associate Professor, Department of Physiology, Michigan State University, East Lansing, Michigan
CARDIOVASCULAR PHYSIOLOGY (Chapters 17–25)

JILL W. VERLANDER, DVM

Division of Nephrology, Hypertension and Transplantation, College of Medicine, University of Florida, Gainesville, Florida
RENAL PHYSIOLOGY (Chapters 39–42)

PREFACE

Physiology is the study of the normal functions of the body—the study of the body's various molecules, cells, and organ systems, and the inter-relationships among them. Because the study of medicine is the study of the abnormal functions of the body, it is essential to understand normal physiology if one is to understand the mechanisms of disease. It is for this reason that physiology and other important sciences basic to medicine are introduced first in the veterinary curriculum.

Physiology is a vast subject, and veterinary students are too busy to learn all that is known about it. We have, therefore, made an effort to limit the concepts presented in this book to those germane to the practice of veterinary medicine. All of the authors are either physiologists and also veterinarians, or physiologists who have had extensive discussions about content with veterinary clinicians.

This book is designed for first-year veterinary students. Its goal is to introduce the student to those principles and concepts of physiology pertinent to the practice of veterinary medicine. Other goals are to introduce the reader to physiopathology and clinical problem-solving techniques and to help the reader understand the relationship between physiology and the practice of veterinary medicine.

This book is designed to be as student-friendly as possible. New concepts in the text are introduced by a declarative statement designed to summarize the essential point. This format also helps the reader survey the chapter or review for an exam. These declarative statements are also listed at the beginning of each chapter as an outline.

Chapters include one or more Clinical Correlations at the end. These are designed to show the reader how knowledge of physiology is applied to the diagnosis and treatment of veterinary patients. They also provide the student with an additional way to think through the principles and concepts presented, and they can serve as a basis for classroom case discussions.

In most chapters, several practice questions and answers are included as another method for students to review the book's content. The brief bibliography for each chapter is designed to lead the reader to more advanced textbooks, assuming that most veterinary students are too busy to read original literature. I welcome suggestions of ways to improve this book in subsequent editions.

I want to thank Dr. Bari Olivier for his help in developing the Clinical Correlations in the cardiovascular physiology chapters. I also want to thank our two illustrators, Bud Kramer and Teri Sexton, and Mary Herdt for her patience and skill as a typist. Finally, I want to thank several members of the W. B. Saunders Company staff for their guidance in what was, for me, a new professional challenge.

JIM CUNNINGHAM

CONTENTS

STEVEN HEIDEMANN

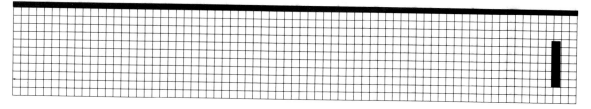

THE CELL

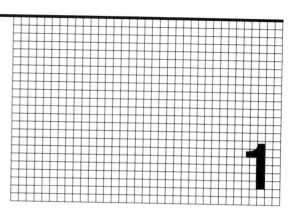

The Molecular and Cellular Basis of Physiological Regulation

1. All physiological change is mediated by proteins
2. Protein function depends on protein shape and shape changes
3. A series of enzymatic reactions converts tyrosine into the signaling molecules dopamine, norepinephrine, and epinephrine
4. Muscle contraction and its initiation and cessation depend on the binding specificity and allosteric properties of proteins
5. Biological membranes are a mosaic of proteins embedded in a phospholipid bilayer

TRANSPORT

1. Only small, uncharged molecules and oily molecules can penetrate biomembranes without the aid of proteins
2. Molecules move spontaneously from regions of high free energy to regions of lower free energy
3. Important transport equations summarize the contributions of the various driving forces
4. Starling's hypothesis relates fluid flow across the capillaries to hydrostatic pressure and osmotic pressure
5. Membrane proteins that serve the triple functions of selective transport, catalysis, and coupling can pump ions and molecules to regions of higher free energy
6. Many membrane proteins selectively facilitate the transport of ions/molecules from high to low electrochemical potential
7. Passive transport of K^+ across the plasma membrane creates an electrical potential
8. Spatial organization of active and passive transport proteins enables material to pass completely through the cell
9. Membrane fusion allows for a combination of compartmentalization and transport of material

INFORMATION TRANSMISSION AND TRANSDUCTION

1. External signaling molecules bind to receptors on the surface of cells, causing a "second message" to be sent to the cytoplasm of the cell
2. Specific physiological information is inherent in the receptor/ligand complex, not in the hormone/neurotransmitter molecule
3. Ca^{2+} transport across plasma and intracellular membranes is an important second messenger
4. Cyclic AMP is produced by activation of a membrane-bound enzyme in response to binding of hormone/neurotransmitter to receptors
5. The receptor-mediated hydrolysis of a rare phospholipid of the plasma membrane produces two different second messengers with different actions
6. Steroid hormones interact with receptors within the cell, not with cell surface receptors

Physiology is the study of the regulation of change within organisms, in this case higher animals. Our understanding of physiology has changed dramatically in the past 20 years as a result of insight into the molecular basis of biological regulation. This chapter summarizes our current understanding of the molecular and cellular basis of that regulation. Most of the principles in this chapter apply to all animal cells. The approach taken is one of functional molecular anatomy. That is, the molecular structure of the cell is examined with particular emphasis on the physiological function, in the intact animal, of the molecules and supramolecular structures. Only those aspects of cell function that illuminate the medical physiology of the higher animals are discussed. The reader is referred to the list of texts at the end of this chapter for more complete coverage of the cell. Some review of basic concepts and vocabulary is presented. However, the discussion assumes that the reader is familiar with the cell and its constituent molecules as presented in courses in general biology and an undergraduate course in biochemistry.

All Physiological Change Is Mediated by Proteins

All physiological change is mediated by a single class of polymeric macromolecules (large molecules), the proteins. Protein function can be subdivided into a number of categories: catalysis, reaction coupling, transport, and structure.

Catalysis is the ability to markedly increase the rate of a chemical reaction without altering the equilibrium of the reaction. The vast ma-jority of biochemical reactions occur at a physiologically useful rate only because of protein catalysts, called *enzymes*. Examples of enzymatic catalysis in the synthesis of a class of physiological regulator molecules, catecholamines, are given later in this chapter.

In *reaction coupling*, two reactions are joined together with the transfer of energy. Energy from a spontaneous reaction (similar to water flowing downhill) is funneled to a nonspontaneous reaction (e.g., sawing wood) so that the sum of the two reactions is spontaneous. That is, the energy liberated by the "downhill" reaction is used to drive the "uphill" reaction. This is the basic function of a motor; i.e., the "downhill" burning of gasoline is coupled with the "uphill" movement of the car. The ability of proteins to couple spontaneous and nonspontaneous reactions allows cells to be chemical motors, using chemical energy to do various jobs of work. One such job of work, the contraction of striated muscle, is discussed later with particular emphasis on the proteins involved.

Proteins provide a pathway for the *transport* of most molecules and all ions into and out of the cell. Transport and transport proteins are discussed more fully after a discussion of the lipid bilayer membrane, the major obstacle to transport.

Proteins that form filaments and that glue cells to each other and to their environment are responsible for the *structure* and organization of cells and of multicellular assemblies (i.e., the tissues and organs of animals). The internal structure of the muscle cell, as well as its ability to do work, is due to the properties of the muscle proteins discussed later.

Catalysis, coupling, transport, and structural functions can be combined on individual protein molecules. As will become apparent, such multifunctional proteins carry out many important physiological functions. Also important is the fact that any of these protein functions can be used to carry information within the cell. Information can be defined as any difference that makes a difference or, more simply, any difference that regulates something. Changes (differences) in enzymatic activity, ion transport, or adhesion to the environment can all "make a difference," signaling the cell that conditions have changed and triggering an appropriate response.

Protein Function Depends on Protein Shape and Shape Changes

Protein function is founded on two molecular characteristics: (1) proteins can bind to other molecules very specifically; and (2) proteins change shape, which in turn alters their binding properties and their function. Protein's binding specificity is the result of their complex three-dimensional structure. Grooves or indentations on the surface of protein molecules, called *binding sites,* permit specific interactions with a molecule of a complementary shape, called the *ligand.* This complementary shape mechanism underlying binding is similar to the shape interaction between a lock and key. Several aspects of the lock and key analogy are worth noting: only a small part of the protein (lock) is engaged in binding; the binding is very specific; and small changes in the shape of the binding site (keyhole) or the shape of the ligand (key) can cause major changes in protein (lock) behavior. Like the lock and key, the complementary shape interaction serves a recognition function; only those molecules with the right shape affect protein function. Unlike the majority of locks, however, proteins frequently have multiple binding sites for multiple ligands.

Thus, the three-dimensional shape of a protein, its *conformation,* determines protein function. Protein shape is due to hydrogen bonding between the amino acids that compose the protein and to the hydrophobic (water-hating) and hydrophilic (water-loving) properties of the constituent amino acids. Hydrogen bonds stabilize the positions of amino acid pairs in the polypeptide (protein) chain. Hydrophobic regions tend to congregate in the middle of a protein away from water, whereas hydrophilic amino acids tend to be found on the protein's outer surface interacting with the abundant cellular water. These same forces are used to hold the ligand in the protein binding site. The position of the ligand in the binding site is stabilized by hydrogen bonds between the ligand and the amino acid side groups of the binding site, just as hydrogen bonds within the polypeptide chain stabilize the shape of the polypeptide. Precisely because the same forces are responsible for the shape of the protein and for its binding properties, shape influences binding and, in turn, binding can influence protein shape. The ability of proteins to change shape is called *allostery* (Greek— other shape).

Allosteric changes in protein conformation arise in three general ways, summarized in Figure 1–1. One way (Fig. 1–1A), just mentioned, is that a protein changes shape depending on which ligands are bound at particular binding sites. The sequence—specific binding→ protein shape change→ change in protein binding properties and protein function→ this change regulates something—is a common molecular mechanism underlying physiological control. This method involves no alteration in the covalent structure of the protein. However, a second method (Fig. 1–1B) of producing conformational changes occurs as a result of a covalent modification of one or more of the amino acid side groups of the protein. By far the most common such change is the covalent addition (esterification) of a phosphate group to the —OH group on the side chain of serine, threonine, or tyrosine residues in the protein. Because the phosphate group is highly charged, phosphorylation of a protein alters hydrogen bonding and other electrostatic interactions within the protein chain, altering its conformation and functional properties. In a third method, some physiologically important proteins change shape in response to the electrical field surrounding the protein (Fig. 1–1C). These respond to a voltage change by altering the position of charged amino acids, thus altering protein shape.

The significance of binding specificity and allostery can be better appreciated with two examples of their role in physiological function. The first example is the role of enzymes in synthesizing three structurally similar signaling molecules. This example shows how binding specificity is important in catalytic function and how allostery underlies the regulation of the synthesis. The second example is more complex, their role in the contraction

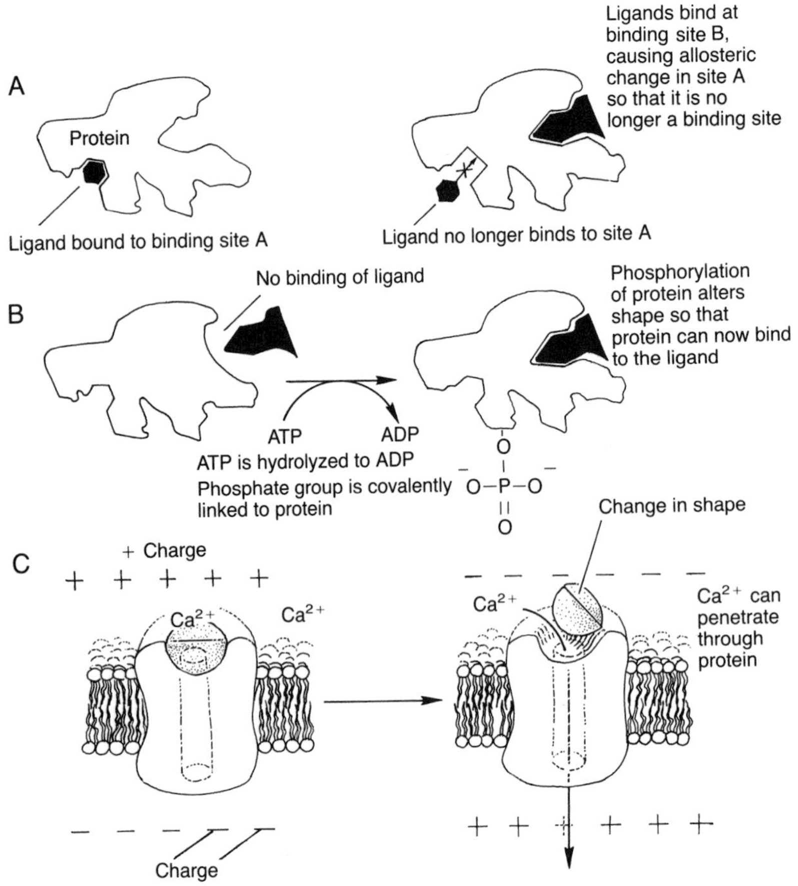

A

Protein

Ligand bound to binding site A

Ligands bind at binding site B, causing allosteric change in site A so that it is no longer a binding site

Ligand no longer binds to site A

B

No binding of ligand

Phosphorylation of protein alters shape so that protein can now bind to the ligand

ATP   ADP
ATP is hydrolyzed to ADP
Phosphate group is covalently linked to protein

$$O-P-O$$

Change in shape

C

+ Charge

+ + + + +

Ca^{2+} Ca^{2+}

Ca^{2+} Ca^{2+} can penetrate through protein

− − − −

Charge

Figure 1–1. Three common mechanisms of allosteric shape change in proteins. (*A*) Ligand binding. Ligand binding to an allosteric site (site B) on a protein changes the protein's conformation such that binding site A is altered; ligand no longer binds at site A because of the binding event at site B. (*B*) Phosphorylation. Addition of a phosphate group to a serine, threonine, or tyrosine residue of a protein alters the protein's conformation, changing its binding characteristics. Shown here is a hypothethical example in which phosphorylation activates an otherwise inactive protein. Some proteins inactivate by this mechanism. (*C*) Voltage-dependent proteins. The conformation of some proteins, particularly ion channels, is altered by the electrical field surrounding the protein. Shown here is the opening (activation) of a voltage-dependent, gated Ca^{2+} channel when the membrane depolarizes.

of muscle. The contraction of muscle shows how proteins can exploit the basic properties of specific binding and allosteric shape change to do more than one job of work at the same time; muscle proteins serve a structural role, serve a catalytic function, and couple the "downhill" hydrolysis of adenosine triphosphate (ATP) to do mechanical work, the "uphill" lifting of weight.

A Series of Enzymatic Reactions Converts Tyrosine into the Signaling Molecules Dopamine, Norepinephrine, and Epinephrine

Figure 1–2 is a diagram of the series of reactions by which the amino acid tyrosine is converted into three different signaling molecules: dopamine, a brain neurotransmitter; norepinephrine, a neurotransmitter of the peripheral autonomic nervous system; and epinephrine, an autonomic neurotransmitter and hormone. Dopamine, norepinephrine, and epinephrine share a similar structure. All con-

tain a phenyl (benzene) ring with two hydroxyl groups (i.e., catechol) and an amine group (hence catecholamines). They are among the large number of molecules that function as neurotransmitters. That is, the electrically coded information sent along nerve cells causes the release of a chemical, the neurotransmitter, at the terminal of the neuron, which is next to a target cell such as another nerve, a muscle, or an endocrine cell. The electrically encoded information of the nerve is transmitted to the target cell by the binding of the neurotransmitter to proteins on the surface of the target cell. Obviously, proper neurotransmitter synthesis is crucial to nervous function and physiological regulation.

In the first step of catecholamine biosynthesis, tyrosine binds to the enzyme tyrosine hydroxylase, which catalyzes the addition of another hydroxyl group to the phenyl group to form dihydroxyphenylalanine, nearly always called *dopa*. This hydroxyl group alters the enzyme–ligand interaction; the key no longer fits the keyhole. Dopa is released from

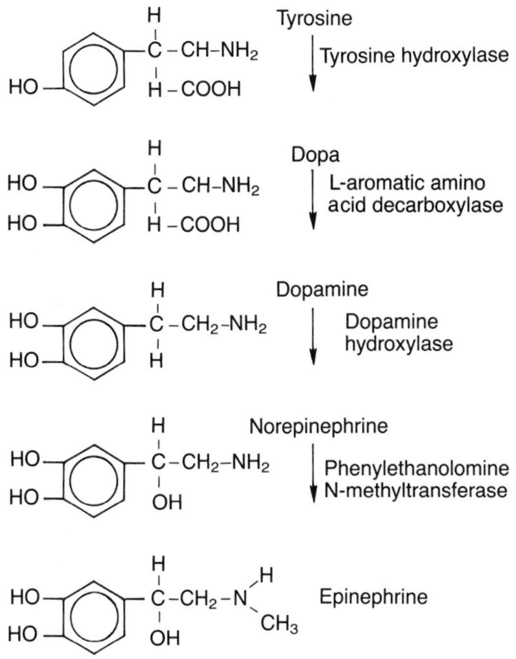

Figure 1–2. Epinephrine biosynthetic pathway. The amino acid tyrosine is metabolized to the neurotransmitters dopamine, norepinephrine, and epinephrine. The diagram shows the names and structural formulae for each compound in the path and the names of the enzymes that catalyze each reaction.

the tyrosine hydroxylase and is then bound by another enzyme, L-aromatic amino acid decarboxylase. As the name implies, this enzyme catalyzes the removal of the carboxyl group, converting dopa to dopamine. Dopamine is converted into norepinephrine by the activity of dopamine hydroxylase, which adds another hydroxyl group on the 2 carbon tail of dopamine. Finally, addition of a methyl group to the amino nitrogen by phenylethanolamine *N*-methyl transferase gives rise to epinephrine (also called adrenalin). Note the binding specificity of the enzymes: whereas the catecholamine structures are all similar to one another, different enzymes bind each one; e.g., epinephrine does not bind to dopamine hydroxylase.

The allosteric properties of one enzyme in this pathway provide an example of physiological regulation. Certain hormones and neurotranmitters cause the phosphorylation of tyrosine hydroxylase, the first enzyme in the pathway, increasing its activity. That is, phosphorylation of the enzyme increases the rate at which it catalyzes the conversion of tyrosine to dopa. Because this step is the slowest in

the pathway, an increase in the activity of this protein increases the net rate of synthesis of all the catecholamines. Regulated decreases in the rate of catecholamine synthesis are achieved by a different allosteric mechanism—binding of end products to the enzyme. Dopamine, norepinephrine, and epinephrine can all bind to tyrosine hydroxylase at a site different than the site for tyrosine. These binding events inhibit the enzymatic activity. The inhibition of the pathway by its own end products makes this a classic case of allosteric control called *end product inhibition*. Many substances regulate their own synthesis by inhibiting an initial enzyme in the pathway. If the cell has enough end product, these products inhibit further synthesis by allosteric changes in the enzyme. This is an example of the following sequence: specific binding→ protein shape change→ change in protein binding properties and protein function→ this change regulates something.

Muscle Contraction and Its Initiation and Cessation Depend on the Binding Specificity and Allosteric Properties of Proteins

There are three types of muscle tissue in vertebrates: skeletal muscle, responsible for the animal's ability to move; cardiac muscle, a muscle type found only in the heart but structurally similar to skeletal muscle; and smooth muscle, which surrounds hollow organs such as blood vessels, gut, and uterus. All three produce tensile force by contracting and shortening the length of the muscle. All three produce contractile force by the binding and the allosteric properties of two proteins, actin and myosin. Starting and stopping the contraction process depends on two additional proteins in skeletal and cardiac muscle, troponin and tropomyosin. Contraction initiation and cessation in smooth muscle depends on a different system with different proteins and is discussed later in this chapter.

Myosin is a large protein, shaped rather like a two-headed golf club. The tail of the myosin molecule corresponds to the shaft of the golf club, and there are two knobs at one end of the tail that, like golf clubs, are called heads. Myosin tails bind specifically to other myosin tails, forming bipolar aggregates called *thick filaments* (Fig. 1–3). Myosin heads specifically bind ATP and another muscle protein, *actin*. Actin binds to itself to form long, thin fila-

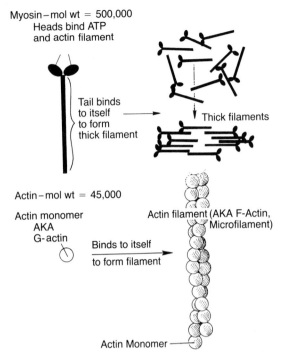

Myosin—mol wt = 500,000
Heads bind ATP
and actin filament

Tail binds
to itself
to form
thick filament

Thick filaments

Actin—mol wt = 45,000

Actin monomer
AKA
G-actin

Actin filament (AKA F-Actin,
Microfilament)

Binds to itself
to form filament

Actin Monomer

Figure 1–3. The assembly of myosin and actin to form filamentous structure. Myosin tails aggregate with one another to form a thick filament, a substructure of striated muscle. Actin monomers (G-actin) are a single polypeptide chain forming a globular protein that can bind to other actin monomers to form actin filament, also called microfilaments. The actin filament is the basic structure of striated muscle thin filaments; thin filaments have troponin and tropomyosin as part of their structure also.

ments, called *thin filaments* in muscle and called *microfilaments* or *F-actin* (filamentous actin) in other cell types (see Fig. 1–3). Actin filaments play an important architectural role

in all animal cells. Animal cells depend on actin filaments for their shape; the actin filaments provide strong threads that can be tied together in various ways to form thick bundles or woven networks. These actin bundles and actin networks are used to support the cell in particular shapes, like ropes holding up the woven fabric of a circus tent.

In muscle, the interaction of myosin, ATP, and actin to produce contraction and force is shown in Figure 1–4.

Step A: ATP binds to a myosin head; in this conformation myosin has little ability to bind to actin.

Step B: An enzymatic activity associated with the myosin head (an ATPase) rapidly causes a partial hydrolysis of ATP to adenosine diphosphate (ADP) and inorganic phosphate (P_i), both of which stay bound to the myosin. With ADP and P_i bound, myosin has a slightly different shape that is able to bind to nearby actin filaments.

Step C: When myosin binds to actin, called *cross-bridging*, the myosin head couples the complete hydrolysis of ATP to a forceful flexing of the head. This allosteric change causes the actin filament to slide past the thick filament. This sliding puts the actin filament under tension, which in turn causes the muscle to contract (shorten) against the load of the muscle (i.e., lifting a weight or pumping out blood). *All muscle contraction depends on sliding of actin and myosin filaments.* This same allosteric change of myosin also alters myosin binding properties so that it releases the ADP and P_i.

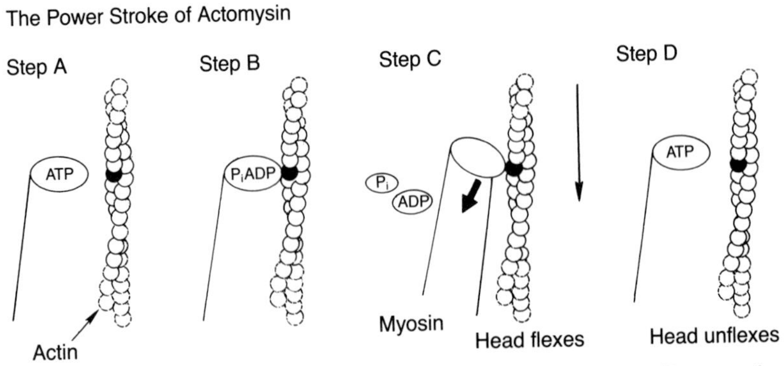

The Power Stroke of Actomysin

Figure 1–4. The power stroke of actomyosin. (*A*) The myosin head has bound to ATP. In this conformation, myosin has little affinity to bind to actin. (*B*) ATP is partially hydrolyzed to ADP and P_i; the hydrolysis is partial because the products remain bound to the myosin head. The change in what is bound to the myosin (ADP and P_i, not ATP) has the conformation of myosin so that it binds to actin with high affinity. (*C*) Hydrolysis is complete, myosin releases ADP and P_i. This change in what is bound at the myosin head causes an allosteric change in the head; it flexes. Because the myosin head is still bound to the thin filament, the flexion causes the thin filament to slide past the thick filament. (*D*) A new ATP molecule binds to the myosin head; as for Step A, myosin had little affinity for actin in this state, and the head releases from the thin filament and unflexes.

Step A

ATP

Actin

Step B

P_iADP

Step C

P_i
ADP

Myosin

Head flexes

Step D

ATP

Head unflexes

Step D: The binding of a new ATP molecule to the myosin head again causes myosin to change shape, the head unflexes and loses its affinity for actin, releasing the cross-bridge, and the cycle can start over. *Rigor mortis* of dead animals is due to a lack of new ATP to bind to myosin heads. In the absence of ATP, myosin heads remain in Step C, i.e., bound to actin. The muscle is stiff because it is completely cross-bridged together.

The actomyosin motor uses the binding and allosteric properties of proteins to (1) create structural filaments capable of withstanding and transmitting mechanical force, (2) catalyze the hydrolysis of ATP, and (3) couple the "downhill" ATP hydrolysis to the "uphill" contraction to produce force. For just the one protein, myosin, there are a number of examples of the characteristic sequence described earlier: specific binding→ protein shape change→ change in protein's binding properties and protein function→ this change makes a difference.

This system of contractile proteins requires some control so that, for example, the heart beats rhythmically and skeletal muscle contraction is coordinated. At the organismal level, muscle contraction is primarily under control by electrical stimulation from nerves or other electrically active cells (see Chapter 5). The transmission of electrical excitation to the actomyosin system is called *excitation-contraction coupling. Excitation-contraction coupling*

in all types of muscle depends on changes in intracellular Ca^{2+} concentration. In skeletal and cardiac muscle, but not smooth muscle, two additional thin filament proteins, *troponin* and *tropomyosin*, are required for this coupling. Troponin binds to tropomyosin and to Ca^{2+}. Tropomyosin is a long, thin protein that binds in the groove of the actin filament (see Fig. 1–3) in such a way that its positions, high in the groove or snuggled down deep in the groove, allow or prevent the myosin head access to the thin filament (Fig. 1–5). Excitation-contraction coupling works as follows:

Step A: Electrical excitation of a muscle cell causes an increase in the intracellular concentration of Ca^{2+}.

Step B: The additional Ca^{2+} binds to troponin, causing an allosteric change in troponin.

Step C: This change is transmitted to the tropomyosin molecule also bound to the troponin. When troponin binds Ca^{2+}, tropomyosin moves in such a way that it exposes the actin site for myosin cross-bridging. As long as troponin binds Ca^{2+}, the muscle contracts by the actomyosin cycle outlined earlier.

Step D: When the Ca^{2+} concentration drops to normal, however, troponin no longer binds Ca^{2+}. This causes tropomyosin to move up in the thin filament groove so that it again blocks the myosin-binding sites on actin. Myosin

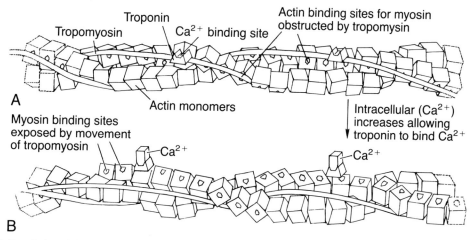

Figure 1–5. Regulation of the actomyosin ATPase and muscle contraction by Ca^{2+}. (*A*) In the absence of high concentrations of Ca^{2+}, tropomyosin sits in the groove of the actin filament to obstruct the binding sites on actin for myosin. (*B*) In the presence of higher Ca^{2+} concentrations, the ion binds to troponin, causing an allosteric change in troponin's interaction with tropomyosin. This allosteric change, in turn, changes the interaction of tropomyosin with the actin filament to expose the myosin-binding sites on actin.

heads can no longer cross-bridge, and muscle contraction stops.

As with the actomyosin motor, striated muscle regulation shows many examples of the specific binding function, e.g., the specific binding of Ca^{2+} to troponin, the binding of tropomyosin to both actin and troponin. The binding of tropomyosin to actin serves not only a regulatory role but also a structural role; the actin filament is stabilized by tropomyosin, making it less likely to disassemble into actin subunits. The change in the binding geometry of tropomyosin that directly regulates myosin access to actin is a good example of the importance of allosteric change and the following sequence: specific binding (Ca^{2+} to troponin) → protein (tropomyosin) shape change→ change in protein's binding properties and protein function → a difference in the position of tropomyosin, which regulates the actomyosin motor.

Biological Membranes Are a Mosaic of Proteins Embedded in a Phospholipid Bilayer

Before continuing the discussion of the molecular basis of physiological control, an additional factor must be introduced. This is the phospholipid bilayer of biological membranes. Phospholipids are molecules that have two long tails of hydrophobic fatty acid and a head containing a charged, hydrophilic phosphate group. Under appropriate aqueous conditions, these molecules spontaneously form an organized membrane structure containing two layers (a bilayer) of phospholipid molecules. In both layers the hydrophilic heads point outward to hydrogen bond with water, and the oily, fatty-acid tails point inward, toward one

another and away from the water. Proteins embedded in this lipid bilayer, called *intrinsic membrane proteins* or just *membrane proteins*, produce the *fluid mosaic* structure of biomembranes shown in Figure 1–6. All biological membranes share this fluid mosaic structure, whether the membrane is the outer plasma membrane separating cytoplasm from extracellular fluid or the membrane surrounding intracellular membranous organelles such as endoplasmic reticulum or lysosomes. It is called a fluid mosaic because of the mosaic of proteins among phospholipids, and because the phospholipid layer is fluid; proteins can move around and diffuse within the plane of the bilayer "like icebergs floating in a phospholipid sea" (the apt phrase of S.J. Singer, one of the originators of the model).

Biological membranes are another crucial molecular structure underlying physiological control. The basic fluid mosaic structure serves four broad functions: (1) compartmentalization, (2) selective transport, (3) information processing and transmission, and (4) organizing biochemical reactions in space.

Compartmentalization is the ability to separate and segregate different regions by composition and function. For example, the lysosome is a membranous organelle within cells that contains hydrolytic (digestive) enzymes that can potentially digest the cell. Indeed, this organelle was called the "suicide sac" by its discoverer, C. DeDuve. The lysosomal membrane compartmentalizes these potentially harmful enzymes, segregating them from the bulk cytoplasm. For example, the rigor mortis that begins shortly after death is transitory because upon death the lysosomes begin to break open, releasing their enzymes; the actomyosin cross-bridges are digested apart.

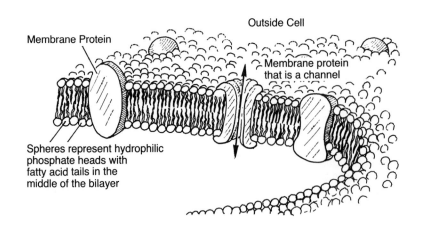

Outside Cell

Membrane Protein

Membrane protein that is a channel

Spheres represent hydrophilic phosphate heads with fatty acid tails in the middle of the bilayer

Figure 1–6. The fluid mosaic model for biomembranes. Biomembranes consist of a lipid bilayer in which are imbedded membrane proteins.

Clearly, the membrane cannot keep a compartment perfectly sealed; material must enter and leave the cell and its internal compartments. Selective transport is due in part to the properties of the phospholipid bilayer but mostly to transport proteins embedded in the membrane. These proteins are characteristically selective in their transport functions; e.g., the protein that serves as the main ion channel underlying neuronal signaling is 15 times more permeable to Na^+ than to K^+. Transport is a major topic of cell physiology and is discussed in more detail later.

If the cells of an organism are to respond to external changes, they must receive information about the state of the outside world. Just as we higher animals have our sensory organs—eyes, ears, nose, and so forth—arrayed on our outside surface, so too cells have most of their information processing and transmission apparatus on their external surfaces. These are intrinsic membrane proteins of the plasma membrane. This is discussed in greater detail later.

At first glance it might seem odd that a fluid membrane could provide spatial organization for biochemical reactions. However, returning to the "icebergs on a phospholipid sea" analogy, random collisions are much more likely for material in the two-dimensional membrane surface than for material moving through the three-dimensional volume of the cytoplasm. This much larger collision probability is exploited by the cell in a number of physiological processes. Membranes can also be fenced off into distinct regions across which there is limited diffusion of membrane proteins. For example, certain cells in the kidney have two membrane regions that are quite distinct with respect to transport proteins. This organization (described in more detail later) is important in the regulation of salt and water balance by the animal.

TRANSPORT

Only Small, Uncharged Molecules and Oily Molecules Can Penetrate Biomembranes Without the Aid of Proteins

Charged particles, i.e., ions, do not pass through a pure phospholipid bilayer because of the inner, hydrophobic region of bilayer. Polar molecules (molecules with no net charge but with electrical imbalances) with a molecular weight greater than about 100 daltons are also unable to pass readily through a pure lipid bilayer, thus excluding all sugar molecules (monosaccharides), amino acids, nucleosides, as well as their polymers—polysaccharide, proteins, and nucleic acids. On the other hand, some crucially important polar molecules, e.g., water and urea, are small enough to pass through the lipid bilayer. Small, moderate, and large-size molecules that are soluble in oily solvents readily pass through a pure lipid bilayer. Physiologically important molecules in this class include O_2, N_2, and the steroid hormones (see Chapters 33 and 45). However, many toxic, synthetic molecules, such as insecticides, are in this category also.

Molecules Move Spontaneously from Regions of High Free Energy to Regions of Lower Free Energy

The majority of biochemicals do not pass readily through a phospholipid bilayer. Transport of this molecular majority requires a protein pathway across the biomembrane. Also needed is a force causing movement along the pathway. Before elaborating on membrane proteins as pathways through the lipid bilayer, the energy factors that drive the transport are considered.

On a planet such as Earth with a considerable gravitational potential, objects fall spontaneously. This is a manifestation of the principle that movement occurs to minimize the potential energy of the object. Indeed, all change in the universe (at scales greater than the subatomic particles) occurs to minimize the potential energy, also called the *free energy*, of the system. The movement of molecules is strongly affected by forces such as concentration, pressure (both part of chemical potential), and voltage (electrical potential). Molecules move spontaneously from a region of higher concentration to lower concentration, from higher to lower pressure, and from higher to lower electrical potential. Each of these factors—concentration, pressure, and electrical potential—is a source of free energy. The transport of a molecule does not depend necessarily on any one factor; rather, the sum of all the free energy contributions is the determinant of transport. The sum of all the free energy contributions on a substance is expressed usually on a per mol basis as the *electrochemical potential*. The electrochemical potential is the free energy of the substance, from all sources, per mol of the substance.

In order for spontaneous transport to occur there must be a difference in the electrochemical potential of the substance between two regions. The two regions are usually two compartments separated by a membrane. This difference in electrochemical potential is called the *driving force.* Typically students have little trouble understanding the direction of spontaneous flow as long as only one factor contributes to the electrochemical potential, pressure, concentration, or voltage. However, understanding physiological transport, both across cells and across tissues, requires an understanding of the contribution of each factor to the driving force. For example, the flow of fluid from the capillaries of the vascular system depends on the balance between both the hydrostatic pressure difference and the concentration difference of solutes (osmotic pressure) across the capillary. Similarly, movement of Na^+ and K^+ ions across the plasma membrane of nerve cells depends on the driving forces contributed by both voltage differences and ion concentration differences across the membrane.

Material moves spontaneously from regions of high electrochemical potential to low electrochemical potential. Such transport is called *diffusion* or *passive transport.* *Net* movement of material, i.e., diffusion, stops when the electrochemical difference between regions equals zero. The state at which the free energy or the electrochemical potential difference is zero is called *equilibrium.* Equilibrium means balance, not equality. Equilibrium is reached when the free energy (electrochemical potential) is balanced; the value on one side is the same as the other. In most cases the source of the free energies on the two sides never becomes equal; the concentrations, the pressure, and the voltages remain different, but their differences balance out so that the sum of the free energy differences is zero.

Equilibrium is a particularly important concept because it describes the state toward which change occurs if no work is put into the system. Once the system reaches equilibrium, no further net change occurs unless some energy is added to the system. The words *net change* are important. Molecules at equilibrium still move and exchange places, but as much goes in one direction as in the other, so there is no net flow of material.

If the cell requires material to move from low to high electrochemical potential, i.e., in the direction away from equilibrium, thus increasing the difference in free energy between two regions, then some driving force, some work, most be provided by some other decrease in free energy. This type of transport is *active transport.* Active transport uses proteins that combine transport and reaction coupling functions; the protein couples the "uphill" movement of material to a "downhill" reaction such as ATP hydrolysis.

Important Transport Equations Summarize the Contributions of the Various Driving Forces

It is worthwhile developing some quantitative aspects of transport, beginning with simple examples and developing equations for the effect of more than one driving force. These equations can be seen as summaries of the physical laws. In most cases, the equations describe phenomena with which we have experience, living in a technological society. In these equations, c stands for concentration, V for volume, P for pressure, and so forth. These are common enough concepts. It is important to think about these equations in real life terms, not as abstract symbols.

One of these equations relates a hydrostatic (pressure) driving force for water movement that just balances a chemical potential driving force. Recall that *osmosis* is the movement of water across a semipermeable membrane in response to the difference in the electrochemical potential of water on the two sides of the membrane (Fig. 1–7). The chemical potential of water is lower in 1 L of water in which is dissolved 2 mmol of NaCl than in 1 L of water in which is dissolved 1 mmol of NaCl. If these two solutions are separated by a pure lipid bilayer, Na^+ and Cl^- ions cannot move to equilibrate the concentration. Rather, the freely permeable water moves from the side with the higher water potential (low concentration of solute) to the side with the lower water potential (higher concentration of solute). This dilutes the 2-mmol solution. However, water movement never produces equal concentrations of salt. Rather, another driving force appears as the water moves. The hydrostatic pressure of water increases on the side to which the water moves, increasing the electrochemical potential of the water on that side. Net water movement stops when the increase in water potential from hydrostatic pressure exactly balances the decrease in water potential from the dissolved salt, so that the

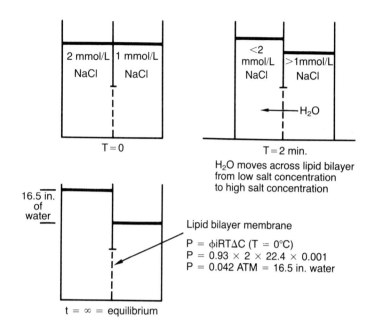

Figure 1–7. Osmosis. At time (t) = 0, two compartments are separated by a lipid bilayer membrane (no transport proteins) that contains salt solutions of differing concentrations. At t = 2 minutes, the salt ions cannot move across the membrane to equilibrate their concentration, but water can move. Water moves from the region of higher water potential (low salt) to the region of lower water potential (high salt). Water continues to pass the lipid bilayer until at t = equilibrium; the difference in the height of water between the two sides creates a difference in pressure that is equal but opposite to the difference in the water potential between the two sides. That is, the free energy difference due to differing salt concentrations is equilibrated by an equal but opposite free energy difference due to pressure.

electrochemical potential becomes equal on both sides of the membrane.

The initial potential difference of water in Figure 1–7 is due to the difference in the concentration of material dissolved in the water. A proper explanation of why the water in a solution has a lower chemical potential than pure water (why water in a concentrated solution has a lower potential than in a dilute solution) is beyond the scope of this chapter. However, readers familiar with the concept of entropy will realize that the disorder of a system increases with the introduction of different particles into a pure substance and with the number of different particles introduced. An analogy would be that a canister with mixed sugar and salt is more disordered, therefore at higher entropy, than a canister with only pure salt or pure sugar. Also, the disorder of the system increases as more sugar is added to salt (up to 50:50); a pinch of sugar in a canister of salt only increases the disorder slightly. Because an increase in entropy causes a decrease in free energy, the free energy of water (solvent) in a solution is decreased as the mole fraction of solute increases.

Osmosis is important to cells and tissues, because generally water can move freely across them whereas much of the dissolved material cannot. Given a concentration difference of some nonpermeable substances, van't Hoff's equation relates how much water pressure is required to bring the system to equilibrium,

i.e., the free energy contributed by a pressure difference across the membrane that exactly balances an opposing free energy contribution due to a concentration difference.

$$P = i \, RT \, \Delta c$$

P = osmotic pressure, the driving force for water movement expressed as an equivalent hydrostatic pressure in atmospheres (1 atm = 15.2 lb/in^2 = 760 mmHg). Osmotic pressure is also symbolized by π to distinguish it from other pressure terms.

i = number of ions formed by dissociating solutes (2 for NaCl, 3 for CaCl$_2$, and so forth)

R = gas constant = 0.082 L atm/mol degree

T = temperature on the Kelvin scale; 0° C = 273°K

(RT is a measure of the free energy of 1 mol of material because of its temperature. At 0° C, RT = 22.4 L atm /mol)

Δc = the difference in the molar concentration of the impermeable substance across the membrane

This equation summarizes a balance of driving forces; P amount of hydrostatic pressure is the same driving force as a particular concentration difference, Δc. The osmotic pressure depends only on the concentration difference of the substance; no other property of the substance need be taken into account. Those phenomena that depend only on concentration, like osmotic pressure, freezing point depression, and boiling point elevation, are called *colligative properties*. Van't Hoff's law is strictly true only for ideal solutions that are approximated in our less than ideal world only by very dilute solutions. Real solutions require a "fudge factor" called the *osmotic coefficient*, symbolized by φ. The osmotic coefficient can be looked up in a table, then plugged into the equation as follows:

$$P = \phi \, i \, RT \, \Delta c$$

The term φic for a given substance represents the osmotically effective concentration of that substance and is often called the *osmolar* or *osmotic concentration*, measured in osm/L. In general, the osmolar concentration of a substance is approximated by the usual concentration times the number of ions formed by the substance; the osmotic coefficient provides a small correction. The osmolarity of a 100-mmol NaCl solution (0.1 mol) is then = 0.93 (φ for NaCl) × 2 ($NaCl \rightarrow Na^+ + Cl^-$) × 0.1 mol = 0.186 osm = 186 mosm.

The equation above summarizes a phenomenon crucial for physiological function. The greater the concentration difference of an impermeable substance across a membrane, the greater is the tendency for water to move to the side of high concentration. Indeed, if you plug some numbers into this equation, you may be surprised at the large pressures required to balance modest concentration differences. For example, an NaCl concentration difference of 0.1 mol (5.8 g/L) is equilibrated by a pressure (4.2 atm) equal to a column of water 141 ft high (divers must be wary of "the bends" when ascending from below 70 ft of water). The importance of this is that a small concentration difference can produce a strong force for moving water. The body makes effective use of this to transport water in many tissues; ions/molecules are transported into or out of a compartment—and water follows by osmosis.

Starling's Hypothesis Relates Fluid Flow Across the Capillaries to Hydrostatic Pressure and Osmotic Pressure

An excellent practical example of how a balance of driving forces is responsible for the flow of water and permeable substances across a semipermeable membrane is the movement of water and ions across the single layer of cells (endothelial cells) that compose blood capillaries. The single cell layer composes, in effect, a semipermeable membrane with different transport qualities than that of authentic lipid-bilayer membranes. The junctions between cells have holes large enough for small molecules and ions to have a pathway for diffusion. Only large molecules, most importantly proteins, are unable to move through the holes. The difference in protein concentration between the blood and the water solution surrounding tissue cells, called the *extracellular fluid* (ECF) or *interstitial fluid*, creates an osmotic pressure for the movement of water with all its dissolved small molecules and ions. This osmotic pressure due to dissolved proteins has a special name: *colloid osmotic pressure* or *oncotic pressure*. Protein is more concentrated in the blood than in the interstitial fluid, producing an oncotic pressure of about 0.02–0.03 atm = 15–25 mmHg, driving water into the capillary. On the basis of this driving force alone, one would expect the capillaries to fill up with water, thus dehydrating the tissue spaces. However, the heart is a pump that exerts a true hydrostatic pressure on the blood, tending to drive the water (and other permeable molecules) out of the capillaries. The net driving force is the algebraic sum of the oncotic pressure difference and hydrostatic pressure difference between the capillaries and the interstitial fluid.

$$\text{net driving force in capillary} = (P_c - P_i) - (\pi_c - \pi_i)$$

P_c = hydrostatic pressure in the capillary

P_i = hydrostatic pressure in the interstitial space (usually near 0)

π_c = oncotic pressure of blood plasma in capillary (approx. 28 mmHg)

π_i = oncotic pressure of interstitial fluid (approx 5 mmHg but depends on the particular tissue)

This equation has enormous relevance to the function of the circulatory system. On the arterial end of capillaries the hydrostatic pressure (P_c) is high, about 35 mmHg. Plugging this number into the equation along with the others, the net pressure in the capillary is + 12 mmHg; fluid is being driven out of the capillary on the arterial side (*capillary filtration*).

The flow of fluid through the resistance of the capillary causes a decline in pressure so that the hydrostatic pressure on the venous side is low, $P_c = 15$ mmHg. The oncotic pressures have not changed, so the net driving force on the venous side is -8 mmHg; there is a net absorption of fluid into the capillary on the venous side (*capillary reabsorption*). This arrangement achieves a major function of the circulatory system; nutrients are delivered to cells on the arteriolar side, and waste products are absorbed from the tissue on the venous side of capillaries.

Pathological alterations in this system emphasize the physiological importance of balance of driving forces for transport. Chronic liver disease occurs with some frequency in horses and dogs, among other mammals. The liver is compromised in its ability to synthesize and secrete a major blood protein, serum albumin. The decline in the concentration of serum albumin lowers the oncotic pressure of the blood. As a result, there is more force to drive fluid out of the capillaries on the arterial side and less driving force for net absorption of fluid on the venous side of capillaries. This causes the tissue spaces of the diseased animals to fill with fluid, a painful and visually obvious symptom called *edema.* The clinical correlation at the end of the chapter provides another example of edema in which increased hydrostatic pressure in the veins and capillaries causes increased capillary filtration and less capillary reabsorption.

Membrane Proteins That Serve the Triple Functions of Selective Transport, Catalysis, and Coupling Can Pump Ions and Molecules to Regions of Higher Free Energy

Van't Hoff's law and Starling's hypothesis dealt with passive transport, i.e., movement of material in the direction of lower electrochemical potential. However, the cell moves many ions/molecules against their electrochemical potential. That is, this selective transport requires the expenditure of energy by the cell. Transport in a direction requiring an expenditure of energy (i.e., input of work) is called *active transport.* Active transport depends on intrinsic membrane proteins that use specific binding and allostery to achieve the dual functions of selective transport and reaction coupling. Many, but by no means all, active transport proteins obtain the energy for transport from ATP hydrolysis; these proteins must function also as enzymes (ATPases).

An important example of active transport is the Na^+, K^+ pump (also known as Na^+, K^+ ATPase). This intrinsic membrane protein consists of four polypeptide chains ($2 \alpha + 2 \beta$) and has a mass of approximately 300,000 daltons. This molecule catalyzes the hydrolysis of ATP and couples the hydrolysis energy to the movement of Na^+ out of the cell and K^+ into the cell. This ion pump creates and maintains a considerable concentration gradient across the cell membrane for both ions (see Table 1–1, table of ionic concentrations in cell, plasma, and extracellular fluid). Figure 1–8 shows our current understanding of this protein's structure and outlines the cycle of binding and conformational changes underlying its transport function. The Na^+, K^+ ATPase pumps 3 Na^+ *out of* the cell and 2 K^+ *into* the cell for each ATP hydrolyzed. These directions of ion pumping cause a high Na^+ concentration outside the cell and a low concentration inside, whereas K^+ concentration is high inside and low outside the cell. The different directions of pumping for the two ions depend on differing binding specificity of the pump protein in the two conformational states. The ability of the protein to couple this transport to the enzymatic breakdown of ATP allows the transport to occur against the concentration gradients, from lower to higher electrochemical potentials for both ions. In the particular case of the Na^+, K^+ pump, the number of transported electrical charges is asymmetric; 3 + charges leave for each 2 + charges that enter. This asymmetry of electrical charge transport means that the Na^+, K^+ pump is *electrogenic,* making a minor contribution to the electrical potential (voltage) across cell membranes, discussed more fully later.

Table 1–1.
CONCENTRATIONS (mmol/L) OF VARIOUS SUBSTANCES IN THE INTRACELLULAR, EXTRACELLULAR, AND PLASMA FLUIDS

	Intracellular	Extracellular	Blood Plasma
Na^+	15	140	142
K^+	150	5	4
Ca^{2+}	0.0001	1	2.5
Mg^{2+}	12	1.5	1.5
Cl^-	10	110	103
HCO_3^-	10	30	27
Phosphate	40	2	1
Glucose	1	5.6	5.6
Protein	4.0	0.2	2.5

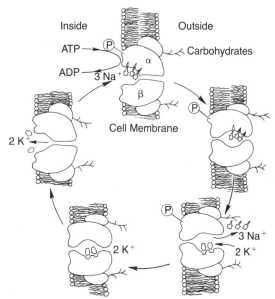

Figure 1–8. A hypothetical transport cycle for the Na$^+$, K$^+$ ATPase. Changes in the conformation of this transport protein driven by ATP hydrolysis and ion-binding events cause 3 Na$^+$ ions to be moved out of the cell against a concentration gradient and 2 K$^+$ ions to be moved into the cell, also against a concentration gradient, for each ATP hydrolyzed. (Redrawn from a diagram by Dr. Seth Hootman.)

Many different intrinsic membrane proteins actively transport a wide variety of ions and molecules against the transported molecules' electrochemical gradient. Many, like the Na$^+$, K$^+$ pump, couple the energy-requiring "uphill" transport with the "downhill" hydrolysis of ATP. However, any potential source of free energy can be coupled to the energy-requiring transport. Indeed, the gradient of Na$^+$ set up by the Na$^+$, K$^+$ pump is itself used frequently as a source of energy. That is, the "downhill" flow of Na$^+$ from outside the cell to the inside is a spontaneous reaction whose energy can be coupled to some "uphill" reaction. For example, the transport of glucose and many amino acids from the food mass in the small intestines into the cells lining the gut is an active transport process and requires a Na$^+$ concentration gradient. Transport proteins in the plasma membrane of intestinal epithelial cells couple the spontaneous diffusion of Na$^+$ into the cell to the inward, energy-requiring transport of the sugar or amino acids. In cells of the proximal tubule of kidney, inward, passive Na$^+$ transport is coupled to the active, outward transport of hydrogen ions (acid).

These examples of transport can be referred to in a number of ways. Because two ions/molecules must be transported together or not at all, such transport is called *co-transport*. Co-transport can involve one process of passive transport (diffusion) with an active transport process, as in the two examples in the preceding paragraph; it can involve two active transport processes, like the Na$^+$, K$^+$ ATPase; or it can involve two diffusion processes. In the first case, the need for co-transport is energetic; the flow of one ion is needed to drive the other. In the two latter cases, the need for co-transport is a restriction based on the binding properties of the transport protein; it cannot bind one without the other. Co-transport proteins that transport both substances in the same direction are called *symports* or *symporters*. The Na$^+$, sugar co-transporter in the gut is a symport. Co-transport proteins that transport the two substances in opposite directions, like the Na$^+$, K$^+$ ATPase or the Na$^+$, H$^+$ transporter of the kidney, are called *antiports* or *antiporters*. Parenthetically, those proteins that transport just a single ion or molecule are called *uniports* or *uniporters*. Active transport at the expense of the energy stored in the Na$^+$ electrochemical gradient across the cell membrane is called *secondary active transport* because of its dependence on the Na$^+$ concentration gradient established by the primary active transport of the Na$^+$, K$^+$ pump.

Many Membrane Proteins Selectively Facilitate the Transport of Ions/Molecules From High to Low Electrochemical Potential

The movement of ions and of medium and large polar molecules requires a protein molecule to serve as a pathway through the obstruction of the phospholipid bilayer. If the movement of the substance is in the natural direction of its electrochemical gradient (movement from high to low), the transport process is called *facilitated diffusion*. The membrane proteins mediating this transport process through the phospholipid bilayer are *channels* or *carriers* (Fig. 1–9). These are distinguished by the extent to which the protein interacts with the transported substance.

Carriers bind the transported substance in the lock and key manner, so there is a site-specific binding of the transported substance to the transport protein. Carrier-mediated transport is typically much slower than chan-

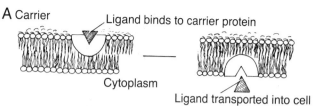

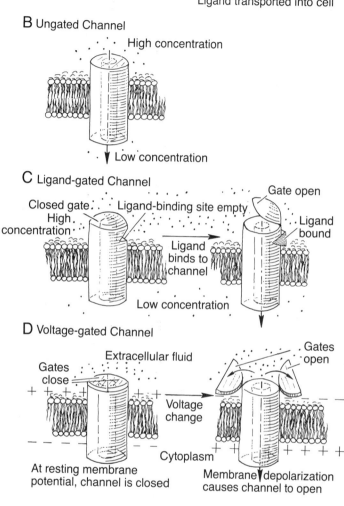

Figure 1–9. Types of transport proteins mediating facilitated diffusion. In all cases the ion moves from a region of high potential (shown here as high concentration) to a region of low potential. (*A*) Carriers. In a few instances material is carried by a transport protein that binds tightly to the material, and the complex moves through the lipid bilayer. (*B*) Ungated channels. Many transport proteins form a pore in the membrane through which ions can permeate. Selectivity of these and other channels is based on the size of the pore and the weak interactions of ions with the atoms lining the pore. (*C*) Ligand-gated channels. The transport protein again forms a pore through the membrane. In the case of gated channels, access of the ion to the pore is controlled by a gate, a substructure of the transport protein that can open and close the pore. In ligand-gated channels the opening and closing of the gate is controlled by the binding of a ligand to the channel. (*D*) Voltage-gated channels are similar to ligand-gated channels except that the opening and closing of the gate is controlled by the electrical field around the channel.

nel-mediated diffusion because of the relatively slow binding and unbinding processes. The Na^+, K^+ pump is an example of a carrier.

Channels can be thought of as protein donuts embedded in the phospholipid bilayer. The hole in the donut is a pore in the membrane through which small ions such as Na^+, K^+, Ca^+, Cl^-, and H^+ are transported. The pore size and the interaction of the transported material with the amino acid side groups lining the pore allow membrane channels to be selective. Only specific molecules or ions can move through a particular channel. Movement of material through channels is nearly as rapid

as diffusion, because the channel does not bind the ion. Some channels are open at all times, like Na^+ channels in the proximal tubule of the kidney. Many channels, however, open or close in response to signals. These latter type are called *gated channels*. The opening and closing of the gates are examples of the allosteric property of proteins. The same signals responsible for allosteric changes in general—ligand binding, phosphorylation, and voltage differences—also control the opening and closing of gated channels, as shown in Figure 1–9.

Channels that open in response to ligand

binding are called *ligand-gated channels.* The nicotinic acetylcholine receptor is a ligand-gated channel found in skeletal muscle membrane directly beneath incoming neurons (nerve cells). This channel is found also in the membrane of neurons in autonomic ganglia. As the name implies, the nicotinic acetylcholine receptor binds to the drug nicotine and the neurotransmitter acetylcholine. In both cases the channel opens in response to ligand binding. This channel plays a key role in transmitting electrical stimulation from neurons to skeletal muscle cells. Briefly, motor neurons release the neurotransmitter acetylcholine in response to the electrical signal coming down the neuron. This acetylcholine binds to and opens the ligand-gated channel on the skeletal muscle. The influx of Na^+ into the muscle cell initiates an electrical response in the muscle, causing the release of Ca^{2+} (through gated channels in the endoplasmic reticulum), in turn causing contraction. (This brief account of neuromuscular transmission, presented only to provide orientation to the function of acetylcholine channel, is expanded in Chapter 4.) In the case of the nicotinic acetylcholine receptor/channel, the specific binding and allosteric properties of the protein serve the dual functions of selective transport across the membrane and information reception and transmission to the muscle cell.

Channels that open in response to voltage changes across the membrane are called *voltage-gated* or *voltage-dependent channels.* This type of channel is largely responsible for the neurons' ability to transmit information along their length and to release neurotransmitter. All voltage-gated channels have a range of membrane potentials that cause them to open; this is the channel's *activation range.* The minimum membrane potential that causes opening is the channel's *threshold.* The activation range and threshold vary from channel to channel, depending on the conformation of the protein and the electrical properties of the amino acid side groups that form the gate of the channel. In addition to an open and closed configuration, many voltage dependent channels have a third conformation, called *inactivated.* Like the closed configuration, the inactivated conformation prohibits the diffusion of ions through the channel. Unlike the closed configuration, it does not open in response to changes in membrane potential. Inactivation can be regarded as an enforced rest period for the channel. Voltage-dependent channels that

do not inactivate have only open and closed conformations, and they take up one or the other conformation, depending on the membrane potential.

In the discussion of protein function, it was pointed out that any of the functions of proteins could be used to transmit information if a difference in the protein function changed the cell. Gated channels, both ligand- and voltage-gated, are ideal candidates for information transmission because they change their function—opening and closing, permitting or stopping transport. Indeed, the sole physiological function of the nicotinic acetylcholine receptor/channel, described earlier, is the transmission of information.

Passive Transport of K^+ Across the Plasma Membrane Creates an Electrical Potential

Cells maintain an electrical potential difference across their plasma membrane. That is, the cell membrane is a battery; if one attaches electrodes to the two ends of a battery or to the inside and outside of a cell, one finds a voltage difference between the two ends or sides. If one provides a path for electrical charges to move—a metal wire containing free electrons in the case of a battery, or a membrane channel through which ions can move in the case of the cell—then an electrical current flows from higher to lower electrical potential. The diversity of battery-powered devices in our society suggests how many ways this electrical potential can be exploited. The physiology of animals also exploits the baseline electrical potential across the plasma membrane, called the *resting membrane potential.* The word resting is added to distinguish the baseline potential from the instantaneous values of membrane potential during the passage of membrane currents.

The resting membrane potential is the indirect result of the concentration gradients of ions across the plasma membrane caused by the activity of the Na^+, K^+ ATPase. Partly, this membrane potential is a result of the asymmetry in numbers of ions pumped by the Na^+, K^+ ATPase. However, most of the membrane potential is due to the passive flow of K^+ through nongated channels (*K^+ leak channels*) in response to the concentration gradient of K^+ (high inside, low outside). This concentration gradient sets up an electrical driving force (voltage) that exactly balances the concentration driving force. The concentration of K^+ inside a mammalian cell is about 150 mmol; outside in the interstitial fluid, it is about 5 mmol. As a result, K^+ tends to diffuse from the cytoplasm through the leak channel to the interstitial fluid. However, when K^+ alone leaves the cytoplasm without an accompanying negative ion, it causes an electrical imbalance. The inside of the cell has negative charges not neutralized by K^+ ions, and the interstitial fluid now has positive K^+ ions not balanced by negative charges. The cell is building an electrical potential difference across the plasma membrane with the cytoplasm being negative relative to the interstitial fluid. This electrical potential driving force increases until it balances the concentration driving force for K^+. This situation is analogous to osmosis: the concentration-driven flow of water across a semipermeable membrane creates a different driving force, pressure, that eventually balances the concentration driving force. Similarly for the resting membrane potential: the concentration-driven flow of K^+ across the semipermeable membrane (semipermeable in the sense that negative ions do not accompany the K^+) creates a different driving force, an electrical voltage, that eventually balances the concentration force. As in the case of osmosis, an equation is used to relate the size of the concentration gradient to the size of the electrical potential that provides an exact balance. This equation is called the *Nernst equation*:

$$E_X = RT/zF \; 1n \; [X_{outside}]/[X_{inside}]$$

E_X = the equilibrium potential for ion X

RT = the gas constant times the absolute temperature

z = electrical valence for the ion, $+1$ for Na^+ and K^+, -1 for Cl^-, and so forth

F = Faraday constant = the number of coulombs of electrical charge in a mole of ions = 96,500 coulombs/mol

[X] = concentration of ion X

A simpler form of this equation can be written by taking advantage of the fact that R and F are constants, T is nearly constant under physiological conditions, and the natural log of a number is 2.3 times the common log of a number ($\log_{10}$).

$$E_X = -60 \; mV/z \; log \; [X_{inside}]/[X_{outside}]$$

mV = millivolts

Because the state of balance between the electrical driving force and the concentration driving force is equilibrium, the value of the electrical potential is called the *equilibrium potential* of the ion. Given the concentrations above for K^+ inside (150 mmol) and outside (5 mmol) the cell, the equilibrium potential for K^+ is:

$$E_K^+ = -60 \; mV/+1 \times log \; 150/5 = -60 \; mV$$
$$log \; 30 = -60 \; mV \times 1.47 = -88.2 \; mV$$

Indeed, the measured resting membrane potential across a human muscle cell is -90 mV.

A number of aspects of this important equation are worth discussing. If the equilibrium potential for a particular ion is the same as the measured membrane potential, the net driving force for the ion is zero. In this case, there is no net movement even in the presence of wide open channels to provide a path through the membrane. For any ionic gradient across a biological membrane, if the measured electrical potential across that membrane is not the equilibrium potential of the ion, there is a driving force for the transport of that ion. If the measured electrical potential has the same sign but is larger in magnitude than the equilibrium potential, the ion flows in the direction of the electrical potential. If the sign is the same but the magnitude lower, then the concentration driving force determines the direction of flow of the ion. If the measured potential is opposite in sign to that of the equilibrium potential, both electrical and concentration forces are acting on the ion in the same direction. In all of these cases, ions permitted to flow (i.e., having an open channel) continue to do so until the concentration potential and electrical potential balance one another and equilibrium is reached or until the channel closes.

It would be reasonable, but incorrect, to assume that the transport of ions required to set up the electrical potential measurably alters the concentration gradient. This is untrue because of the large amount of energy required to separate electrical charges. The separation of charge arising from the transport of a few ions balances the energy of quite substantial concentration gradients. Indeed, so few ions move that they cannot be measured by chemical means. Thus, electrical, not chemical, measurements are used routinely to assess transport of ions in cells. The measurable voltage changes caused by immeasurably small concentration changes of ions means also that the electrical phenomena at the membrane persist for many hours, even if the Na^+, K^+ ATPase is inactivated by a toxin. That is, an existing concentration gradient of K^+ would require hours to dissipate at the rate of K^+ leakage characteristic of the plasma membrane. Using the membrane battery analogy, the Na^+, K^+ ATPase is a battery recharger. One's portable radio does not require the minute-to-minute services of a battery recharger. Enough energy is stored in the battery to operate the radio for an appreciable period, although the battery recharger is needed ultimately. Similarly, enough energy is stored in the K^+ concentration gradient to maintain the membrane potential for a period of time. The Na^+, K^+ ATPase is not required on a minute-to-minute basis, although it is needed ultimately to maintain the concentration gradient on which the resting membrane potential depends.

Spatial Organization of Active and Passive Transport Proteins Enables Material to Pass Completely Through the Cell

Although macromolecules and biomembranes clearly underlie physiological function, many phenomena of the intact animal emerge that are not initially apparent as a simple sum of parts. One interesting example is the spatial organization of plasma membrane transport proteins so that ions move across the cell from one ECF compartment to another. This *transcellular transport* is important in the kidney (see Chapter 40). The plasma membrane of the epithelial cells in the proximal tubules of the kidney contains two distinct regions. The apical membrane regions face the lumen of the tubule and the fluid that will become urine, and the basolateral regions are near the capillaries and the blood. The apical surface contains ungated protein channels for Na^+ whereas the basolateral surface contains Na^+, K^+ ATPase molecules. The membrane proteins in one region are prevented from diffusing into the other by membrane structures (called tight junctions). Na^+ diffuses into the cell on the apical surface from the urine-like fluid driven by both the concentration gradient and the resting membrane potential. Once inside the cell, the Na^+ is pumped out the basolateral surface, essentially into the blood, by the Na^+, K^+ ATPase. This allows the kidney to reabsorb and thus conserve Na^+. As

long as the Na^+, K^+ ATPase remains restricted to the basolateral surface and the passive channel to the apical membrane, Na^+ can move through the cell from the urine-like fluid in the tubule to the blood in the capillaries. If either protein should lose its spatial restriction, Na^+ would be transported into and out of the cell on the same surface, merely consuming ATP with no net transport of Na^+ from lumen to capillary.

Membrane Fusion Allows for a Combination of Compartmentalization and Transport of Material

Impermeable molecules can be transported across the cell membrane as carriers or channels by means other than membrane proteins. This method involves using membrane itself as a carrier compartment. The lipid bilayer of biological membranes shares a basic similarity of structure with soap bubbles. As with soap bubbles, small vesicles of biomembrane (essentially membrane bubbles) can fuse to form larger membrane surfaces. A large membrane surface can also pinch off (requiring fusion of two membrane surfaces) into small vesicles. When these processes occur at the plasma membrane they are called *exocytosis* and *endocytosis*, respectively (Fig. 1–10). When these processes occur at internal membrane sites, the process is referred to as *membrane fusion*, whatever the direction. Membrane fusion underlies a good deal of membrane vesicle traffic around the cell. This traffic creates intracellular vesicles, renews plasma membrane by adding newly synthesized membrane, and also transports material within the cell and across the plasma membrane. Because the transport is compartmentalized within a membrane bubble, the transported material can be targeted specifically to one or another region of the cell. Also, particular changes can occur during transport only in that particular vesicle compartment.

Exocytosis and endocytosis are crucial in the transport of cholesterol (Fig. 1–11). Cholesterol is an essential lipid component of many animal biomembranes; the plasma membrane lipids of animals are about 15% cholesterol and 60% phospholipids. Cholesterol is also the starting material for the synthesis of the entire group of hormones called *steroids* (see Chapter 32). Cholesterol can be synthesized by animals and is also absorbed by meat-eating animals from their diet. Because cholesterol is

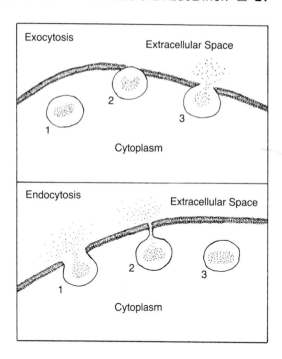

Figure 1–10. Two membrane fusion processes: exocytosis and endocytosis. In exocytosis, a membrane-bound vesicle from the cytoplasm (*1*) makes contact and fuses with the plasma membrane (*2*). As the vesicle membrane becomes continuous with the plasma membrane, the contents of the vesicle are released to the extracellular space (*3*). In endocytosis, some material from the extracellular space is surrounded by plasma membrane (*1*), which continues to invaginate until the edges are able to fuse (*2*), thus pinching off a vesicle from the plasma membrane (*3*). Membrane fusion can occur between any two compartments within cells separated by lipid bilayer membrane, not only between the cytoplasm and extracelluar space as shown here.

soluble in oil, it passes from food through the plasma membrane without protein mediation into the cells of the gut lining. However, transport of dietary cholesterol through the circulatory system requires that cholesterol molecules form a complex with a protein molecule to form low density lipoproteins (LDLs). In order to take up cholesterol from the circulation, cells bind the LDLs to intrinsic membrane proteins that act as LDL receptors. The receptor-LDL complex then diffuses in the plane of the membrane into specific regions to form coated pits. The coated pit is taken into

the cytoplasm by endocytosis, as shown in Figure 1–11. In addition to the transport function, *receptor-mediated endocytosis* functions also to concentrate extracellular material prior to internalization. The coated pit is not taken into the cell until it has collected the LDLs from a far larger volume of ECF than the cell could "drink." The membrane vesicles formed by this endocytosis fuse subsequently to become an endosome. The endosome compartment becomes acidic, which causes dissociation of the LDL and the receptor. Through unknown means, the endosome is then able to further

Figure 1–11. Processes of membrane fusion involved in cholesterol uptake by cells. Starting at the left, an LDL-containing cholesterol binds to an LDL-receptor protein of the plasma membrane and is endocytosed, forming an endosome. The receptor is detached from its LDL ligand in the endosome. The LDL portion of the endosome fuses with a lysosome to digest the LDL and produce free cholesterol while the receptor-containing portion of the endosome pinches off a vesicle to return to the plasma membrane, thus recycling the receptor. (Redrawn from Alberts B, et al: Molecular Biology of the Cell. New York, Garland Publishing, 1983.)

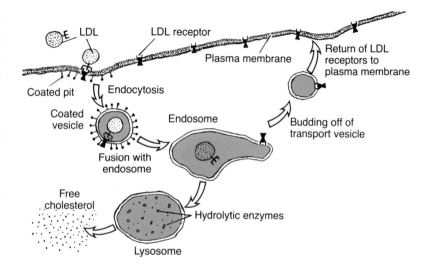

separate and compartmentalize the receptor from the LDL. Membrane vesicles containing the now vacated LDL receptors return to the plasma membrane and fuse by exocytosis. The LDL receptor is recycled to the plasma membrane to pick up more LDL. Experimental evidence suggests that a single LDL receptor molecule can cycle between the plasma membrane and endosomal vesicles more than 100 times before losing its activity. Meanwhile, the LDL moiety is segregated to another endosomal vesicle, which fuses with the lysosome. The lysosome contains hydrolytic enzymes, thus allowing the internalized LDL to be digested. The cholesterol is now available to the cell for steroid synthesis or incorporation into membrane.

Other molecules are recycled by endocytosis also. For example, released catecholamine neurotransmitters discussed earlier are endocytosed back into the neuron that released them, saving the neuron the effort of manufacturing new neurotransmitter. Not all endocytosed molecules are recycled. Many are broken down after their endosome fuses with a lysosome. Indeed, as described later, this is one method of regulating receptor number on the plasma membrane.

INFORMATION TRANSMISSION AND TRANSDUCTION

External Signaling Molecules Bind to Receptors on the Surface of Cells, Causing a Second Message to Be Sent to the Cytoplasm of the Cell

The LDL receptor is involved in the transport of material into cells. Many other *receptors* never get into the cell. Rather, these receptors are intrinsic proteins of the plasma membrane whose task is to transmit and transduce information to the cell from the extracellular environment without the receptor or its signaling molecule getting into the cell. Receptors distinguish among the large number of external signaling molecules (various hormones, neurotransmitters, growth factors, and so forth) through the usual protein mechanism of highly specific binding. As shown in Figure 1–12, binding of the hormone/neurotransmitter to the receptor causes an allosteric change in the receptor conformation that in turn can (1) open (or, less commonly, close) a ligand-gated channel, or (2) activate (or, less commonly, inactivate) a ligand-dependent enzyme activity. The receptor molecule may itself be the enzyme or channel, as in the case of the acetylcholine receptor discussed earlier. Frequently, as shown in Figure 1–12, the receptor is a distinct protein that then activates the channel or enzyme. Figure 1–12 is a simplified view of such an information transduction system that shows the receptor diffusing in the plane of the membrane and colliding with and activating membrane channels or membrane-associated enzymes. Activation occurs only if the receptor is in the hormone/neurotransmitter-bound shape, i.e., activation requires the hormone/receptor complex (see Fig. 1–12). The signal carried by the hormone/neurotransmitter is communicated to the cell through a series of "differences that make a difference." As shown later, there are more steps in this series than shown in Figure 1–12.

After binding of the external signal to the receptor, the ensuing change in ion channel or enzyme function can alter the membrane potential or cause certain molecules/ions to change their concentration in the cytoplasm. Those ions and molecules that are linked to receptor-ligand binding are called *second messengers*. A second messenger is an ion or molecule that carries the information *within* the cytoplasm of a cell in response to a signal on the outside surface of a cell, such as the binding of a hormone, to a neurotransmitter or to an electrical event (the first message). One of the major advances in our understanding of the molecular basis of physiological signaling is the realization that there are only a few second messenger systems within animals cells. These are (1) changes in Ca^{2+} concentration within the cytoplasm as a result of transport of Ca^{2+} through gated channels; (2) changes in the concentration *cyclic AMP (cAMP)*, a special hydrolytic breakdown product of ATP; and (3) increases in the concentration of inositol triphosphate in the cytoplasm and increases in the concentration of diacylglycerol in the plasma membrane, both as a result of the breakdown of a rare membrane phospholipid, *phosphotidyl inositol 4,5 bisphosphate (PIP$_2$)*.

There are a much larger number of different hormones, neurotransmitters, and growth factors than second messengers. This means that several receptor-mediated events are converted into the same intracellular signal. How does the cell sort out this information? Different cells respond differently to the same sec-

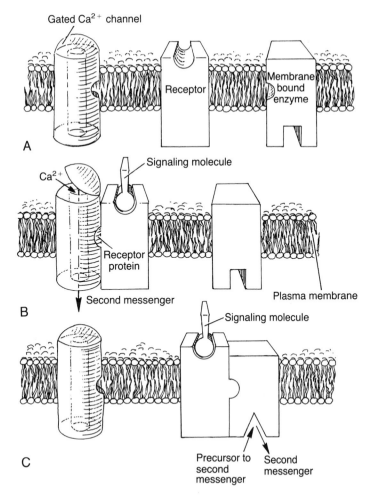

Figure 1–12. A simplified diagram of receptor-mediated information transduction via second messengers. (*A*) The plasma membrane of virtually all animal cells contains receptors, receptor-mediated ion channels, and receptor-mediated enzymes. (*B*) A signaling molecule, e.g., a neurotransmitter (the first message), binds to its receptor, altering the receptor's affinity for a gated Ca^{2+} channel. The binding of the neurotransmitter/receptor complex changes the conformation of the gated channel, opening the gate, permitting the inward diffusion of Ca^{2+}. The increased cytoplasmic Ca^{2+} is the second messenger that stimulates a change in cytoplasmic physiology appropriate for the signaling molecule. (*C*) A signaling molecule, e.g., a hormone (the first message), binds to its membrane receptor, altering the receptor's affinity for a membrane-associated enzyme. The binding of the hormone/receptor complex causes an allosteric change in the enzyme, activating its enzymatic activity. This activity synthesizes a molecule, which acts as a second messenger, stimulating a cytoplasmic response appropriate for the hormone.

ond messenger ion/molecule as a result of the specialized function and makeup of that cell, i.e., the differentiated state it achieved during the development of the animal. Muscle cells respond differently to an increase in $[Ca^{2+}]$ than nerve cells do because the two cells have different proteins that are responsible for their specialized tasks. That is, muscle-specific proteins respond differently than neuron-specific proteins to an increase in Ca^{2+}.

Specific Physiological Information Is Inherent in the Receptor/Ligand Complex, Not the Hormone/Neurotransmitter Molecule

Before discussing the three second messenger systems in more detail, it is useful to elaborate on some important points about the nature and regulation of the information transfer between the external signal molecule and receptor. Further reading in this book provides ample evidence that the same hormone and especially neurotransmitter molecule can bind to different receptors. These different receptor-binding events send different information to the cell from the same external signal molecule. For example, acetylcholine is bound by two different receptors, the nicotinic ion channel described earlier and the muscarinic receptor, which is not an ion channel and sends completely different information to the cell. The hormone/neurotransmitter itself does not contain any specific information; rather, it is a simple signal, like the phone ringing. One must answer the phone to get the information. The information content of the hormone/neurotransmitter is really contained in the three-dimensional shape of the receptor molecule. The change in the shape of the receptor on binding the hormone/neurotransmitter is the specific message to the cell.

Cells can make themselves more or less sensitive to the signal of the hormone/neurotransmitter. For example, most cells respond to a prolonged period of exposure to hormone/

neurotransmitter by reducing their sensitivity to that molecule. One way is to internalize the receptors by endocytosis, fuse the endosome with a lysosome, and digest the receptor. Typically, receptor number is decreased by endocytosis in response to a sustained high concentration of ligand. This is called *down regulation* of the receptor. This process allows the cell to adapt to high ligand concentrations; receptor-ligand interaction is a true chemical equilibrium. The proportion of receptor-ligand complexes, which determines physiological response, depends on the concentration of both receptors and ligands. In the presence of a high ligand concentration, a decrease in receptor number returns the binding equilibrium to the normal proportion of bound/unbound receptors. This allows the cell to respond to increases and decreases in ligand even at high concentrations of ligand. Another way of regulating the response to a hormone/neurotransmitter is to alter the binding function of the receptor, e.g., by phosphorylating it, so that its affinity for the ligand is reduced or increased.

Ca^{2+} Transport Across Plasma and Intracellular Membranes Is an Important Second Messenger

The transport of Ca^{2+} ions through gated channels across the plasma membrane and across intracellular membranes (e.g., endoplasmic reticulum) is a major second messenger system for physiological information transfer. The available evidence suggests that the major role of Ca^{2+} *within* cells is as a physiological signal. In the extracellular compartment, the major physiological function of Ca^{2+} is to be the principal mineral of bone. One example of Ca^{2+} as a second messenger, the role of Ca^{2+} in regulating the actomyosin ATPase of muscle, has already been discussed. Ca^{2+} is an excellent ion for use as a second messenger, because the cytoplasmic concentration of Ca^{2+} is extremely low, about 10^{-7} mol/L in a resting cell. Increases in intracellular Ca^{2+} concentration can be (1) detected easily because the background noise is so low, and (2) achieved easily because the [Ca^{2+}] in the ECF and in some cellular compartments, such as the endoplasmic reticulum and mitochondria, is 10^4 higher than in the cytoplasm (see Table 1–1). Thus, there is an enormous driving force for Ca^{2+} into the cytoplasm under most conditions.

Increased Ca^{2+} concentration in the cytoplasm alters cellular function by binding to any of several Ca^{2+} binding proteins that serve as control proteins. Troponin is one Ca^{2+} binding protein already mentioned. Reviewing the example of striated muscle contraction from the point of view of Ca^{2+}: Ca^{2+} (second messenger) diffuses through gated channels in the endoplasmic reticulum (sarcoplasmic reticulum) of muscle in response to electrical events (first message) on the plasma membrane of the muscle cell. The diffusion of Ca^{2+} from the concentrated storehouse of the sarcoplasmic reticulum increases [Ca^{2+}] in the cytoplasm of the muscle cell, where it binds to troponin. Upon binding Ca^{2+}, troponin changes its interaction with tropomyosin, which now moves to allow myosin heads access to the actin of the thin filament. The actomyosin ATPase is activated and muscle contraction ensues.

Calmodulin is a Ca^{2+}-binding protein that plays an important control function in nearly all animal cells. Like troponin, calmodulin binds Ca^{2+} when the cytoplasmic [Ca^{2+}] increases. The Ca^{2+}/calmodulin complex activates a large number of different cellular processes. In most cases, but not all, the Ca^{2+}/calmodulin complex binds to and activates an enzyme. One such enzyme, a protein kinase, is involved in the release of neurotransmitter from nerve endings. In response to electrical activity on the plasma membrane of a neuron, the voltage-dependent Ca^{2+} channels at the terminal of a neuron open to allow the facilitated diffusion of Ca^{2+} into the cytoplasm. The increase in cytoplasmic [Ca^{2+}] causes it to bind to calmodulin. The Ca^{2+}/calmodulin complex in turn binds to and activates an enzyme, a Ca^{2+}/calmodulin–dependent protein kinase. This enzyme catalyzes the hydrolysis of ATP and couples it to the simultaneous phosphorylation of other proteins:

$$\text{ATP} + \text{protein} \xrightarrow{\text{Ca}^{2+}\text{calmodulin–dependent}} \text{ADP} + \text{protein phosphate}$$

In this case the phosphorylated protein causes exocytosis of synaptic vesicles (membrane vesicles full of neurotransmitter) at the plasma membrane, releasing the neurotransmitter into the narrow space separating the neuron from its target cell (the synaptic cleft).

Excitation/contraction coupling in smooth muscle was not discussed with the other muscle types earlier because it is mediated through calmodulin. Stimulation of smooth muscle causes an increase in the intracellular $[Ca^{2+}]$, causing calmodulin to bind Ca^{2+}. The $Ca^{2+}/$calmodulin complex activates a special protein kinase—myosin kinase. This enzyme catalyzes the hydrolysis of ATP and couples it to the phosphorylation of polypeptide chains in the heads of myosin molecules (see Fig. 1–3). This phosphorylation increases the affinity of the myosin heads for actin filaments; cross-bridging to actin ensues, and myosin strokes past the thin filament producing filament sliding, contraction, and force.

Cyclic AMP Is Produced by Activation of a Membrane-Bound Enzyme in Response to Hormone/Neurotransmitter Binding to Receptors

Changes in the activity of membrane-associated enzyme activities is an important mechanism of transmitting information across the cell membrane. Binding of a signaling molecule to receptors on the extracellular face of the plasma membrane changes the activity of an enzyme located on the cytoplasmic face. The enzyme catalyzes a breakdown reaction; one or more of the breakdown products released into the cytoplasm are second messengers. One important such second messenger system, and the first to have been discovered, is the hydrolytic breakdown of ATP to $3',5'$ adenosine monophosphate, or cAMP, by the enzyme adenyl cyclase. Cylic AMP is the second messenger, and adenyl cyclase is turned on or off as a result of the binding of various hormones and neurotransmitters to cell surface receptors.

As summarized in Figure 1–13, three distinct membrane proteins interact to produce cAMP: (1) any of several receptors, (2) a regulatory protein that binds guanosine triphosphate (GTP) (called the *G protein*), and (3) the catalytic protein that actually hydrolyzes ATP to cAMP. Their interaction provides an example of the ability of biomembranes to organize biochemical reactions in space. The likelihood of three proteins' colliding and thus being able to interact is much greater in the two-dimensional ''phospholipid sea'' than in the three-dimensional cytoplasm.

A large number of different hormones/neurotransmitters that bind to different membrane receptors use cAMP to transmit information across the membrane. Receptors and their hormones/neurotransmitters that use cAMP as

their second messenger include β-*adrenergic receptors* that bind epinephrine or norepinephrine, increasing cAMP production and providing important regulation to nearly all tissues. The starvation message carried by the binding of *glucagon* to its receptor (see Chapter 32) is carried to the cytoplasm by an increase in cAMP. *Antidiuretic hormone (ADH)* binding to its receptors in kidney cells uses cAMP to regulate urine production (see Chapter 41). A number of therapeutic drugs bind to these same receptors and mimic or prevent the physiological action of the hormone/neurotransmitter that normally binds to the receptor.

After ligand binding, the ligand-receptor complex is able to bind to and activate the regulatory G protein (see Fig. 1–13B). The G protein, in turn, changes shape and binds to the catalytic subunit, altering its shape and regulating its ability to bind ATP, and hydrolyzes the catalytic subunit to cAMP (see Fig. 1–13C). There are two types of G proteins in the adenyl cyclase system. The G_s (s for stimulatory) activates the catalytic subunit; this is the G protein shown in Figure 1–13. A different G protein, G_i, inhibits adenyl cylase when activated. Some diseases are the result of the binding of bacterial toxins to the G proteins. Cholera symptoms result from the binding of the toxin of the bacteria *Vibrio cholera* to the G_s protein, and the irreversible activation of the G_s protein, which in turn irreversibly activates the catalytic subunit. Pertussis (whooping cough) toxin binds irreversibly to and activates G_i, thus inactivating the enzymatic activity.

As suggested by the inhibitory G protein, regulated decreases in cAMP concentrations are an important part of the cAMP second messenger system. There are two mechanisms for such decreases: decreasing the rate of cAMP production, or eliminating cAMP after formation. The former is achieved by G_i inhibiting the catalytic subunit. Certain inhibitory receptors specifically interact with G_i. Opium and drugs derived from it, such as codeine and morphine, are examples of signaling molecules that bind to inhibitory receptors, activate G_i, and inhibit production of cAMP. Other examples are norepinephrine and epinephrine acting through α_2-adrenergic receptors. Recall that these same neurotransmitters activated adenyl cyclase when bound to β-adrenergic receptors. This is another example of the principle that the receptor-ligand complex contains the information, not the hor-

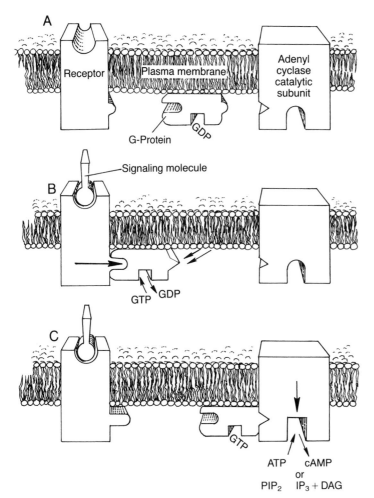

A

Receptor
Plasma membrane
Adenyl cyclase catalytic subunit
G-Protein
GDP

B

Signaling molecule
GTP GDP

C

GTP
ATP   cAMP
or
PIP₂   IP₃ + DAG

Figure 1–13. Receptor-mediated information transduction by the plasma membrane involves a regulatory G protein for many second messengers. Shown here is the classic example of adenyl cyclase, although PIP₂ and some ion channels are regulated similarly also. (*A*) Membrane receptor and enzyme similar to Figure 1–12 is shown along with the G protein. The G protein has three binding sites, one for the hormone/receptor complex, one for GTP and guanosine diphosphate (GDP), and one for the catalytic protein of adenyl cyclase. (*B*) Binding of the signaling molecule stimulates an allosteric change in the receptor protein *(single arrow)*, allowing it to bind to the G protein. The binding of the receptor complex stimulates an allosteric change in the G protein such that GDP is released and GTP is bound by the G protein. In turn, the binding of GTP causes an allosteric change in the G protein *(double arrows)*, allowing it to bind to the catalytic subunit. (*C*) The binding of the GTP/G protein to the catalytic subunit causes an allosteric change in the catalytic subunit such that ATP can now bind to its active site and be hydrolyzed to cAMP. If the catalytic subunit were phospholipase C, its activation would permit the hydrolysis of PIP₂ to IP₃ and DAG, as shown in Figure 1–14.

mone/neurotransmitter itself. The elimination of cAMP after formation is regulated by the enzyme *cyclic nucleotide phosphodiesterase.* This enzyme hydrolyzes the 3' ester bond of the phosphate to the sugar to produce plain 5'AMP. Phosphodiesterase is a Ca^{2+}/cal-modulin–activated enzyme, so in many cells the activities of the Ca^{2+} and cAMP second messenger systems antagonize one another.

The increase or decrease in cAMP concentrations affects cell function through cAMP's interaction with a particular protein kinase. This protein kinase is called *cAMP-dependent protein kinase* or *protein kinase A.* It is completely distinct from the Ca^{2+}/calmodulin–dependent protein kinase discussed earlier. However, the basic outline of action is similar. Protein kinase A is activated by binding cAMP. The higher the concentration of cAMP in a cell, the greater the number of active protein kinase A molecules. The activated kinase binds to proteins and ATP, hydrolyzing the ATP and phospho-

rylating the protein. As several examples have shown, this phosphorylation alters the activity of the target protein, altering its particular characteristic function—catalysis, transport, coupling, and so forth.

Mammals respond to a stressful stimulus by increasing the force of heart contraction, among other physiological effects. This increase in force demonstrates the role of cAMP as a second messenger and shows that physiological control is based on allosteric changes in proteins. The stressful stimulus causes the adrenal medulla to release epinephrine to the blood, and sympathetic nerves release norepinephrine to the heart. Both catecholamines bind to β-adrenergic receptors on the cardiac muscle cells. The receptor-ligand interaction stimulates adenyl cyclase, increasing intracellular [cAMP], thus increasing protein kinase A activity. Protein kinase A phosphorylates voltage-dependent Ca^{2+} channels in the cardiac muscle plasma membrane. In the phosphorylated state, these channels remain open somewhat longer in response to membrane potentials above threshold. Consequently, more Ca^{2+} enters the cell for a given electrical stimulation than at lower levels of cAMP. The increase in Ca^{2+} allows more troponin to bind Ca^{2+}; more tropomyosin moves out of the way of myosin heads, causing more cross-bridging and more force production.

The Receptor-Mediated Hydrolysis of a Rare Phospholipid of the Plasma Membrane Produces Two Different Second Messengers with Different Actions

The most recently discovered second messenger system differs from either Ca^{2+} or cAMP in that *two* distinct second messenger molecules are produced as a result of an enzymatic activation by a single receptor-ligand complex. Phosphotidyl inositol is a membrane phospholipid that can accept additional phosphate groups by reaction with the —OH groups on the inositol (see Fig. 1–14). PIP_2 is the membrane phospholipid that is broken down to produce two important second messengers. PIP_2 is hydrolyzed to *diacylglycerol (DAG)* and *inositol trisphosphate (IP₃)* by a receptor-mediated enzyme, called phospholipase C or phosphodiesterase (completely dis-

tinct from the cyclic nucleotide phosphodiesterase) or phosphoinositidase. Although many distinct processes are controlled through the PIP_2 path, it plays a particularly important role in control of growth and of receptor-mediated secretion. The effect of acetylcholine acting through muscarinic receptors (*not* the nicotinic receptor/ion channel of the nerve-muscle synapse) is often transmitted and transduced through activation of the PIP_2 pathway.

The events involved in the receptor-mediated production of IP_3 and DAG from PIP_2 are rather similar to those in the production of cAMP. The membrane system appears to consist of three distinct intrinsic membrane proteins: (1) any of several different receptors, including the muscarinic acetylcholine receptor and the receptors for some growth factors; (2) a regulatory GTP-binding protein, similar but not identical to G_s of the cAMP pathway; and (3) the hydrolytic enzyme phospholipase C/phosphodiesterase/phosphoinositidase. A hormone/neurotransmitter or growth factor binds to the receptor, forming a receptor-ligand complex. This complex activates the G protein that in turn activates the hydrolytic enzyme. At present, only a stimulatory G activity for phosphoinositidase is known; there is no evidence for an inhibitory G activity in this system.

The activation of the hydrolytic enzyme in-

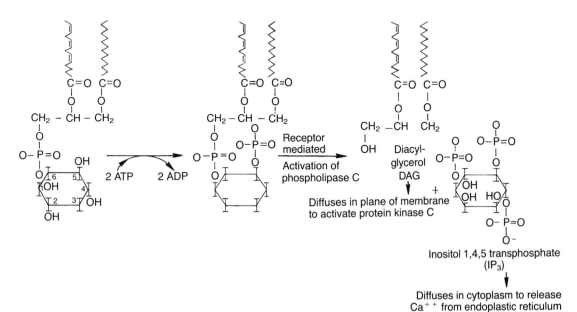

Figure 1–14. Inositol phosphate metabolism. A membrane lipid shown to the left, phosphotidyl inositol, is phosphorylated to PIP_2 (phosphotidyl inositol 4,5 bisphosphate), which upon receptor-mediated activation of phospholipase C is hydrolyzed to DAG and IP_3.

creases the concentration of IP_3, which is water-soluble and so diffuses through the cytoplasm. IP_3 binds to and opens ligand-gated Ca^{2+} channels in the endoplasmic reticulum. This releases Ca^{2+} from that high $[Ca^{2+}]$ compartment into the cytoplasm. Ca^{2+} thus becomes, in a manner of speaking, the third messenger in this system, though this term is not in widespread use. The ensuing increase in cytoplasmic $[Ca^{2+}]$ affects cellular function by the same mechanisms outlined earlier for Ca^{2+} as a second messenger; e.g., binding to calmodulin, the Ca^{2+}/calmodulin complex in turn activating various enzyme activities. In receptor-mediated secretion, for example, the binding of acetylcholine to muscarinic receptors in the pancreas (the organ that secretes digestive enzymes) causes an increase in PIP_2 breakdown and an increase in cytoplasmic IP_3. The IP_3 opens ligand-gated Ca^{2+} channels in the endoplasmic reticulum, and intracellular $[Ca^{2+}]$ increases. The process then becomes similar to the release of neurotransmitter. Calmodulin binds Ca^{2+} and the complex activates a protein kinase that causes exocytosis of secretory vesicles (membrane bubbles full of secretory product) with the plasma membrane, releasing the enzymes into an extracellular space that is contiguous with the gut.

DAG is produced also upon activation of phosphoinositidase, but it is not at all soluble. DAG diffuses in the plasma membrane, binding to and activating membrane-associated protein kinase, protein kinase C (PKC). Protein kinase C is not an intrinsic membrane protein and can bind reversibly to the cytoplasmic face of the plasma membrane. PKC phosphorylates other proteins and changes their activity. Because of the membrane-bound character of the enzyme, most evidence indicates that PKC phosphorylates membrane proteins such as receptors and ion channels, regulating their function. In the case of the secretory response to some hormone/neurotransmitter stimulus, PKC generally acts separately but additively with IP_3 to produce the response. However, much interest focuses on longer-term effects of PKC activation, particularly its role in growth control and cancer. A class of chemicals long known to promote the onset of cancer, phorbol esters, is a potent substitute for DAG at activating PKC. Also, overproduction of PKC by tissue culture cells induced by genetic engineering methods causes a loss of growth control by the cells. This effect is consistent with the evidence that

the receptors for some growth factors (extracellular polypeptides that act as cell division hormones) act through the PIP_2 pathway.

Steroid Hormones Interact With Receptors Within the Cell, Not With Cell Surface Receptors

Recall that steroid hormones are soluble in oily solvents and are able to diffuse through the lipid bilayer without the mediation of transport proteins. This is true also of the hydrophobic hormones of the thyroid gland. Consequently, the receptors for steroid and thyroid hormones are soluble proteins within the target cell. The steroid hormone diffuses from the blood into the cell and binds to its receptor, and the hormone/receptor complex is, as in previous examples, the physiologically active entity that ultimately triggers a cellular response. However, because the signaling molecule itself can get into the cell, steroids do not require a second messenger; the hormone/receptor complex is itself active within the cytoplasm (Fig. 1–15). Steroid and thyroid hormones have a wide variety of physiological effects, including sexual development, control of reproduction, control of growth and metabolism, and salt and water balance.

These effects are produced when the expression of particular genes is turned on by the binding of the hormone/receptor complex to specific regions of the cell's DNA. That is, these hormones regulate which genes will be transcribed into RNA, regulate the rate of transcription, and regulate some post-transcriptional events involved in protein synthesis by the ribosomes. Steroid and thyroid hormone receptors help select which of the genetically encoded information in the cell is to be translated into a polypeptide chain and how much of that polypeptide is made. Different steroids bind to different receptors, as for other signaling molecules, although the different steroid receptors are similar to one another. The hormone/receptor complex, but not the ligand-free receptor, is able to pass through the nuclear membrane where it binds to specific sequences of DNA. Each different hormone/receptor complex binds to one or more regions of DNA specific for that particular complex. This binding stimulates the transcription of the particular gene into RNA, usually within minutes. As in the other instances of protein function, the shape of the hormone/receptor complex is responsible for

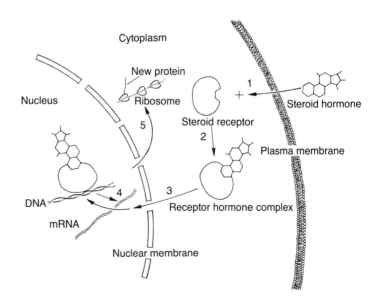

Figure 1–15. The mechanism of action of steroid hormones. (*1*) Steroid hormone penetrates the lipid bilayer passively because of the steroid's oil solubility. (*2*) Inside the cell the steroid binds to a cytoplasmic receptor. (*3*) The hormone/receptor complex enters the nucleus and binds to regulatory sequences of DNA. (*4*) This initiates transcription of a steroid-responsive gene to produce messenger RNA (mRNA). (*5*) The mRNA is transported to the cytoplasm, where it is translated into a polypeptide that alters cell physiology.

the specificity of binding of the complex to particular sequences of DNA.

The activity of many steroid hormones is complex, the synthesis of a number of different gene products being stimulated by one type of hormone/receptor complex. A relatively simple example of this mechanism of steroid action is the action of aldosterone. Aldosterone is a steroid secreted by a particular group of cells in the adrenal cortex (see Chapter 40) in response to a reduction in blood volume. Aldosterone's target cells are the epithelial cells of the kidney whose function is the transcellular ion transport discussed earlier. Aldosterone enters the cytoplasm of these cells and binds to its receptor, and the hormone/receptor complex migrates to the nucleus, where it stimulates the synthesis of two proteins. One is the passive Na^+ channel protein for the apical (urine) face of the cell and the other is a protein that stimulates the activity of the Na^+, K^+ ATPase on the basolateral (blood) surface of the cell. The increased number of Na^+ channels and increased pumping mean that more Na^+ can be resorbed from the urine-like fluid and transported into the blood. The increase in Na^+ concentration of the blood causes an osmotic absorption of water from the intracellular compartment to the blood, thus increasing blood volume. The increased Na^+ in the blood also causes thirst (Chapter 41); this water intake increases blood volume as well.

CLINICAL CORRELATION

PERIPHERAL EDEMA

HISTORY □ You examine a 2-year-old cow that has been grazing on a poor-quality pasture. The owner states that she seems to have a poor appetite, walks slowly, and stands apart from the rest of the herd. She has developed swelling beneath the skin of her brisket and ventral thorax.

CLINICAL EXAMINATION □ On clinical examination you find a listless cow standing in a pasture littered with various metal objects. Examination of the cardiovascular system reveals distended jugular veins and abnormal heart sounds characterized by irregular sloshing sounds throughout the cardiac cycle that drastically muffle the first and second heart sounds. Subcutaneous edema (swelling) can be seen throughout the chest and abdomen but most prominently in the dependent ventral areas of the thorax. Pushing on these swollen areas leaves a dent (pitting edema).

COMMENT □ This is a characteristic history of a cow with *hardware disease*. The cow, grazing on a pasture littered with metal debris, swallows nails, wire, and so forth. Because these objects are heavier than the rest of the feed, they drop into the reticulum, a stomach chamber located just caudal to the diaphragm and heart. With the contractions of the reticulum, a metal object migrates through the reticular wall, diaphragm, and pericardium, leading to an inflammatory response in the pericardium (pericarditis). As inflammatory exudate fills the pericardial sac; it muffles the heart sounds, and if gas is present in the exudate, a sloshing sound may be heard on auscultation. As this exudative fluid fills the pericardial sac, it limits the pumping efficiency of the heart by limiting its filling during diastole and by obstructing venous return to the heart (see Chapter 20). The result is backward failure of the heart causing increased hydrostatic pressure in the veins and capillaries. As the capillary hydrostatic pressure rises, capillary filtration is favored over reabsorption, and water leaves the capillary and accumulates in the interstitial space. This accumulated interstitial fluid, primarily as the result of increased capillary filtration, is seen clinically as edema. The other common cause of edema is decreased capillary colloidal osmotic pressure from low serum protein. However, this does not usually play a part in hardware disease.

TREATMENT □ Treatment includes surgical removal of the foreign object and antibiotic treatment for the pericarditis. However, in such an advanced case as mentioned here, often treatment is not completely successful.

Bibliography

Alberts B, et al: Molecular Biology of the Cell, 2nd ed. New York, Garland Publishing, 1989.
A first-class survey of cell biology at a level similar to that here. Chapters 3, 6, and 12 are particularly relevant to this chapter.
Darnell J, Lodish H, Baltimore D: Molecular Cell Biology. New York, Scientific American Books, 1986.
Similar to Alberts, et al. Chapters 15 and 16 are particularly relevant to this chapter.
Schramm M, Selinger Z: Message transmission: Receptor controlled adenylate cyclase system. Science 225:1350–1356, 1984.
An advanced review of our understanding of this important second messenger system.
Miller RJ: G proteins flex their muscle. Trends in Neuroscience 11:3–6, 1988.
A brief review of G proteins for nonspecialists.

PRACTICE QUESTIONS FOR CHAPTER 1

1. Increasing the extracellular [K$^+$] will

a. have no effect on the resting membrane potential.
b. cause the resting membrane potential to decrease (i.e., cause the inside to become less negative with respect to the outside).
c. cause the resting membrane potential to increase (i.e., cause the inside to become more negative with respect to the outside).
d. increase the concentration potential for K$^+$ across the plasma membrane.
e. require the Na$^+$, K$^+$ pump to work harder to pump K$^+$.

2. G proteins are similar to receptors in that both

a. bind extracellular signaling molecules.
b. interact directly with adenyl cyclase catalytic subunits.
c. have activated and inactivated states dependent on ligand binding.
d. are extracellular protein molecules.
e. directly activate a protein kinase activity.

3. Which of the following statements concerning intracellular Ca^{2+} is *false?*

a. It is a second messenger for hormones and neurotransmitters.
b. It is responsible for excitation contraction coupling in smooth muscle.
c. An increase in its concentration in a nerve terminal stimulates the release of neurotransmitter.
d. It activates protein kinase A.
e. Its concentration is increased in the presence of IP$_3$.

4. If, in a particular capillary bed, the plasma oncotic pressure were to increase and hydrostatic pressure remained constant,

a. more blood plasma would filter from the capillaries.
b. the transport effect would be similar to decreasing hydrostatic pressure.
c. one would suspect a deficiency in blood protein levels.
d. one would suspect an increase in extracellular fluid protein concentrations.
e. fluid reabsorption on the venous side of the capillary bed would decline.

5. Substance x is found to be at much higher concentration on the outside of a cell than in the cytoplasm, yet no transport of x from the extracellular fluid to the cytoplasm occurs. Which of the following statements is *inconsistent* with this state of affairs?

   a. Substance x has the same electrochemical potential outside and inside the cell.
   b. Substance x is large, is poorly soluble in oil, and has no transport proteins in the membrane.
   c. Substance x is an ion and the measured membrane potential is the equilibrium potential calculated by the Nernst equation.
   d. Substance x is a steroid molecule.
   e. Substance x is actively transported from the cell to the ECF.

JAMES G. CUNNINGHAM

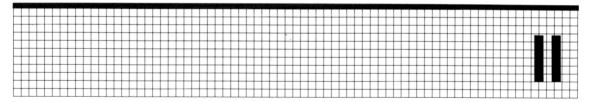

NEUROPHYSIOLOGY

2

Introduction to the Neuromuscular System

1. The neuron is the major functional unit of the nervous system
2. The mammalian nervous system is divided into two subsections, the central nervous system and the peripheral nervous system

The nervous system is the first multicellular system included in this book because it is one of the major coordinating systems of the body and because many concepts included with the nervous system are needed to understand other systems of the body.

Because most clinical signs in veterinary neurology involve abnormal movement (e.g., seizures, paralysis), the physiology of posture and locomotion is emphasized in the following chapters. Veterinary ophthalmology has become an extensive subspecialty, so the physiology of vision is emphasized also. Understanding the autonomic nervous system is essential to understanding much pharmacology and the reflex control of many of the body's most critical functions. Similarly, understanding the blood-brain barrier and the cerebrospinal fluid (CSF) system is essential to understanding the central nervous system's (CNS) homeostasis and the diagnostic CSF tap. The electroencephalogram (EEG) and sensory evoked potentials are described because of their emerging clinical importance in veterinary medicine. Because of space limitations,

only those basic physiological concepts essential to the practice of veterinary medicine are emphasized. For a more expansive study of neuromuscular physiology, the reader may refer to the several monographs mentioned in the bibliographies.

The Neuron Is the Major Functional Unit of the Nervous System

The major functional unit of the nervous system is the neuron, or nerve cell, a cell type whose shape varies considerably with its location in the nervous system. Nearly all neurons have an information-receiving area of the cell membrane, usually called its *dendrite*; a cell body containing the organelle for most cell metabolic activity; an information-transmitting extension of the cell membrane called an *axon*; and a presynaptic terminal to the axon.

The other cell type in the nervous system is the glial cell (Greek—glue), playing largely a structural role. Glial cells do not produce action potentials.

The Mammalian Nervous System Is Divided into Two Subsections, the Central Nervous System and the Peripheral Nervous System

The CNS is divided into the brain and spinal cord (Table 2–1). A series of protective bones surround the entire CNS. The brain is surrounded by the skull, and the spinal cord is surrounded by a series of cervical, thoracic, and lumbar vertebrae and ligaments. These vertebrae are aligned so that they form a functional canal or conduit through which the spinal cord passes; some degree of flexion is possible between each vertebrae.

The peripheral nervous system is divided into motor (efferent) and sensory (afferent) subsystems. Within the motor peripheral nerves are somatic motor neurons, which carry action potential commands from the CNS to synaptic junctions at skeletal muscles, and the autonomic nervous system's motor neurons, which carry action potentials, through an intermediate synapse, to synapses at smooth muscle, cardiac muscle, and some exocrine glands. Sensory peripheral nerves bring action potential messages to the CNS from peripheral receptors. It is the responsibility of these receptors to transduce some environmental energy (e.g., light, sound, stretch of a muscle) into action potentials that travel to the CNS and to encode the intensity of this energy's stimulation of the receptor by increasing the frequency of action potentials as the intensity of stimulation increases. Sensory nerves carrying action potentials from receptors such as the photoreceptors of the eye, auditory receptors of the ear, or stretch receptors of the skeletal muscle would be classified as somatic sensory peripheral nerves. Receptors located within the chest and abdomen send action potentials to the CNS along visceral sensory peripheral nerves.

Table 2–1
ORGANIZATION OF THE NERVOUS SYSTEM

1. Central nervous system (CNS)
   A. Brain
   B. Spinal cord
2. Peripheral nervous system (PNS)
   A. Efferent (motor)
      (1) Somatic—skeletal muscle
      (2) Automatic—cardiac muscle
                       smooth muscle
                       exocrine gland
   B. Afferent (sensory)
      (1) Somatic
      (2) Visceral

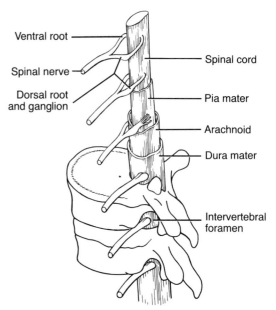

Figure 2–1. The spinal cord and the three layers of the meninges within the vertebral canal. Sensory action potentials enter the spinal cord along axons in the dorsal roots. Motor action potentials exit the spinal cord along axons in the ventral roots. (Redrawn from Gardner E: Fundamentals of Neurology, 3rd ed. Philadelphia, WB Saunders, 1959.)

Within the spinal canal, sensory and motor peripheral nerves are separated; sensory nerves enter the spinal cord through the dorsal nerve roots whereas the motor nerves exit the spinal cord through the ventral roots (Fig. 2–1).

The entire CNS is surrounded by three protective layers called meninges (Fig. 2–1). The innermost layer, lying next to the CNS, is called the pia mater. The pia mater consists of a single layer of fibroblast cells joined to the outer edge of the brain and spinal cord. The middle layer, called the arachnoid, is so named because it looks like a spider's web. The arachnoid is a thin layer of fibroblast cells that traps CSF between it and the pia mater (subarachnoid space). The outermost meningeal layer is the dura mater. It consists of a much thicker layer of fibroblast cells that serve to protect the CNS. Within the brain cavity of the skull, the dura mater is fused often with the inner surface of the bone.

CSF is a clear, colorless fluid found within the subarachnoid space, the central canal of the spinal cord, and the ventricular system of the brain (see Chapter 14). It is produced primarily in the ventricles of the brain, it flows down a pressure gradient from the ventricles to the subarachnoid space, and from this space it passes into the venous system. It is a dynamic fluid, being replaced several times daily. CSF serves as a shock absorber for the CNS during abrupt body movement.

The brain can be divided roughly into a lower and upper brain. The lower brain consists of the medulla, pons, mesencephalon, diencephalon, cerebellum, and basal ganglia and is responsible for much subconscious coordination, such as the control of blood pressure, respiratory rate, and equilibrium. The upper brain consists of the cerebral cortex and is responsible for much conscious activity. Some more detailed anatomy of the brain is presented later as necessary to understand the physiology of posture and locomotion.

Bibliography

Berne RM, Levy MN (eds): Physiology, 2nd ed. St Louis, CV Mosby, 1988, pp 69–76.

Guyton AC: Textbook of Medical Physiology, 7th ed. Philadelphia, WB Saunders, 1986, pp 546–549.

Kandel ER, Schwartz JH (eds): Principles of Neural Science, 2nd ed. New York, Elsevier, 1985, pp 3–24.

Willis WD, Grossman RG: Medical Neurobiology, Neuroanatomical and Neurophysiological Principles Basic to Clinical Neuroscience, 3rd ed. St Louis, CV Mosby, 1981, pp 1–26.

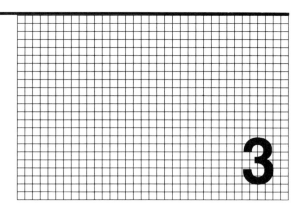

The Neuron

1. Neurons have four distinct anatomical regions
2. Nerve cell membranes contain a resting electrical membrane potential
3. The resting membrane potential is the result of three major determinants
4. The resting membrane potential can be changed by synaptic signals from a presynaptic cell
5. Action potentials begin at the axon's initial segment and spread down the entire length of the axon

There are two classes of cells in the nervous system: the neuron (or nerve cell) and the neuroglial cell (or glia). The neuron is the basic functional unit of the nervous system. The large number of neurons and their interconnections give the nervous system its complexity. There are approximately 10 billion neurons in the average vertebrate nervous system, far more neurons in a nervous system than people on Earth, and 10–50 times more glial cells, the cells that provide firmness and structure for the central nervous system (CNS). The numbers of cells in the nervous system are huge, but knowing their common elements makes understanding them easier.

Neurons Have Four Distinct Anatomical Regions

A typical neuron has four morphologically defined regions (Fig. 3–1): the dendrites, the cell body (also called the soma or perikaryon), the axon, and the presynaptic terminals to the axon. These four anatomical regions are important to the four major electrical and chemical responsibilities of neurons: receiving sig-

nals from neighboring neurons, integrating these often-opposing signals, transmitting electrical impulses some distance along the axon, and signaling an adjacent cell at the presynaptic terminal. Three organelles are common in nerve cell bodies: the nucleus; the endoplasmic reticulum, upon which secretory and membrane proteins are synthesized; and the Golgi apparatus, which carries out the processing of secretory and membrane components. The cell body usually gives rise to several branch-like extensions, called *dendrites*, whose surface area and extent far exceed those of the cell body. The dendrites serve as the major receptive apparatus of the neuron to receive signals from neighboring neurons. The cell body also gives rise to the *axon*, a tubular process that is often long (over 1 m in some large animals). The axon is the conducting unit of the neuron, transmitting an electrical impulse (the action potential) from its initial segment at the cell body to the other end of the axon at the presynaptic terminal. Axons lack ribosomes and, therefore, cannot synthesize proteins. Instead, macromolecules are synthesized in the cell body and are carried

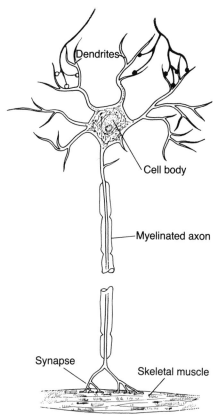

Figure 3–1. A typical neuron has four functionally important regions. The dendrites receive signals from neighboring neurons, the cell body integrates these signals, the axon transmits action potentials some distance along the cell, and the presynaptic terminal signals adjacent cells.

along the axon to the presynaptic terminals by a process called *axoplasmic transport*. Large axons are surrounded by a fatty insulating coating called *myelin*. In the peripheral nervous system, myelin is formed by Schwann's cells, specialized glial cells that wrap around the axon much like toilet paper wrapped around a broomstick. The myelin sheath is interrupted at regular intervals by sites called *nodes of Ranvier*.

Axons branch near their ends into several specialized endings called *presynaptic terminals*. These presynaptic terminals transmit a chemical signal to an adjacent cell, usually another nerve or muscle cell. The site of contact of the presynaptic terminal with the adjacent cell is called the *synapse*. It is formed by the presynaptic terminal of one cell (presynaptic cell), the receptive surface of the adjacent cell (postsynaptic cell), and the space between these two cells, the *synaptic cleft*. The presynaptic terminals of an axon usually contact the recep-

tive surface of the adjacent nerve cell, on one of its dendrites, but sometimes this contact is made on the cell body or occasionally on the terminal end of another cell's axon (for presynaptic inhibition). Presynaptic terminals contain *synaptic vesicles* that contain a chemical transmitter prior to its release into the synaptic cleft.

Nerve Cell Membranes Contain a Resting Electrical Membrane Potential

Nerve cells, like other cells of the body, have an electrical charge that can be measured across their outer cell membrane (*resting membrane potential*). However, the electrical membrane potential in nerve and muscle cells is unique in that its magnitude can be changed as the result of synaptic signaling from neighboring cells or within a receptor as a response to transduction of some environmental energy. When a nerve or muscle's membrane potential is reduced sufficiently, a further and dramatic change in the membrane potential occurs, called an action potential; this action potential spreads along the entire length of the nerve axon.

Understanding the origins of the resting electrical membrane potential is complicated, particularly quantitatively. In qualitative terms, however, the resting membrane potential is the result of the differential separation of charged ions, especially Na^+ and K^+, across the membrane and the resting membrane's differential permeability to these ions diffusing back down their concentration gradients (see also Chapter 1). Even though the net concentration of positively and negatively charged ions is similar in the intracellular and extracellular fluids, an excess of positively charged cations accumulates immediately outside the cell membrane, and an excess of negatively charged anions accumulates immediately inside the cell membrane (Fig. 3–2). This makes the inside of the cell negative with respect to the outside of the cell. The magnitude of the resulting electrical difference across the membrane varies from cell to cell, ranging from about 40 to 75 mV, and is commonly about 75 mV in mammalian nerve cells. Because we arbitrarily take the extracellular fluid to be 0 mV, the resting membrane potential is -75 mV, more negative on the inside than on the outside.

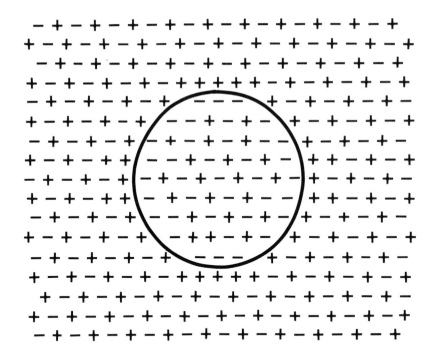

Figure 3–2. The concentration of positively and negatively charged ions is similar in both the intracellular and extracellular spaces. However, more positively charged ions accumulate immediately outside the cell membrane and more negatively charged ions accumulate immediately inside the nerve membrane.

The Resting Membrane Potential Is the Result of Three Major Determinants

Three major factors cause the resting membrane potential.

1. *The Na^+, K^+ pump.* Cell membranes have an energy-dependent pump that pumps Na^+ ions out of the cell and K^+ ions into the cell against their concentration gradients. The pump itself generates some of the resting membrane potential, because it pumps three molecules of Na^+ out for every two molecules of K^+ into the cell, thus concentrating positively charged cations outside the cell.

2. *Differential permeability of the membrane to diffusion of ions.* The resting membrane is much more permeable to K^+ ions than to Na^+ ions. Therefore, positively charged K^+ cations are allowed to diffuse out of the cell through nongated leak channels back down their concentration gradient until the resulting electrical membrane potential reaches an equilibrium with the driving force of the K^+ concentration gradient. This further contributes to the buildup of positive charges immediately outside the membrane. Because the resting membrane is almost completely impermeable to Na^+ ions, once pumped out of the cell, Na^+ cannot diffuse back into the cell, even though both the electrical and concentration gradients for Na^+ would drive Na^+ ions back into the cell if the sodium channels in the resting membrane were open. (See Chapter 1 for a more complete discussion of ion channels.)

3. *Negatively charged anions trapped in the cell.* Many intracellular anions are macromolecules synthesized within the neuron and are too big to get back out through the cell's plasma membrane. Therefore, they are trapped within the cell and attracted to the inner surface of the membrane by the accumulated positive charges just outside the cell.

These three determinants—the Na^+, K^+ pump, the differentially permeable membrane, and the trapped intracellular anions—are the primary source of the resting membrane potential. The magnitude of this potential can be predicted by the Nernst and Goldman equations, and the reader is referred to Chapter 1 and to books in the bibliography for a more quantitative understanding of the resting membrane potential.

There are a number of important clinical implications to our discussion of the resting membrane potential. The Na^+, K^+ pump requires energy in the form of adenosine triphosphate (ATP), which is derived from the intracellular metabolism of glucose and oxygen. Because the neuron cannot store either glucose or oxygen, anything that deprives the nervous system of either substrate leads to serious clinical neurological deficits. Fortunately, hormones and other forces maintain serum glucose and oxygen within narrow limits. Because Na$^+$ and K$^+$ are the primary ions determining the resting membrane potential (Cl$^-$ ions align themselves passively along the membrane as a result of the charge established by Na$^+$ and K$^+$), it is essential that serum levels of Na$^+$ and K$^+$ be regulated carefully. The endocrine system (Chapter 33) and kidney (Chapter 40) maintain serum Na$^+$ and K$^+$ within narrow limits. Anything altering serum levels of either ion beyond normal limits also leads to potentially severe neurological deficits.

The Resting Membrane Potential Can Be Changed by Synaptic Signals from a Presynaptic Cell

Although most cells of the body have a resting membrane potential, nerve and muscle cells are unique in that their membrane potential can be altered by a synaptic signal from an adjacent cell. Even though there are billions of synapses in the nervous system, there are basically only two ways that a presynaptic signal can alter the postsynaptic electrical potential: it can decrease or increase its magnitude. Whether a synapse results in a decreased or increased postsynaptic potential depends on the nature of the chemical transmitter in the presynaptic vesicle and on the nature of the receptor to that chemical transmitter in the postsynaptic membrane.

If a chemical synaptic transmission leads to a reduction in the postsynaptic membrane potential as compared with the resting level (e.g., from −75 mV to −55 mV), the postsynaptic potential change is said to be an *excitatory postsynaptic potential* or EPSP (Fig. 3–3A). It is

called excitatory because each such synaptic transmission increases the chances that an action potential will originate at the initial segment of the nerve's axon. When the magnitude of the membrane potential is reduced to a smaller quantity (e.g., from −75 mV to −55 mV) by such an EPSP, the membrane is said to be *depolarized*, or more accurately, hypopolarized. This hypopolarization of the postsynaptic membrane results from the interaction of the chemical transmitter from the presynaptic nerve and its appropriate receptor on the postsynaptic membrane. This interaction causes ligand-gated Na$^+$ channels to open, thus allowing Na$^+$ ions to diffuse into the neuron down both sodium's concentration and its electrical gradient. Because the presynaptic chemical transmitter is destroyed quickly at the postsynaptic membrane, this postsynaptic potential change is transient, lasting only a few milliseconds. The magnitude of the change in this postsynaptic potential is greatest at the synapse. Although the hypopolarization spreads over the nerve cell membrane, it decreases with distance from the originating synapse, much as the waves created by throwing a stone into a lake decrease with distance from the place where the stone fell.

If instead the presynaptic transmitter's interaction with the postsynaptic receptor results in further opening of the membrane's K$^+$ channels, then K$^+$ ions diffuse out of the cell even faster than usual, and an increase (hyperpolarization) in the postsynaptic membrane potential is the result. Such hyperpolarization of the postsynaptic membrane is called an *inhibitory postsynaptic potential* (IPSP) (Fig. 3–3B), because each such transmission makes it less likely that an action potential will result

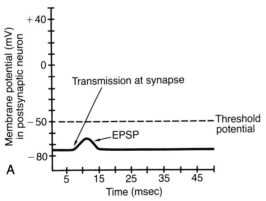
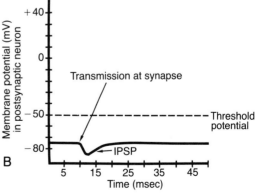

Figure 3–3. Postsynaptic potentials. (*A*) An excitatory postsynaptic potential (EPSP) resulting from an excitatory presynaptic transmitter drives the membrane potential toward threshold. (*B*) An inhibitory postsynaptic potential (IPSP) resulting from an inhibitory presynaptic transmitter drives the membrane potential away from threshold.

at the nerve axon's initial segment. As with EPSPs, IPSPs also spread over the neuron's membrane, and the hyperpolarization decreases with distance from the originating synapse.

Action Potentials Begin at the Axon's Initial Segment and Spread Down the Entire Length of the Axon

Excitatory or inhibitory postsynaptic potentials are the result, on the postsynaptic membrane, of an action potential and synaptic transmission from a presynaptic cell. However, these postsynaptic potentials decrease in magnitude as they spread along the postsynaptic cell membrane. Because many nerve and muscle cells are long, the cell needs a mechanism for sending an electrical signal from its information-receiving end on the postsynaptic dendritic and soma membrane to the information-transmitting zone at the end of the often lengthy axon. This is accomplished by an explosive event called an *action potential*, which begins at the axon's initial segment, as the result of competing EPSP and IPSP forces, and spreads down the length of the axon without decreasing in magnitude.

At the axon's initial segment, the arriving EPSPs and IPSPs are averaged. EPSPs open voltage-gated Na^+ channels (see Chapter 1), allowing some Na^+ ions to rush into the cell, while IPSPs open voltage-gated K^+ channels, allowing more K^+ to exit the cell. If only a few EPSPs or IPSPs arrive at the initial segment, its membrane potential is not changed sufficiently to cause an action potential. However, if EPSPs far outnumber IPSPs, the initial segment's membrane potential is reduced substantially. If this reduction in the membrane potential is sufficient to reach an important *threshold* level for the voltage-gated Na^+ channels, an action potential develops.

The action potential is characterized by explosive changes in the membrane potential; first, a dramatic and swift depolarization of the membrane potential occurs in which the inside of the cell actually becomes more positive than the outside, followed by a more gradual repolarization of the membrane. The depolarization phase of the action potential is caused by the extensive opening of voltage-gated Na^+ channels and the consequent influx of Na^+ ions. As the action potential's depolarization phase continues, the Na^+ channels close gradually and the K^+ channels open

gradually, allowing even more K^+ ions to exit. This brings depolarization to a halt and allows repolarization to occur. As repolarization continues, the membrane potential returns temporarily beyond its resting level to a hyperpolarized state and then eventually returns to its resting state. The whole action potential takes about 1–2 milliseconds (ms) in most nerves, but longer in many muscle cells. Figure 3–4 illustrates this sequence of events.

Perhaps an analogy would be helpful to understand these difficult concepts. Imagine the resting nerve membrane as a toilet. Like the nerve, the toilet has stored potential energy by filling the tank at the back of the toilet. (The nerve has done so by generating the resting membrane potential.) If the handle of the toilet is pushed down only briefly, some water runs into the toilet, but the flush cycle is not completed. (This is much like an EPSP without the action potential.) However, if the handle is held down long enough, a critical threshold is reached, the flush cycle is triggered, and it must run its course, including the refilling of the tank, before another flush cycle can be started. This flush cycle is like the action potential. It is triggered once a critical hypopolarization threshold is reached. It must run its course, including re-establishing the resting membrane potential before another action potential can be initiated. Because the flush cycle takes a finite amount of time, only a limited number of flush cycles can be completed in an hour, even if you flushed the toilet again each time the tank refilled. Simi-

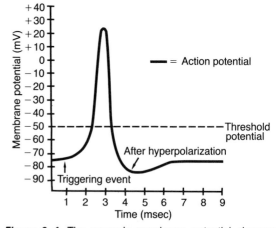

Figure 3–4. The neuron's membrane potential changes dramatically during an action potential. It depolarizes first well beyond threshold and then repolarizes again to its original resting potential. (Redrawn from Sherwood L: Human Physiology: From Cells to Systems. St. Paul, West Publishing Co., 1989, p 95.)

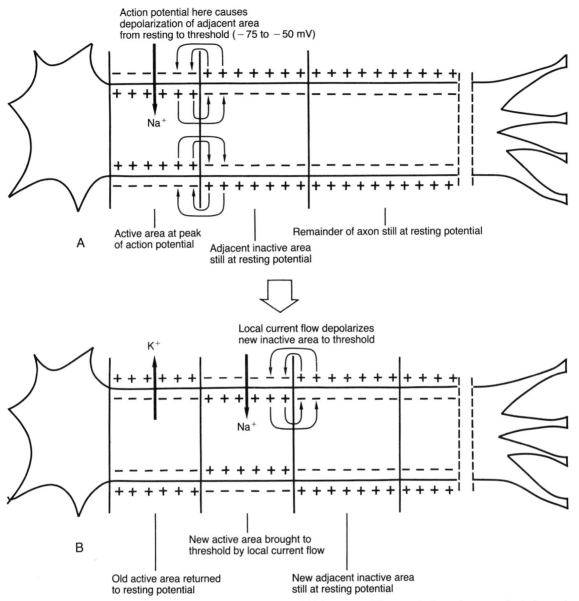

Action potential here causes
depolarization of adjacent area
from resting to threshold (-75 to -50 mV)

Na$^+$

A Active area at peak
of action potential

Adjacent inactive area
still at resting potential

Remainder of axon still at resting potential

Local current flow depolarizes
new inactive area to threshold

K$^+$

Na$^+$

B Old active area returned
to resting potential

New active area brought to
threshold by local current flow

New adjacent inactive area
still at resting potential

Figure 3–5. The action potential, first generated in the axon's initial segment (A), spreads down the unmyelinated axon by triggering an action potential in the immediately adjacent membrane (B). (Redrawn from Sherwood L: Human Physiology: From Cells to Systems. St. Paul, West Publishing Co., 1989, p 99.)

larly, because the action potential also has a finite duration, there is a limit to the number of action potentials per second that can be generated on a nerve.

The action potential spreads from its origin at the initial segment down the axon. The dramatic action potential depolarization of the initial segment's membrane causes voltage-gated Na$^+$ channels to open in the immediately adjacent axon membrane. This causes an action potential to develop there, which triggers a similar cycle in its adjacent membrane,

and so on down the axon. In this way an action potential spreads from the axon's initial segment down to the presynaptic terminal at the axon's far end (Fig. 3–5).

The speed with which the action potential is conducted down the axon varies. In a small unmyelinated axon, the conduction velocity is relatively slow (e.g., 0.5 m/second), but conduction velocities of greater than 70 m/second (so that a distance nearly as long as a football field is traveled in 1 second) are known to occur in large myelinated nerve axons. This

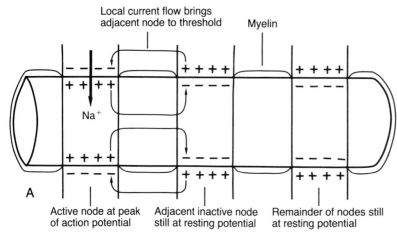

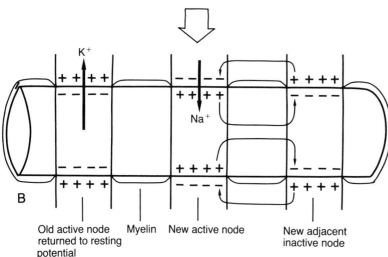

Figure 3–6. Saltatory conduction of action potentials in myelinated axons (*A → B*) is faster than action potential conduction in unmyelinated axons, because the action potential functionally jumps from node to node. (Adapted from Sherwood L: Human Physiology: From Cells to Systems. St. Paul, West Publishing Co., 1989.)

occurs because the action potential functionally jumps from node to node owing to the influence of the myelin and the greater concentration of voltage-gated Na^+ channels at the nodes of Ranvier (Fig. 3–6).

CLINICAL CORRELATION

HYPOGLYCEMIA

HISTORY □ You examine an 8-year-old boxer dog whose owner complains that the dog experiences seizures, weakness, and confusion near the time he is fed.

CLINICAL EXAMINATION □ The dog's physical examination, including his neurological examination, was within normal limits. His fasting serum glucose was 29 mg/dL (normal is 70–110 mg/dL) and the ratio between serum insulin and serum glucose was markedly elevated.

COMMENT □ Neurons are dependent primarily on oxygen and glucose as metabolites for ATP energy production, and neurons cannot store appreciable quantities of glucose. ATP is needed for maintenance of the normal electrical membrane potential. Deprived of adequate glucose, and hence ATP, the brain malfunctions, commonly with seizures, weakness, and confusion. These signs were more common at the time of feeding because insulin's release is stimulated, either by eating or psychologically in anticipation of eating.

In this case, the insulin to glucose ratio is elevated, probably owing to an insulin-secreting tumor of the pancreas. Because insulin facilitates glucose's transport through cell membranes, too much insulin results in the transfer of too much serum glucose to the cytoplasm of other cells of the body, thus depriving the brain's neurons of this essential metabolite.

TREATMENT □ Insulinomas can usually be found and removed from the pancreas surgically. However, a high rate of metastasis with this tumor means that other tumor sites may remain, in the liver and elsewhere, to overproduce insulin.

Bibliography

Berne RM, Levy MN (eds): Physiology, 2nd ed. St Louis, CV Mosby, 1988, pp 22–45, 55–65.
Guyton AC: Textbook of Medical Physiology, 7th ed. Philadelphia, WB Saunders, 1986, pp 101–120.
Kandel ER, Schwartz JH (eds): Principles of Neural Science, 2nd ed. New York, Elsevier, 1985, pp 49–86.
Willis WD, Grossman RG: Medical Neurobiology, Neuroanatomical and Neurophysiological Principles Basic to Clinical Neuroscience, 3rd ed. St Louis, CV Mosby, 1981, pp 1–48.

PRACTICE QUESTIONS FOR CHAPTER 3

1. In treating critically ill patients with intravenous fluids, which two ions are most important to the nerve membrane potential?

   a. Na^+ and Cl^-
   b. K^+ and Cl^-
   c. Ca^{2+} and Cl^-
   d. K^+ and Ca^{2+}
   e. Na^+ and K^+

2. The energy required by the Na^+, K^+ nerve membrane pump is derived from ATP. In the neuron, this energy results from the nearly exclusive metabolism of oxygen and

   a. amino acids.
   b. fatty acids.
   c. glucose.
   d. glycogen.
   e. proteins.

3. If the frequency of IPSPs on a nerve membrane decreases while the frequency of EPSPs remains the same, what will happen to the action potentials on the nerve cell membrane?

   a. Frequency of action potentials increases
   b. Frequency of action potentials decreases
   c. Frequency of action potentials remains unchanged
   d. Action potentials would be eliminated
   e. Action potentials would be conducted with increased velocity

4. During an excitatory postsynaptic potential in a nerve membrane, which of the following is the most important ion flow?

   a. Sodium ions diffuse out of the cell.
   b. Sodium ions diffuse into the cell.
   c. Potassium ions diffuse out of the cell.
   d. Potassium ions diffuse into the cell.
   e. None of the above

5. Choose the *incorrect* statement below:

   a. Conduction velocity of action potentials is slower in myelinated than in unmyelinated nerves.
   b. Conduction velocity of action potentials is faster in myelinated than in unmyelinated nerves.
   c. In saltatory conduction of action potentials, the action potential jumps from node to node (nodes of Ranvier).
   d. Action potentials are of equal magnitude at the beginning and at the end of an axon.

4

The Neuromuscular Synapse

1. The anatomy of the neuromuscular synapse is specialized for one-way communication
2. Action potential on the presynaptic nerve triggers an action potential on the muscle through the release of acetylcholine

Nerves communicate with each other and with other cells of the body, such as muscle or secretory cells. Such communication occurs between cells at specialized junctions called *synapses,* a word taken from the Greek word for junction, or to bind tightly. Synaptic transmission between cells can be either electrical or chemical. At electrical synapses, ionic current flows between pre- and postsynaptic cells as the mediator for transmission. More commonly, synaptic transmission is mediated by a chemical messenger. Released from the presynaptic cell by the arriving action potential, this chemical messenger diffuses to the postsynaptic cell membrane, where it binds with a receptor, thus initiating the postsynaptic potential change. The best understood of these chemical synapses is the synapse between a motor neuron and a skeletal muscle cell—the neuromuscular synapse. This is the synapse discussed in this chapter. Other synapses are discussed in subsequent chapters.

The Anatomy of the Neuromuscular Synapse Is Specialized for One-Way Communication

The motor neuron (later to be called the α lower motor neuron) comes into close apposition with the skeletal muscle cell at a specialized junction called the neuromuscular synapse (Fig. 4–1). This synapse has a presynaptic (nerve) side, a narrow space between the nerve and muscle, called the synaptic cleft, and a postsynaptic (muscle) side.

The presynaptic portion of the synapse is made up of the terminal portion of the motor neuron, whose axon extends from the central nervous system (CNS) to the muscular cell to signal muscular contraction. This synaptic, transmitting end of the axon contains a large number of synaptic vesicles that contain the chemical transmitter substance—in this case acetylcholine. These vesicles are clustered around an active zone of the presynaptic mem-

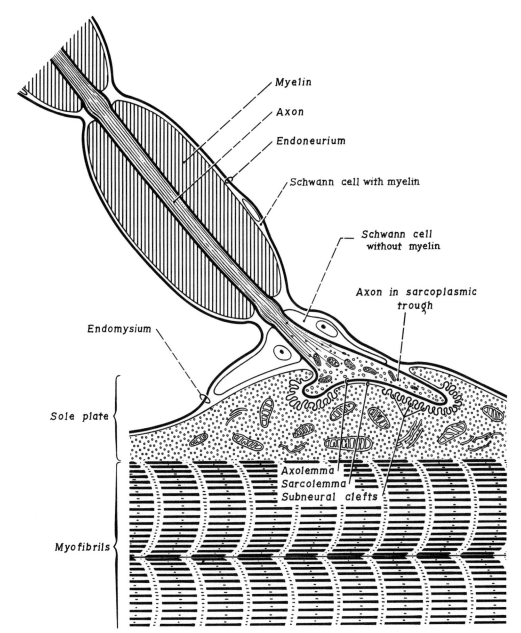

Figure 4–1. The neuromuscular synapse has a presynaptic (nerve) side, a narrow space between the nerve and muscle called the synaptic cleft, and a postsynaptic (muscle) side. (From De Lahunta A (ed): Veterinary Neuroanatomy and Clinical Neurology, 2nd ed. Philadelphia, WB Saunders, 1983.)

brane, adjacent to the postsynaptic junctional folds. The presynaptic nerve terminal also contains mitochondria, an indication of the active metabolism that takes place in the nerve cytoplasm as acetylcholine is synthesized before it is absorbed into the synaptic vesicles.

The presynaptic (nerve) and postsynaptic (muscle) cell membranes are separated by a narrow space from 20 to 30 nm wide, called

the synaptic cleft. The cleft contains extracellular fluid and a basal lamina of spongy reticular fibers.

The postsynaptic cell membrane has several specialized features that facilitate synaptic transmission. The membrane has a series of invaginations, called junctional folds, that increase the surface area of the postsynaptic membrane. Receptors to the acetylcholine neurotransmitter are located on the postsynaptic membrane at the mouth of these junctional folds.

Because the neurotransmitter is found only on the presynaptic nerve side of the synapse, transmission can go from nerve to muscle only, not in the reverse direction.

An Action Potential on the Presynaptic Nerve Triggers an Action Potential on the Muscle Through the Release of Acetylcholine

The function of the neuromuscular synapse is to transmit an action potential message unidirectionally between a motor nerve and a skeletal muscle cell with a frequency and timing established by the nervous system. The arrival of an action potential along the motor nerve triggers the release of the acetylcholine transmitter, which then binds with receptors on the postsynaptic muscle cell membrane, resulting in the genesis of an action potential along the muscle cell.

An action potential on a motor nerve arises at its initial axon segment, then spreads along the entire axon, eventually arriving at its terminal, presynaptic end (see Chapter 3). As the action potential arrives at the presynaptic membrane, in the presence of sufficient Ca^{2+} ions, many of the acetylcholine-containing synaptic vesicles fuse with the presynaptic membrane, open, and release their acetylcholine into the synaptic cleft. Following transmitter release, the vesicle membrane is recycled back into the presynaptic nerve cytoplasm to be refilled with acetylcholine from the cytoplasm.

Acetylcholine then diffuses across the synaptic cleft. Arriving at the postsynaptic membrane, acetylcholine binds with a transmitter-specific receptor, which controls ligand-gated ion channels in the postsynaptic muscle membrane (see Chapter 1).

As acetylcholine binds with its postsynaptic receptor, ligand-gated Na^+ channels are opened, and Na^+ ions diffuse into the muscle cell, triggering an action potential on the muscle cell membrane (see Chapter 3). Acetylcholine is allowed to bind with its receptor only briefly before it is destroyed by the enzyme acetylcholinesterase.

This enzyme, located on the postsynaptic membrane, inactivates acetylcholine by cleaving it into acetyl and choline molecules. Because the neurotransmitter is destroyed soon after its binding with the muscle membrane receptor, and more transmitter will not be available to attach to the receptors in sufficient quantities until another nerve action potential occurs, there is a roughly 1:1 ratio between action potentials on the nerve and muscle cell membranes.

As seen in the next chapter, action potentials on the muscle cell membrane lead to contraction, or mechanical shortening, of the muscle cell. When this contraction is combined with the shortening of many muscle cells, movement of the body occurs.

CLINICAL CORRELATION

MYASTHENIA GRAVIS

HISTORY ☐ You examine a 5-year-old female German shepherd whose owner states that the dog becomes progressively weak with exercise. The owner states also that recently, just after eating, the dog has begun to vomit food in formed, cylindrically shaped boluses.

CLINICAL EXAMINATION ☐ All physical examination abnormalities were referable to the neuromuscular system. After resting, the dog's neurological examination was within normal limits. But with even moderate exercise, the dog became progressively weak, particularly in the front legs. Intravenous injection of an acetylcholinesterase inhibitor, edrophonium (TENSILON), eliminated all clinical signs of weakness. Radiographs of the chest revealed an enlarged esophagus and thymus.

COMMENT ☐ The history, enlarged esophagus, and response to an acetylcholinesterase inhibitor confirm the diagnosis of myasthenia gravis (grave muscle weakness). This is caused by a failure of transmission at the neuromuscular synapse. This transmission failure is due to antibodies produced by the body against its own acetylcholine receptors. Receptors complexed with these abnormal antibodies cannot cause the depolarization of the postsynaptic membrane in the time acetylcholine normally has to work at the synapse. Acetylcholinesterase inhibitors allow acetylcholine to build up at the synapse, facilitating normal transmission.

The large amount of skeletal muscle in the dog's esophagus explains its enlargement from paralysis. These patients often vomit formed boluses of food shortly after eating.

Myasthenia gravis is associated often with mediastinal masses, usually of the thymus, which may be a source of either the antireceptor antibodies or the antigen.

TREATMENT □ Spontaneous remissions are common. Until then, oral daily acetylcholinesterase inhibitors are given.

Bibliography

Berne RM, Levy MN (eds): Physiology, 2nd ed. St Louis, CV Mosby, 1988, pp 46–52.
Guyton AC: Textbook of Medical Physiology, 7th ed. Philadelphia, WB Saunders, 1986, pp 136–139.
Kandel ER, Schwartz JH (eds): Principles of Neural Science, 2nd ed. New York, Elsevier, 1985, pp 87–107, 176–185.
Lance JW, McLeod JG: A Physiological Approach to Clinical Neurology, 3rd ed. London, Butterworths, 1981, pp 46–70.
Willis WD, Grossman RG: Medical Neurobiology, Neuroanatomical and Neurophysiological Principles Basic to Clinical Neuroscience, 3rd ed. St Louis, CV Mosby, 1981, pp 49–85.

PRACTICE QUESTIONS FOR CHAPTER 4

1. At the somatic neuromuscular synapse, Ca^{2+} ions are necessary to

   a. bind the transmitter with the postsynaptic receptor.
   b. facilitate diffusion of the transmitter to the postsynaptic membrane.
   c. split the transmitter in the cleft, thus deactivating the transmitter.
   d. fuse the presynaptic vesicle with the presynaptic membrane, thus releasing the transmitter.
   e. metabolize the transmitter within the presynaptic vesicle.

2. A drug that would prevent the release of acetylcholine at the neuromuscular synaptic junction would cause what, if any, clinical signs?

   a. Convulsions and excess muscle contractions
   b. Paralysis
   c. No effect on an animal's movement

3. The neurotransmitter between the α motor neuron and the extrafusal skeletal muscle fiber is

   a. norepinephrine.
   b. acetylcholine.
   c. epinephrine.
   d. γ amino butyric acid.
   e. dopamine.

4. You examine a dog that can walk briefly but tires quickly and, after a few minutes of walking, is unable to rise until she rests for several minutes. She is bright, alert, and responsive. Neurological examination after the dog has rested is essentially within normal limits. Intravenous infusion of an acetylcholinesterase-inhibiting drug eliminated the clinical signs of fatigue. Where is the most likely location for this dog's pathology?

   a. Brain
   b. Neuromuscular junction
   c. Thoracolumbar spinal cord
   d. Lower motor neurons to the front leg(s)
   e. Lower motor neurons to the hind leg(s)

5. Several drugs compete with acetylcholine for the postsynaptic receptor at the neuromuscular junction. If you overdosed your patient with one of these competitive drugs, what would the antidote have to do at the synapse?

   a. Decrease the release of acetylcholine
   b. Decrease the effectiveness of acetylcholinesterase
   c. Decrease synaptic Ca^{2+}
   d. Increase the postsynaptic membrane potential
   e. None of the above

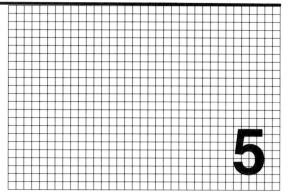

5

The Physiology of Muscle

1. All movement is the result of contraction of skeletal muscles across a movable joint
2. There are several levels of organization in any skeletal muscle
3. Action potentials on the sarcolemma spread to the interior of the cell along the transverse tubules
4. The sliding of actin along the myosin molecule results in physical shortening of the sarcomere
5. The action potential on the sarcolemma is coupled to the contraction mechanism through the release of Ca^{2+} from the sarcoplasmic reticulum
6. Muscles change their strength of contraction by varying the number of active motor units
7. The electromyogram is the clinical measurement of the electrical behavior within a skeletal muscle
8. Most skeletal muscle fibers can be divided into either fast-contracting or slow-contracting fibers
9. The structure of cardiac and smooth muscle differs from that of skeletal muscle
10. The role of calcium ions in excitation-contraction coupling in cardiac and smooth muscle differs from that in skeletal muscle

There are three types of muscle in the body: skeletal, cardiac, and smooth muscle. Skeletal muscle makes up about 40% of the body, and smooth muscle and cardiac muscle make up nearly 10% more. Because most veterinary patients with disease of the neuromuscular system exhibit abnormalities of movement, it is important to understand how skeletal muscle functions and how it is controlled by the nervous system. Abnormalities of cardiac muscle and smooth muscle feature prominently in many other clinical disorders and in pharmacological mechanisms also.

This chapter explains the physiology of skeletal muscle. Brief comparisons with cardiac and smooth muscle are made also. Cardiac muscle is mentioned more extensively in chapters on the cardiovascular system, and the role of smooth muscle in other body systems is mentioned numerous times throughout this book.

All Movement Is the Result of Contraction of Skeletal Muscles Across a Movable Joint

All body movement is the result of contraction of skeletal muscle. Skeletal muscle consists of a central fleshy contractile portion and two tendons—one on each end of the muscle. The muscle and its tendons are arranged in the body so that they originate on one bone and insert on a different bone while spanning a joint. As the muscle contracts, shortening the distance between the origin and insertion tendons, the bones move with respect to each other, bending at the joint (Fig. 5–1). When activated by the motor nerve, a skeletal muscle can only shorten. Most joints have a muscle on both sides, both to decrease its angle (flexion) and to increase its angle (extension). All

movement performed by an animal is the result of contraction of skeletal muscles across a movable joint. It is important, then, to understand the anatomy and physiology of skeletal muscle before the discussion of how the nervous system choreographs the contraction of groups of muscle cells in order to perform purposeful movement.

There Are Several Levels of Organization in Any Skeletal Muscle

Figure 5–2 illustrates the several levels of organization in a typical skeletal muscle. Each muscle belly seen during dissection is made up of varying numbers of muscle cells (usually called muscle fibers) that span the several inches between the origin and insertion tendons. They range between 10 and 80 μm in diameter and contain multiple mitochondria and other intracellular organelles. The outer limiting membrane is called the sarcolemma. It consists of a true cell membrane, called the plasma membrane, and an outer polysaccharide layer that attaches to the tendons at the cells' extremities. Each muscle cell is innervated by only one nerve ending, located near the middle of the fiber.

Each muscle fiber is made up of successively smaller subunits (see Fig. 5–2). Muscle fibers each contain several hundred to several thousand *myofibrils* arranged in parallel along its length, like a handful of spaghetti. Each myofibril is made up of a series of repeating *sarcomeres*, the basic contractile unit of the muscle fiber.

The sarcomere has a disc at each end called the Z disc. The sarcomere contains four types of large, polymerized protein molecules responsible for muscular contraction. Numerous thin protein filaments, called *actin*, are attached to the Z discs and extend toward the center of the sarcomere like parallel fingers pointing at each other. Each actin filament consists of two strands of actin protein and two strands of *tropomyosin* protein wound together as a helix. Also located intermittently along the tropomyosin molecules are globular protein molecules called *troponin*, which have an affinity for calcium ions. Suspended between the actin filaments are thicker *myosin* protein filaments. Myosin also consists of protein helixes and contains intermittent crossbridges that interact with actin to shorten the sarcomere.

Located in parallel to the myofibrils are

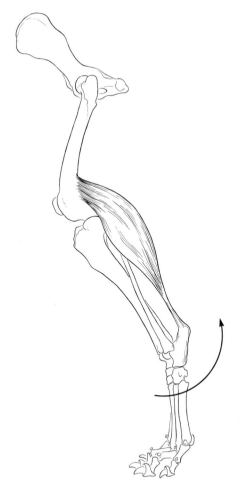

Figure 5–1. All noticeable movement is the result of contraction (shortening) of a skeletal muscle attached across a movable joint.

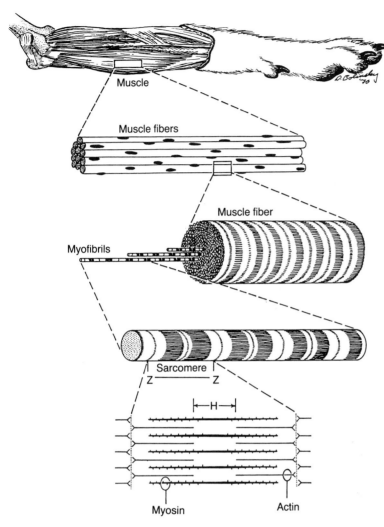

Figure 5–2. There are several levels of organization in a typical skeletal muscle.

numerous long endoplasmic reticula called the *sarcoplasmic reticula* in muscle cells (Fig. 5–3). They sequester calcium ions in relaxed muscle.

Located between sarcoplasmic reticula, but perpendicular to the long axis of the muscle fiber, are the *transverse tubules* (see Fig. 5–3). These tubules traverse the diameter of the muscle cell from one side of the sarcolemma to the other, much like piercing a sausage with a nail perpendicular to its long axis. These tubules are filled with extracellular fluid. They are important because they allow the muscle cells' action potential to be transmitted to the interior of the cell.

Action Potentials on the Sarcolemma Spread to the Interior of the Cell Along the Transverse Tubules

Skeletal muscle cells have a resting membrane potential like that of nerve, a membrane potential that can be excited by synaptic transmission at the neuromuscular junction (see Chapter 4). It is at the neuromuscular junction that action potentials are generated. Once an action potential is generated at the synapse near the center of the muscle fiber, it spreads in both directions along the length of the fiber by mechanisms similar to action potential spread in unmyelinated nerve axons. In contrast to those on axons, however, action potentials on the sarcolemma are also transmitted to the interior of the cell along the transverse tubules. This allows the action potential to reach the sarcoplasmic reticula even in the innermost regions of the muscle fiber. The consequences of the action potential's arrival at the sarcoplasmic reticulum is discussed later when the coupling of excitation (the action potential) with contraction (shortening) of the sarcomeres is examined.

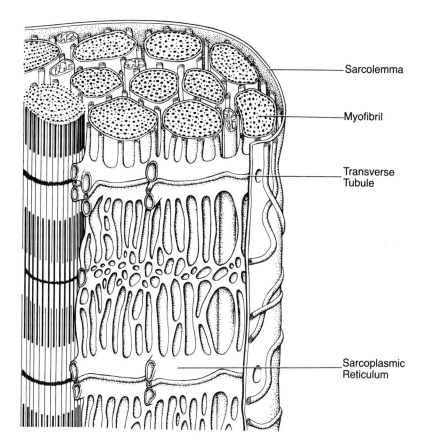

Sarcolemma

Myofibril

Transverse Tubule

Sarcoplasmic Reticulum

Figure 5–3. A three-dimensional diagram of skeletal muscle showing the juxtaposition of myofibrils, transverse tubules, and sarcoplasmic reticula. (Adapted from Leeson TL, Leeson CR, and Paparo AA (eds): Text/Atlas of Histology. Philadelphia, WB Saunders, 1988.)

The Sliding of Actin Along the Myosin Molecule Results in Physical Shortening of the Sarcomere

Figure 5–4 illustrates the sarcomere in the relaxed state and in its shorter, contracted state. The sarcomere is changed from its relaxed state to the shorter, contracted state when calcium ions become available to the sarcomere. In the presence of calcium ions and a sufficient source of adenosine triphosphate (ATP), actin and myosin molecules slide over one another, thus shortening the sarcomere. Because each myofibril is made up of a series of repeating and connected sarcomeres, the net result is the physical shortening of the distance between the two ends of the muscle. A detailed molecular explanation of this sliding filament mechanism of sarcomere shortening is not known, but several portions of the process have now been established. At several points along the actin molecule, there are active sites that chemically interact with the head of the myosin molecule. In the absence of calcium ions, these sites are either inhibited or covered by the tropomyosin molecules in their helix. But in the presence of calcium, which binds with troponin, the tropomyosin molecule is in some way changed so that these active actin sites are freed to react with the myosin molecules. In some poorly understood way, these reactions cause actin and myosin to "walk along" each other in order to shorten the sarcomere. In the absence of calcium, this "walk-along" bonding no longer occurs, and relaxation results.

The Action Potential on the Sarcolemma Is Coupled to the Contraction Mechanism Through the Release of Ca^{2+} from the Sarcoplasmic Reticulum

At rest, calcium ions are pumped out of the sarcoplasmic fluid and into the sarcoplasmic reticulum by an energy-dependent pump. This leaves too low a concentration of calcium in the sarcomere to allow contraction. However, as an action potential spreads along the cell surface and into the muscle fiber along the transverse tubules, it arrives eventually in the

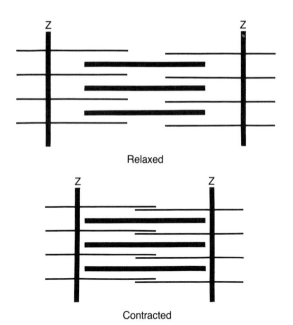

Figure 5–4. The sliding of actin along the myosin molecule results in the physical shortening (contraction) of the sarcomere.

neighborhood of the sarcoplasmic reticulum. The arrival of the action potential at the sarcoplasmic reticulum causes the release of calcium ions, which diffuse down their concentration gradient out of the sarcoplasmic reticulum and into the fluid bathing the sarcomere. These calcium ions then trigger contraction. As the action potential passes, calcium is pumped again into the sarcoplasmic reticulum, and relaxation results. This cycle is known as *excitation-contraction coupling*.

Muscles Change Their Strength of Contraction by Varying the Number of Active Motor Units

A *motor unit* is defined as one motor neuron and all the muscle fibers that it innervates. Even though each muscle fiber is innervated by only one neuron, each motor neuron's axon branches as it reaches the muscle and innervates several muscle fibers. The ratio of nerve to muscle fiber varies with the function of the muscle. For example, large antigravity muscles (see Chapter 9) like the quadriceps femoris and gastrocnemius muscles have several hundred muscle fibers innervated by each motor nerve. Muscles requiring little strength but discrete control, like the muscles that control the position of the eyes, may have less than ten muscle fibers for each motor axon.

The nervous system can call upon a muscle to contract with greater force primarily by increasing the number of motor units that contract at any one time (called *spatial summation*). Force of contraction can be increased also by increasing the frequency of contraction within a motor unit (called *temporal summation*). A muscle contracts by gradually increasing and then decreasing the number of active motor units. As seen in Chapter 9, this choreography is the responsibility of the central nervous system (CNS).

In skeletal muscle, the nervous system can command that some percentage of motor units be contracting all the time (although not the same motor units), thus continually shortening the distance between the origin and insertion tendon. When contraction of a whole muscle belly occurs without relaxation, the muscle is said to be in *tetany*. Tetanization of cardiac muscle would be fatal, because heart muscle must relax to allow cardiac filling before it contracts to pump out the blood. Later in this chapter, it is shown how cardiac muscle prevents tetany.

The Electromyogram Is the Clinical Measurement of the Electrical Behavior within a Skeletal Muscle

As an action potential spreads along a muscle fiber, a small portion of the electrical current generated spreads away from the fiber, even to the overlying skin. Electrodes placed on the skin or inserted into the muscle belly can record a summated electrical potential when the muscle contracts. Such a measurement is called an *electromyogram* and is for skeletal muscle what the electrocardiogram (ECG) is for cardiac muscle. The measurement of the electromyogram is useful when trying to determine whether weakness or paralysis is due to disease in the skeletal muscle, neuromuscular junction, motor neuron, or CNS.

Most Skeletal Muscle Fibers Can Be Divided into Either Fast-Contracting or Slow-Contracting Fibers

Skeletal muscle fibers with short contraction times are sometimes called *fast twitch fibers*. They tend to be larger, have extensive sarcoplasmic reticula for rapid release of calcium ions, and have less extensive blood and mitochondrial supplies, because aerobic metabolism is less important. Fast twitch fibers are well adapted for jumping, sprinting, and other brief, powerful movements.

By contrast, *slow twitch fibers* are smaller muscle fibers, have a rich blood and mitochondrial supply, and have a great deal of myoglobin, an iron-containing and oxygen-storing protein similar to hemoglobin. These fibers rely more heavily on oxidative metabolism and are better adapted for the continual contraction of antigravity extensor muscles.

Because slow twitch muscles have more myoglobin, they are sometimes called red muscle, whereas fast twitch fibers are called white muscle. Usually, a muscle belly is made up of a blend of these two types, the proportions varying depending on the muscle's use. This blend can be changed with exercise, such as in an athlete training for a different type of sports event.

The Structure of Cardiac and Smooth Muscle Differs from That of Skeletal Muscle

Like skeletal muscle, *cardiac muscle* is striated and contains sarcoplasmic reticula and myofibrils with actin and myosin subunits forming the fundamental contractile component. Cardiac muscle contains transverse tubules also, but cardiac muscle differs from skeletal muscle in some important ways. Cardiac muscle cells are shorter than those of skeletal muscle and are connected to each other through end-to-end *intercalated discs*. Action potentials can spread from one cardiac muscle cell to another across these intercalated discs without the need for any nerve transmission. In fact, as explained in Chapter 18, action potentials arise spontaneously in specialized cardiac muscle cells and then spread throughout a large population of cardiac muscle cells as if they were a functional syncytium. The frequency of such action potentials, and the force of the resulting contraction, are influenced by the autonomic nervous system, but such innervation is not necessary for action potential genesis.

Smooth muscle cells are much smaller and shorter than skeletal muscle cells. They do not contain transverse tubules, presumably because their actin and myosin molecules are close enough to the outer cell membrane to be influenced directly by the sarcolemma's action potential and transmembrane diffusion of Ca^{2+} ions.

Some smooth muscle cell tissues, usually called *visceral smooth muscle,* have gap junctions between cells and operate like a functional syncytium with cell-to-cell action potential transmission much as in cardiac muscle. This type of smooth muscle is described more fully in Chapter 27. Another type of smooth muscle cell tissue, usually called *multiunit smooth muscle,* has completely separate muscle cells, each of which receives autonomic innervation. Multiunit smooth muscle can be found, for example, in the iris and ciliary body of the eye, where precise control of muscular contraction is needed. Visceral smooth muscle is common in the gastrointestinal tract and other organs of the thoracic and abdominal cavities.

The Role of Calcium Ions in Excitation-Contraction Coupling in Cardiac and Smooth Muscle Differs from That in Skeletal Muscle

Contraction of both cardiac and smooth muscle cells results from the sliding together of actin and myosin protein filaments just as in skeletal muscle. This sliding of actin over myosin requires ATP and does not occur unless Ca^{2+} ions are present, again as in skeletal muscle. But the origins of the intracytoplasmic Ca^{2+} ions that permit contraction differ. In skeletal muscle Ca^{2+} is sequestered in the sarcoplasmic reticulum. With the arrival of the action potential along the sarcolemma and transverse tubule, Ca^{2+} is released from the sarcoplasmic reticulum and diffuses out into the cytoplasm, where it triggers contraction. With the passage of the action potential, Ca^{2+} is pumped back into the sarcoplasmic reticulum, and the muscle relaxes. In skeletal muscle, little if any extracellular Ca^{2+} is needed for contraction. However, in cardiac and smooth muscle, both extracellular and sarcoplasmic reticulum Ca^{2+} ions are important in triggering contraction. Both muscle types contain sarcoplasmic reticulum with sequestered Ca^{2+}, although they are less well developed in smooth muscle. With the arrival of the action potential along the cell membrane (and the T tubules in cardiac muscle), slow channels are opened to Ca^{2+}, allowing the influx of extracellular Ca^{2+} ions. This second source of calcium supplements the sarcoplasmic reticulum Ca^{2+} in triggering contraction. If drugs called *calcium channel blockers* are used to block the entry of extracellular Ca^{2+} ions, the force of contraction is reduced. Once the action potential has passed, muscle relaxation is accomplished by pumping cytoplasmic Ca^{2+}

back into the sarcoplasmic reticula and through the sarcolemma into the extracellular space.

Bibliography

Berne RM, Levy MN (eds): Physiology, 2nd ed. St Louis, CV Mosby, 1988, pp 315–356.
Guyton AC: Textbook of Medical Physiology, 7th ed. Philadelphia, WB Saunders, 1986, pp 120–153.
Kandel ER, Schwartz JH (eds): Principles of Neural Science, 2nd ed. New York, Elsevier, 1985, pp 196–208.
Lance JW, McLeod JG: A Physiological Approach to Clinical Neurology, 3rd ed. London, Butterworths, 1981, pp 63–70.

PRACTICE QUESTIONS FOR CHAPTER 5

1. The number of extrafusal muscle fibers in each motor unit would be lowest in which of the following muscles?

   a. Quadriceps
   b. Triceps
   c. Gluteal muscles
   d. Muscles for moving the human fingers
   e. Muscles for wagging the canine tail

2. Action potentials in skeletal muscle cells trigger the release from the sarcoplasmic reticulum of what ion critical to the muscle's contractile process?

   a. Ca^{2+}
   b. Na^+
   c. K^+
   d. Cl^-
   e. HCO_3^-

3. A gross skeletal muscle belly can be made (by the CNS) to contract more forcefully by

   a. causing more of its motor units to contract simultaneously.
   b. increasing the amount of acetylcholine released during each neuromuscular synaptic transmission.
   c. increasing the frequency of action potentials in the α motor neuron's axon.
   d. both a and c
   e. both b and c

4. Choose the *incorrect* statement below:

   a. The muscle fiber and nerve cell membranes are similar because they both have a resting membrane potential.
   b. A whole muscle, such as the gastrocnemius muscle, can be made to contract more forcefully by increasing the number of motor units contracting.
   c. The muscle membrane's transverse tubular system transmits the action potential to the interior of the cell.
   d. The muscle cell membrane transmits action potentials by saltatory conduction.
   e. The shortening of a skeletal muscle during contraction is due to the sliding together of actin and myosin filaments.

5. Which of the following is NOT a part of a motor unit?

   a. The α motor neuron
   b. The neuromuscular synapse
   c. Extrafusal muscle fibers
   d. The sarcomere
   e. The intrafusal muscle fiber

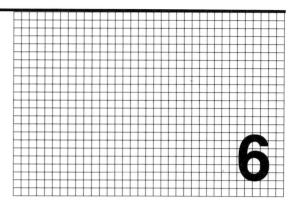

The Concept of a Reflex

1. A reflex arc contains five fundamental components
2. Reflex arcs are either segmental or intersegmental
3. Reflexes are widespread in the nervous system and underlie a major portion of the neurological examination of a patient

The reflex arc is fundamental to the physiology of posture and locomotion as well as to the clinical examination of the nervous system. The word *reflex* comes from the Latin word *reflectere*, which means to bend backward. A reflex arc, in a sense, is reflected off the central nervous system (CNS). A reflex can be defined as an involuntary, qualitatively unvarying response of the nervous system to a stimulus. The anatomy and function of a reflex arc are programmed genetically and are fully developed at birth.

A Reflex Arc Contains Five Fundamental Components

All reflex arcs contain five basic components (Fig. 6–1). If any one of these five components malfunctions, the reflex response will be altered.

1. All reflex arcs begin with a *receptor*. Receptors vary widely within the body, but all share a common function: they transduce some environmental energy and convert that energy into action potentials, the only language the nervous system understands. For example, receptors of the retina transduce light; those in the skin transduce heat, cold, pressure, and so forth; muscle spindle receptors transduce stretch. Many other types of receptors also transduce some particular form of environmental energy. Once transduction occurs, action potentials are generated along sensory nerves at a frequency proportional to the intensity of the energy transduced. This proportionality between the intensity with which the receptor is stimulated and the frequency of the resulting sensory nerve action potentials is called *frequency coding* and is the way the receptor communicates to the CNS the intensity of light, heat, stretch, and so forth that it has transduced.

2. The next component in a reflex arc is a *sensory nerve* (afferent nerve). These nerves carry action potentials from the receptor to the CNS. They enter the spinal cord by way of the dorsal roots.

3. The third component of a reflex arc is a *synapse* in the CNS. Actually, for most reflex arcs, more than one synapse occurs. However, a few reflex arcs are monosynaptic, like those that come from the muscle spindle.

4. The fourth component is a *motor nerve* (efferent nerve) carrying action potentials from

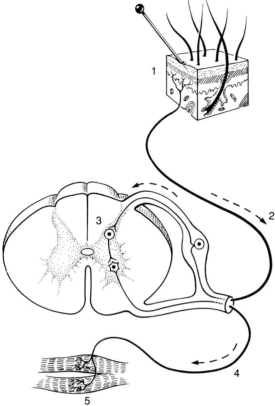

Figure 6–1. A reflex arc contains five fundamental components: *(1)* a receptor, *(2)* a sensory neuron, *(3)* one or more synapses in the CNS, *(4)* a motor neuron, and *(5)* a target organ, usually a muscle. (Used with permission from De Lahunta A (ed): Veterinary Neuroanatomy and Clinical Neurology. Philadelphia, WB Saunders, 1983, p 60.)

the CNS to the target (effector) organ. Motor nerves leaving the spinal cord depart by way of the ventral roots.

5. The last component is some *target organ* (effector organ) that causes the reflex response. Usually this is a muscle like the skeletal muscles of the quadriceps muscle of the leg, in the case of the knee jerk (muscle stretch) reflex, or like the smooth muscle of the iris, in the case of the pupillary light reflex.

Reflex Arcs Are Either Segmental or Intersegmental

A *segmental reflex* is one in which the reflex arc passes through only a small segment of the CNS. The muscle stretch reflex and the pupillary light reflex are examples of segmental reflex, because they use only a small segment of either the spinal cord or brainstem. An *intersegmental reflex* is one in which multiple segments of the CNS are utilized. Conscious

proprioception response is a good example of this type, because sensory action potentials may enter as far away as the lumbar spinal cord and yet travel all the way to the cerebral cortex before the motor response is generated. The motor response returns along roughly the same intersegmental route.

Reflexes Are Widespread in the Nervous System and Underlie a Major Portion of the Neurological Examination of a Patient

Reflex arcs are ubiquitous in the nervous system and are the basis of much of an animal's subconscious response to its environment. Much of a veterinarian's clinical examination of the nervous system involves evoking reflex responses, e.g., the pupillary light reflex, muscle stretch (knee jerk) reflex, and flexor reflex.

If any of these five components malfunctions, the expected reflex response will not occur. It is important to know the general anatomy, physiology, and expected normal clinical response of the common reflexes in order to carry out a neurological examination so that lesions can be localized. Several such reflexes are discussed in some detail in subsequent chapters of this book.

Bibliography

Berne RM, Levy MN (eds): Physiology, 2nd ed. St Louis, CV Mosby, 1988, pp 199–214.
Guyton AC: Textbook of Medical Physiology, 7th ed. Philadelphia, WB Saunders, 1986, pp 606–618.
Lance JW, McLeod JG: A Physiological Approach to Clinical Neurology, 3rd ed. London, Butterworths, 1981, pp 73–98.
Oliver JE, Hoerlein BF, Mayhew IG (eds): Veterinary Neurology. Philadelphia, WB Saunders, 1987, pp 7–48.
Willis WD, Grossman RG: Medical Neurobiology, Neuroanatomical and Neurophysiological Principles Basic to Clinical Neuroscience, 3rd ed. St Louis, CV Mosby, 1981, pp 168–181.

PRACTICE QUESTIONS FOR CHAPTER 6

1. Which of the following is NOT a necessary part of a reflex arc?

   a. Receptor
   b. Sensory (afferent) nerve
   c. Internuncial (connector) nerve

d. Motor nerve
e. Target (responding) organ

2. Which of the following is NOT a function of a receptor?

   a. Transduction of light into action potentials by the retina
   b. Transduction of sound into action potentials by the cochlea
   c. Transduction of action potentials from the motor neuron into physical shortening by skeletal muscle
   d. Transduction of painful stimuli into action potentials by free nerve endings of the skin

3. When the intensity with which a receptor is stimulated is increased, what happens to the frequency of action potentials along the sensory nerve from that receptor?

a. Increases
b. Decreases
c. No change

4. Which of the following is NOT an example of a segmental reflex?

   a. Muscle stretch reflex
   b. Pupillary light reflex
   c. Conscious proprioception reflex

5. An intersegmental reflex arc is one in which

   a. no receptor is present.
   b. axons in the arc traverse many segments of the CNS.
   c. neurons are unmyelinated.
   d. only smooth muscle is the target organ.

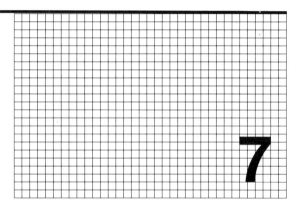

7

Skeletal Muscle Stretch Receptors

1. The muscle spindle stretch receptor is an encapsulated, specialized muscle fiber with separate motor and sensory innervations
2. The muscle spindle conveys information about muscle length to the central nervous system
3. Action potentials along the spindle sensory nerve lead reflexly to contraction of the extrafusal muscles
4. The central nervous system can control spindle sensitivity directly through the γ motor neurons
5. The Golgi tendon organ is a stretch receptor located in the tendons of the muscle and senses tension in the tendon

Movement, characteristic of all animals, is one of the qualities that separate animals from plants. An animal's movement must oppose gravity and should be purposeful. Such movement, the end product of skeletal muscle contraction, is initiated and coordinated by the central nervous system (CNS) through its control of the motor unit (see Chapter 5). In order for the CNS to control the appropriateness of body movement, it must assess the effect of gravity on the many muscles of the body, and it must detect any discrepancy between the movement it intends to command and the movement that actually occurs. Once such discrepancies are detected, appropriate adjustments can be made.

In this context it should not be surprising that mammals have evolved two important receptor systems in their skeletal muscles to detect the result of the muscle's attempt to carry out a CNS command and to assess the effect of gravity on the body. These two receptors are the *muscle spindle* and the *Golgi tendon organ* (Fig. 7–1). The muscle spindles, arranged in parallel to the contracting skeletal muscle fibers, provide information about muscle length. The Golgi tendon organ, arranged in series with the contracting skeletal muscle fibers, detects muscle tension. The anatomy and physiology of these two receptor systems are discussed in this chapter. How the CNS uses the information gathered from these receptors in coordinating posture and locomotion is discussed in Chapter 9.

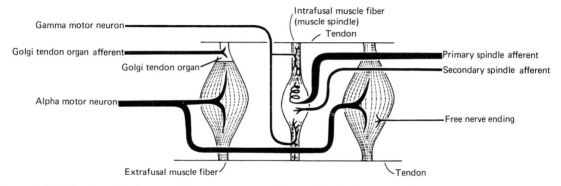

Figure 7–1. Skeletal muscles have two important receptors, the muscle spindle and the Golgi tendon organ. The intrafusal muscle fibers (muscle spindle) are in parallel with the extrafusal muscle fibers; the Golgi tendon organ is in series with the extrafusal fibers. (From Kandel ER, Schwartz JH: Principles of Neural Science, 2nd ed. Copyright 1985 by Elsevier Science Publishing Company, Inc.)

The Muscle Spindle Stretch Receptor Is an Encapsulated, Specialized Muscle Fiber with Separate Motor and Sensory Innervations

The muscle spindle is an encapsulated group of several slender and specialized skeletal muscle fibers (Fig. 7–2). Because their capsule is spindle-shaped (or fusiform), these muscles are called *intrafusal muscle fibers,* and the receptor is called the muscle spindle. They are too few, small, and weak to contribute directly to the shortening of a gross muscle, but their contraction has a dramatic effect on the receptor. The muscle fibers that cause physical shortening of the muscle (the majority of muscle fibers in a muscle belly) are called *extrafusal muscle fibers.* Extrafusal muscle fibers span the length of the gross muscle from origin to insertion tendon. Intrafusal muscle fibers and their capsules are much shorter but are functionally connected to both tendons through the connective tissue of the muscle.

Intrafusal muscle fibers have contractile proteins at their polar ends, but none in their middle, equatorial region. Therefore, their polar ends can contract, but their equatorial, fluid-filled middle region cannot. The spindle sensory (afferent) nerve arises from this equatorial region and carries action potentials from the spindle to the CNS by way of the peripheral nerves. The contractile, polar regions of the intrafusal muscle are innervated by their own separate motor nerves, called γ *motor neurons.* Extrafusal muscle fibers, those muscle fibers that cause the physical shortening of the muscle, receive a different nerve supply within the motor unit. They are called α *motor neurons.* With few exceptions, γ motor neurons go only to intrafusal muscle fibers and α motor neurons go only to the extrafusal muscle fibers.

There are two subtly different types of intrafusal fibers, spindle sensory neurons, and γ motor neurons within the spindle, but their functional difference in detecting muscle length is not important enough to mention here.

The Muscle Spindle Conveys Information about Muscle Length to the Central Nervous System

The only way in which action potentials can be generated along the spindle sensory nerve is by stretching (lengthening) the middle, equatorial segment of the intrafusal muscle fiber. However, this equatorial segment can be lengthened in two different ways. First, because the intrafusal muscle fibers lie parallel to the larger extrafusal fibers and are functionally connected to both the origin and insertion tendons (see Fig. 7–1), anything that would cause lengthening of the whole muscle would also stretch the equatorial region of the spindle's intrafusal muscle fiber. A change in body position due to gravity would be an example of movement that would usually cause extensor muscle lengthening. The second way in which the intrafusal muscle's equatorial region can be lengthened is by the contraction of the polar ends of the intrafusal muscle itself—something it does in response to γ motor nerve stimulation.

Regardless of which way the intrafusal muscle's central region is lengthened, action potentials are generated along the spindle sen-

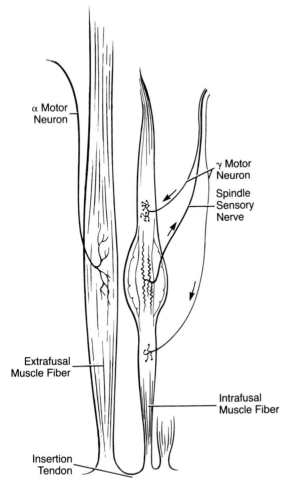

α Motor
Neuron

γ Motor
Neuron

Spindle
Sensory
Nerve

Extrafusal
Muscle Fiber

Intrafusal
Muscle Fiber

Insertion
Tendon

Figure 7–2. The muscle spindle receptor is an encapsulated group of specialized muscle cells with a separate set of motor and sensory nerves. The muscle spindle detects and sends to the CNS information about muscle length and changes in muscle length.

sory nerve in direct proportion to the amount of lengthening of the middle of the intrafusal muscle. These sensory nerves can detect not only a change in length during the dynamic phase of muscle lengthening, but also the steady state length of the muscle as the animal holds the joint still.

Action Potentials Along the Spindle Sensory Nerve Lead Reflexly to Contraction of the Extrafusal Muscles

Action potentials are generated on the spindle sensory nerve at a frequency proportional to the degree of lengthening of the spindle's equatorial region. They are transmitted to the CNS where they make an excitatory, mono-

synaptic connection with the α motor neurons that return to the extrafusal fibers of the same muscle. This leads to contraction of the extrafusal motor units in that muscle, which in turn results in a shortening of the muscle spindle's equatorial region. This shuts off the action potentials from the spindle receptor. (This is a classic negative feedback system.)

You can try this on any animal or human by striking the patellar tendon with a blunt object. This is the insertion tendon of the quadriceps muscle. Because this tendon goes over a "pulley" (the patella), hitting this tendon results in a longitudinal stretch of the whole quadriceps muscle, thus also stretching the muscle spindles. Action potentials from the spindle receptor go to the lumbar spinal cord, by way of the dorsal roots, and cause excitatory postsynaptic potentials (EPSPs) on the α motor neurons of the motor units that return to the quadriceps muscle. This causes contraction of the quadriceps muscle and an extension of the knee joint, which is an example of the *muscle stretch reflex*, or *myotatic reflex*. When it is applied to the quadriceps muscle, it is called the knee jerk reflex, but the mechanisms are present in all muscles. However, this is the easiest muscle from which to evoke the stretch reflex, because it is one of the few whose tendon goes over a sesamoid pulley before inserting on the next bone. Because of the pulley under the tendon, a lateral deflection of the tendon, as from a reflex hammer, results in a longitudinal stretch of the muscle—hence, the reflex. Hitting other tendons only moves the muscle belly laterally and does not easily result in the stretch reflex. Therefore, in the clinical neurological examination of most animals, the knee jerk reflex is the most commonly evoked muscle stretch reflex.

Of course, this system has not evolved to teach you to use a reflex hammer, but among other things, it allows the CNS to know when the muscle is stretched by change in body position. Later we shall see many other functions of the muscle spindles.

The Central Nervous System Can Control Spindle Sensitivity Directly Through the γ Motor Neurons

As mentioned earlier, contraction of the extrafusal muscle fibers is controlled by the larger α motor neurons; intrafusal muscle fibers are controlled by the smaller γ motor neurons. Gamma motor neurons innervate the intrafusal muscle fibers at their polar ends, the regions containing contractile protein. Action potentials on the γ motor neurons cause shortening of the polar regions of the spindle's intrafusal muscles, but not the equatorial region, because this middle section is devoid of contractile protein. Instead, the equatorial portion stretches.

The significance of γ innervation to the intrafusal muscle fibers is much debated, but there are many probable functions for this unique motor innervation of a receptor. As the gross muscle shortens owing to extrafusal muscle contraction, simultaneous contraction of the intrafusal fibers, due to γ motor nerve stimulation, allows the spindle receptor to remain sensitive to sudden stretches of the gross muscle over the entire range of its length. The CNS can initiate contraction of the extrafusal fibers reflexly by way of the γ motor neurons using what is known as the γ loop. The γ loop consists, in sequence, of the γ motor nerve; the intrafusal muscle fiber, including the equatorial receptor portion; the spindle sensory nerve with its monosynaptic excitatory synapse; the α motor neuron back to the same muscle; and the extrafusal muscle fibers. Chapter 9 shows how simultaneous coactivation of both the α and γ motor neurons allows the brain to test the initial load on a muscle and to test whether the amount of contraction intended by the brain was that which actually occurred. It is because of these many important roles of the muscle spindle in posture and locomotion that they have been emphasized here.

The Golgi Tendon Organ Is a Stretch Receptor Located in the Tendons of the Muscle and Senses Tension in the Tendon

Each Golgi tendon organ is a slender capsule within the tendon in series with 15–20 extrafusal skeletal muscle fibers (Fig. 7–3). Each tendon organ has an afferent, sensory nerve that carries action potentials to the CNS. The Golgi tendon organ has no motor innervation.

Because the Golgi tendon organ is in series with the extrafusal fibers, when they contract

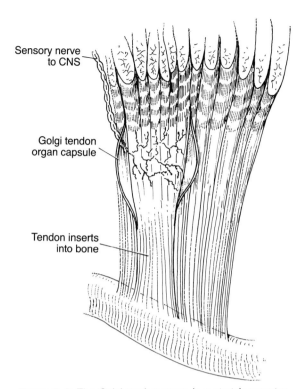

Figure 7–3. The Golgi tendon organ is a stretch receptor located in the tendons of skeletal muscle. It detects tension in the tendon and sends information about this tension to the CNS.

the tendon organ is stretched and action potentials are sent to the CNS along the sensory nerve at a frequency proportional to the tension developed by the muscle. By contrast, the muscle spindle is in parallel with the extrafusal muscle fibers, and when they contract the spindle reduces its action potential frequency.

When action potentials along the spindle sensory nerve reach the CNS, as mentioned before, they cause reflex EPSP stimulation to the α motor neurons returning to that same muscle. Action potentials along the sensory nerves from the Golgi tendon organ have the opposite effect. They cause inhibitory postsynaptic potentials (IPSPs) on the α motor neuron, thus reducing extrafusal muscle fiber contraction.

These two skeletal muscle stretch receptors provide the CNS with vital information about muscle length (the spindle) and muscle tension (the Golgi tendon organ). Such information is essential if the CNS is to adequately coordinate posture and locomotion.

CLINICAL CORRELATION

FEMORAL NERVE MONONEUROPATHY

HISTORY □ You examine an 8-year-old male golden retriever. The owner complains that the dog cannot bear weight on his right rear leg.

CLINICAL EXAMINATION □ Physical examination deficits are limited to the right rear leg, where you find that the quadriceps femoris muscles of this leg are much smaller than those of the left rear leg. The dog cannot bear weight on the right rear leg because the right quadriceps femoris muscles are paralyzed. When you tap on the left patellar tendon with a reflex hammer, the knee briskly extends (the knee jerk or muscle stretch reflex). However, when you tap on the right patellar tendon, no movement occurs.

COMMENT □ The quadriceps femoris muscle group is one of the major antigravity muscle groups of the leg causing the stifle joint (knee joint) to extend. The paralysis in this animal's quadriceps muscle is the reason he cannot bear weight on the leg. The small size of the right quadriceps muscle is due to atrophy, or muscle wasting, which in turn is due to the loss of the α motor neuron to the extrafusal muscle fibers in the quadriceps muscle belly (see Chapter 8). This would also cause a loss of the muscle stretch reflex, because even though the spindle sensed the stretch of the muscle belly caused by either gravity or the reflex hammer, the α motor neuron returning to the quadriceps muscle is unable to signal the muscle to contract, hence completing the reflex arc. This syndrome could occur if the femoral nerve was damaged by a tumor or trauma. If the pathology were in the peripheral nerve rather than only in the ventral roots, then there would likely be some sensory loss in addition to the motor deficits.

TREATMENT □ This is a femoral nerve mononeuropathy. Its treatment would depend on the cause of the nerve damage.

Bibliography

Berne RM, Levy MN (eds): Physiology, 2nd ed. St Louis, CV Mosby, 1988, pp 199–210.
Guyton AC: Textbook of Medical Physiology, 7th ed. Philadelphia, WB Saunders, 1986, pp 606–613.
Kandel ER, Schwartz JH (eds): Principles of Neural Science, 2nd ed. New York, Elsevier, 1985, pp 451–455.
Willis WD, Grossman RG: Medical Neurobiology, Neuroanatomical and Neurophysiological Principles Basic to Clinical Neuroscience, 3rd ed. St Louis, CV Mosby, 1981, pp 128–133.

PRACTICE QUESTIONS FOR CHAPTER 7

1. As the distance between the origin and insertion tendons is increased (the muscle is stretched), what happens to the frequency of action potentials along the sensory nerve from the muscle spindle in that muscle?

   a. Increase
   b. Decrease
   c. No change

2. Activation of the Golgi tendon organ leads to

   a. EPSPs to the α motor neuron that returns to that muscle.
   b. EPSPs to the α motor neuron innervating the antagonist muscle.
   c. EPSPs to the α motor neuron innervating the antagonist muscle.
   d. IPSPs to the α motor neuron that returns to that muscle.
   e. IPSPs to the γ motor neuron innervating that antagonist muscle.

3. The muscle spindle receptor in skeletal muscle can be stimulated to generate action potentials by

   a. contraction of the extrafusal fiber.
   b. contraction of the intrafusal fiber.
   c. passive stretch of the whole muscle.
   d. stimulation of the γ motor neuron.
   e. b, c, and d

4. Which of the following situations will NOT lead to action potentials on the sensory nerve coming from the muscle spindle?

   a. Contractions of the extrafusal muscle fibers in the muscle antagonistic to the muscle in which the spindle is being recorded

b. Contraction of the intrafusal muscle fibers within the recorded spindle
c. Contraction of the extrafusal muscle fibers in the muscle in which the spindle is being recorded
d. Passive stretch of the muscle in which the spindle is being recorded
e. Stimulation of the γ motor neuron to the muscle in which the spindle is being recorded

5. Which of the following is NOT a component of the γ loop to an extensor muscle?

a. Alpha motor neuron to the extensor muscle
b. Gamma motor neuron to the extensor muscle
c. Muscle spindle in the extensor muscle
d. Extrafusal muscle fiber of the extensor fiber
e. Alpha motor nerve of the antagonistic flexor muscle

8

Concept of Lower and Upper Motor Neurons and Their Malfunction

1. The lower motor neuron is classically defined as the α motor neuron
2. Disease of lower motor neurons causes stereotypical clinical signs
3. Upper motor neurons are in the central nervous system
4. Signs of upper motor neuron disease differ from those of lower motor neuron disease

The majority of veterinary patients with neurological disease display some abnormality of posture and locomotion spanning a range from weakness or paralysis to spasticity, rigidity, and convulsions. The goal of the diagnostic process is deciding where such a patient's lesion is located and what the lesion is. Central to diagnostic logic in neurology is deciding whether the patient's lesion is located in the lower motor neurons or upper motor neurons. (The two other possible locations of lesions causing movement disorders are the neuromuscular junction and skeletal muscle.) This chapter defines lower and upper motor neurons, because these concepts are useful in understanding the physiology of posture and locomotion and will be essential in later neurology courses.

Malfunctions of these two neuron populations are described briefly also.

The Lower Motor Neuron Is Classically Defined as the α Motor Neuron

The concept of a lower motor neuron is decades old in neurology. The α motor neuron is classically defined as that neuron whose cell body and dendrites are located in the central nervous system (CNS) and whose axon extends out through the peripheral nerves to synapse with the extrafusal skeletal muscle fibers. This is the final common pathway through which the CNS channels commands to the extrafusal skeletal muscle. This definition predates the discovery of γ motor neurons that innervate muscle spindles, and some would include γ motor neurons in the definition of lower motor neurons. Yet all the clinical signs caused by lower motor neuron disease can be explained by the loss of the α motor neuron.

Disease of Lower Motor Neurons Causes Stereotypical Clinical Signs

Regardless of the pathological basis for disease of lower motor neurons, a stereotypical set of clinical signs results in the skeletal muscles they innervate.

1. *Paralysis.* Disease of the α motor neurons usually prevents the nerve's action potentials from reaching the neuromuscular junction. Therefore, despite the brain's intention to command the muscle to contract, the message cannot get to the muscle, and paralysis is the result. In fact, such paralysis is usually so complete that the adjective flaccid is used to describe the paralysis in which no muscle contraction occurs.

2. *Atrophy.* Atrophy means the shrinking or wasting of skeletal muscle mass distal to the lower motor neuron lesion. This occurs within days of the injury to the nerve. The origins of this atrophy are controversial. Some physiologists believe that nerves produce nutrients transmitted across the synapse and needed for the muscle's health. Lack of such nutrients, due to the loss of the lower motor neuron, would then lead to atrophy. (The word atrophy comes from the Greek word meaning "without food," so Greek philosophers may have been particularly farsighted in choosing this term.) However, other physiologists now believe that it is simply a matter of the frequency with which the muscle is stimulated, because denervation atrophy can be prevented largely by electrical stimulation of the muscle itself.

3. *Loss of segmental reflexes.* Segmental reflexes (see Chapter 6) require the α motor neuron in the reflex arc in order for the reflex response to occur. Hence, such reflexes as the muscle stretch reflex and toe-pinch withdrawal (nociceptive) reflex will not occur, because the motor nerve portion of the arc is gone.

Because diseases of the motor nerve occur often in a mixed peripheral nerve that contains sensory nerve axons also, there may be loss of sensory modalities. This sensory loss is not strictly speaking, a lower motor neuron sign.

Upper Motor Neurons Are in the Central Nervous System

Upper motor neurons are all the neurons of the CNS that influence the lower motor neuron. In the next chapter, upper motor neurons are subdivided into three subsystems: the py-

ramidal system, the extrapyramidal system, and the cerebellum. For now, think of upper motor neurons as multineuronal systems beginning in the brain but sending axons down the spinal cord to synapse with the lower motor neurons.

Signs of Upper Motor Neuron Disease Differ from Those of Lower Motor Neuron Disease

Lesions of upper motor neurons cause clinical signs that are significantly different from those produced by lower motor neuron disease.

1. *Inappropriate movement.* In contrast to the inevitable paralysis of lower motor neuron disease, lesions of upper motor neurons cause a variety of movement disorders depending on the location of the lesion.

Spinal cord disease usually causes various degrees of weakness, whereas disease of the brain may cause seizures, rigidity, circling gaits, inability of the animal to know the position of limbs (proprioceptive deficits), and other inappropriate movements. A more precise description of this general category is presented in the chapters on the brain's control of posture and locomotion, on the cerebellum, and on the vestibular apparatus.

2. *No atrophy.* Because the lower motor neuron is intact, the muscle does not atrophy. (Modest disuse atrophy may develop much later.)

3. *Retained segmental reflexes.* Because the neuronal circuit or the segmental reflex arc (see Chapter 6) is not interrupted in upper motor neuron disease, reflexes such as the muscle stretch and toe-pinch withdrawal reflexes are retained, whereas in lower motor neuron disease, segmental reflexes are lost.

The following clinical correlations illustrate common examples of lower and upper motor neuron disease. Be sure to understand these concepts and why these dogs have the clinical signs they do before reading Chapter 9.

CLINICAL CORRELATIONS

LOWER MOTOR NEURON DISEASE

HISTORY □ A 2-year-old male German shorthaired pointer dog was admitted to the local veterinary clinic. His vaccinations were current, and there was no history of contributing prior illness.

A few days prior to admission, the dog had had a fight with a skunk. For 48 hours prior to admission an ascending paralysis developed characterized by weakness, then paralysis of first the back legs, and then the front legs. No barking was noticed during the illness. He was able to control his bladder and bowel and to move his head.

CLINICAL EXAMINATION □ On admission, the dog was unable to bear weight on any of his four legs. Other than an elevated respiratory rate, physical examination deficits were limited to the nervous system. He was able to eat, drink, and move his head. A dense paralysis was noted in all legs, and no motor response could be elicited to toe pinch or tapping the quadriceps tendon. There was widespread atrophy of the muscles of all four legs as well as those of the thorax and abdomen. The dog did seem to be aware of painful stimuli. There were no cranial nerve deficits. Routine blood cell counts and serum chemistry were within normal limits.

COMMENT □ Generalized atrophy, paralysis, and loss of segmental reflexes indicate widespread, bilateral loss of lower motor neuron function. Fortunately, the disease has spared the muscles of the head and the diaphragm, although the elevated respiratory rate indicates an attempt to compensate for paralysis of some of the respiratory muscles. A clinical diagnosis of polyradiculoneuritis (or coonhound paralysis) was made. This disease is preceded often by the bite of another animal. Pathological changes are found predominately in the ventral roots of the spinal cord where the axons of the lower motor neurons leave the spinal cord. The dorsal roots are usually spared; hence this dog's apparent ability to feel pain. The clinical signs are those of widespread lower motor neuron disease. The syndrome resembles Guillain-Barré syndrome in humans, and both syndromes have been suggested to be autoimmune in origin.

TREATMENT □ Animals with this form of paralysis usually recover spontaneously. Good nursing care is essential during the illness.

UPPER MOTOR NEURON DISEASE

HISTORY □ A 5-year-old male dachshund is brought to a local veterinary clinic. His vacci-

nation history is current and he has had no contributing past medical or surgical illnesses. Two days prior to his admission he seemed in pain. Throughout the next day he became progressively weak in his hind legs.

CLINICAL EXAMINATION □ Physical examination abnormalities were limited to the nervous system. The dog was bright, alert, responsive, and able to bear weight normally on his front legs. However, he was weak and unsteady on his hind legs. No atrophy was apparent. All cranial nerve reflexes were normal, as were the spinal segmental reflexes of both front and hind legs. Intersegmental responses were normal in the front legs but absent in the hind legs. Such responses include conscious proprioception of a paw's being placed upside-down while supporting the animal's weight. Normally an animal realizes the paw is in an unusual position and returns the paw to the correct, pads-down position. Failure to do this promptly indicates a lesion somewhere along the sensory or motor routing for this response. This routing includes the peripheral nerves for that limb, the spinal cord rostral to that limb on the same side, and the contralateral brain.) Complete blood count and serum chemistry analysis were within normal limits.

COMMENT □ The absence of atrophy and the retention of segmental reflexes in the affected limbs indicate that the lower motor neurons, neuromuscular junction, and skeletal muscle are normal and that this is an upper motor neuron disease. Because only the hind limbs are affected by weakness and proprioceptive deficits, the cervical spinal cord and brain must be normal, as motor commands to the front legs are transmitted reliably. Therefore, the lesion must be between the front and hind limbs. This is a typical history and clinical presentation for a dog with a herniated intervertebral disc.

TREATMENT □ Treatment and prognosis depend on the severity of the spinal cord trauma. Medical management is aimed at reducing edema, vasospasm, and other metabolic consequences of the disease that make the damage to the spinal cord worse. When surgery is indicated by the severity of the trauma, its goal is to relieve spinal cord compression. With appropriate medical and surgical management many dogs recover useful spinal function.

Bibliography

Berne RM, Levy MN (eds): Physiology, 2nd ed. St Louis, CV Mosby, 1988, pp 85–86, 225–226, 348–351.

Guyton AC: Textbook of Medical Physiology, 7th ed. Philadelphia, WB Saunders, 1986, pp 134–135, 617–618, 629–631, 638.

Kandel ER, Schwartz JH (eds): Principles of Neural Science, 2nd ed. New York, Elsevier, 1985, pp 196–208, 440–442.

Lance JW, McLeod JG: A Physiological Approach to Clinical Neurology, 3rd ed. London, Butterworths, 1981, pp 46–73.

Smith LH, Thier SO (eds): Pathophysiology—The Biological Principles of Disease, 2nd ed. Philadelphia, WB Saunders, 1985, pp 1004–1009.

PRACTICE QUESTIONS FOR CHAPTER 8

1. You examine a dog that is unable to stand and bear weight on the right rear leg. The right rear leg is much smaller in diameter than the left rear leg. Pinching the toe on the left rear leg results in withdrawal of the left rear leg, but pinching the toe on the right rear leg results in no movement of the right rear leg. Conscious proprioception response to the left rear leg is normal but to the right rear leg is absent. Where is this dog's pathology?

   a. Lower motor neuron to the right rear leg
   b. Lower motor neuron to the left rear leg
   c. Upper motor neuron to the right rear leg
   d. Upper motor neuron to the left rear leg
   e. Neuromuscular synapse of the right rear leg

2. You examine a dog that is bright, alert, and responsive. She can stand and bear weight on both her front legs, but she cannot stand or bear any weight on her back legs. Her knee-jerk and toe-pinch withdrawal reflexes are normal in all four legs. There is no atrophy. Conscious proprioception response is normal in the front legs but absent in both rear legs. Injecting acetylcholinesterase-inhibiting drugs caused no change in the clinical signs. Where is the dog's pathology?

   a. Brain
   b. Cervical spinal cord (spinal cord of the neck)
   c. Spinal cord between the front and rear legs (thoracolumbar spinal cord)

   d. Lower motor neurons to the rear legs
   e. Neuromuscular junction

3. You examine a dog that is bright, alert, and responsive but unable to stand on any of its four legs. Toe-pinch and knee-jerk local (segmental) reflexes are normal in all four legs. There is no atrophy. Conscious proprioception response is absent in all four legs. Injecting an acetylcholinesterase-inhibiting drug does not change the clinical signs. Where is this dog's pathology?

   a. Brain
   b. Cervical spinal cord (spinal cord in the neck)
   c. Spinal cord between the front and rear legs (thoracolumbar spinal cord)
   d. Lower motor neurons to all four legs
   e. Neuromuscular junction

4. You are presented with a horse that is unable to stand or support any weight on his hind legs. You electrically stimulate both the sciatic and femoral nerves with a sufficient stimulus, but neither stimulation results in muscular contraction. However, direct stimulation of both the gastrocnemius and quadriceps femoris muscles of the rear leg results in muscular contraction. From these observations, what do you logically conclude to be the location of this horse's pathology?

   a. Upper motor neurons to the rear legs
   b. Lower motor neurons to the rear legs
   c. Neuromuscular synapses of the rear legs
   d. Muscles of the rear legs
   e. Either b or c

5. You examine a cat that cannot bear weight on her hind legs. She is bright, alert, and responsive. Atrophy is present in the back legs. Cranial nerve reflexes are within normal limits, as are segmental reflexes and conscious proprioception to the front legs. Knee-jerk and toe-pinch withdrawal reflexes were absent in the hind legs. What is the most likely location for this cat's pathology?

   a. Brain
   b. Cervical spinal cord
   c. Thoracolumbar spinal cord
   d. Lower motor neurons to the front leg(s)
   e. Lower motor neurons to the hind leg(s)

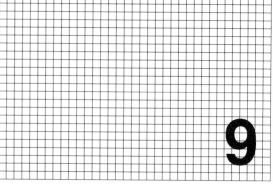

9

The Brain's Control of Posture and Locomotion

1. The central nervous system can be divided into six anatomical regions
2. The pyramidal system consists of three major axon pathways descending from the cerebral cortex
3. Pyramidal system axons originate from particular regions of the cerebral cortex
4. The pyramidal system initiates voluntary, discrete, often learned movements
5. Pyramidal system axons influence both α and γ lower motor neurons
6. Lesions in the pyramidal system cause contralateral weakness and loss of proprioception
7. The extrapyramidal system has four major tracts descending from the brainstem to influence spinal lower motor neurons
8. The extrapyramidal system maintains postural muscle tone in proximal, antigravity extensor muscles
9. The role of the basal ganglia is poorly understood
10. The cerebral cortex plays a role in extrapyramidal system function
11. Clinical syndromes resulting from extrapyramidal system lesions include either rhythmic or nonrhythmic movement disorders

Movement can be divided into two general forms. The first is a largely learned, voluntary, conscious, and skilled form, usually mediated by flexor muscles. The second is a postural, antigravity muscle tone that is generally subconscious, involuntary, and the result of extensor muscle contraction. The skilled, flexor-mediated movement results from fairly discrete contraction of a few muscle groups often distal to the spinal column. Antigravity, postural muscle tone results from the continuing contraction of larger groups of extensor muscles often located closer to the spinal column.

Unlike the sensory system, which takes physical energy and transforms it into neural information, the motor system takes neural information and transforms it into physical energy. Remember that all movement is the result of the contraction of varying numbers of extrafusal skeletal muscle fibers within vary-

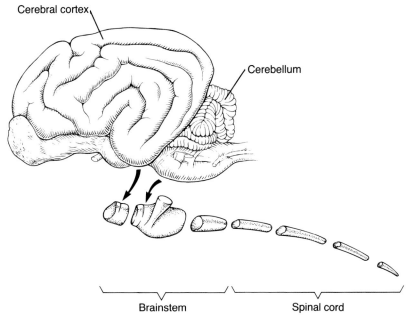

Figure 9–1. The CNS has an axial organization with the phylogenetically oldest part (the spinal cord) being caudal and the newest part (the cerebral cortex) being rostral. The CNS can be divided into six major regions: the spinal cord, medulla, pons, midbrain, diencephalon, and cerebral hemispheres.

ing numbers of motor units. These extrafusal muscle fibers do not contract until commanded to do so by the α lower motor neuron. The α motor neuron in turn does not send such an action potential command until signaled to do so by descending upper motor neurons from the brain. Hence, the α motor neuron is the final common neural pathway by which the brain can initiate the extrafusal muscle contractions that result in both voluntary and antigravity movements.

Initiating the learned, skilled, voluntary movement is largely the responsibility of a subgroup of upper motor neurons called the *pyramidal system.* Responsible for initiating antigravity, postural extensor muscle tone is held by the upper motor neurons that constitute the *extrapyramidal system.* A third subgroup of upper motor neurons, those of the *cerebellum,* helps to coordinate movement initiated by either the pyramidal or extrapyramidal system. It constantly compares the intended movement with the actual movement and makes appropriate adjustments. The cerebellum is discussed in Chapter 11. Before we discuss the pyramidal and extrapyramidal systems, however, we must first mention some general principles of neuroanatomy.

The Central Nervous System Can Be Divided into Six Anatomical Regions

The central nervous system (CNS) has an axial organization; the phylogenetically oldest part (the spinal cord) is caudal and the newest portions (the cerebral cortex) are rostral. The CNS can be divided into six major regions (Fig. 9–1).

1. The *spinal cord* is the most caudal region in the CNS. As mentioned in Chapter 2, it receives action potentials along sensory, dorsal root axons from receptors in the skin, muscles, tendons, joints, and visceral organs. It contains the cell bodies and dendrites of the lower motor neurons whose axons exit through the ventral roots to reach skeletal muscles. The spinal cord also contains axons carrying sensory information to the brain and motor commands from the brain to the lower motor neurons. The spinal cord is continued rostrally as the *brainstem,* which consists of the next three major regions of the CNS.

2. The *medulla* is the most rostral extension of the spinal cord, resembling it in many ways. It also contains several cranial nerve motor nuclei and centers for controlling the respiratory and cardiovascular systems.

3. The *pons* lies rostral to the medulla and contains the cell bodies of large numbers of neurons in a two-neuron chain that relays information from the cerebral cortex to the *cerebellum*. The cerebellum is not a part of the brainstem but is usually grouped with the pons because of its position dorsal to the pons in the posterior fossa. The cerebellum is important in coordination of movement and motor learning.

4. The *midbrain* lies rostral to the pons and is important to eye movement and subconscious postural control. Each region of the brainstem contains axon tracts carrying action potentials back and forth between the spinal cord and the rostral brain. The brainstem also contains the *reticular formation*, a net-like complex of many small neurons that regulate consciousness and modify spinal reflexes.

5. The *diencephalon* contains the *thalamus*, a relay station for sensory systems projecting into the cerebral cortex, and the *hypothalamus*, which regulates the autonomic nervous system and hormone secretion of the pituitary gland.

6. The *cerebral hemispheres* are made up of the cerebral cortex and the basal ganglia. Collectively called the cerebrum, these structures are associated with higher motor and sensory functions and with consciousness.

The CNS surrounds a system of interconnected cavities called ventricles that contain cerebrospinal fluid (see Chapter 14).

The sensory, motor, and consciousness systems of the brain have several distinct pathways arranged in parallel. For instance, both the visual and auditory systems have separate, parallel systems, and the motor system has the parallel pyramidal and extrapyramidal tracts. Each of these pathways contains synaptic relay stations along their routes and are usually topographically organized. Most pathways are crossed for unknown reasons.

Keeping these principles in mind allows a better understanding of the anatomy and function of the pyramidal and extrapyramidal systems. It also helps in appreciating the complexity of this remarkable evolutionary biological achievement.

The Pyramidal System Consists of Three Major Axon Pathways Descending from the Cerebral Cortex

All axons within the pyramidal system originate from neurons located in layer V of the cerebral cortex. These pyramidal upper motor neuron axons then extend to terminations in three different regions of the CNS. Like most axon tracts within the CNS, they are named for their sites of origin and termination.

The longest of the three pyramidal system tracts, the *corticospinal tract*, begins in the cerebral cortex and ends in the contralateral spinal cord (Fig. 9–2). Along its route, it descends from the cerebral cortex through the internal capsule, diencephalon, mesencephalon, and pons. When it gets to the medulla oblongata, about 90% of corticospinal tract axons cross to the opposite side of the nervous system and continue descending to end near lower motor neurons on the contralateral side of the spinal cord. The remaining 10% of the axons descend ipsilaterally into the spinal cord, but most of these axons also cross at a segmental level before influencing lower motor neurons. As the corticospinal axons descend through the medulla oblongata, they pass through a section of the ventral medulla that looks like a pyramid when seen in cross section. This is probably the origin of the term *pyramidal* system. The extrapyramidal system, described later, is so named because, as its axons travel through the medulla oblongata, they pass outside the pyramids.

The second of the pyramidal system tracts to leave the cerebral cortex is the *corticobulbar tract*. These axons follow the same route as for the corticospinal tract axons, but they terminate in the brainstem. Hence, they influence brainstem lower motor neurons to muscles of the head, whereas the corticospinal tract influences spinal lower motor neurons.

The third and last of the pyramidal system's descending axon tracts is the *cortico-pontine-cerebellar tract* system. It too begins in the cerebral cortex and descends into the brainstem to reach the pons, where it synapses with a second neuron whose axons sweep up predominately to the contralateral cerebellar cortex (see Chapter 11). This is the only pyramidal system axon tract that does not influence lower motor neurons directly. Its role is to inform the cerebellum of movement intended by the cerebral cortex so that, if that is not the actual movement, the cerebellum can make appropriate adjustments.

Pyramidal System Axons Originate from Particular Regions of the Cerebral Cortex

Even though all axons of the pyramidal system originate from neurons in layer V of

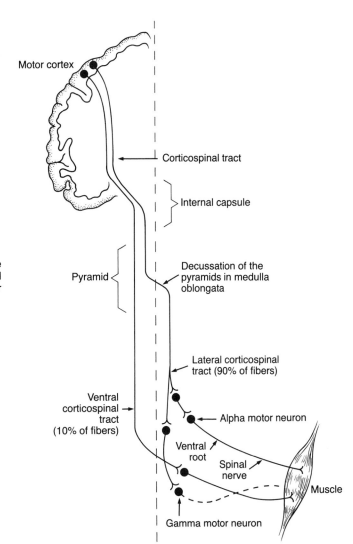

Figure 9–2. The corticospinal tract begins in the cerebral cortex and ends in the contralateral spinal cord to influence both α and γ lower motor neurons.

the cerebral cortex, not all regions of the cerebral cortex give rise to pyramidal system axons. The cerebral cortex, as seen grossly from a lateral view, is anatomically subdivided into four major regions, or lobes: the frontal, parietal, occipital, and temporal lobes (Fig. 9–3). The cerebral cortex is functionally subdivided also. The pyramidal system arises disproportionately from the *motor cortex*, a limited area of the parietal cortex. In humans, the motor cortex is located just rostral to the central sulcus and therefore is called the precentral gyrus. The motor cortex's boundaries are less well understood in most animals, but it is located generally in the region of the cruciate sulcus.

Pyramidal tract axons arise also from three other cortical areas: from an area just rostral to the motor cortex, called the *premotor cortex;* from the *parietal sensory cortex;* and from a *supplementary motor cortex* on the medial surface of the parietal lobe.

These origins of the pyramidal system axons have been discovered using both anatomical and electrophysiological techniques. Retrograde axonal degeneration can be traced up into the cortex following sectioning of the pyramids of the medulla oblongata. The presence or absence of movement of the contralateral body can be observed also following electrical stimulation of the cerebral cortex. These latter electrical stimulation studies have been best developed in humans, in whom surgical removal of epileptogenic cortical lesions must often be preceded by electrical stimulation studies to be sure essential areas of the cortex are left intact. Similar studies have been done on several species of animals.

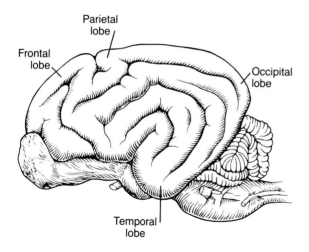

Figure 9–3. The cerebral cortex, as seen grossly from the lateral view, is anatomically subdivided into four major regions and lobes: the frontal, parietal, occipital, and temporal lobes. The cerebral cortex is functionally divided also, and the pyramidal system arises disproportionately from the motor cortex, a limited area of the parietal cortex.

Phylogenetically, the corticospinal and corticobulbar tracts first appeared in mammals. The higher the mammal phylogenetically, the more sophisticated the motor representation becomes in the motor cortex. This parallels the increasing ability to carry out skilled, voluntary movement. Hence, in higher mammals, and particularly in primates, a distorted somatotopic representation of the body can be found in the motor cortex. It disproportionately represents muscles of the body responsible for skilled, learned movements. In Figure 9–4 you can see the case of the phylogenetically highest mammal, the human, in whom muscles for the hand and mouth are disproportionately represented because these are the muscles needed for grasping and for speech. The motor cortex of the cat is shown also.

The distribution of corticospinal tract axons within the spinal cord is influenced by phylogeny also. In primates and carnivores, corticospinal axons go to both the front and rear legs, whereas in horses, most go only to the front legs.

The Pyramidal System Initiates Voluntary, Discrete, Often Learned Movements

The pyramidal system initiates skilled, learned, voluntary movement through its influence on lower motor neurons of the contralateral body. Extrafusal muscle fibers responsible for bringing about such movement tend to be flexor muscles of joints distal to the spine. It is not known how the various areas of the cerebral cortex interact before sending

their final action potential commands down the pyramidal tract axons. It seems likely that, before the cerebral cortex can send a command to the lower motor neuron, a motor plan of action must be designed. Such a plan would have to select a sequence of muscular contractions designed to accomplish the desired movement, and it would have to specify how much each muscle must contract. It seems likely that the premotor cortex and supplementary motor cortex play important roles in generating such a plan, perhaps in concert with the basal ganglia. The posterior parietal sensory cortex probably also plays an important role in providing spatial information for targeting movement and for some error correction, although the cerebellum and the muscle spindle reflex circuit are likely more important in error correction. This complex interplay of interconnected portions of the cerebral cortex results ultimately in a final action potential command sent down the corticospinal and corticobulbar tract axons to influence the contralateral lower motor neurons. A carbon copy of this command of intended movement is sent also to the cerebellum along the corti-pontine-cerebellar tract. Here it is compared with the cerebellum's knowledge of what movement is actually occurring so that any appropriate adjustments can be made.

Pyramidal System Axons Influence Both α and γ Lower Motor Neurons

The corticospinal tract axons descend the neuraxis to influence lower motor neurons in the contralateral spinal cord; corticobulbar

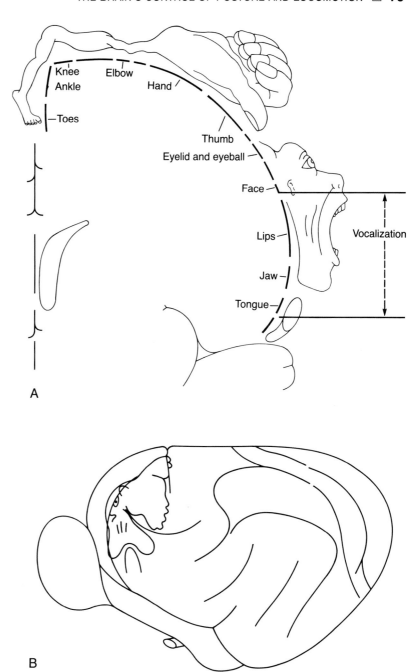

Figure 9–4. The map of the motor cortex, noting the origins of axons going to the skeletal muscles of the body, is a disproportionate representation of the body's shape. Note that in the phylogenetically highest mammal, the human *(A)*, muscles of the hand and mouth are disproportionately represented because these muscles are needed for grasping and for speech. The motor cortex of a cat *(B)* is shown also. *(A,* Redrawn from Penfield W, Rasmussen T: The Cerebral Cortex of Man. New York, Macmillan, 1950; used with permission from Berne RM, Levy MN: Physiology, 2nd ed. St. Louis, CV Mosby, © 1988. *B,* From Prosser CL: Comparative Animal Physiology, 3rd ed. New York © 1988. Reprinted by permission of John Wiley & Sons, Inc., 1988.)

tract axons influence lower motor neurons of the brainstem, usually on the contralateral side. This influence is exerted over both α and γ lower motor neurons (see Chapter 7), usually through short interneurons in the immediate neighborhood of the lower motor neuron. (Some direct, monosynaptic connections to the lower motor neuron are found in primates.)

The simultaneous activation of both α and γ lower motor neurons is known as *coactiva-*tion. These synaptic influences over the α motor neuron allow the pyramidal tract axons to command the intended movement by causing contraction of the appropriate extrafusal muscle fibers. The role of the simultaneous coactivation of the γ motor neuron to the intrafusal muscle fiber, however, is less clear. One likely function of this coactivation is to cause shortening of the intrafusal muscle fiber along with extrafusal muscle fiber. The spindle would shorten along with the whole muscle and therefore would maintain its sensitivity to muscle stretch regardless of the overall length of the muscle.

An error-correction or servo-assist function for coactivation of the γ motor neurons has been proposed also but is less well accepted by physiologists. In this role, the coactivation of γ motor neurons would lead to additional excitatory postsynaptic potentials (EPSPs) on the α motor neuron, by way of the γ loop, if the initial pyramidal tract stimulation of the α motor neuron failed to cause the intended amount of extrafusal fiber contraction. If the initial stimulation of the α motor neuron motor unit was sufficient, the intended shortening would occur and no servo-assist would be necessary from the γ loop. However, if the initial α stimulation of extrafusal fibers was not sufficient to cause the desired contraction, coactivation of the γ motor neurons would have caused shortening of the intrafusal fibers even though the spindle itself had not shortened. This would lead to more reflex EPSPs onto the α motor neuron by way of the γ loop. In this way, through coactivation the local, segmental γ loop reflex circuit helps accomplish the intended contraction if the initial α motor neuron stimulation from the pyramidal system was insufficient. This would occur if the load opposing contraction was underestimated by the cerebral cortex. Such coactivation would work much like the power-steering in a car, in which a compressor in the motor adds power to the driver's turning of the steering wheel when large resistance is encountered by the tires.

Coactivation of the γ lower motor neuron may also serve to inhibit the antagonist muscles through reflex inhibitory postsynaptic potentials (IPSPs) (see Chapter 7), but it seems more likely that this is accomplished directly by the pyramidal system neurons through inhibitory interneurons to these antagonist motor units.

Lesions in the Pyramidal System Cause Contralateral Weakness and Loss of Proprioception

The severity of the deficits resulting from lesions of the pyramidal system varies with the evolutionary development of the animal. In primates, such as humans, in whom the pyramidal system is developed extensively, pyramidal tract lesions cause a dense weakness of the contralateral body. Such one-sided weakness is called *hemiparesis* and is most extensive in the hand and facial muscles. In most veterinary species, the pyramidal system is not as well developed, and pyramidal system lesions cause much less severe contralateral weakness and almost no alteration of gait. However, pyramidal upper motor neuron lesions in veterinary species do cause important postural response deficits in the contralateral limbs. An example is the *conscious proprioception response*. This is the ability of an animal to return its paw to a normal, pads-down posture when the paw is turned upside-down. This response requires the animal's conscious awareness that the paw is upside-down (proprioception), and then requires that the animal be able to respond consciously by returning the paw to its normal posture. This latter motor response requires the integrity of the upper motor neurons of the corticospinal tract. When these corticospinal tract neurons are damaged, the animal is slow to return its paw to a normal posture. In addition, toes tend to be dragged on the ground as the leg is drawn forward in normal gait. Noting these conscious proprioception response deficits and other subtle gait changes is important in localizing lesions within the CNS.

The Extrapyramidal System Has Four Major Tracts Descending from the Brainstem to Influence Spinal Lower Motor Neurons

The pyramidal system has a relatively simple neuroanatomy. Its three tracts begin in the cerebral cortex and end in the spinal cord, the brainstem, and the cerebellum. With the exception of the pyramidal system's corticospinal tract, all other descending upper motor neuron axon tracts that influence spinal lower motor neurons begin in the brainstem. These are all part of the much more complex *extrapyramidal system*.

The extrapyramidal system has four major descending axon tracts that leave the brainstem to influence spinal lower motor neurons. Like most other tracts in the CNS, they are named for the places at which they begin and end. The first is the *reticulospinal tract*, which begins in the reticular activating system in the middle of the medulla oblongata, pons, and midbrain. It ends on or near a diffuse population of spinal, mostly γ lower motor neurons to more proximal extensor muscles. The second, the *vestibulospinal tract,* begins in the medullary vestibular nuclei and ends on a similarly diffuse population of γ and α spinal neurons. The third, the *tectospinal tract,* begins in the visual tectum and ends on the lower motor neurons of the rostral spinal cord. The fourth extrapyramidal descending tract is the *rubrospinal tract.* It begins in the red nucleus and ends on lower motor neurons to somewhat more distal extensor muscles. Each of these extrapyramidal tracts is influenced by other parts of the brain.

The Extrapyramidal System Maintains Postural Muscle Tone in Proximal, Antigravity Extensor Muscles

The responsibility of the extrapyramidal system is to maintain subconscious postural antigravity muscle tone. This muscle tone is found in extensor muscles whose contraction opposes gravity's pull on the body toward the earth. It is generally found in more proximal muscle groups located near the spinal column. By contrast, the pyramidal system, as mentioned earlier, initiates voluntary movement in more distal, usually flexor muscles. These two systems must work together, because voluntary movement requires postural adjustments. Much of the coordination between these two upper motor neuron systems is done by the cerebellum. In the paragraphs that follow, the function of the separate, descending extrapyramidal tracts is described to illustrate how the tracts contribute to the general function of antigravity muscle tone.

The *reticulospinal tract* originates in the reticular activating system found in the medial medulla oblongata, pons, and midbrain. The reticular activating system, often called the reticular formation, is a complex of small, netlike neurons that anatomically are an extension of the spinal cord into the brainstem. Once thought to be a diffuse and fairly nonspecific system, it is now known to contain a number of functionally specific nuclei. One such functionally specific set of neurons are those giving rise to the reticulospinal tract. Many neurons of the reticular formation are tonically active, both as the result of stimulation from ascending, sensory axons with branches into the reticular formation, and as the result of intrinsic activity of reticular formation neurons themselves.

This tonic activity within the reticular formation gives rise to action potentials departing

rostrally into the cerebral cortex to cause general arousal, the absence of which leads to coma, and caudally along the reticulospinal tract to influence particularly γ lower motor neurons. Figure 9–5 illustrates two subsections of the reticular formation, areas 4 and 5, giving rise to the reticulospinal axons. Action potentials on axons from the more rostral area 5 cause EPSPs in γ motor neurons to antigravity extensor muscles. Through the γ loop (see Chapter 7), the extrafusal muscle fibers of these muscles are reflexly made to contract, resulting in postural muscle tone. Action potentials along axons from the more caudal area 4 cause IPSPs in γ motor neurons to antigravity extensor muscles. Both areas 4 and 5 are influenced by the more rostral basal ganglia and cerebral cortex, which tend to reduce the EPSP-producing facilitation of area 5 and stimulate the IPSP-producing inhibition from area 4. Action potentials descending from these two areas to cause an appropriate blend of EPSPs and IPSPs within the γ loop of extensor antigravity muscles are the major origin of postural muscle tone.

Some muscle tone is contributed also by action potentials along the *vestibulospinal tract* axons. These axons arise from the vestibular nuclei in the medulla oblongata and descend to influence some α but mainly γ lower motor neurons to proximal antigravity muscles. Vestibular nuclei neurons are also tonically active as the result of tonic sensory axon input from the inner ear's vestibular system (see Chapter 10). As changes in head position are detected

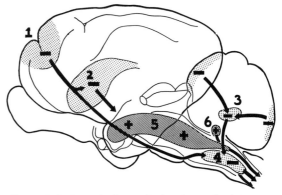

Figure 9–5. Areas in the cat brain where stimulation produces facilitation *(plus signs)* or inhibition *(minus signs)* of stretch reflexes: *(1)* motor cortex; *(2)* basal ganglia; *(3)* cerebellum; *(4)* reticular inhibitory area; *(5)* reticular facilitatory area; *(6)* vestibular nuclei. (Reproduced, with permission, from Lindsley DB, Schreiner LH, Magoun HW: An electromyographic study of spasticity. J Neurophysiol 12:197, 1949.)

by the vestibular system receptors, the vestibulospinal tract neurons make appropriate adjustments in postural muscle tone to maintain the desired balance.

The functions of these two extrapyramidal system neuron tracts can be better understood by considering the mechanisms of the clinical state called *decerebrate rigidity*. This condition occurs occasionally as the result of severe rostral brain disease. It also results from surgical transection of the brain at the midbrain level, as discovered by the famous British neurophysiologist Charles Sherrington. This transection functionally disconnects the EPSP-producing reticulospinal tract and vestibulospinal tract from more rostral brain areas that reduced their output. The result is an overactive reticulospinal tract and vestibulospinal tract, causing an excess of EPSPs on γ motor neurons to antigravity muscles. The animal assumes a hobbyhorse–like posture often so rigid that it stands in a fixed position. Because this rigidity is the result of overactive γ loop stimulation of the antigravity motor units, if the dorsal roots in one leg of a decerebrate rigid animal are cut, the rigidity is abolished in that leg. Had the overstimulation along the reticulospinal and vestibulospinal tracts led directly to the α extensor motor neuron, cutting the dorsal roots would not have abolished the rigidity. (However, cutting the ventral roots would have abolished such rigidity.) It is by these and other observations on the decerebrate animal that we know postural muscle tone is mediated primarily by the vestibulospinal and reticulospinal tracts, causing a blend of EPSPs and IPSPs on the γ loop to proximal, extensor antigravity muscles.

These mechanisms cause the muscle contraction necessary for antigravity muscle tone, but not the to-and-fro rhythmicity of walking and running. This oscillation in motor neurons is added by interneurons of the spinal cord. It may be these spinal interneurons that are affected by distemper virus, causing the characteristic chorea in some dogs with clinical distemper. The rhythmicity of walking and running is generated by spinal interneurons influencing the lower motor neurons.

The *tectospinal tract*, the third of the extrapyramidal descending tracts, begins in the visual tectum of the midbrain (superior colliculus) and ends in the cervical spinal cord. It is important in the reflex coordination of the head and eye movements while watching a moving object.

The *rubrospinal tract*, the last of the major descending extrapyramidal tracts, begins in the red nucleus of the midbrain and influences spinal lower motor neurons, particularly those to more distal muscles. The red nucleus receives axons from the motor cerebral cortex. The function of the rubrospinal tract is poorly understood, and its ablation apparently leads to little dysfunction.

The Role of the Basal Ganglia Is Poorly Understood

The *basal ganglia* are a group of nuclei deep within the cerebral hemispheres. They include a bilateral set of three large subcortical nuclei: the caudate nucleus, the putamen, and the globus pallidus. They receive inputs from the cerebral cortex and, among other places, project outputs back to the motor and premotor cortices. The basal ganglia region is one of the most poorly understood areas of the brain. The basal ganglia appear to play a role in planning of movement initiated by the pyramidal and possibly the extrapyramidal system. They may play a role also in coordinating some rhythmic movements, because lesions of the basal ganglia often give rise to rhythmic, tremorous movement disorders.

The Cerebral Cortex Plays a Role in Extrapyramidal System Function

As suggested by Figure 9–5, the cerebral and cerebellar cortices also influence the extrapyramidal system. Presumably the cerebral cortex adds a sense of purposefulness to posture and locomotion controlled by the extrapyramidal system by choosing, as an example, the general direction and speed with which to walk or run.

Clinical Syndromes Resulting from Extrapyramidal System Lesions Include Either Rhythmic or Nonrhythmic Movement Disorders

Focal lesions of the extrapyramidal system cause abnormal, involuntary movements, alterations in muscle tone, and disturbed posture. Such movement disorders are divided usually into rhythmic and nonrhythmic movement disorders. Rhythmic extrapyramidal disorders include what is known as a *nonintention tremor*. This is a tremor that is worse when the patient is at rest and becomes better when the patient intends to move. (A cerebellar tremor gets worse with intended movement and is called an *intention tremor*.) An example of a rhythmic extrapyramidal movement disorder is Parkinson's tremor in humans, and an apparently related condition is star thistle poisoning in horses. In each case, there is a nonintention tremor of muscles of prehension—the hand in humans and the muzzle in horses. In both syndromes, there is a lesion of the substantia nigra, a brainstem structure that projects dopamine-secreting axons to the globus pallidus of the basal ganglia. At least in the human case, it appears that the loss of these dopaminergic neurons is important in the mechanism of the disease, because giving dopamine precursor, which crosses the blood-brain barrier, reduces the clinical signs.

An example of a nonrhythmic extrapyramidal movement disorder is the decerebrate rigidity described earlier in this chapter.

CLINICAL CORRELATION

FOCAL LESION OF THE MOTOR CORTEX

HISTORY □ You examine an 11-year-old female boxer dog. Her vaccination history is current. She had an adenocarcinoma of the mammary gland removed 6 months prior to your examination.

The owner states that over the past few days the dog has become progressively weak in the left front and left rear leg and occasionally stands with the left front paw upside-down. On the previous day, the dog suffered a seizure.

CLINICAL EXAMINATION □ On physical examination of the patient you find several routine old-age changes and the results of the mammary surgery. You find also that the dog seems drowsy and is weak on the left front and left rear legs. She has a conscious proprioception response deficit of both the left front and left rear legs. Radiographic study of the chest reveals metastatic, neoplastic lesions in the lungs.

COMMENT □ The conscious proprioception response is tested by turning the animal's paw upside-down while gently supporting her weight. A normal dog senses (conscious proprioception) that the paw is upside-down and returns it to the normal pads-down posture (motor response). This is called a response, rather than a reflex, because it involves a degree of conscious control. This particular response requires skin and joint receptors and the peripheral nerve in the tested leg, and the sensory neuron tracts that ascend toward the brain along the ipsilateral (same side) spinal cord. They cross to the contralateral (opposite side) of the brain in the brainstem and end in the contralateral cerebral cortex. As the animal becomes consciously aware that the paw is in an unusual position, action potentials are sent back down the corticospinal tract to the lower motor neurons of the muscles of the leg, causing the paw to be returned to the normal position. With some thought to the wiring diagram of this response, you can imagine that conscious proprioception deficits of the left front and left rear legs could be caused by a lesion of either the left cervical spinal cord or the right motor cortex. The fact that this dog developed seizures (a brain disease) at about the same time suggests that this dog's lesion is in the right cerebral cortex. The brain is a common site for metastasis, and the radiographic lung lesions suggest that the mammary tumor has spread to the right brain. The lung contains the first capillary bed that a metastatic cancer cell is likely to encounter when it enters the venous system of the mammary gland. Some cells stop here and grow.

TREATMENT □ Usually dogs with metastatic mammary carcinomas are not treated except to make them more comfortable.

Bibliography

Berne RM, Levy MN (eds): Physiology, 2nd ed. St Louis, CV Mosby, 1988, pp 196–280.

Guyton AC: Textbook of Medical Physiology, 7th ed. Philadelphia, WB Saunders, 1986, pp 619–651.

Kandel ER, Schwartz JH (eds): Principles of Neural Science, 2nd ed. New York, Elsevier, 1985, pp 429–442, 478–534.

Lance JW, McLeod JG: A Physiological Approach to Clinical Neurology, 3rd ed. London, Butterworths, 1981, pp 101–191.

Oliver JE, Hoerlein BR, Mayhew IG (eds): Veterinary Neurology. Philadelphia, WB Saunders, 1987, pp 47–53.

Smith LH, Thier SO (eds): Pathophysiology—The Biological Principles of Disease, 2nd ed. Philadelphia, WB Saunders, 1985, pp 1036–1072.

Willis WD, Grossman RG: Medical Neurobiology, Neuroanatomical and Neurophysiological Principles Basic to Clinical Neuroscience, 3rd ed. St Louis, CV Mosby, 1981, pp 347–403.

PRACTICE QUESTIONS FOR CHAPTER 9

1. In order to increase muscle tone (continued contraction of some percentage of muscle fibers) in the body's antigravity muscles, the extrapyramidal system must

   a. increase the IPSPs to γ motor neurons of flexor muscles.
   b. increase the EPSPs to γ motor neurons of extensor muscles.
   c. increase the IPSPs to γ motor neurons of extensor muscles.
   d. increase the EPSPs to γ motor neurons of flexor muscles.
   e. increase the EPSPs to α motor neurons of flexor muscles.

2. Decerebrate rigidity theoretically may be abolished by

   a. removing the cerebellum.
   b. cutting the cervical spinal cord completely in two (complete transection).
   c. removing the cerebral cortex.
   d. cutting the dorsal (posterior) roots.
   e. Either b or d

3. The pyramidal system, in general, initiates what form of movement?

   a. Antigravity movement
   b. Postural muscle tone
   c. Skilled, mostly flexor movement
   d. Tremulous movement
   e. None of the above

4. You are presented with a dog with a dense weakness and conscious proprioceptive reflex deficit of his left front and left back legs. A single site of pathology could cause these signs if it were located in the

   a. left cervical spinal cord.
   b. left cerebral cortex.
   c. right cerebral cortex.
   d. Either a or b
   e. Either a or c

5. The corticospinal tract simultaneously coactivates both the α and the γ lower motor neurons. If the initial coactivation fails to be sufficient to cause shortening of the whole muscle belly, the sensory fibers from the muscle spindle of that muscle belly will have what influence on the α motor neurons to the same muscle?

   a. Add EPSPs
   b. Add IPSPs
   c. Have no influence
   d. Add presynaptic inhibition
   e. Either b or d

10

The Vestibular System

1. The vestibular system is a bilateral receptor system located in the inner ear
2. Specialized regions of the vestibular system contain receptors
3. The semicircular canals detect rotary acceleration and deceleration of the head
4. The utricle and saccule detect linear acceleration and deceleration and static position of the head in space
5. The vestibular system provides sensory information for reflexes involving spinal motor neurons, the cerebellum, and extraocular muscles of the eye
6. Vestibular reflexes coordinate head and eye movements to maximize visual acuity during movements of the head

In order to coordinate posture and locomotion, the brain needs to know not only what movement it intends to command, but also what movement the body is actually performing. Chapter 7 describes the muscle spindle, an important source of information for the brain about body position and movement. Another important source of information is the vestibular system. This is a bilateral receptor system, located in the inner ear, that informs the brain about the position and motion of the head in space.

The vestibular system is a common site of pathology. Lesions of the vestibular system cause in most veterinary species a similar syndrome characterized by head tilt, compulsive rotary movements such as circling or rolling, and nystagmus—a spontaneous, oscillating movement of the eyes.

In order to understand how such clinical signs arise and the importance of the vestibular system to the physiology of movement, its anatomy and function are studied first.

The Vestibular System Is a Bilateral Receptor System Located in the Inner Ear

The inner ear, or labyrinth, is made up of two parts: the bony labyrinth and the membranous labyrinth. The *bony labyrinth* is a system of tunnels through the petrous temporal bone of the skull. The bony labyrinth houses both the vestibular system and the receptor for hearing, the *cochlea* (see Chapter 16). Within the bony labyrinth is the *membranous labyrinth* (Fig. 10–1), so named because it is made up of thin membranes of epithelium. This epithelial membrane is specialized at some locations to become the sensory receptor cells. The membranous labyrinth is separated from the bony labyrinth by a fluid called *perilymph*. The membranous labyrinth is filled with a fluid called *endolymph*.

Each vestibular portion of the labyrinth consists of two major sets of structures: three *semicircular canals* located at approximately

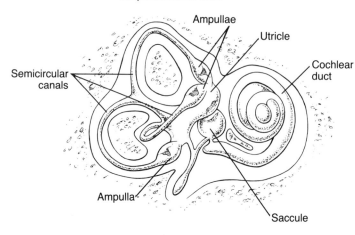

Temporal bone of skull

Ampullae

Utricle

Semicircular canals

Cochlear duct

Ampulla

Saccule

Figure 10–1. The bilateral inner ear contains receptor systems for hearing (cochlea) and for sensing the position of the head (vestibular system or labyrinth). The vestibular system on each side of the head contains three semicircular canals, a utricle, and a saccule.

right angles to each other, and a pair of saclike structures called the *utricle* and *saccule.*

Specialized Regions of the Vestibular System Contain Receptors

Each structure within the vestibular system has a region of epithelial lining that has become specialized into a set of receptor cells called *hair cells* (Fig. 10–2). Each hair cell has several hair-like projections into the endolymph and is innervated at its base by a sensory afferent nerve that carries action potentials to the brainstem. The hair-like projections from all of the hair cells within any one vestibular structure are bound together by a gelatinous mass so that displacement of this gelatinous mass causes all the hair cell projections to bend in the same direction. In the utricle and saccule, this gelatinous mass also contains calcium carbonate crystals called *otoliths.* These otoliths are more dense than the endolymph and are deflected by gravity.

At rest, sensory nerves innervating vestibular hair cells transmit action potentials spontaneously at about 100 spikes/second (Fig. 10–3). When the hair cell projections are bent in one direction, the hair cells depolarize, and the action potential frequency increases. When bent in the opposite direction, hair cell mem-

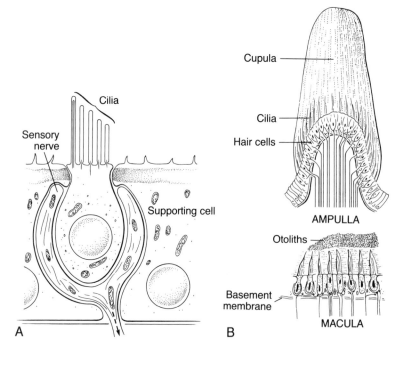

Cilia

Sensory nerve

Supporting cell

A

Cupula

Cilia

Hair cells

AMPULLA

Otoliths

Basement membrane

MACULA

B

Figure 10–2. Each vestibular structure has a region of epithelial cells that are specialized as receptor cells or hair cells *(A).* Those in the semicircular canals are clustered in a region called the ampulla where all the cilia are glued together by a gelatinous mass called the cupula *(B).* The hair receptor cells of the utricle and saccule are clustered in the region called the macula. Their gelatinous masses contain calcium carbonate crystals called otoliths.

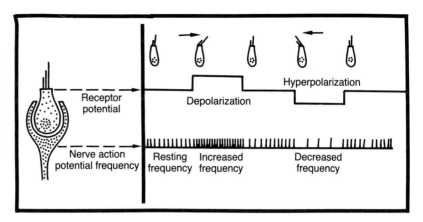

Figure 10–3. At rest, sensory nerves innervating vestibular hair cells transmit action potentials spontaneously at about 100 spikes/second. When hair cell cilia are deflected in one direction, the action potential frequency increases; when they are deflected in the opposite direction, the frequency decreases.

branes hyperpolarize, and the sensory nerve spike frequency decreases. Therefore, displacement of the hair cell projections in either direction can be detected by the brain as either an increase or a decrease from the resting action potential frequency. How the brain uses this information to detect the direction of head movement is described later.

The Semicircular Canals Detect Rotary Acceleration and Deceleration of the Head

Three semicircular canals are located within each inner ear (Fig. 10–4). They are positioned at approximately right angles to each other, and both ends of each fluid-filled canal terminate in the utricle. Each semicircular canal has an enlargement, called the *ampulla,* near its junction with the utricle. The ampulla contains the hair cell receptor system, called the *cupula,* whose hair cells and sensory nerves are attached to its base and whose gelatinous mass attaches to the roof of the ampulla (Fig. 10–5).

When the head begins to turn in a rotary direction (acceleration), the semicircular canal rotates with the head, but the endolymph's acceleration lags behind that of the canal owing to inertia. This relative difference in the rate of acceleration of the semicircular canal and its enclosed endolymph causes a displacement of the gelatinous mass in the ampulla and therefore a bending of the hair cells, thus changing the firing rate of their sensory nerves. The opposite happens with deceleration.

Semicircular canals, located on both sides of the head but in roughly the same plane, work as a pair to provide the brain with information about the direction and nature of head move-

ment. For instance, a clockwise rotary acceleration of the head would cause bending of the directionally sensitive hair cell projections in one of the semicircular canals on each side of the head. However, the sensory nerve from one side of the head would carry an increased action potential frequency, whereas that of the other side would carry a decreased action

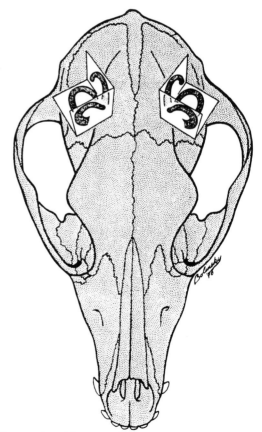

Figure 10–4. Three semicircular canals are located on each side of the head and detect rotary acceleration and deceleration of the head.

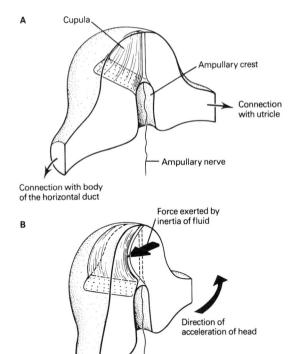

Figure 10–5. The ampullae of the semicircular canals contain a hair cell receptor system. *(A)* The ampullary crest of the horizontal canal. *(B)* Displacement of the cupula by flow of endolymph caused by head movement. (Reprinted by permission of the publisher from Kandel ER, Schwartz JH (eds): Principles of Neural Science, 2nd ed. Copyright 1985 by Elsevier Science Publishing Company, Inc.)

potential frequency. The brain has learned to interpret that reciprocal change in sensory action potential frequency as resulting from clockwise or counterclockwise acceleration or deceleration in a given plane of movement. In this way, the bilateral system of six semicircular canals detects the direction of both rotary acceleration and deceleration of the head and alerts the brain for appropriate reflex response.

The Utricle and Saccule Detect Linear Acceleration and Deceleration and Static Position of the Head in Space

In the utricle and saccule, the hair cell receptor is called the *macula*. Its filamentous projections also extend up into the endolymph and are bound together by a gelatinous mass. In these structures, the gelatinous mass also contains calcium carbonate crystals called *otoliths*. These otoliths are more dense than the endolymph and hence sink toward the earth's center in response to gravity. This gravita-

tional force on the otoliths in the gelatinous mass results in a bending of the hair cells and thus a change in frequency of action potentials along the sensory nerve fibers. Because the hair cells of the utricle and saccule are not all oriented in the same direction, the pattern of action potential firing varies depending on differing head positions. In this way, the utricle and saccule can inform the brain about the stationary position of the head. Astronauts in low gravitational settings get relatively little information from their utricles and saccules about their stationary head position and must rely more heavily on visual and other sensory cues to detect head position.

The Vestibular System Provides Sensory Information for Reflexes Involving Spinal Motor Neurons, the Cerebellum, and Extraocular Muscles of the Eye

Action potentials from vestibular receptors arrive in the medulla along axons of the eighth cranial nerve. Nearly all these axons synapse in the vestibular nuclear complex—a bilateral group of four distinct nuclei occupying a substantial portion of the medulla beneath the fourth ventricle. From here, second-order neurons project to three important areas of the nervous system. The vestibulospinal tract, part of the extrapyramidal system, provides excitatory facilitation to γ and some α motor neurons of antigravity muscles (see Chapter 9). Other neurons project to the cerebellum, especially the flocculonodular lobe, where they provide valuable information necessary for the coordination of movement. A third vestibular influence is over the movements of the eyes.

Vestibular Reflexes Coordinate Head and Eye Movements to Maximize Visual Acuity During Movements of the Head

Vestibular reflex control of the extraocular muscles of the eye coordinates eye and head movements. As the head turns, the eyes remain fixed on the field of vision for as long as possible. Imagine that a dog is seated on a piano stool, and you rotated him in clockwise fashion to the right. As you rotate him slowly to the right, his eyes would rotate in his head slowly to the left so that the eyes remained fixed on the same field of vision as long as possible. As the eyes reach the limit of their leftward excursion, they swiftly move to the right, in the direction of the head movement, until they fix on a new field of vision. If the head is still rotating, the cycle is repeated. This allows the animal time to interpret a field of vision despite rotation of the head. This reflex requires normal sensory input from the semicircular canals, the medial longitudinal fasciculus in the brainstem, and the integrity of the motor units in the extraocular muscles. Of course, this reflex can be overwhelmed if head rotation is too fast. Similarly, if the head is tilted to one side, the eyes rotate in the opposite direction, helping to maintain the visual field in the horizontal plane.

These vestibular movements of the eyes, normal with head movement, appear occasionally under pathological conditions even when the head is straight and at rest. Unilateral pathology of one of the vestibular systems results in abnormal, asymmetrical action potential frequencies to the brainstem. This causes spontaneous, oscillating movements of the eyes, even when the head is at rest. This condition is known as *nystagmus* and usually has fast and slow directional components owing to the normal vestibular reflex control of the eyes. Transient nystagmus can be seen also if a spinning animal or person is suddenly stopped. For a brief period of time, inertia of the endolymph causes it to continue rotating even though the head has stopped. This causes overstimulation of the vestibular eye reflexes, and hence the transient nystagmus. (Humans report dizziness during this time. Try it carefully on a friend and look for post-rotatory nystagmus and ask for subjective impressions.)

A persisting head tilt and compulsive circling or rolling often accompany nystagmus in acute vestibular disease in animals, presumably also associated with abnormal, asymmetrical action potential inputs from the vestibular systems on either side of the head.

CLINICAL CORRELATION

VESTIBULAR SYNDROME

HISTORY □ A 3-year-old male cocker spaniel is brought to your clinic. The owner states that for the previous 2 days, the dog has held his right ear lower than his left ear. He also tends to walk in circles, clockwise to the right. You have treated this dog previously for an infection of the outer ear.

CLINICAL EXAMINATION □ On physical examination of the dog you find that the outer ear infection persists. You also confirm the owner's complaint that the dog persistently tilts his head with the right ear down and circles to the right; you find that he has a horizontal nystagmus. The rest of your physical examination is within normal limits.

COMMENT □ Head tilt, circling, and nystagmus constitute a common constellation of clinical signs often called the *vestibular syndrome.* It results from pathology in the vestibular system, usually in the membranous labyrinth. It is due frequently to the extension of an infection from the outer and middle ear to the labyrinth of the inner ear. This results in an abnormal balance of action potential frequencies between the normal and abnormal sides of the vestibular system, causing asymmetric stimulation of the ocular and postural reflex mechanisms normally controlled by the vestibular nuclei.

TREATMENT □ When such labyrinthitis is due to bacterial infection, treatment with appropriate antibiotics is often effective in eliminating the clinical signs by returning the peripheral receptor to its normal function.

Bibliography

Berne RM, Levy MN (eds): Physiology, 2nd ed. St Louis, CV Mosby, 1988, pp 179–188.

Guyton AC: Textbook of Medical Physiology, 7th ed. Philadelphia, WB Saunders, 1986, pp 619–626.

Kandel ER, Schwartz JH (eds): Principles of Neural Science, 2nd ed. New York, Elsevier, 1985, pp 584–596.

Lance JW, McLeod JG: A Physiological Approach to Clinical Neurology, 3rd ed. London, Butterworths, 1981, pp 246–254.

Oliver JE, Hoerlein BR, Mayhew IG (eds): Veterinary Neurology. Philadelphia, WB Saunders, 1987, pp 361–362.

Smith LH, Thier SO (eds): Pathophysiology—The Biological Principles of Disease, 2nd ed. Philadelphia, WB Saunders, 1985, pp 1117–1121.

Willis WD, Grossman RG: Medical Neurobiology, Neuroanatomical and Neurophysiological Principles Basic to Clinical Neuroscience, 3rd ed. St Louis, CV Mosby, 1981, p 307–314.

PRACTICE QUESTIONS FOR CHAPTER 10

1. The receptor system detecting rotary acceleration and deceleration of the head is located in the

a. utricle.
b. saccule.
c. semicircular canal.
d. cochlea.
e. retina.

2. Astronauts in the low gravity environment of the moon are most likely to have malfunctions of what sensory system?

a. Muscle spindle
b. Retinal photoreceptor
c. Golgi tendon organ
d. Utricle and saccule
e. Olfaction

3. The semicircular canals of the vestibular receptor system detect

a. rotary acceleration of the head.
b. linear acceleration of the head.
c. the static position of the head.
d. whether the visual image is fixed on the retina.

e. the relative position of the head with respect to the visual horizon.

4. You are presented with a dog with a head tilt, compulsive circling, and nystagmus. The most likely site of this dog's pathology is the

a. cerebellar hemisphere.
b. cerebral cortex.
c. vestibular system.
d. cervical spinal cord.
e. facial (seventh cranial) nerve.

5. Nystagmus, as a clinical sign, is usually a sign of pathology in the

a. cerebral cortex.
b. reticular activating system.
c. spinal cord.
d. vestibular system.
e. oculomotor nerves.

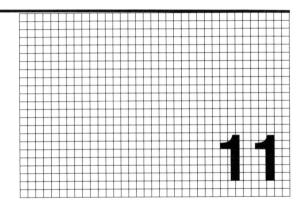

The Cerebellum

1. The cerebellum constantly compares the intended movement with the actual movement and makes appropriate adjustments
2. Cerebellar histology and phylogeny give clues to cerebellar function
3. The vestibulocerebellum helps coordinate balance and eye movements
4. The spinocerebellum helps coordinate muscle tone and movement
5. The cerebrocerebellum helps coordinate the planning of limb movements
6. The cerebellum plays a role in motor learning
7. Cerebellar disease causes abnormalities of movement

The preceding chapters describing the physiology of posture and locomotion discuss the function of lower motor neurons—the final common pathway through which the central nervous system (CNS) can initiate and control movement through the contraction of skeletal muscle. The pyramidal system and the extrapyramidal system are described next as two of the three major subgroups of upper motor neurons that influence the lower motor neuron. The extrapyramidal system is responsible for involuntary antigravity movement caused largely by contraction of proximal extensor muscles. The pyramidal system is responsible for more skilled, learned, voluntary movements caused by contraction of distal flexor muscles. This chapter describes the function of the cerebellum, the third upper motor neuron subgroup.

The cerebellum, which is Latin for "little brain," is located caudal to the cerebral cortex and dorsal to the brainstem (Fig. 11–1). Although it constitutes only 10% of the total brain, it contains over half of all the brain's neurons. It has a highly regular, three-layered,

cortical histology, suggesting that each cerebellar region may perform a similar task with differing afferent inputs from various regions of the nervous system.

The cerebellum is not necessary for sensation or movement. Muscle strength remains largely intact with complete destruction of the cerebellum. But the cerebellum plays a crucial role in the coordination of movement initiated by other parts of the brain. Lesions of the cerebellum lead to major clinical deficits in the grace with which movement is accomplished.

The Cerebellum Constantly Compares the Intended Movement with the Actual Movement and Makes Appropriate Adjustments

In performing the essential role of choreographer of motor commands, the cerebellum first receives information from the pyramidal and extrapyramidal systems about the movement it has commanded. It also receives information from muscle spindles, the vestibular system, and other sensory receptors about the

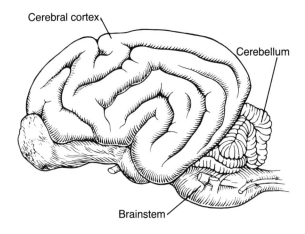

Cerebral cortex

Cerebellum

Brainstem

Figure 11–1. The cerebellum, which in Latin means *little brain,* is located caudal to the cerebral hemispheres and dorsal to the brainstem. (Redrawn from Miller ME, Christiansen GC, Evans HE: The Anatomy of the Dog. Philadelphia, WB Saunders, 1964.)

movement the body is actually performing. When this intended movement and actual movement are not the same, the cerebellum's job is to carry out the adjustments necessary to make them the same. For example, if the brain intends that a cat move its mouth to a piece of food in a dish, but sensory receptors inform the cerebellum that the trajectory of the head will cause the mouth to miss the dish, the cerebellum makes appropriate adjustments in the output of the pyramidal and extrapyramidal systems to correct the head's trajectory.

This chapter describes cerebellar histology and phylogenetic anatomy as clues to cerebellar function. Movement disorders resulting from lesions of the cerebellum are described as further clues to the function of this part of the brain.

Cerebellar Histology and Phylogeny Give Clues to Cerebellar Function

The cerebellum occupies most of the posterior cranial fossa. It is composed of an outer mantle of gray matter called the cerebellar cortex, inner white matter consisting of axons arriving and departing from the cortex, and three pairs of deep cerebellar nuclei within the white matter.

The cortex throughout the cerebellum consists of three layers and only five types of neurons: stellate, basket, Golgi, granule, and Purkinje's cells (Fig. 11–2). The outermost layer is the *molecular layer* and consists primarily of granule cell axons, known as parallel fibers; dendrites of neurons located in deeper layers; and scattered inhibitory interneurons—the stellate and basket cells. The middle *Purkinje's cell layer* consists of the large cell bodies of Purkinje's neurons. Axons of the Purkinje's neurons go to the deep cerebellar nuclei. They are the only output neurons of the cerebellar cortex and are all inhibitory. The innermost *granular cell layer* contains a vast number of small granular cells and occasional Golgi cells.

The primary input axons to the cerebellum are the mossy fiber and climbing fiber axons. They are both excitatory. They cause excitatory postsynaptic potentials (EPSPs) within the cerebellar cortex and, through collateral axons, within the deep cerebellar nuclei. The primary input/output circuit of the cerebellum consists of the climbing and mossy fiber stimulation to the deep cerebellar nuclei, whose output in turn modifies the pyramidal and extrapyramidal systems (Fig. 11–3). However, the output of the deep cerebellar nuclei is itself modified by inhibition from Purkinje's cell axons. The Purkinje's cell inhibition of deep cerebellar nuclei results from the cerebellar cortex's integration of mossy and climbing fiber inputs with its motor memory. Even though the cortical synaptology is now understood, just how the cerebellum remembers motor patterns and modifies the output of the deep nuclear neurons is not known. Because the cortical histology is similar throughout the cerebellum, it seems likely that similar modulation processes occur regardless of the cerebellar region. However, inputs from and outputs to different parts of the nervous system would render different motor results. Therefore, it is useful to examine the three major phylogenetically different divisions of cerebellum.

The cerebellum can be divided into three distinct regions from both a functional and a phylogenetic perspective (Figs. 11–4 and 11–5). The *vestibulocerebellum* occupies the flocculonodular lobe. Its afferents come from the

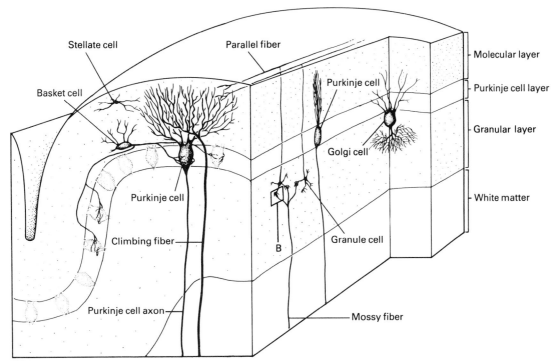

Figure 11–2. Five types of neurons are organized into three layers in the cerebellar cortex. A single cerebellar folium is sectioned vertically, in both longitudinal and transverse planes, to illustrate the general organization of the cerebellar cortex. (Reprinted by permission of the publisher from Kandel ER, Schwartz JH: Principles of Neural Science, 2nd ed. Copyright 1985 by Elsevier Science Publishing Company, Inc.)

vestibular nuclei of the medulla, and it projects back to them. Because this part of the cerebellum was the first to appear in vertebrate evolution, it is sometimes called the archicerebellum. The *spinocerebellum* extends rostrocaudally through the medial portion of the cerebellum. It receives afferents from the periphery, especially the spinal cord. Its outputs project primarily to the extrapyramidal, brainstem nuclei. Because this part of the cerebellum appeared next in evolution, it is sometimes referred to as the paleocerebellum. The *cerebrocerebellum* occupies the lateral cerebellar hemispheres. Its inputs are exclusively with the cerebral cortical pyramidal system by way of the corticopontine cerebellar system (see Chapter 9), and its outputs project back to the cerebral cortex by way of the thalamus. Because this is the phylogenetically newest part of the cerebellum, it is often referred to as the neocerebellum.

The Vestibulocerebellum Helps Coordinate Balance and Eye Movement

The vestibulocerebellum receives most of its afferent input from the vestibular system and the visual system. Its efferent output returns to the vestibular nuclei where it influences balance, controlled by the vestibulospinal tract, and the coordination of head and eye movement.

The Spinocerebellum Helps Coordinate Muscle Tone and Movement

The spinocerebellum receives sensory inputs by way of the spinal cord from muscle and cutaneous receptors. It also receives input from the visual, auditory, and vestibular systems. Its outputs, by way of its deep cerebellar nuclei, are to the extrapyramidal system. Here, when the actual movement being accomplished is not the movement intended by the extrapyramidal system, the spinocerebellum makes the appropriate adjustments. In doing so, it helps to control both the execution of movement and muscle tone.

The Cerebrocerebellum Helps Coordinate the Planning of Limb Movements

The cerebrocerebellum receives its inputs from the motor and sensory cerebral cortices

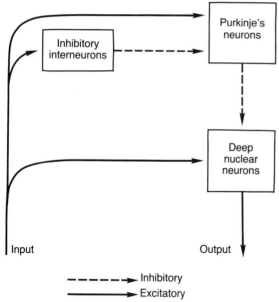

Figure 11–3. The input-output organization of the cerebellum involves inhibitory modification of excitatory input.

phylogenetic addition to the brain during primate evolution. Presumably this is linked to the primate's ability to coordinate finger movements and the mouth and tongue movements necessary for speech.

It is generally believed that this area of the cerebellum plays an important role in the preparation, or planning, of movement, whereas the spinocerebellum helps coordinate the execution of movement.

The Cerebellum Plays a Role in Motor Learning

There is now substantial evidence that the primary cerebellar circuit is the excitatory input of the climbing and mossy fibers on the deep cerebellar nuclei and their outputs to the extrapyramidal and pyramidal systems. In turn, these deep cerebellar nuclei are modified by the inhibitory Purkinje's cell axons from the cerebellar cortex, cells also stimulated by climbing and mossy fiber afferents. This collateral Purkinje's cell influence on the deep nuclei can be modified by motor experience. Hence, as you learn a motor skill, such as riding a bicycle, you have to concentrate on what you are doing. But after the skill is learned, presumably in large measure by the cerebellum, the coordination of these motor patterns is taken over by the cerebellum and

by way of the corticopontine-cerebellar system (see Chapter 9). This area of the cerebellum receives no information from peripheral receptors. Its outputs return to the motor and premotor cerebral cortices by way of the thalamus. The dramatic growth of the cerebrocerebellum and cerebral cortex was the major

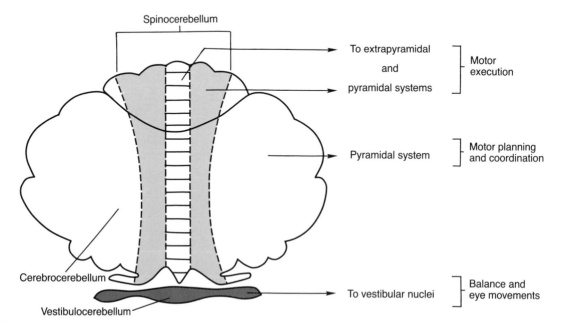

Figure 11–4. The cerebellum can be divided into three distinct regions from both a functional and phylogenetic perspective. This figure illustrates these three regions and regions of the brain to which their outputs project. (Redrawn from Kandel ER, Schwartz JH: Principles of Neural Science, 2nd ed. Copyright 1985 by Elsevier Science Publishing Company, Inc.)

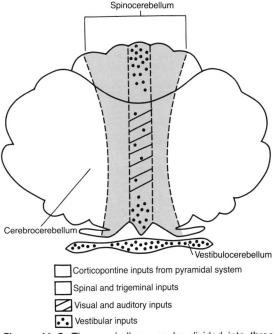

Corticopontine inputs from pyramidal system

Spinal and trigeminal inputs

Visual and auditory inputs

Vestibular inputs

Figure 11–5. The cerebellum can be divided into three distinct regions from both a functional and phylogenetic perspective. This figure illustrates these three regions and the area of the nervous system from which sensory axons project. (Redrawn from Kandel ER, Schwartz JH: Principles of Neural Science, 2nd ed. Copyright 1985 by Elsevier Science Publishing Company, Inc.)

you can concentrate on other things while riding your bike.

Cerebellar Disease Causes Abnormalities of Movement

The cerebellum constantly compares the intended movement with the actual movement and makes appropriate adjustments. In cerebellar disease, these appropriate adjustments are not made, resulting in a variety of movement disorders. Affected animals often place their paws far apart *(wide-based gait)* and walk in an incoordinated fashion *(ataxia)* reflecting the inability of the vestibulocerebellum and spinocerebellum to coordinate balance and movement of the axial skeleton. Affected animals also have various degrees of *dysmetria* (inappropriate measure of muscular contraction). In animals, this is often manifested as difficulty in bringing the muzzle to a fixed point in space, such as a food dish, and exaggerated "goose stepping" walking movements. *Intention tremor* is also common in cerebellar disease. This is an oscillating movement disorder (tremor) that is worse when the

animal is intending to move. Unlike the tremors of the extrapyramidal system (see Chapter 9), intention tremors are much less severe when the animal is relaxed and not moving and are worse when a movement is being performed. In animals, intention tremors seem worse in the head and axial (proximal) antigravity muscles. If the vestibular cerebellum is involved, nystagmus may also be seen (see Chapter 10).

The clinical syndrome resulting from cerebellar disease is one of many examples in which the mechanism of disease can be understood by knowing normal physiology.

CLINICAL CORRELATION

CEREBELLAR HYPOPLASIA

HISTORY ☐ An 11-week-old female barn kitten is brought to your clinic for examination. The owner states that this kitten and several others in the litter have been incoordinated since they began to walk.

CLINICAL EXAMINATION ☐ Physical examination abnormalities are limited to the nervous system. The kitten is bright, alert, and responsive and seems to be of normal size for her age. All cranial nerve and spinal segmental reflexes and intersegmental responses are within normal limits. There is no atrophy. The kitten is incoordinated (ataxic) when she moves and tends to raise her front paws higher than normal when walking ("goose stepping" hypermetria). She has a wide-based gait with her paws held far apart. There are coarse, rhythmic movements of her head and proximal antigravity muscles that are absent at rest and worse when she is attempting a precise movement such as getting her head to a food dish (intention tremor). Her complete blood count and serum chemistries are within normal limits.

COMMENT ☐ This kitten demonstrates classic signs of cerebellar disease. It is the job of the cerebellum to constantly compare the intended movement with the actual movement and, where these are not the same, make the appropriate adjustments. When the cerebellum cannot do this, movement disorders characterized by wide-based gaits, ataxia, dysmetria, and intention tremor occur. These movement disorders are worse with precise movement and nearly absent at rest.

In this kitten's case, her clinical signs are likely due to cerebellar hypoplasia in which the cerebellum never developed completely *in utero.* The *in utero* infection of feline panleukopenia virus results in destruction of the actively dividing granule cells, with an underdevelopment (hypoplasia) of the granular cell layer of the cerebellum. Purkinje's cells may be affected also. Barn cats are often poorly vaccinated for this disease, and often several kittens in a litter are affected.

TREATMENT □ There is no treatment for cerebellar hypoplasia because of this *in utero* virus infection. It is not a progressive disease, and if kept in a fairly safe environment, the kitten can have a normal life span.

Bibliography

Berne RM, Levy MN (eds): Physiology, 2nd ed. St Louis, CV Mosby, 1988, pp 227–238.

Guyton AC: Textbook of Medical Physiology, 7th ed. Philadelphia, WB Saunders, 1986, pp 638–648.

Kandel ER, Schwartz JH (eds): Principles of Neural Science, 2nd ed. New York, Elsevier, 1985, pp 502–521.

Lance JW, McLeod JG: A Physiological Approach to Clinical Neurology, 3rd ed. London, Butterworths, 1981, pp 191–219.

Oliver JE, Hoerlein BR, Mayhew IG (eds): Veterinary Neurology. Philadelphia, WB Saunders, 1987, pp 197–198.

Smith LH, Thier SO (eds): Pathophysiology—The Biological Principles of Disease, 2nd ed. Philadelphia, WB Saunders, 1985, pp 1068–1072.

Willis WD, Grossman RG: Medical Neurobiology, Neuroanatomical and Neurophysiological Principles Basic to Clinical Neuroscience, 3rd ed. St. Louis, CV Mosby, 1981, pp 368–385.

PRACTICE QUESTIONS FOR CHAPTER 11

1. A tremor (abnormal, rhythmic movement) that is worse when the patient is performing a precise movement than when at rest is likely due to an abnormality of the

   a. cerebral cortex.
   b. extrapyramidal system.
   c. cerebellum.
   d. vestibular system.
   e. γ lower motor neurons.

2. Which of the following is among the necessary sources of sensory information for the cerebellum?

   a. Muscle spindle
   b. Vestibular system
   c. Visual system
   d. All of the above
   e. None of the above

3. Loss of the cerebellum causes conscious proprioception response deficits.

   a. True
   b. False

4. Loss of the cerebellum causes loss of the muscle stretch reflex.

   a. True
   b. False

5. Cats with congenital malformations of the cerebellum often have ataxia, intention tremor, and wide gait.

   a. True
   b. False

The Autonomic Nervous System and Adrenal Medulla

1. The autonomic nervous system differs from the somatic motor system in at least two important ways
2. The autonomic nervous system has two major subdivisions
3. The sympathetic nervous system arises from the thoracolumbar spinal cord
4. The parasympathetic nervous system arises from the brainstem and spinal cord
5. Most autonomic neurons secrete either acetylcholine or norepinephrine as a neurotransmitter
6. Acetylcholine and norepinephrine have different postsynaptic receptors
7. There are general differences in sympathetic and parasympathetic function
8. The autonomic nervous system participates in many homeostatic reflexes
9. Preganglionic neurons are influenced by the brain
10. Loss of autonomic neurons results in the hypersensitivity of the target organ to transmitter

The autonomic nervous system is a part of the nervous system that is generally not under conscious control. It is for this reason that Langley named this segment of the nervous system *autonomic*, from two Greek words meaning self-governing or independent.

The autonomic nervous system is usually defined as a peripheral motor system innervating smooth muscle, cardiac muscle, and some glandular tissue, although it is subject to reflex and cerebral control. It regulates such subconscious body functions as blood pressure, heart rate, intestinal motility, and the diameter of the eye's pupil.

This system has a unique anatomy, synaptic transmission, and effect on its various target organs. It is the site of action of a large number of drugs and is essential for homeostasis. This chapter describes the general anatomy and function of the autonomic nervous system. The autonomic nervous system's specific effect on particular target organs is described in the chapters for each of the body's systems.

93

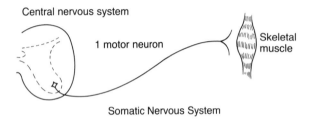

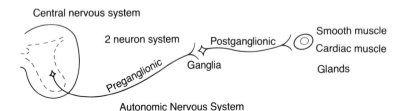

Autonomic Nervous System

Figure 12–1. The autonomic nervous system differs from the somatic nervous system in the number of nerves it has in the peripheral nervous system. The somatic nervous system has one nerve whose cell body is located in the CNS and whose axon extends, uninterrupted, to the skeletal muscle where the first peripheral chemical synapse occurs. By contrast, the autonomic nervous system has two peripheral nerves. The first, called a *preganglionic nerve*, also has its cell body in the CNS, but its axon innervates a second neuron in the chain, called the *postganglionic nerve*. Its cell body is in a peripheral structure called a *ganglion*.

The Autonomic Nervous System Differs from the Somatic Motor System in at Least Two Important Ways

The autonomic nervous system differs from the somatic motor system in its target organ and in the number of neurons in its peripheral circuit. The somatic motor system innervates skeletal muscle. Skeletal muscle is that muscle responsible for all movements of the body as described in Chapters 4 and 5. By contrast, the autonomic nervous system innervates smooth muscle, cardiac muscle, and some glands (Table 12–1). Cardiac muscle is the muscle of the heart (see Chapter 18). Smooth muscle is the muscle in blood vessels, most of the gastrointestinal (GI) tract, the bladder, and other hollow visceral structures.

The autonomic nervous system differs also in the number of nerves it has in the peripheral nervous system (Fig. 12–1). The somatic nervous system has one nerve whose cell body is located in the central nervous system (CNS) and whose axon extends, uninterrupted, to the skeletal muscle, where the first peripheral chemical synapse occurs. By contrast, the autonomic nervous system has two peripheral nerves. The first, called a *preganglionic nerve*, also has its cell body in the CNS, but its axon

Table 12–1
TWO SUBDIVISIONS OF THE MOTOR NEURONS IN THE PERIPHERAL NERVOUS SYSTEM

1. Somatic motor nerves	—Skeletal muscle
2. Autonomic motor nerves	—Cardiac muscle
	—Smooth muscle
	—Exocrine gland

innervates a second neuron in the chain, called the *postganglionic nerve*. Its cell body is in a peripheral structure called a *ganglia*. A ganglia is defined as a collection of nerve cell bodies outside the CNS. As another example, remember the dorsal root ganglia along sensory nerves leading to the spinal cord. There are chemically mediated synapses both between the pre- and postganglionic neurons and between the postganglionic nerve and its target organ. The autonomic nervous system differs also in the amount of myelin along the peripheral axons—postganglionic neurons are usually unmyelinated—and in a few other, less important ways.

The Autonomic Nervous System Has Two Major Subdivisions

The autonomic nervous system is divided into two major subdivisions on the basis of the anatomical origin of their preganglionic neurons and on the basis of their synaptic transmitters with the target organ. These two subdivisions are the *sympathetic nervous system* and the *parasympathetic nervous system*.

The Sympathetic Nervous System Arises from the Thoracolumbar Spinal Cord

The sympathetic nervous system generally has short preganglionic and long postganglionic axons. Preganglionic axons of the sympathetic nervous system leave the spinal cord by way of the ventral roots of the first thoracic through the third or fourth lumbar spinal nerves (Fig. 12–2). For this reason, it is often

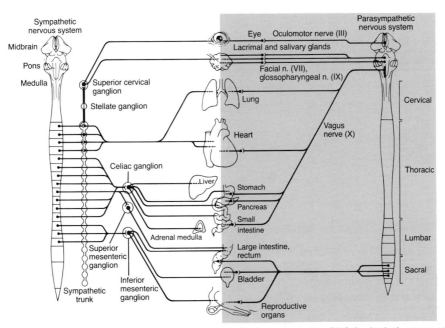

Figure 12–2. This figure illustrates the site of origin of preganglionic axons in the CNS for both the sympathetic nervous system (left) and the parasympathetic nervous system (right). Several sites of projection of postganglionic axons are shown also. (From Kandel ER, Schwartz JH: Principles of Neural Science, 2nd ed. Copyright 1985 by Elsevier Science Publishing Company, Inc., New York.)

called the *thoracolumbar system.* They pass through a communicating branch to enter the *paravertebral sympathetic ganglion chain,* where most synapse with a postganglionic neuron (Fig. 12–3). These postganglionic axons extend

then to one of the hollow visceral organs or re-enter the spinal nerves to extend to more distal structures. A few preganglionic axons pass through the paravertebral ganglia to synapse with postganglionic neurons in more

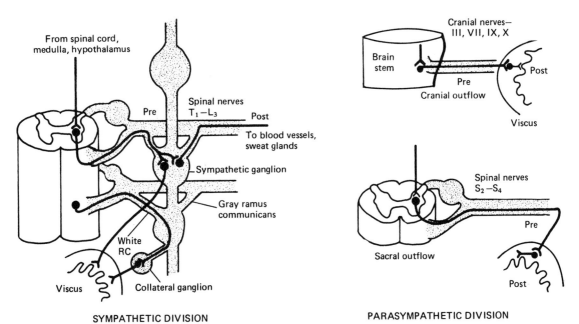

Figure 12–3. Autonomic nervous system. *Pre,* preganglionic neuron; *Post,* postganglionic neuron; *RC,* communicating branch. (From Ganong WF: Review of Medical Physiology, 13th ed. Norwalk, Appleton & Lange, 1987.)

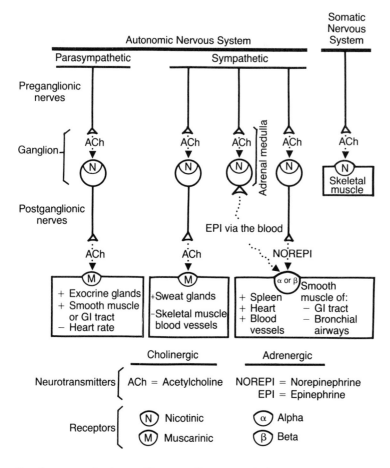

Figure 12–4. Classification of autonomic and somatic nerves with respect to their transmitter or mediator released, their postsynaptic receptors, and their general effect on the effector organ. Acetylcholine, released from the presynaptic membrane, can stimulate either a muscarinic or a nicotinic postsynaptic receptor, depending on the particular location of the synapse. Similarly, norepinephrine can stimulate either α or β receptors, again depending on the location of the synapse.

distal *prevertebral ganglia,* usually named for neighboring blood vessels.

The adrenal medulla is a special variation on this anatomical theme. A few sympathetic, preganglionic axons extend all the way to the adrenal medulla, where they synapse with rudimentary postganglionic neurons that make up the adrenal medullary secretory cells. These vestigial postganglionic neurons secrete their transmitter substance directly into the circulating blood. The transmitter substance, acting like a true hormone, is carried by the blood to all tissues of the body.

The Parasympathetic Nervous System Arises from the Brainstem and Spinal Cord

The parasympathetic nervous system generally has long preganglionic and short postganglionic axons. Preganglionic axons of the parasympathetic system leave the CNS by way of cranial nerves three, seven, nine, and ten, and by way of several sacral spinal nerves. For this reason, it is called the *craniosacral*

system (see Fig. 12–2). The long preganglionic axons pass to parasympathetic ganglia in or near the target organ, where they synapse with short postganglionic neurons. (In the GI system, postganglionic neurons have an extensive network called the *intrinsic nervous system.* It is described in Chapter 26.)

Most Autonomic Neurons Secrete Either Acetylcholine or Norepinephrine as a Neurotransmitter

As you will recall from Chapter 4, acetylcholine is the neurotransmitter at the somatic neuromuscular synapse. Acetylcholine is also the neurotransmitter at all autonomic ganglia (Fig. 12–4), although there is evidence that dopamine-secreting ganglionic interneurons may play a role in sympathetic ganglia also. The neurotransmitter secreted by parasympathetic, postganglionic neurons is also acetylcholine. Acetylcholine-releasing synapses are often called *cholinergic.* Most anatomically sympathetic, postganglionic neurons secrete *norepinephrine*. However, anatomically sympathetic, postganglionic neurons to blood vessels of skeletal muscle produce vasodilation and secrete acetylcholine, as do sympathetic, postganglionic nerves to sweat glands in some species. Norepinephrine-releasing synapses are often called *adrenergic*.

In the case of the adrenal medulla, innervating preganglionic axons release acetylcholine, but the vestigial, postganglionic neurons of the adrenal medullary tissue release both epinephrine and norepinephrine into the circulating blood.

It is important that, once released, the neurotransmitter not linger in the synaptic cleft. The neurotransmitter must be either destroyed in the cleft or dissipated so that the postsynaptic membrane can recover its resting potential and be ready for the next synaptic transmission. Because some synapses can transmit impulses up to several hundred times per second, neurotransmitter destruction must occur quickly. In the case of acetylcholine, acetylcholinesterase destroys the transmitter in the cleft. In the case of norepinephrine, however, simple diffusion and reuptake by the presynaptic neuron are the most likely ways its effect on the postsynaptic membrane is terminated.

Acetylcholine and Norepinephrine Have Different Postsynaptic Receptors

The neurotransmitters secreted by the autonomic nervous system all stimulate their target organ by first binding with a postsynaptic receptor. These receptors are proteins in the cell membrane. When the transmitter binds with the postsynaptic receptor, the membrane's permeability to selected ions is changed, and the postsynaptic membrane potential either increases or decreases with a resulting change in the probability of action potentials in the postsynaptic cell.

Acetylcholine stimulates two different receptors (see Fig. 12–4). These are *muscarinic* and *nicotinic* receptors. Muscarinic acetylcholine receptors are found on all the target cells stimulated by postganglionic parasympathetic neurons and cholinergic postganglionic neurons of the sympathetic nervous system. Nicotinic receptors are found at all synapses between pre- and postganglionic neurons and at the somatic neuromuscular junction.

Muscarinic receptors were named because they are stimulated by muscarine, a toadstool poison. Muscarine does not stimulate nicotinic receptors. Nicotine stimulates the nicotinic receptors but not muscarinic receptors. Of course, acetylcholine stimulates both. Different drugs block each receptor. For example, atropine blocks muscarinic receptors whereas curare blocks nicotinic receptors.

There are two major types of adrenergic receptors, called α and β receptors. The β receptors are further subdivided into β_1 and β_2 receptors, on the basis of the effect of adrenergic blocking and stimulating drugs.

There Are General Differences in Sympathetic and Parasympathetic Function

Although both the sympathetic and parasympathetic systems are important for homeostasis—maintaining the constancy of the interval environment—there are some important general differences in their function.

In physical and some emotional stress, the sympathetic system discharges as a unit, resulting in widespread stimulation of the body. This causes an increase in heart rate and blood pressure, the dilation of the pupil of the eye, elevation in blood glucose and free fatty acids, and an increased state of arousal. All of these widespread effects are useful in responding to an emergency. (Cannon called the sympathetic [noradrenergic] system the "fight or flight" system.) The effect of sympathetic discharge is not only widespread but lasts longer than parasympathetic (cholinergic) discharge because of the prolonged circulation of epinephrine and norepinephrine. Indeed, the adrenal medulla's secretion of epinephrine and norepinephrine into the circulating blood provides prolonged adrenergic stimulation to the entire body, even to some tissues that do not have direct sympathetic, postganglionic stimulation.

Even though the adrenergic system usually has a widespread effect, it is also capable of discrete control of particular organs. For example, the dilator smooth muscle in the iris causes enlargement of the pupil in low ambient light without more widespread effects on the body.

By contrast, the parasympathetic (cholinergic) system is more discrete in its effects on particular organs and more concerned with the vegetative aspects of daily living. For ex-

Table 12–2
RESPONSES OF EFFECTOR ORGANS TO AUTONOMIC NERVE IMPULSES AND CIRCULATING CATECHOLAMINES*

Effector Organs	Cholinergic Impulses Response	Noradrenergic Impulses	
		Receptor Type	*Response*
Eye			
Radial muscle of iris	—	α	Contraction (mydriasis)
Sphincter muscle of iris	Contraction (miosis)		—
Ciliary muscle	Contraction for near vision	β	Relaxation for far vision
Heart			
S-A node	Decrease in heart rate; vagal arrest	β_1	Increase in heart rate
Atria	Decrease in contractility and (usually) increase in conduction velocity	β_1	Increase in contractility and conduction velocity
A-V node and conduction system	Decrease in conduction velocity; A-V block	β_1	Increase in conduction velocity
Ventricles	—	β_2	Increase in contractility and conduction velocity
Arterioles			
Coronary, skeletal muscle, pulmonary, abdominal viscera, renal	Dilation	α β_2	Constriction Dilation
Skin and mucosa, cerebral, salivary glands	—	α	Constriction
Systemic veins	—	α β_2	Constriction Dilation
Lung			
Bronchial muscle	Contraction	β_2	Relaxation
Bronchial glands	Stimulation	?	Inhibition (?)
Stomach (monogastric)			
Motility and tone	Increase	α, β_2	Decrease (usually)
Sphincters	Relaxation (usually)	α	Contraction (usually)
Secretion	Stimulation		Inhibition (?)
Intestine			
Motility and tone	Increase	α, β_2	Decrease
Sphincters	Relaxation (usually)	α	Contraction (usually)
Secretion	Stimulation		Inhibition (?)
Gallbladder and ducts	Contraction		Relaxation

ample, cholinergic stimulation assists digestion and absorption of food by increasing gastric secretion, increasing intestinal motility, and relaxing the pyloric sphincter. For this reason the parasympathetic nervous system is sometimes called the *anabolic* or *vegetative* nervous system.

Many organs of the body have both sympathetic (adrenergic) and parasympathetic (cholinergic) innervation, each with a reciprocal effect. For example, adrenergic stimulation increases heart rate, whereas cholinergic decreases heart rate. Adrenergic stimulation enlarges pupillary diameter, whereas cholinergic stimulation causes pupillary constriction.

Table 12–2 gives a more complete listing of the response of various organs to adrenergic and cholinergic stimulation.

The Autonomic Nervous System Participates in Many Homeostatic Reflexes

Many of the body's visceral functions are regulated by *autonomic reflexes*. Like reflex arcs in the somatic nervous system (see Chapter 6), autonomic reflex arcs also include a sensory side to the arc including a visceral receptor, a sensory nerve often called a *visceral afferent* nerve, and one or more synapses in the CNS. The autonomic nervous system is usually defined as the peripheral, motor pre- and postganglionic neurons. Visceral afferent neurons are usually not included in this definition, but are generally essential parts of the autonomic reflex arc.

Autonomic reflexes are extremely common and are described in detail for each body

Table 12–2
RESPONSES OF EFFECTOR ORGANS TO AUTONOMIC NERVE IMPULSES AND CIRCULATING CATECHOLAMINES* *Continued*

Effector Organs	Cholinergic Impulses Response	Noradrenergic Impulses	
		Receptor Type	*Response*
Urinary bladder			
Detrusor	Contraction	β	Relaxation (usually)
Trigone and sphincter	Relaxation	α	Contraction
Ureter			
Motility and tone	Increase (?)	α	Increase (usually)
Uterus	Variable†	α, β$_2$	Variable
Male sex organs	Erection	α	Ejaculation
Skin			
Pilomotor muscles	—	α	Contraction
Sweat glands	Generalized secretion	α	Slight, localized secretion‡
Spleen capsule	—	α	Contraction
		β$_2$	Relaxation
Adrenal medulla	Secretion of epinephrine and norepinephrine		—
Liver	—	α, β$_2$	Glycogenolysis
Pancreas			
Acini	Increased secretion	α	Decreased secretion
Islets	Increased insulin and glucagon secretion	α	Decreased insulin and glucagon secretion
		β$_2$	Increased insulin and glucagon secretion
Salivary glands	Profuse, water secretion	α	Thick, viscous secretion
		β$_2$	Amylase secretion
Lacrimal glands	Secretion		—
Juxtaglomerular cells	—	β$_1$	Increased renin secretion
Pineal gland	—	β	Increased melatonin synthesis and secretion

*Adapted from Weiner N, Taylor P: Neurohumoral Transmission: The Autonomic and Somatic Motor Nervous Systems. In Gilman AG, Goodman LS, Rall TW, Murad F: Goodman and Gilman's The Pharmacological Basis of Therapeutics, 7th ed. New York, Macmillan, 1985.
†Depends on stage of estrous cycle, amount of circulating estrogen and progesterone, pregnancy, and other factors.
‡On palms of human hands and in some other locations (adrenergic sweating).

system in later chapters of this book. A few are described briefly here as examples.

Control of Blood Pressure. Stretch receptors in the internal carotid artery and the aorta detect systemic blood pressure. As blood pressure rises above normal limits, sympathetic, adrenergic vasoconstrictor nerves are inhibited and blood pressure falls back to within normal limits. (Why this does not happen in hypertensive humans is the subject of much contemporary research.)

Pupillary Light Reflex. When a flashlight is shown into an animal's eye, light stimulates photoreceptors in the retina (see Chapter 13). Sensory action potentials are then transmitted to the brainstem along the optic nerve where, through several interneurons, parasympa-

thetic, cholinergic neurons stimulate the constrictor smooth muscle of the iris. This causes the pupillary diameter to become smaller.

Gastric secretion of digestive fluids in anticipation of food, and the emptying of the rectum and bladder in response to filling, are but a few of the many other automatic reflexes that are described in more detail throughout this book.

Preganglionic Neurons Are Influenced by the Brain

Much as the lower motor neuron of the somatic system is influenced by the upper motor neuron (see Chapter 8), the preganglionic autonomic neuron is influenced also by

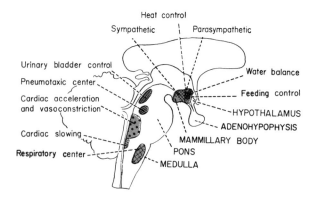

Figure 12–5. Autonomic control centers of the brain stem. (From Guyton AC: Textbook of Medical Physiology, 7th ed. Philadelphia, WB Saunders, 1986.)

CNS axons descending from the brainstem, hypothalamus, and even the cerebral cortex. Many brainstem nuclei are known to influence preganglionic neurons in order to control particular visceral functions. Figure 12–5 illustrates several such centers. In turn, each of these brainstem centers can be influenced by the hypothalamus and cerebral cortex, creating a complex system of upper motor neurons within the CNS that helps coordinate autonomic reflexes and directly influence action potential frequency within preganglionic neurons. As we learn more about these central systems controlling the autonomic nervous system, we may find that they play an important role in such diseases as hypertension and various GI diseases.

Loss of Autonomic Neurons Results in the Hypersensitivity of the Target Organ to Transmitter

When the postganglionic neuron to a target organ is lost, the smooth muscle of that organ becomes hypersensitive to any transmitter circulating in the blood. For example, the arterioles of the skin are usually under some adrenergic tone resulting in some vasoconstriction. If the postganglionic, adrenergic neuron to the skin is destroyed, vasodilation occurs. However, if norepinephrine is injected into the blood supply to this area of skin, a dramatic (hypersensitive) vasoconstriction occurs. This is thought to be due, at least in part, to an increase in postsynaptic α receptors at the denervated synapse. Why these receptors should increase in numbers is not known.

CLINICAL CORRELATION

HORNER'S SYNDROME

HISTORY □ A 7-year-old male golden retriever is brought to your clinic for examination. The owner states that during the past 3 weeks, the dog has become progressively weak in his left front leg and now cannot bear weight on this limb. The owner has noticed also that the dog's left upper eyelid seems to be droopy.

CLINICAL EXAMINATION □ Physical examination abnormalities are limited to the nervous system. The dog is bright, alert, and responsive. Except for the left front leg, cranial nerve and spinal segmental reflexes and all intersegmental responses are within normal limits. The dog cannot bear weight on the left front leg, and it is atrophied. No segmental reflexes (e.g., toe-pinch withdrawal) or intersegmental responses (e.g., conscious proprioception) can be elicited from the left front leg. The left upper eyelid droops lower than the right upper lid, and the left pupil is smaller than the right pupil. The left nictitating membrane (third eyelid) is prolapsed out over part of the cornea, and the left eye seems sunken into the orbit more than the right eye.

COMMENT □ This dog has a lesion of his left brachial plexus, probably a neoplasm. It has caused a lower motor neuron syndrome to the left front leg with atrophy, paralysis, and loss of reflexes. The tumor has damaged the preganglionic neurons of the left sympathetic nervous system as they leave the first two thoracic segments on their way toward the eye. Loss of the sympathetic innervation to the region of the eye causes a small pupil (miosis), droopy upper eyelid (ptosis), a sunken eye (enophthalmus), and a prolapsed nictitating membrane. This constellation of clinical signs is called Horner's syndrome, first named by a Swiss ophthalmologist in 1869. Sympathetic preganglionic neurons pass through the brachial plexus (where they were damaged in this dog) and ascend in the vagosympathetic trunk to synapse with the postganglionic neurons in the cranial cervical ganglia. The postganglionic cell axons then go to the region of the eye where they innervate the dilator smooth muscle cells of the iris. When they are paralyzed, the constrictor fibers of the iris are unopposed, and miosis is the result. The sympathetic nervous system also innervates several smooth muscle fibers that lift the upper eyelid and help position the nictitating membrane and the eye within the socket. Because the preganglionic fibers are relatively exposed in the neck, they are commonly damaged. Horner's syndrome can occur also as a result of damage to either the postganglionic neurons or the neurons that descend from the hypothalamus to the rostral thoracic cord to control the preganglionic neurons.

TREATMENT □ Treatment involves removing the cause of sympathetic nerve damage.

Bibliography

Berne RM, Levy MN (eds): Physiology, 2nd ed. St Louis, CV Mosby, 1988, pp 280–296.

Gilman AG, Goodman LS, Rall TW, Murad F (eds): Goodman and Gilman's The Pharmacological Basis of Therapeutics, 7th ed. New York, Macmillan, 1985, pp 66–99.

Guyton AC: Textbook of Medical Physiology, 7th ed. Philadelphia, WB Saunders, 1986, pp 686–700.

Lance JW, McLeod JG: A Physiological Approach to Clinical Neurology, 3rd ed. London, Butterworths, 1981, pp 263–285.

Smith LH, Thier SO (eds): Pathophysiology—The Biological Principles of Disease, 2nd ed. Philadelphia, WB Saunders, 1985, pp 1121–1137.

PRACTICE QUESTIONS FOR CHAPTER 12

1. Choose the *incorrect* statement below:

   a. A ganglia is a collection of nerve cell bodies outside the CNS.
   b. Acetylcholine is the chemical transmitter at the parasympathetic, postganglionic-to-target organ synapse.
   c. Sympathetic postganglionic neurons are usually longer than those of the parasympathetic system.
   d. The adrenal medulla secretes mostly norepinephrine and relatively little epinephrine.
   e. Atropine blocks acetylcholine transmission at the parasympathetic, postganglionic end organ.

2. The chemical transmitter substance between pre- and postganglionic neurons of the sympathetic component of the autonomic nervous system is

   a. norepinephrine.
   b. acetylcholine.
   c. epinephrine.
   d. dopamine.
   e. γ aminobutyric acid.

3. The neurotransmitter at the sympathetic postganglionic-to-target organ synapse is

   a. norepinephrine.
   b. epinephrine.
   c. acetylcholine.
   d. dopamine.
   e. γ aminobutyric acid.

4. A drug such as atropine that blocks parasympathetic, postganglionic neurons to the eye leads to

   a. an abnormally constricted pupil but normal focusing ability for near vision.
   b. an abnormally dilated pupil but normal focusing ability for near vision.
   c. an abnormally constricted pupil and poor ability to focus on near objects.
   d. an abnormally dilated pupil and poor ability to focus on near objects.
   e. no change in either pupillary diameter or focusing ability.

5. Horner's syndrome is caused by the loss of

   a. sympathetic innervation to the eye.
   b. parasympathetic innervation to the eye.
   c. the acetylcholine transmitter.
   d. acetylcholinesterase.
   e. the smooth muscle of the iris.

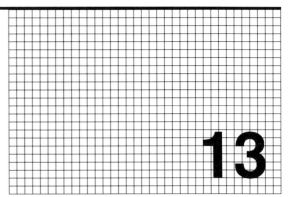

The Visual System

1. The eye's anatomy is adapted to the eye's role as a visual receptor
2. Through the process of accommodation, the lens changes shape to focus images from various distances onto the retina
3. The vertebrate retina consists of five major cell types
4. The fovea solves a distortion problem found in other areas of the retina
5. Pigment behind the retina either absorbs or reflects light, depending on the animal's habits
6. Photoreception occurs in the rods and cones
7. The electrical response of the photoreceptor to light is transmitted to the ganglion cells by the bipolar cells
8. The electroretinogram records the electrical response of the retina to a flashing light
9. Ganglion cell axons transmit action potentials to the visual cortex by way of the lateral geniculate nucleus
10. The diameter of the pupil is controlled by the autonomic nervous system
11. The retina, optic nerve, and autonomic nerve supply to the pupil can be tested with a flashlight
12. Aqueous humor determines intraocular pressure

The visual system is the sensory modality an animal can least afford to loose. It is also a sensory system commonly involved in clinical pathology. Indeed, a whole discipline of veterinary ophthalmology has developed in recent years. Hence, this chapter is devoted to the visual system.

The eyes are complex sense organs that are basically an extension of the brain. They evolved from primitive light-sensing spots on the surface of invertebrates and in some species have developed many remarkable variations, providing special advantages in various ecological niches. Each eye has a layer of receptors, a lens system for focusing an image

on these receptors, and a system of axons for transmitting action potentials to the brain. This chapter describes the way these and other components of the eye work.

The Eye's Anatomy Is Adapted to the Eye's Role as a Visual Receptor

Figure 13–1 shows the anatomy of the normal eye in the horizontal plane. The white, outer protective layer encasing most of the eyeball is called the *sclera*. It is modified anteriorly into a clear, stratified squamous epithelial layer called the *cornea*. In the posterior two-thirds of the eye, the sclera is lined with

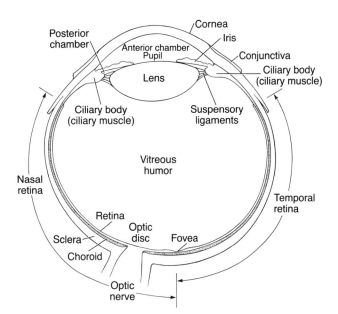

Figure 13–1. Schematic diagram of a horizontal section through the right eye as viewed from above. (Redrawn with permission from Walls GL: The Vertebrate Eye and Its Adaptive Radiation. Cranbrook Institute of Science, Bull. 19, 1942.)

a vascular and pigmented layer called the *choroid.* Inside the choroid is the retina, the layer containing the photoreceptors.

As light enters the eye, it enters a compartment called the *anterior chamber.* The anterior and *posterior chambers* are filled with a clear, water-like fluid called *aqueous humor.* Separating the anterior and posterior chambers is a diaphragm of varying size called the *iris.* The iris is a pigmented structure containing dilator and constrictor smooth muscle fibers arranged to vary the diameter of the *pupil,* the hole in the iris through which light passes on its way to the retina. Behind the iris is the *lens.* The lens is suspended in the eye by the *suspensory ligaments.* Suspensory ligaments attach to the lens and to the *ciliary body,* a muscular structure at the base of the iris. Behind the lens is a chamber filled with a gelatinous fluid called the *vitreous humor.* Behind the vitreous humor is the neural retinal layer. The retina is interrupted at a point where axons of the retina's ganglion cell layer leave the retina on the way to the brain. This point, the *optic disc,* is a recognizable structure when examining the eye with an ophthalmoscope. The optic disc gives rise to the optic nerve, a cranial nerve so rich in axons that there are more axons in both optic nerves than in all the dorsal roots of the spinal cord.

Also visible with the ophthalmoscope, on the surface of the retina, are the *retinal blood vessels* (Fig. 13–2). These are a network of arteries and veins that enter the retina at the optic disc and provide much of the nutrition

to the retina. Vessels of the choroid provide the remaining nutrition to the retina. Examining retinal vessels often provides valuable clues to pathology elsewhere in the cardiovascular system.

Thanks to pressure generated by the aqueous humor and the inelasticity of the sclera and cornea, the globe of the eye is basically spherical.

The lacrimal gland, located near the lateral canthus of the eye, produces tears in response to parasympathetic nerve stimulation. Tears then flow over the cornea and are drained into the nose by the nasolacrimal duct. A regular flow of tears across the cornea is essential to the health of the cornea.

Through the Process of Accommodation, the Lens Changes Shape to Focus Images from Various Distances onto the Retina

When a camera focuses the images of objects at various distances from the film, the distance between the lens and the film is changed. The eye focuses images by changing the shape of the lens, not by changing the distance between the lens and the retina.

Figure 13–3 shows the primary structures responsible for accommodation. The lens of the eye is made up of an elastic *lens capsule* containing a jelly-like substance. If the eye's lens were taken out of the eye, it would assume a spherical shape owing to the elasticity of its capsule, much like filling a balloon with jelly. When suspended in the relaxed

DORSAL

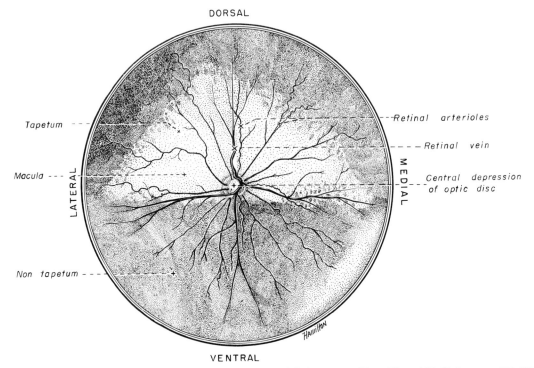

Tapetum

Retinal arterioles

Retinal vein

Macula

LATERAL

MEDIAL

Central depression
of optic disc

Non tapetum

VENTRAL

Figure 13–2. Ocular fundus of the right eye as viewed with an ophthalmoscope. (From Evans HE, Christensen GC: Miller's Anatomy of the Dog, 2nd ed. Philadelphia, WB Saunders, 1979.)

eye, however, the elasticity of the suspensory ligaments pulls on the equator of the lens, causing it to flatten in its anterior-posterior dimension. This flattened, less convex lens causes less refraction of light rays and allows the focus onto the retina of objects more than 20 feet away. To focus the image of objects

closer to the eye, however, the lens must assume a more spherical convex shape. This is accomplished by the contraction of the ciliary muscles of the ciliary body. This contraction of the ciliary muscle is much like the contraction of a sphincter and decreases the inner diameter of ciliary body. In turn, this

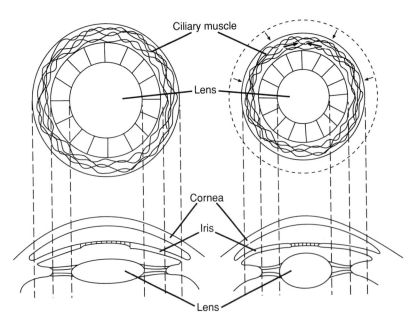

Ciliary muscle

Lens

Cornea

Iris

Lens

Figure 13–3. Primary ocular structures responsible for accommodation. The shape of the lens is shown when the ciliary muscle is relaxed (left) and contracted (right).

Figure 13–4. Horse's ramp-shaped retina, which provides a longer focal length for viewing downward *(F₁)* than for viewing along the axis of the eye *(F₂)*. This means that, within limits, lower, nearer objects are automatically in focus without the use of accommodation. (Redrawn from Prince JH, et al: Anatomy and Histology of the Eye and Orbit in Domestic Animals. Springfield, IL, Charles C Thomas, 1960.)

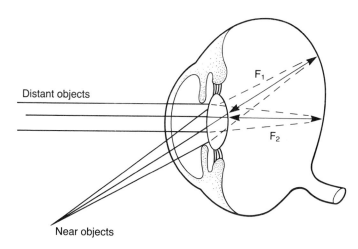

moves the attachments of the suspensory ligaments to a new position closer to the lens and decreases the pull on the equator of the lens. The result of the inherent elasticity of the lens capsule is a more spherical lens with more light refraction that focuses onto the retina the image of nearer objects. The more contraction of the ciliary muscle, the more spherical the lens becomes. Horses have a ramp-shaped retina (Fig. 13–4), allowing some degree of focusing on near objects without changing the shape of the lens, achieved by changing the posture of the head, because the distance between the lens and the stimulated area of the retina would vary.

In humans, as the lens ages, it becomes less elastic and tends to remain less convex, even when the ciliary muscles contract. Many people older than 40 years of age need reading glasses to help their less elastic lens focus on near objects.

The lens should be clear and free of opacities. However, in *cataracts*, the lens becomes more opaque, causing random refraction of light and blurred vision, often eventually leading to blindness.

The Vertebrate Retina Consists of Five Major Cell Types

Unlike somatic receptors of the skin, the retina is not a peripheral end organ but rather a part of the central nervous system (CNS). Skin receptors are derived from conventional ectoderm. The retina is derived from neuroectoderm, a specialized portion of the ectoderm giving rise to the brain. For this reason, the retina is a fairly complex extension of the brain capable of an initial interpretation of the visual image.

The vertebrate retina consists of five major cell types: photoreceptor cells, bipolar cells, horizontal cells, amacrine cells, and ganglion cells (Fig. 13–5).

There are two types of photoreceptor cells: *rods* and *cones*. Both rods and cones make direct synaptic connection with the interneurons called *bipolar cells*, which connect the

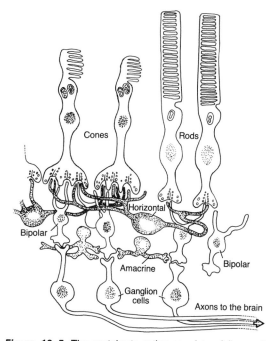

Figure 13–5. The vertebrate retina consists of five major cell types: photoreceptor cells (either rods or cones), bipolar cells, horizontal cells, amacrine cells, and ganglion cells. (Redrawn from Kandel ER, Schwartz JH: Principles of Neural Science, 2nd ed. New York, Elsevier Science Publishing Company, Inc., 1985, p 352.)

receptors with the ganglion cells. Ganglion cell axons carry action potentials to the brain through the optic nerves.

Modifying the flow of information at the synapses between the photoreceptors, bipolar cells, and ganglion cells are two interneuron cell types: the horizontal cells and the amacrine cells. The horizontal cells mediate lateral interactions between the photoreceptors and bipolar cells. The amacrine cells mediate lateral interactions between the bipolar cells and the ganglion cells.

The Fovea Solves a Distortion Problem Found in Other Areas of the Retina

Throughout most of the retina, light rays travel through ganglion cells, bipolar cells, and occasionally amacrine and horizontal cells before reaching the photoreceptors. Although these inner cell types are relatively transparent, they still cause some distortion of light rays.

The *fovea* is an area of the retina designed specially to minimize this distortion. It is located at the back of the retina, where light rays would fall from more distant objects (Fig. 13–6). In the fovea, the inner ganglion and

bipolar cells are pushed aside, allowing light rays direct access to the photoreceptors.

Just nasal to the fovea is the *optic disc*. The optic disc is the origin of the optic nerve where ganglion cell axons gather to leave the retina. There are no photoreceptors in the optic disc, so this area is called the *blind spot.*

Pigment Behind the Retina Either Absorbs or Reflects Light, Depending on the Animal's Habits

In animals that rely heavily on acute, daylight vision, there is a dark pigment in the epithelial layer behind the photoreceptors and in the choroid. This pigment absorbs light that has passed by the photoreceptors without stimulating them. If such light were reflected back into the retina, the sharpness of the visual image would be blurred. However, in nocturnal animals these pigmented layers contain a reflecting pigment and are called the *tapetum.* This allows the retina to make optimum use of what light it gets, but at the expense of visual acuity. Reflection of light off the tapetum causes the familiar "night shine" from nocturnal animals' eyes.

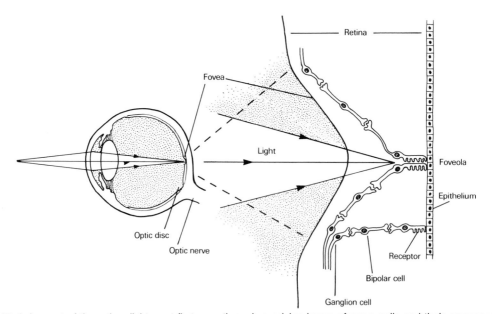

Figure 13–6. In most of the retina, light must first pass through overlying layers of nerve cells and their processes before it reaches the photoreceptors. However, in the center of the fovea, an area termed the foveola, these proximal neural elements are shifted to the side; therefore, light has a direct pathway to the photoreceptors in this region. An enlarged drawing of the back of the retina is shown on the right. (Reprinted with permission of the publisher from Kandel ER, Schwartz JH: Principles of Neural Science, 2nd ed. Copyright 1985 by Elsevier Science Publishing Company, Inc.)

Photoreception Occurs in the Rods and Cones

The anatomies of the photoreceptors, rods and cones, are similar, but with some important differences. Both cell types are divided into three parts: a synaptic terminal, an inner segment, and an outer segment (Fig. 13–7). The synaptic terminal synapses with the bipolar cells. The inner segment includes the nucleus, mitochondria, and other cytoplasmic structures. The inner and outer segments are connected by a microtubule-containing cilium. The outer portions are specialized for photoreception. They contain an elaborate array of stacked membranous discs whose membranes contain visual photopigments.

These discs are regularly being formed near the cilium and phagocytized by the pigmented epithelium. Loss of this normal turnover in the outer segment may be important in several retinal diseases. Photopigments are made up of a protein called an *opsin* and *retinal,* an aldehyde of vitamin A. When light hits the photoreceptor, the photopigment is transformed, leading to a change in the membrane potential of the photoreceptor. Unlike most receptor cell membranes that hypopolarize with stimulation, photoreceptors hyperpolarize when struck by light. In the case of rods, the photopigment is called *rhodopsin.* In the dark eye, many Na^+ channels remain open, allowing for leakage of Na^+ ions into the rod,

which lowers the electrical membrane potential. When photons of light strike rhodopsin, the retinal is transformed in a way that leads, through a second messenger, to a closing of many Na^+ channels. The result is a hyperpolarization of the receptor cell membrane and a decrease in transmitter released at the synapse with the bipolar cell. Although not as well understood, photoreception in cones results apparently from a similar breakdown of cone opsin and a hyperpolarization of the cones' electrical membrane potential.

Rods are adapted for night vision. They are highly sensitive to light of all wavelengths, not selective of the direction from which light comes, and are highly convergent, through bipolar cells, on individual ganglion cells.

Cones, found in many animals, are adapted to acute, daylight color vision. They have a lower sensitivity to light, are directionally sensitive, and in the fovea are linked with almost equal numbers of ganglion cells. According to the *Young-Helmholtz theory,* animals with color vision have inherited at least two, and in higher mammals three, different types of cones. Each is maximally sensitive to one of the three primary colors: red, green, and blue. Any perceived color can be interpreted as being made up of some proportion of these three primary colors. Individuals who lack one or more of these cone types due to faulty genetic transmission are color blind to a par-

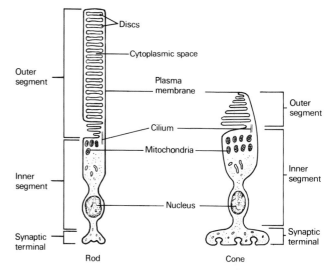

Figure 13–7. The two types of photoreceptors, rods and cones, have characteristic structures. Both rod cells and cone cells are differentiated into inner and outer segments connected by a cilium. The inner segments of both cell types contain the nucleus and most of the cell's biosynthetic machinery and are continuous with the synaptic terminals. The outer segments of the membranous discs contain the light-transducing apparatus. The membranous discs in the outer segments of rod cells are separated from the plasma membrane, whereas the discs of cone cells are not. (Adapted from O'Brien DF: The Chemistry of vision. Science 218:961–966, 1982. Reprinted by permission of the publisher from Kandel ER, Schwartz JH: Principles of Neural Science, 2nd ed. Copyright 1985 by Elsevier Science Publishing Company, Inc.)

ticular spectrum of color. Such color blindness is linked to the X chromosome.

The extent to which various veterinary species perceive color is the subject of much debate. Some mammals have only rods and are presumably color blind. Most mammals have some cones, but whether this provides them with color vision is debated. On the other hand, some birds, lizards, turtles, frogs, and teleost fish are said to have color vision. Only primates are known to have the classic color vision with which we, as humans, are familiar.

The Electrical Response of the Photoreceptor to Light Is Transmitted to the Ganglion Cells by the Bipolar Cells

The hyperpolarizing response of the rods and cones to light influences bipolar cells by a chemically mediated synapse. In turn, the bipolar cell influences action potential frequencies in the ganglion cell axons on their way to the brain. Horizontal cells influence bipolar cells, and amacrine cells influence ganglion cells to make it easier for the brain to detect contrast between brightness and darkness and to distinguish contour. A more detailed description of the synaptic and membrane changes in the chain of transmission within the retina is beyond the scope of this book. To learn more about the many interesting and unusual phenomena occurring in the retina, the reader should refer to the bibliography at the end of this chapter.

The Electroretinogram Records the Electrical Response of the Retina to a Flashing Light

The *electroretinogram* (ERG) is a clinical electrophysiological recording from the cornea and skin near the eye. It records the electrical response of the retina to a light flashed into the eye. It has three waves: the A wave, primarily corresponding to the activation of visual pigment and photoreceptors; the B wave, primarily caused by the response of retinal bipolar cells; and a slower C wave, thought to originate in the pigment epithelium.

Ganglion Cell Axons Transmit Action Potentials to the Visual Cortex by Way of the Lateral Geniculate Nucleus

In order for the image, created in the retina by the visual field, to reach consciousness, the image must be re-created in the visual cerebral cortex. Figure 13–8 shows the visual pathway by which the axons of the ganglion cells project to the lateral geniculate nucleus and by which the lateral geniculate nucleus axons project to the visual cortex. Note that ganglion cell axons from the temporal retina travel along the *optic nerve* to the *optic chiasm* and then project ipsilaterally to the *lateral geniculate nucleus* on the same side of the brain. Ganglion cell axons from the nasal retina come to the optic chiasm and cross to the contralateral geniculate nucleus on the opposite side of the brain. From there, both lateral geniculate nuclei project to the *visual cortex* in the posterior region of the cerebral cortex by way of the *optic radiations*. Remember that light rays arising in the lateral, peripheral field of vision would enter the near eye and cross to stimulate photoreceptors and ganglion cells of the nasal retina. Those light rays that can get around the nose to enter the far eye stimulate cells of the temporal retina. By reviewing the visual pathway map (Fig. 13–8) you can see that an image arising in your left lateral field of vision would be registered in the right visual cortex. Images arising from your right lateral field of vision would register in your left visual cortex.

A lesion in the right optic radiations (lesion 3 on the map) would cause a loss of vision in the left lateral visual field. A lesion at the optic chiasm (lesion 2 on the map) would cause bilateral loss of far lateral, peripheral vision (tunnel vision). A lesion in the right optic

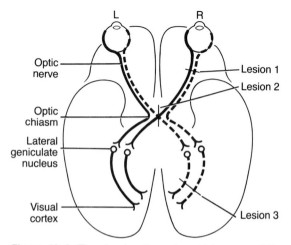

Figure 13–8. The visual pathway by which axons of the ganglion cells project to the lateral geniculate nucleus and axons from the lateral geniculate nucleus project to the visual cortex.

nerve (lesion 1 on the map) would cause loss of vision from the right eye just like closing only that eye.

The Diameter of the Pupil Is Controlled by the Autonomic Nervous System

The iris of the eye contains two sets of smooth muscle fibers. One set, arranged in a circular pattern around the pupil, causes the pupil to constrict (get smaller) when they contract. These constrictor fibers are innervated by preganglionic, parasympathetic nerves found in the oculomotor cranial nerve, Postganglionic neurons begin in the ciliary ganglion, just behind the eye, and secrete acetylcholine as the neurotransmitter. The other smooth muscle fibers of the iris are arranged radially from the pupil, like spokes of a wheel. When these radial smooth muscle fibers contract, they cause the pupil to get larger (dilate). These dilator fibers are innervated by the sympathetic nervous system. Sympathetic, preganglionic neurons begin in the first two thoracic segments and course cranially in the vagosympathetic nerve trunk of the neck. Postganglionic axons begin in the cranial cervical ganglion in the anterior neck and course to the region of the eye where they innervate the dilator fibers of the iris, the muscle that helps lift the upper eyelid, and the muscle that helps keep the "third eyelid" in place at the medial canthus of the eye; the sympathetic postganglionic axons innervate sweat glands and vascular smooth muscle to the face also.

The Retina, Optic Nerve, and Autonomic Nerve Supply to the Pupil Can Be Tested with a Flashlight

When a light is shined into the eye, the pupil of that eye constricts. This is called the *direct pupillary light reflex*. The flashlight triggers the photoreception mechanism leading to the ganglion cell action potentials transmitted along the optic nerve. Some of the ganglion cell axons go to the pretectal region of the brain that, in turn through interneurons, stimulates the preganglionic parasympathetic neurons of the oculomotor nerve. Through stimulation of the postganglionic neurons, these cause constriction of the pupil by stimulating the constrictor smooth muscle fibers of the iris. A normal direct pupillary light reflex tests the integrity of the retina, the ipsilateral sec-

ond and third cranial nerves, a limited region of the brainstem, and the iris. This system also crosses the midline in the brainstem, so that when a light is shined into one eye, not only does the pupil on the same side constrict (direct pupillary light reflex) but also the contralateral pupil constricts. This is called the *indirect pupillary light reflex*. It also requires the integrity of the contralateral oculomotor (third) cranial nerve.

Aqueous Humor Determines Intraocular Pressure

Aqueous humor is a clear liquid found in the anterior and posterior chambers of the eye. Its rate of production and absorption is sufficiently high to replace the entire chamber's volume several times a day.

Aqueous humor is secreted by the ciliary process, which is a system of finger-like processes on the ciliary body of the posterior chamber. It is thought to be formed by the active transport of sodium, chloride, and possibly bicarbonate ions into the posterior chamber. This establishes an osmotic gradient causing water to flow passively into the posterior chamber.

Aqueous humor flows from the posterior to the anterior chamber through the pupil. Flow is caused by a pressure gradient established by the active process of formation in the posterior chamber.

Aqueous humor is then absorbed into the venous system at the angle between the cornea and the iris. This absorption is driven by a pressure gradient and is assisted, at least in many species, by a system of trabeculae and canals. If this absorption into the venous system is obstructed, intraocular pressure increases because production of aqueous humor continues. This pathological increase in intraocular pressure is called *glaucoma*. As intraocular pressure exceeds intravascular pressure in the blood supply to the retina, blindness results.

CLINICAL CORRELATION

HOMONOMOUS HEMIANOPSIA

HISTORY ☐ You examine a 10-year-old male German shepherd whose owner complains that the dog has begun recently to bump into objects with the left side of his face and has had two seizures. The seizures were characterized by turning of the head to the left and stiffening of the left front leg.

CLINICAL EXAMINATION ☐ Physical examination abnormalities are limited to the nervous system. When presented with a maze of unfamiliar objects in the examination room, the dog clearly collides with objects as if he does not see from his left side. He seems somewhat weak in his left front leg. He is otherwise bright, alert, and responsive. His cranial nerve and spinal segmental reflexes are within normal limits, as are his intersegmental, conscious proprioception responses for his right front and right rear legs. However, the conscious proprioception responses for his left front and left rear legs are quite prolonged.

COMMENT ☐ This dog's history and neurological examination abnormalities are common in dogs with brain tumors. This dog has a tumor (neoplasm) arising from the meninges over his right posterior cerebral cortex. It is in this posterior (occipital) cortex that the visual image is interpreted from the visual field of the left side (see Fig. 13–8). It is also in the right cerebral cortex that the conscious proprioception response for the left legs is interpreted. His seizures feature turning the head to the left and transient rigidity of the left front leg because the seizure activity arose from the cerebral cortex at the site of the tumor and spread to the right motor cortex but remained limited to the cerebral cortex on the right side. Because the pyramidal system's corticospinal tract controlling the muscles of the left neck and left front leg arise in the right motor cortex (see Chapter 9), seizure activity causes the transient head turning and left leg stiffness.

TREATMENT ☐ This dog has a meningioma of the right posterior cerebral cortex. Surgical removal was not attempted in this case.

Bibliography

Berne RM, Levy MN (eds): Physiology, 2nd ed. St Louis, CV Mosby, 1988, pp 93–134.
Guyton AC: Textbook of Medical Physiology, 7th ed. Philadelphia, WB Saunders, 1986, pp 700–733.
Kandel ER, Schwartz JH (eds): Principles of Neural Science, 2nd ed. New York, Elsevier, 1985, pp 344–395.
Lance JW, McLeod JG: A Physiological Approach to Clinical Neurology, 3rd ed. London, Butterworths, 1981, pp 220–237.
Oliver JE, Hoerlein BR, Mayhew IG (eds): Veterinary Neurology. Philadelphia, WB Saunders, 1987, pp 171–175.
Smith LH, Thier SO (eds): Pathophysiology—The Biological Principles of Disease, 2nd ed. Philadelphia, WB Saunders, 1985, pp 1098–1111.

PRACTICE QUESTIONS FOR CHAPTER 13

1. A patient whose left pupil diameter is smaller than normal, whose left upper eyelid droops, and whose left eye is sunken into the socket likely has a lesion of which of the following structures?

   a. Left oculomotor nerve
   b. Left vagosympathetic nerve trunk
   c. Right oculomotor nerve
   d. Right vagosympathetic nerve trunk
   e. Optic chiasm

2. Your friend, a member of the football team, is trying without much success to explain the cause for the team's recent scoring trend. A variety of implausible explanations are proposed until he mentions that he is progressively losing peripheral vision from the sides of both his visual fields and has frequent headaches. You recommend that he go see a neurologist because he likely has a lesion in his

   a. left optic nerve near the eye.
   b. right optic nerve near the eye.
   c. cerebral cortex.
   d. optic chiasm.
   e. Both a and b

3. You examine a patient's pupillary light reflexes. Shining a light into the left eye produces both a positive direct and an indirect pupillary response. However, shining the light into the right eye produces neither a direct nor an indirect pupillary response. This patient's pathology is located in which of the following structures?

   a. Left optic nerve
   b. Right optic nerve
   c. Left oculomotor nerve

d. Right oculomotor nerve
e. Left optic cortex

4. You are presented with a dog that is bumping into objects with the left side of his face as if he did not see them. Direct and indirect pupillary light reflexes are normal in both eyes. Where is the most likely location for this dog's pathology?

   a. Left optic nerve
   b. Right optic nerve
   c. Left cerebral cortex

d. Right cerebral cortex
e. Left oculomotor nerve

5. You examine a patient whose right pupil is larger than the left pupil. Where in the autonomic innervation of the eyes could the pathology be located?

   a. Left parasympathetic
   b. Right parasympathetic
   c. Left sympathetic
   d. Right sympathetic
   e. Either b or c

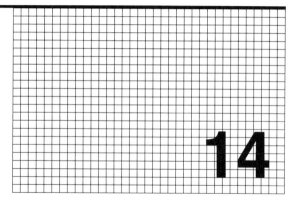

Cerebrospinal Fluid, Blood-Brain Barrier

1. Cerebrospinal fluid has many functions
2. Most cerebrospinal fluid is formed at the choroid plexus
3. Cerebrospinal fluid flows down a pressure gradient through a predictable anatomical route
4. Cerebrospinal fluid is absorbed into the venous system
5. Hydrocephalus is an increased volume of cerebrospinal fluid in the skull
6. Permeability barriers exist between blood and brain

Cerebrospinal fluid (CSF) is a clear fluid present in the ventricles of the brain, the central canal of the spinal cord, and the subarachnoid space. It has almost no blood cells and little protein. Its rate of formation, flow, and absorption is sufficiently high to cause its replacement several times daily. Sampling its pressure, cell count, and levels of various biochemical constituents is a common diagnostic procedure called a *spinal tap*. Injecting radiopaque dyes into the subarachnoid space is the basis of a common neuroradiographic technique called a *myelogram*. Obstruction of flow of CSF is a common cause of hydrocephalus. An understanding of the formation, flow, and absorption of CSF is essential to an understanding of these diagnostic procedures and the pathophysiology of hydrocephalus.

Cerebrospinal Fluid Has Many Functions

One of the most important functions of CSF is to cushion the brain, protecting it against

blows to the head. The specific gravities of the brain and CSF are similar. Because of this similar specific gravity, the brain floats in the fluid.

Because CSF is in equilibrium with the brain's extracellular fluid, it also helps maintain a constant extracellular environment for the brain's neurons and glial cells.

The CSF may serve also as a conduit for some of the brain's polypeptide hormones and other substances.

Most Cerebrospinal Fluid Is Formed at the Choroid Plexus

The majority of CSF is formed by the *choroid plexus*. These are small, cauliflower-like growths that stick out into the CSF of all four ventricles (Fig. 14–1). They consist of tufts of capillaries covered by a thin epithelial layer.

As with aqueous humor, the secretion of CSF depends primarily on the active transport of sodium ions into the ventricles. This sets

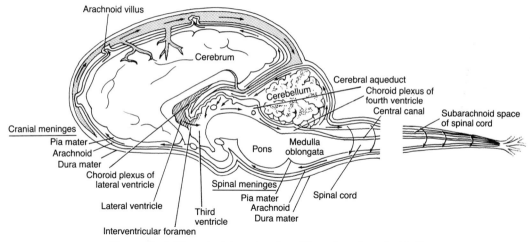

Figure 14–1. Sites of origin and routes of flow of cerebrospinal fluid.

up an osmotic and charge gradient causing water, chloride, and some other ions to flow passively into the ventricle.

Some CSF is secreted by the ependymal lining elsewhere in the ventricular system. Small amounts also diffuse into the ventricles from the perivascular spaces.

It is important to remember that because formation of CSF is an active, energy-dependent process, its formation is independent of either CSF pressure or blood pressure. Therefore, if CSF pressure or general intracranial pressure were to rise owing to an obstruction to flow or a space-occupying mass, for instance, CSF formation would continue.

Cerebrospinal Fluid Flows Down a Pressure Gradient Through a Predictable Anatomical Route

CSF flows, by bulk flow, down a pressure gradient from its site of formation at the choroid plexus through the ventricular system and subarachnoid space into the venous system (see Fig. 14–1). Fluid formed in the *lateral ventricles* passes into the *third ventricle* through the interventricular foramina (foramen of Monro). Here it mixes with fluid formed in the third ventricle. From the third ventricle it passes through the *cerebral aqueduct* (aqueduct of Sylvius) into the *fourth ventricle*. Fluid in the fourth ventricle passes into the *subarachnoid space* through foramina of Luschka and Magendie. Once in the subarachnoid space, some of the fluid passes down along the spinal cord; most passes up over the convexity of the brain, where it is absorbed into the venous system.

The pressure, cell count, and chemical con-stituents of CSF can be sampled by placing a styletted spinal needle into the subarachnoid space. Anatomically, the most convenient place to do this varies with species. In humans, it is usually done in the lumbar spinal column, because the human cauda equina is located near the first lumbar vertebra, and we have five lumbar vertebrae. This provides a relatively large subarachnoid space in the human midlumbar spinal column from which to sample. However, in most veterinary species, the cauda equina ends near the sixth or seventh lumbar vertebrae, leaving only a small subarachnoid space. Instead, most veterinary spinal taps are performed by sampling from the subarachnoid space between the skull and the first cervical vertebra in anesthetized animals. Here the subarachnoid space is called the *cisterna magna* (big cistern) and is much deeper than other portions of the subarachnoid space. Spinal taps provide valuable information about such neuropathology as intracranial space-occupying masses and inflammation.

Cerebrospinal Fluid Is Absorbed into the Venous System

CSF is absorbed into the venous system. Most of the fluid is absorbed through *arachnoid villi* (Fig. 14–2), which are small, finger-like projections of the arachnoid membrane through the walls of venous sinuses in the dura. How absorption occurs at the arachnoid villi is not clear. It appears to be pressure dependent, but whether fluid flows into the venous system through a membrane (a closed

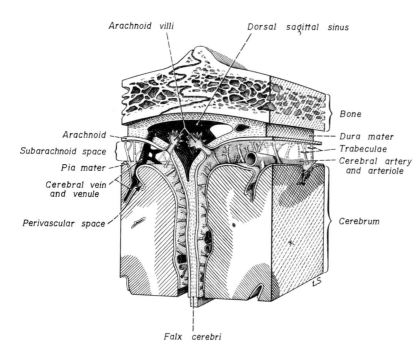

Arachnoid villi

Dorsal sagittal sinus

Bone

Arachnoid

Subarachnoid space

Pia mater

Cerebral vein and venule

Perivascular space

Dura mater

Trabeculae

Cerebral artery and arteriole

Cerebrum

Falx cerebri

Figure 14–2. Cerebrospinal fluid is absorbed into the venous system largely through arachnoid villi. (From De Lahunta A (ed): Veterinary Neuroanatomy and Clinical Neurology, 2nd ed. Philadelphia, WB Saunders, 1983.)

system), through tubules (an open system), or through vacuoles is still a subject of debate.

In normal animals, CSF pressure is regulated primarily by its absorption at the arachnoid villi, because formation is independent of pressure. CSF pressure would be slightly higher than venous pressure then, and obstruction of the venous return from the head causes CSF pressure to rise almost immediately. In some pathological states, such as with brain tumors or meningitis, CSF can increase dramatically.

Hydrocephalus Is an Increased Volume of Cerebrospinal Fluid in the Skull

Hydrocephalus is defined as an increased CSF volume in the skull, usually an increased ventricular volume. In theory, hydrocephalus could be caused by too much fluid production at the choroid plexus, obstruction to its flow, or impaired absorption at the arachnoid villi. In practice, overproduction seems rare whereas obstruction to flow seems more common, particularly at such vulnerable sites as the cerebral aqueduct and the exits from the fourth ventricle. Impaired absorption also occurs secondary to meningitis or hemorrhage, presumably by cellular debris obstructing the exit from the arachnoid villi. The pathogenesis of many cases of hydrocephalus is not known. A common form of treatment, at least in humans, is to surgically implant a tube that

shunts CSF into the atria of the heart or into the peritoneal cavity, thus relieving episodes of increased CSF pressure and preventing brain damage.

Permeability Barriers Exist Between Blood and Brain

Many dyes, once injected into the blood, stain other tissues of the body but not the brain. Capillaries in most tissues allow these dyes to escape into the interstitial space whereas capillaries of the brain do not. In most capillaries (Fig. 14–3) water-soluble compounds leave the capillaries through open clefts between capillary endothelial cells, and exchange is relatively unrestricted. However, in brain capillaries, passage through intercell clefts is blocked by tight junctions, and exchange of blood solutes is highly selective. Many substances, such as large proteins, toxins, and most drugs, are excluded from the brain, whereas others, such as glucose and many amino acids, penetrate easily by specific, carrier-mediated mechanisms. Cerebral capillaries have a greater number of mitochondria and are surrounded by a layer of glial astrocytic end-feet, although the importance of these end-feet to the blood-brain barrier is controversial.

The blood-brain barrier functions to carefully preserve a stable environment for the neurons and glia of the CNS. As Claude Ber-

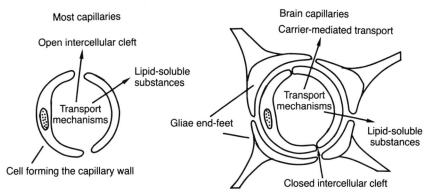

Figure 14–3. Blood-brain barrier. Unlike most capillaries of the body, cells of brain capillary walls are joined by tight junctions that prevent passage of material between the cells. All materials leaving brain capillaries must pass through the cells forming the capillary wall.

nard pointed out in the last century, homeostasis, or constancy of the internal environment, was a precondition for autonomous life. It is not surprising that the brain, the master choreographer of autonomous life, should have a special mechanism for protecting its internal environment from toxins and other outside dangers. Unfortunately for the veterinarian, often it also prevents many antibiotics and other drugs from reaching the brain, particularly drugs with low lipid solubility or drugs bound to plasma proteins.

The blood-brain barrier is apparently not effective in the hypothalamus. This is important, because the hypothalamus helps to control serum osmolality, glucose, and other critical blood parameters and needs to sense the levels of many serum solutes.

CLINICAL CORRELATION

INCREASED INTRACRANIAL PRESSURE

HISTORY ☐ You examine a 9-year-old female boxer. The owner states that recently the dog has seemed more drowsy than usual and had what you recognize to be a generalized tonic-clonic seizure the preceding night.

CLINICAL EXAMINATION ☐ Physical examination of the dog reveals a hard, nodular mass of the mammary gland. Other deficits are referable to the nervous system and are characterized by apparent drowsiness and confusion and by a conscious proprioception response deficit of the right front and right rear legs. Lateral radiographs of the chest reveal metastatic, neoplastic lesions in the lungs. The CSF pressure,

as measured with a manometer through a needle placed in the cisterna magna, is 310 mm CSF. (The normal CSF pressure in dogs is less than 180 mm CSF.)

COMMENT ☐ This is a typical case of a dog with a neoplasm of the mammary gland that has spread first to the lungs, which contain the first capillary bed filter encountered by tumor cells as they invade the venous system, and then to the brain. As the tumor mass increases within the fixed encasement of the cranial vault, cerebrospinal and other fluid volumes are displaced. Some loss of myelin may compensate temporarily for the expanding intracranial mass, but eventually the expanding tumor, encased in the skull, causes an increase in intracranial pressure, which is reflected in an increased CSF pressure in the cisterna magna. In measuring this pressure, the dog is anesthetized and a styletted spinal needle is placed in the cisterna magna. The stylette is removed, and a rigid glass or plastic tube (manometer) is attached by way of a right angle, three-way valve. CSF rises up the manometer to a height proportional to intracranial pressure. Its height is measured off the millimeter graduations marked on the tube.

The proprioception response deficits of the right front and right rear legs result from a focal, asymmetrical lesion of the left cerebral cortex. The seizure also resulted from this mass. With the mammary mass, the metastatic lesions in the lungs, asymmetrical neurological signs, seizures, and the elevated CSF pressure, it is reasonable to conclude that this dog has an intracranial neoplasm that probably spread from the mammary gland to the lungs and the brain.

TREATMENT □ Any treatment in this case would be futile.

Bibliography

Guyton AC: Textbook of Medical Physiology, 7th ed. Philadelphia, WB Saunders, 1986, pp 374–377.

Kandel ER, Schwartz JH (eds): Principles of Neural Science, 2nd ed. New York, Elsevier, 1985, pp 837–844.

Oliver JE, Hoerlein BF, Mayhew IG (eds): Veterinary Neurology. Philadelphia, WB Saunders, 1987, pp 195–197.

Smith LH, Thier SO (eds): Pathophysiology—The Biological Principles of Disease, 2nd ed. Philadelphia, WB Saunders, 1985, pp 1017–1029.

Willis WD, Grossman RG: Medical Neurobiology, Neuroanatomical and Neurophysiological Principles Basic to Clinical Neuroscience, 3rd ed. St Louis, CV Mosby, 1981, pp 227–229.

PRACTICE QUESTIONS FOR CHAPTER 14

1. A drug that would prevent the active transport of Na^+ ions out of cells would lead to

   a. an increased production of both CSF and aqueous humor.
   b. a decreased production of both CSF and aqueous humor.
   c. an increased production of CSF but a decreased production of aqueous humor.
   d. a decreased production of CSF but an increased production of aqueous humor.
   e. no change in the production of either CSF or aqueous humor.

2. You are performing a spinal tap on an anesthetized dog and measuring CSF pressure. While measuring the pressure, you occlude the jugular veins. What would you expect to happen to the CSF pressure?

   a. Pressure would increase
   b. Pressure would decrease
   c. No change in pressure would occur

3. Obstruction of the flow of CSF at the cerebral aqueduct (aqueduct of Sylvius) would lead to dilatation (enlargement) of the

   a. lateral ventricles.
   b. fourth ventricles.
   c. central canal of the spinal cord.
   d. subarachnoid space.
   e. cauda equina.

4. CSF is formed at the

   a. arachnoid villi.
   b. aqueduct of Sylvius.
   c. choroid plexus.
   d. subarachnoid space.

5. Many dyes injected into the venous system can penetrate most tissues of the body, but not the brain.

   a. True
   b. False

15

The Electroencephalogram and Sensory Evoked Potentials

1. All areas of the cerebral cortex share a common histology
2. The electroencephalogram has become a common clinical technique
3. The collective behavior of cortical neurons can be studied noninvasively by using macroelectrodes on the scalp
4. Stimulation of sensory tracts can be recorded as evoked potentials

When many excitable cells are present in a living tissue, their electrical behavior can be detected by macroelectrodes placed on the body at a distance from these cells. Several clinically important electrophysiological diagnostic procedures rely on this concept.

Underlying these procedures is a theory called *volume condition.* This theory describes the spread of ionic currents within the extracellular fluid from a group of nerve or muscle cells to more distant points in the body like the skin. These ionic currents can be measured from the skin. Their wave form is characteristic of the tissue from which they arise. The best known of these electrophysiological recordings is the electrocardiogram from heart muscle (Chapter 19). The electromyogram from

skeletal muscle (Chapter 5) and electroretinogram (Chapter 13) are other examples.

This chapter introduces two other clinical electrophysiological techniques: the *electroencephalogram* (EEG) and *sensory evoked potentials*, particularly *brainstem evoked responses* (BSER). But first, one must understand more about the histology and electrophysiology of the cerebral cortex.

All Areas of the Cerebral Cortex Share a Common Histology

Different regions of the cerebral cortex have different functions. For example, the motor cortex (Chapter 9) projects to the brainstem and spinal cord to initiate skilled, learned, conscious movement. The occipital cortex processes visual information received from the retina of the eye (see Chapter 13). The temporal cortex processes similar information from the ear (see Chapter 16). Yet, even though different cortical regions have different functions, their histology is basically the same. This suggests that cortical, synaptic processing of information is similar in all regions, and what makes differing regions different is the origin of their input signals and the destination of their output signals.

The cerebral cortex contains several different cell types, but most fall into two major classes: *pyramidal cells* and *stellate cells* (Fig. 15–1). These cells are arranged in six layers. The pyramidal cells, so called because their cell bodies are shaped like pyramids, have cell bodies located in deeper layers with their dendrites projecting up to the pial surface of the cortex, where they spread out within layer I. Pyramidal cell axons project to other parts of the central nervous system (CNS) and are the major output signal of the cerebral cortex. Pyramidal cells are generally excitatory at their axon's synapse. Stellate cells, so named because of their star-like appearance, are interneurons within the cortex and can be either excitatory or inhibitory. Sensory inputs arise from specific nuclei of the lateral thalamus and project to layer IV. Interneurons from other parts of the cortex project to layers I and II.

As with other regions of the brain, the cerebral cortex contains about ten times more *glial cells* than neurons. Three types of glia are present in the cortex: astrocytes, oligodendrocytes, and microglia. They do not develop action potentials and are not thought to play a role in signaling. They probably take up excess potassium ions, neurotransmitter, and toxins from the extracellular space. They may also help stabilize the position of the neurons; hence, the origin of the term glia or "glue."

The Electroencephalogram Has Become a Common Clinical Technique

It has been known since the 1930s that a fluctuating electrical voltage reflecting brain activity could be recorded from macroelec-

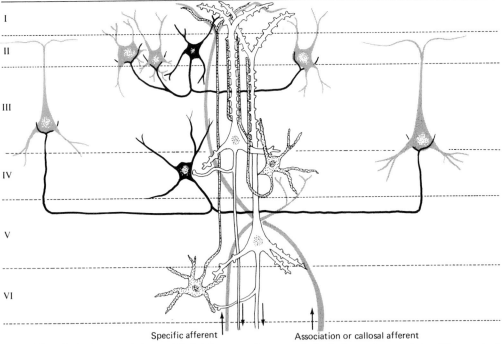

Specific afferent   Association or callosal afferent

Figure 15–1. The principal neuron types and their interconnections are similar in the various regions of the cerebral cortex. Note that the two large pyramidal cells (white) in layers III and V receive multiple synaptic contacts from the star-shaped interneuron (stellate cell, stippled) in layer IV. Basket cell (black) inhibition is directed to the somata of cortical neurons. Major input to the cortex derives from specific thalamic nuclei (specific afferents) and is directed mostly to layer IV; association and callosal input (association and callosal afferents) are in large part directed to more superficial layers. (Reprinted by permission of the publisher from Kandel ER, Schwartz JH: Principles of Neural Science, 2nd ed. Copyright 1985 by Elsevier Science Publishing Company, Inc.)

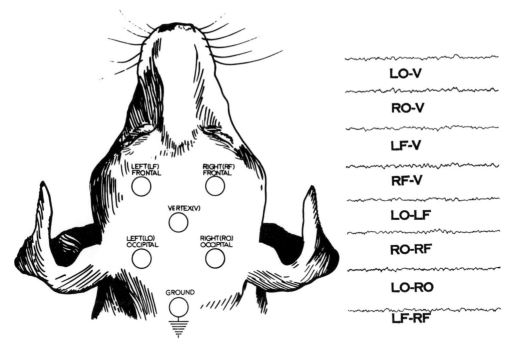

Figure 15–2. Points of electrode attachment for recording the EEG. Recordings obtained from a combination of the lead points are shown. (From Oliver JE, Hoerlein BF, Mayhew IG (eds): Veterinary Neurology. Philadelphia, WB Saunders, 1987.)

Illustration continued on following page

trodes on the scalp. Such a recording is known as an *electroencephalogram*. The frequency of the wave form recorded varies inversely with its amplitude. Both frequency and amplitude change with changes in levels of arousal (Fig. 15–2). An alert animal has a fairly high frequency, low amplitude EEG whereas a more relaxed animal has a slower frequency, higher amplitude EEG. A sleeping animal usually begins sleep exhibiting a slow wave, high amplitude EEG. Paradoxically, there are periods of high frequency, low amplitude EEG during the sleep cycle. Four frequency ranges have been given names: α (8–13 Hz), β (13–30 Hz), δ (0.5–4 Hz), and θ (4–7 Hz).

During the past four decades this technique has been applied clinically. Abnormal EEG activity has been associated empirically with several brain diseases. In human neurology, EEGs have commonly been used to classify the epilepsies, localize lesions, and more recently to help define brain death. EEGs have not been as widely used in veterinary medicine but still hold promise for veterinary neurology.

Where do these scalp recordings originate and what do they have to do with brain function?

The Collective Behavior of Cortical Neurons Can Be Studied Noninvasively by Using Macroelectrodes on the Scalp

The scalp EEG records a fluctuating voltage resulting from changes in postsynaptic potentials in thousands of neurons below the electrode. Each change in voltage has a polarity.

By convention, changes in voltage measured by extracellular electrodes such as those on the scalp have a standard direction of pen deflection. When the voltage change is in a positive direction, the deflection is down; when in a negative direction, the deflection is up (Fig. 15–3). The polarity of the voltage change at the scalp depends on the nature and location of the postsynaptic potential change. If an excitatory postsynaptic potential (EPSP) occurs in a deep cortical layer, positive ions (e.g., Na^+) enter the cell there while other positive ions exit the cell nearer to the pial surface (Fig. 15–3. For simplicity, only one cell is indicated.) This results in a positive voltage change at the scalp macroelectrode. If the EPSP occurs at the pial surface (Fig. 15–3), the voltage recorded from the scalp is negative. The polarity of these changes would be re-

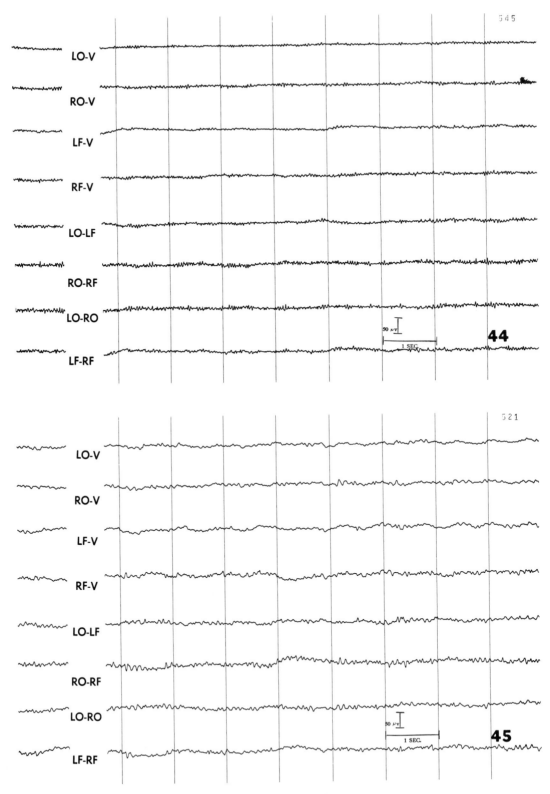

Figure 15–2 Continued

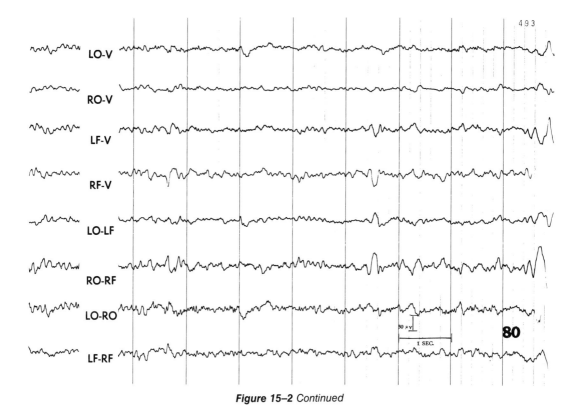

Figure 15–2 *Continued*

versed for inhibitory postsynaptic potentials (IPSPs).

Voltage changes recorded from the scalp are the result of the summated extracellular voltage changes due to the postsynaptic potentials of a large number of active cortical neurons, because the voltage change from any one neuron is too small to see. Action potentials contribute little to the EEG with scalp electrodes.

The amplitude (height) of voltage fluctuations in the scalp-recorded EEG is a function of how many cortical cells are changing their postsynaptic potentials in the same direction at the same time. Because a high amplitude voltage change would result from a large number of neurons firing synchronously, a high amplitude slow frequency EEG is said to be a *synchronized EEG*. When neurons are firing more or less at random, a low amplitude, high frequency EEG results. This EEG is said to be a *desynchronized EEG*.

The frequency with which EEG voltage changes occur is largely set by medial thalamic nuclei and the reticular activating system through their diffuse connections to the cerebral cortex.

The voltage changes recorded from the scalp

result from summated changes in the postsynaptic potentials of large numbers of cerebral cortical neurons. The amplitude and frequency of these changes are influenced by the medial thalamus and the brainstem reticular activating system. However, there are large areas of the brain and the spinal cord that are not reflected in the EEG. There are other clinical electrophysiological recordings that can help examine the function of these areas.

Stimulation of Sensory Tracts Can Be Recorded as Evoked Potentials

Synaptic activity in a sensory pathway can be recorded from the scalp by a technique using computerized averaging that averages out the more random background EEG activity and averages in the electrical response to multiple stimulations of a sensory system. Such signals are called *sensory evoked potentials*.

Because scalp macroelectrodes can more easily record the EEG electrical signals generated from the closer cerebral cortical cells, these higher voltage signals must be eliminated or they would mask the sensory evoked potentials. Because the background EEG sig-

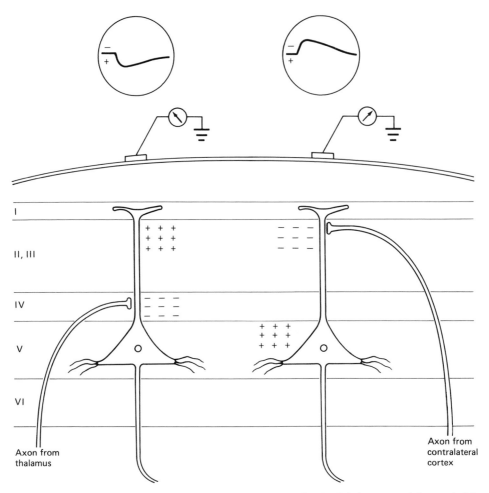

Figure 15–3. Scalp recordings and underlying synaptic mechanisms. On the left is a potential recorded from a scalp electrode following activation of thalamic inputs. The terminals of thalamocortical neurons make excitatory connections on cortical neurons predominantly in layer IV. Thus, the site of inward current flow (sink) is in the superficial cortical layers. Because the recording electrode is located on the scalp, it is closer to the site of outward current flow than inward current flow and, therefore, records a positive potential. By convention, and unlike intracellular recordings, a positive extracellularly recorded potential is a downward deflection. On the right is a potential recorded from an excitatory input from a callosal neuron in the contralateral cortex. The axons of callosal neurons terminate in the superficial cortical layers. A negative potential (upward deflection) is recorded because the electrode is closer to the site of inward current flow than that of the outward flow. (Reprinted by permission of the publisher from Kandel ER, Schwartz JH: Principles of Neural Science, 2nd ed. Copyright 1985 by Elsevier Science Publishing Company, Inc.)

nals are relatively random, a computer can average them together and functionally erase them from the recording. In addition, the computer averages sensory evoked potential signals time-locked to multiple stimulations of a sensory pathway. In this way, scalp macro-electrodes can be used to record electrical events generated in brain locations at a great distance from the recording electrode. For this reason, these sensory evoked potentials are often called *far field potentials.*

One such sensory evoked potential is the *brainstem auditory evoked potential* or BSAER. This clinical electrophysiological procedure re-cords the brainstem electrical events for 10 milliseconds (ms) following a click stimulus to the ear (Fig. 15–4). Usually seven waves are recorded, thought to be generated by brain-stem synaptic relay points in the auditory pathway. Recordings longer than 10 ms are sometimes taken. These later waves reflect cortical response to auditory stimulation. BSAER is being used in animals and humans to assess brainstem function in general and auditory function in particular.

Other sensory evoked potentials can be re-corded from the visual system, the somatosen-sory system, and other sensory modalities.

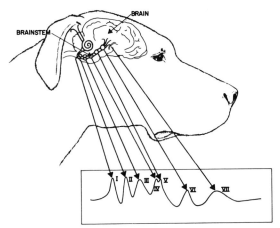

Figure 15–4. Brainstem auditory evoked response. Idealized diagram of wave forms recorded by signal averaging. Neural elements that are believed to sequentially generate the auditory waves: wave I—cochlea, spiral ganglia, and CN VIII; wave II—cochlear nuclei; wave III—nucleus of the trapezoid body; waves IV and V—lateral lemniscus and lemniscal nuclei and caudal colliculus, respectively (these two waves are frequently combined to form one wave); wave VI—medial geniculate body; wave VII—auditory radiations. Positive is upward. (From Oliver JE, Hoerlein BF, Mayhew IG (eds): Veterinary Neurology. Philadelphia, WB Saunders, 1987.)

CLINICAL CORRELATION

BRAIN TUMOR

HISTORY □ You examine a 13-year-old Boston terrier. The owner states that during the past 3 weeks the dog has had seizures of increasing frequency characterized by turning his head to the right, rigidity of the right front and right hind legs, collapsing to the ground, and urination. More recently, he has seemed weak, drowsy, and confused. He tends to walk in circles and seems weak on the right front leg.

CLINICAL EXAMINATION □ Important physical examination deficits are referable to the nervous system. The dog seems weak, drowsy, confused, and unsteady in his gait. He tends to walk in counter-clockwise circles to the left. His cranial and spinal segmental reflexes are within normal limits. His conscious proprioception response is abnormal in the right front leg and normal in the other three legs (see Chapter 6). His EEG reveals that over the left parietal cortex the dominant frequency is slower than over the rest of the brain, and the amplitude is higher. Occasional bursts of electrical spiking activity

can be seen also from the area of the left parietal cortex.

COMMENT □ This is an old dog, with a recent history of progressive, asymmetrical brain disease. This suggests a focal intracranial lesion, perhaps a brain tumor. A focal lesion is further confirmed by the EEG. Brain tumors within the cerebral hemispheres often cause focal slowing of the EEG frequency with increased amplitude. This is called a *slow wave focus*. The tumor itself is electrically silent, but its effect on the surrounding cerebral cortex is to cause slowing and the intermittent bursts of electrical spikes that are seizure activity within the cortex. Between seizures these spikes can still be seen with the EEG, but they do not spread widely enough within the cortex to cause a clinical seizure. During a clinical seizure, this abnormal electrical activity spreads more widely to incorporate normal brain, causing the various motor and other events of the seizure. Why such spikes only occasionally spread to incorporate more distant parts of the brain to cause seizures, and why seizures stop, is still unknown.

TREATMENT □ Many forms of seizure disorders can be managed successfully by removing the underlying cause, or the frequency of the seizures can be reduced with antiepileptic medication. In this dog's case, the cause is likely a brain tumor, for which there is no cure.

Bibliography

Berne RM, Levy MN (eds): Physiology, 2nd ed. St Louis, CV Mosby, 1988, pp 266–268.
Guyton AC: Textbook of Medical Physiology, 7th ed. Philadelphia, WB Saunders, 1986, pp 669–670.
Kandel ER, Schwartz JH (eds): Principles of Neural Science, 2nd ed. New York, Elsevier, 1985, pp 640–647.
Oliver JE, Hoerlein BF, Mayhew IG (eds): Veterinary Neurology. Philadelphia, WB Saunders, 1987, pp 111–144, 168–176.
Smith LH, Thier SO (eds): Pathophysiology—The Biological Principles of Disease, 2nd ed. Philadelphia, WB Saunders, 1985, pp 147–148.
Willis WD, Grossman RG: Medical Neurobiology, Neuroanatomical and Neurophysiological Principles Basic to Clinical Neuroscience, 3rd ed. St Louis, CV Mosby, 1981, pp 445–447.

PRACTICE QUESTIONS FOR CHAPTER 15

1. The EEG is the measurement from the scalp of predominantly what neural event?

a. Presynaptic inhibition in the cerebral cortex
b. Postsynaptic potentials in the cerebral cortex
c. Action potentials in the cerebral cortex
d. Flow of CSF in the lateral ventricles

2. A lesion in which of the following brain structures would have NO influence over the EEG?

a. Cerebral cortex
b. Medial thalamus
c. Internal capsule
d. Cerebellum
e. Reticular activating system

3. Which of the following statements is NOT true about the normal EEG?

a. The EEG should be similar in both cerebral hemispheres.
b. The EEG should be flat in a dead patient.
c. Sleep is often characterized by a slow frequency, high amplitude EEG.
d. The left cerebral cortex usually has a much slower frequency than the right cerebral cortex.

4. The brainstem auditory evoked potential requires the averaging out of the basic EEG before it can be recorded.

a. True
b. False

5. A brain tumor may cause focal slowing of the EEG from the brain tissue immediately surrounding the tumor.

a. True
b. False

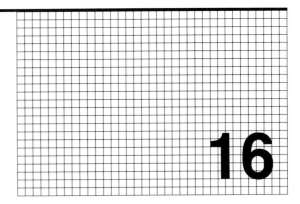

Hearing

1. Sound waves are alternating phases of condensation and rarefaction of molecules in the external environment
2. External and middle ears funnel sound waves to the cochlea
3. The cochlea is located in the inner ear
4. The cochlea transduces sound waves to action potentials in the eighth cranial nerve
5. Action potentials from the cochlea are transmitted up through the brainstem to the cerebral cortex
6. Deafness results from an interruption in the hearing process

Hearing is an important sensory modality. Many mammalian species have a particularly acute sense of hearing. Fortunately the auditory system is not often a site of pathology in veterinary medicine except for occasional congenital defects. Nevertheless, hearing is sufficiently important to warrant a brief discussion of its physiology.

Sound Waves Are Alternating Phases of Condensation and Rarefaction of Molecules in the External Environment

Sound waves are longitudinal vibrations of molecules in the external environment characterized by alternating phases of condensation and rarefaction. Sound is the sensation produced when these alternating changes in pressure strike the tympanic membrane. A plot of these changes in pressure on the tympanic membrane per unit time is a series of waves (Fig. 16–1). Such movements in the environment are usually called sound waves. Generally, the *loudness* of the sound is correlated with the *amplitude* of a sound wave; the

pitch is correlated with the *frequency* of the waves per unit time. The loudness of a sound is usually quantified using the *decibel scale*, which expresses the intensity of the sound as compared to the intensity of a standard sound.

External and Middle Ears Funnel Sound Waves to the Cochlea

The external ear and canal funnel sound waves to the *tympanic membrane (eardrum)* (Fig. 16–2). The eardrum is a membrane between the external and middle ears. The middle ear is an airfilled cavity in the temporal bone and is connected to the nasopharynx by the auditory (eustachian) tube. Three *auditory bones* (ossicles)—the malleus, incus, and stapes—are connected to each other and are located in the middle ear. They transfer vibrations of the eardrum to the oval window, a membranous separation between the middle and inner ears. Two small skeletal muscles are located in the middle ear also. Their contraction alters the transfer of vibration between the eardrum and the oval window.

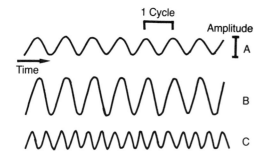

Figure 16–1. Characteristics of sound waves. *A* is the record of a pure tone. *B* has a greater amplitude and is louder than *A*. *C* has the same amplitude as *A* but a greater frequency, and its pitch is higher.

The Cochlea Is Located in the Inner Ear

The inner ear (labyrinth) contains two receptor systems: the vestibular system, which detects the position of the head, and the *cochlea*, a receptor for hearing. The inner ear consists of the *bony labyrinth* and, within the bony labyrinth, the *membranous labyrinth*. The bony labyrinth is a series of tunnels within the petrous temporal bone. Inside these tunnels, surrounded by a fluid called *perilymph*, is the membranous labyrinth. The membranous labyrinth follows the contour of the bony labyrinth and contains *endolymph*. This "tunnel within a tunnel" design continues within both the vestibular and cochlear systems.

The cochlear portion of the labyrinth is a coiled tube. Two membranes, the basilar and Reissner's, divide it into three chambers *(scalae)* throughout its length (Fig. 16–3). The upper and lower scalae contain perilymph and connect with each other at the distal end. The middle scala, the scala media, contains endolymph. Along the floor of the scala media, on the basilar membrane, lies the hair cell receptor system called the *organ of Corti*, which transduces sound waves into action potentials. The organ of Corti contains thousands of

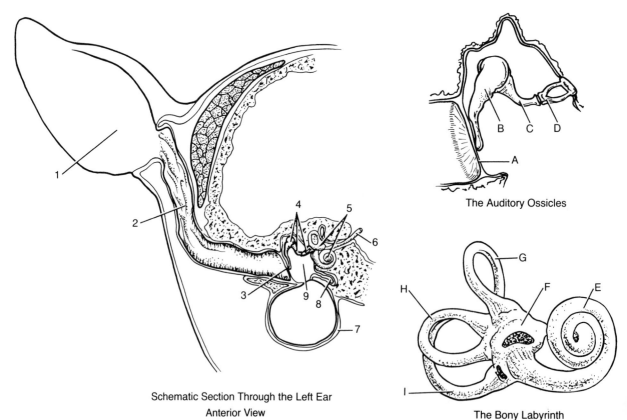

Schematic Section Through the Left Ear
Anterior View

The Auditory Ossicles

The Bony Labyrinth

Figure 16–2. Schematic sections through the left ear; the auditory ossicles; the bony labyrinth. (Reprinted with permission from *Atlas for Applied Veterinary Anatomy*, 2nd edition, by Robert Getty © 1964 by Iowa State University Press, Ames, Iowa 50010.)

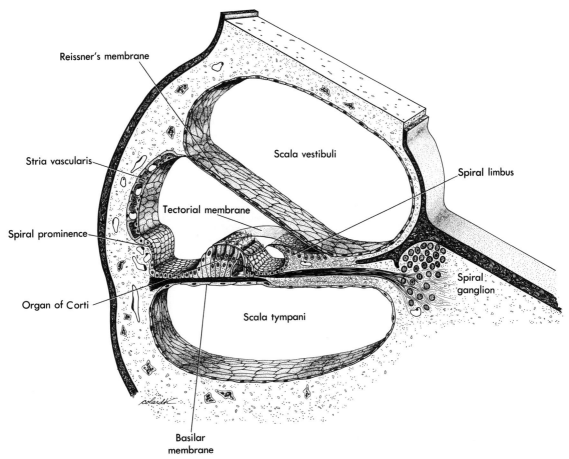

Figure 16–3. Schematic representation of a section through one of the turns of the cochlea. (With permission from Bloom W, Fawcett DW: A Textbook of Histology, 10th ed. Philadelphia, WB Saunders, 1975.)

hair cell receptors that respond to sound waves and give rise to action potentials in the sensory afferent nerves, which carry action potentials along the eighth cranial nerve to the brainstem's cochlear nucleus.

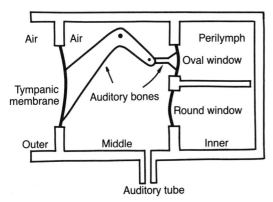

Figure 16–4. Diagrammatic representation of the transmission of vibrations from the outer to the inner ear. (Redrawn from Lippold OCJ, Winton FR: Human Physiology, 6th ed. New York, Churchill Livingstone, 1972.)

The Cochlea Transduces Sound Waves to Action Potentials in the Eighth Cranial Nerve

Sound waves in the external environment cause vibrations of the tympanic membrane. These vibrations are transmitted through the middle ear by the auditory bones and result in similar vibrations of the oval window. This sets up a series of traveling waves in the perilymph of the scala vestibuli that, in turn, cause vibrations in the basilar membrane. A diagrammatic representation of this transmission is found in Figure 16–4. The organ of Corti hair cells along the basilar membrane respond to these traveling waves by generating action potentials along the eighth cranial nerve. Hair cells at differing locations along the basilar membrane are thought to respond to different frequencies of traveling waves (pitch). Loudness is transduced as the intensity with which a given site on the basilar membrane is stimulated.

Action Potentials from the Cochlea Are Transmitted Up Through the Brainstem to the Cerebral Cortex

Action potentials arising in the cochlea travel along the eighth cranial nerve to the cochlear nuclei in the medulla oblongata. From here, action potentials are transmitted to the ipsilateral and contralateral cerebral cortices by way of various brainstem routings including the inferior colliculus and the medial geniculate body. Conscious perception of sound and the perception of its location of origin occur in the cerebral cortex.

Deafness Results from an Interruption in the Hearing Process

Clinical *deafness* may result from a loss of sound transmission in the external or middle ear, called *conduction deafness*, or from malfunction of the cochlear hair cells or nerve pathways, called *nerve deafness*. In veterinary medicine, deafness in young animals is usually caused by a congenital defect in the cochlea, frequently linked with white coat color.

CLINICAL CORRELATION

CONGENITAL DEAFNESS

HISTORY ☐ An almost completely white, male Dalmatian pup is brought to you, the owner complaining that the pup does not appear to hear anything.

CLINICAL EXAMINATION ☐ Your physical examination reveals an apparently normal, healthy Dalmatian pup except for an apparent deafness. He does not seem to respond to voice commands or loud noises. His vestibular and all other neurological reflexes are within normal limits. A brainstem auditory evoked response was flat, suggesting the brain had not received any signal from the cochlea.

COMMENT ☐ Congenital deafness is fairly common in dogs and other animals with white coat color. It is usually caused by the partial or complete absence of the cochlea and occasionally absence of other neural elements of the auditory pathway. This is known as nerve deafness and is usually present at birth (congenital). Why it is linked to white coat color is unknown, but the pattern suggests that it is a genetically determined failure of the cochlea to develop, usually on both sides bilaterally.

Bibliography

Berne RM, Levy MN (eds): Physiology, 2nd ed. St Louis, CV Mosby, 1988, pp 158–178.

Guyton AC: Textbook of Medical Physiology, 7th ed. Philadelphia, WB Saunders, 1986, pp 734–744.

Kandel ER, Schwartz JH (eds): Principles of Neural Science, 2nd ed. New York, Elsevier, 1985, pp 396–408.

Lance JW, McLeod JG: A Physiological Approach to Clinical Neurology, 3rd ed. London, Butterworths, 1981, pp 242–246.

Oliver JE, Hoerlein BF, Mayhew IG (eds): Veterinary Neurology. Philadelphia, WB Saunders, 1987, pp 198–199.

Smith LH, Thier SO (eds): Pathophysiology—The Biological Principles of Disease, 2nd ed. Philadelphia, WB Saunders, 1985, pp 1113–1116.

Willis WD, Grossman RG: Medical Neurobiology, Neuroanatomical and Neurophysiological Principles Basic to Clinical Neuroscience, 3rd ed. St Louis, CV Mosby, 1981, pp 314–323.

PRACTICE QUESTIONS FOR CHAPTER 16

1. Which of the following cranial nerves transmits sound to the brain?

    a. Cranial nerve II
    b. Cranial nerve VII
    c. Cranial nerve VIII
    d. Cranial nerve X

2. A fusion of the auditory bones of the middle ear would likely have what effect on hearing?

    a. Improve hearing
    b. Reduce hearing
    c. Have no effect on hearing

3. If the hair cell receptors were missing from the cochlea, what would the animal experience?

    a. Paralysis
    b. Deafness
    c. Blindness
    d. Anesthesia (lack of all sensation)

4. When the frequency of sound waves increases, this is perceived as

    a. increased pitch.
    b. decreased pitch.
    c. increased loudness.
    d. decreased loudness.

ROBERT B. STEPHENSON

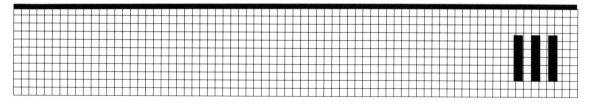

CARDIOVASCULAR PHYSIOLOGY

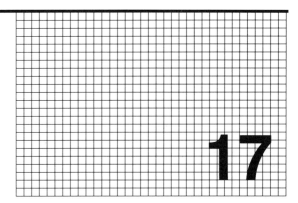

Overview of Cardiovascular Function

1. Knowledge of normal cardiovascular function is the basis for understanding and treating cardiovascular dysfunction
2. Bulk flow and diffusion are the two modes of transport used by the cardiovascular system
3. Diffusion is rapid only over short distances, so every metabolizing cell in the body must be close to a capillary carrying blood by bulk flow
4. The pulmonary and systemic circulations are arranged in series, but the various organs within the systemic circulation are arranged in parallel
5. Cardiac output is the volume of blood pumped each minute by the left ventricle
6. The perfusion pressure for the systemic circulation is much greater than the perfusion pressure for the pulmonary circulation
7. Each type of blood vessel has physical properties suited to its particular function
8. Blood is a suspension of cells in liquid

Knowledge of Normal Cardiovascular Function Is the Basis for Understanding and Treating Cardiovascular Dysfunction

Cardiovascular physiology is the study of the function of the heart and the blood vessels. It was not until 1628 that William Harvey, the father of cardiovascular physiology, set forth the proof that the heart propels blood through the blood vessels in a circulatory pattern. Before that time it was thought that blood flowed out of the heart into the blood vessels and then returned to the heart by backward flow in a tidal fashion, in much the same way that air flows first into the lungs and then back out. Today we take for granted the fact that

the cardiovascular system is a *circulatory system*, not a tidal system. However, William Harvey was so impressed by the complexity of blood flow that he thought initially the motions of the heart and the blood could be comprehended only by God. Generations of veterinary students since Harvey's time have tended to agree with his assessment. The goal in the following pages is to identify the most basic and important principles of normal cardiovascular function and to explain them in a way that best prepares the student to diagnose and treat *cardiovascular dysfunction* (cardiovascular disease).

Cardiovascular dysfunction is encountered often in veterinary practice. Cardiovascular diseases are frequently life-threatening. Therefore, a thorough knowledge of cardiovascular function and dysfunction is vital to the practicing clinician. Some cardiovascular diseases are *primary*, in that the basic disease process affects the cardiovascular system directly. An example of primary cardiovascular dysfunction is hemorrhage, which is obviously life-threatening. Primary cardiovascular disease can be either *congenital* (present at birth) or *acquired* (developed after birth). Myocarditis is an acquired condition in which a viral or bacterial infection inflames and weakens the heart tissue. Congenital heart defects are common in certain breeds of dogs and horses. Although the heart with a congenital defect or with myocarditis may pump an adequate amount of blood when the animal is at rest, it usually cannot deliver the increased blood flow required by the tissues during exercise. The patient exhibits exercise intolerance.

Parasites are another common cause of acquired cardiovascular dysfunction. Heartworms in dogs lodge in the right ventricle and pulmonary artery, where they impede the flow of blood. Blood worms *(Strongylus vulgaris)* in horses lodge in the mesenteric arteries and decrease the blood flow to the intestine. Intestinal motility, secretion, and absorption become depressed, and the horse exhibits signs of gastrointestinal (GI) distress *(colic)*. The condition of inadequate blood flow to any tissue is called *ischemia*. Persistent ischemia leads to permanent tissue damage *(infarction)*.

In many other disease states, although the cardiovascular system is not the primary target of the disease, secondary cardiovascular complications become the most serious and life-threatening aspect. Examples of secondary cardiovascular dysfunctions include the loss of water and electrolytes from the blood stream as a result of persistent diarrhea, vomiting, or burns. Even if blood volume is not depleted to dangerously low levels in these conditions, the concentrations of electrolytes (e.g., K^+ and Ca^{2+}) in the blood often become so abnormal that cardiac arrhythmias result. The abnormalities of body fluid composition can be made worse if incorrect fluid therapy is given. Incorrect fluid therapy can lead also to an accumulation of excess fluid in the tissues of the body, which is called *edema*. If the excess fluid gathers in the lung tissue, the condition is called *pulmonary edema*. Pulmonary edema occurs also in shock-lung syndrome, in which the permeability of lung blood vessels increases. Water, electrolytes, and plasma proteins leave the blood stream and accumulate in the lung tissue and airways. This pulmonary edema impairs the normal exchange of oxygen and carbon dioxide between the blood stream and the airway and can lead to death.

Shock-lung syndrome primarily affects the pulmonary circulation, but other kinds of shock depress the cardiovascular system generally. *Hemorrhagic shock* is a cardiovascular collapse caused by severe blood loss. *Cardiogenic shock* is caused by failure of the heart to pump an adequate amount of blood. *Septic shock* is caused by bacterial infections in the blood stream *(bacteremia)*. *Endotoxic shock* occurs when endotoxins (bacterial wall fragments) enter the blood stream. This often happens when the intestinal mucosa becomes damaged. For example, bacterial enteritis causes the intestinal epithelium to break down, and endotoxins from the intestine enter the blood stream. These endotoxins cause the body to produce substances that depress the heart. Cardiac output and blood pressure decrease. Renal failure, respiratory failure, severe depression, and death follow.

Anesthetic overdose is another common clinical problem in which the most serious and life-threatening symptoms are the secondary cardiovascular complications. Most anesthetics depress the central nervous system (CNS), and the resulting abnormalities in the neural signals to the heart and the blood vessels can depress cardiac output and lower blood pressure. Some anesthetics, the barbiturates in particular, also depress the pumping ability of the heart directly. There are many other examples of primary and secondary cardiovascular dysfunction, but the ones mentioned here illustrate the importance of cardiovascular dysfunction in veterinary medicine.

The remainder of this chapter mentions the general features of the cardiovascular system. Each element of the cardiovascular system is considered in detail in subsequent chapters. Finally, function and dysfunction of the cardiovascular system are summarized by describing the overall effects of heart failure, hemorrhage, and exercise.

Bulk Flow and Diffusion Are the Two Modes of Transport Used by the Cardiovascular System

The primary function of the cardiovascular system can be summarized in one word—*transport*. Cardiovascular transport is essential. If the heart stops and circulation ceases, unconsciousness results within about 30 seconds and irreversible damage to the brain and other sensitive body tissues occurs within a few minutes. The blood transports the metabolic substrates needed by every cell of the body, including oxygen, glucose, amino acids, fatty acids, and various lipids. The blood also carries metabolic waste products away from each cell of the body and delivers them to the lung, kidney, or liver, where they are eliminated. These waste products include carbon dioxide, lactic acid, the nitrogenous wastes of protein metabolism, and heat. Although heat is not a material waste product, its transport by the cardiovascular system to the body surface is essential, because tissues deep within the body would otherwise become overheated during rapid metabolism.

The cardiovascular system also transports hormones, which are blood-borne messengers released by an organ and carried to distant organs, where they alter organ function. For example, insulin is released by cells of the pancreas and carried by the blood to all cells of the body, where it promotes the uptake of glucose. Adrenalin (a mixture of epinephrine and norepinephrine) is released into the blood stream by the adrenal medulla during periods of stress. The epinephrine and norepinephrine circulate to various body organs, where they have effects that prepare a threatened animal for fight or flight. These effects include an increase in heart rate and cardiac contractility, a dilation of skeletal muscle blood vessels, an increase in blood pressure, and increased glycogenolysis.

Finally, the blood transports water and electrolytes, including sodium, potassium, calcium, hydrogen, bicarbonate, and chloride. The kidneys are the organs primarily responsible for maintaining normal water and electrolyte composition in the body. The kidneys accomplish this by altering the electrolyte concentrations in blood as it flows through the kidneys. The altered blood then circulates to all other organs in the body, where it affects the water and electrolyte content in the intracellular and extracellular fluids of each tissue.

Two modes of transport are used in the cardiovascular system. The first of these is *bulk flow*, which is the movement of fluid through tubes (in this case the movement of blood through blood vessels). The primary advantage of bulk flow is that it is rapid over long distances. For example, blood pumped into the aorta reaches all parts of the body within 2–3 seconds. Transport requires energy, and

the source of energy for bulk flow is a hydrostatic pressure difference. Unless the pressure at one end of a blood vessel is less than the pressure at the other end, flow will not occur. The difference in pressure between two points in the circulation is called the *perfusion pressure*. Perfusion means "flow through." Perfusion pressure, which causes blood to flow through a blood vessel, should be distinguished carefully from *transmural pressure*, which refers to the hydrostatic pressure difference between the blood within a blood vessel and the interstitial fluid outside the blood vessel. To summarize, perfusion pressure is the pressure difference *along the length* of a blood vessel; it is the driving force for bulk flow of blood. Transmural pressure is the pressure difference *across the wall* of a blood vessel. Transmural pressure is also called *distending pressure*, because it is the pressure difference that pushes out on the wall of a blood vessel.

Diffusion is the second mode of transport in the cardiovascular system. Diffusion is the primary mechanism by which substances move from the blood stream into the interstitial fluid or vice versa. *Interstitial fluid* is the extracellular fluid that bathes each cell of a tissue. The source of energy for diffusion is a concentration difference. A substance diffuses from the blood stream, across the wall of a capillary, and into the interstitial fluid only if the concentration of the substance is higher in the blood than in the interstitial fluid. If the concentration of a substance is higher in the interstitial fluid than in the blood, and if the capillary wall is permeable to the substance, then the substance diffuses from the interstitial fluid into the capillary blood. It is important to distinguish diffusion, in which a substance moves passively from an area of high concentration toward an area of low concentration, from active transport, in which substances are forced to move in a direction opposite to their concentration gradient. In general, substances are not transported actively across the walls of capillaries.

Diffusion Is Rapid Only Over Short Distances, So Every Metabolizing Cell in the Body Must Be Close to a Capillary Carrying Blood by Bulk Flow

An example illustrates how the two types of transport (bulk flow and diffusion) are used in the cardiovascular system. Consider the transport of oxygen from the lung to a neuron in the brain. With each inspiration, fresh air containing oxygen moves by bulk flow through the trachea, bronchi, and bronchioles into the alveolar air sacs (Fig. 17–1). The wall of each *alveolus* is covered with a meshwork of capillaries, which carry bulk flow of blood. These capillaries bring blood close (within 0.2 μm) to the air in the alveoli (1 micron = 1 μm = 0.001 mm). The blood that returns from the body tissues to the lungs has a lower oxygen concentration than the alveolar air, so oxygen diffuses rapidly from the alveoli into the blood stream. A large dog has about 300 million alveoli, and the alveoli have a huge total surface area (about 130 sq m). The large surface available for diffusion and the short distance between the alveolar air and the capillary blood both promote rapid diffusion. In the blood, about 1% of the oxygen is carried in solution, but most of it is bound to the protein *hemoglobin* in the red blood cells. Each 100 mL

of normal blood can carry 20 mL of oxygen bound to hemoglobin. The oxygen is carried then by the bulk flow of the blood from the lungs to the heart. The heart pumps this oxygenated blood out into the arteries, which deliver it to all parts of the body, including the brain. Capillaries in the brain bring the oxygenated blood close to the brain neurons, which need the oxygen in order to carry on their metabolism. Metabolism depletes the oxygen within the neurons, so the oxygen concentration inside neurons is low. Therefore, a concentration gradient exists for the diffusion of oxygen from the capillary blood to the interstitial fluid and from the interstitial fluid into the *intracellular fluid* of the neurons. The process of diffusion occurs within a few seconds if the capillary is close to the neuron.

Diffusion is rapid, but only over short distances. Each brain neuron must be within 100 μm of a capillary carrying bulk flow of blood if diffusion is to deliver oxygen rapidly enough to sustain normal metabolism in the neuron. Diffusional exchange over distances up to 100 μm typically takes only 1–5 seconds. If the distance involved were a few millimeters, diffusion would take minutes to occur. For oxygen to diffuse a few centimeters through body fluid would take hours. Therefore, normal life processes require that every metabolizing cell of the body be within about 100 μm of a capillary carrying bulk flow. If this condition is interrupted by a blood clot (*thrombus*) in an artery that delivers bulk flow to a particular region of a tissue, then the blood flow in that region decreases, a condition called *ischemia.* Severe ischemia leads to tissue damage and eventually to tissue death, which is called *necrosis.* An area of tissue damage or death caused by interruption of normal blood flow is called an *infarct*. A cerebral infarct causes the condition commonly known as *stroke*. An infarct in the heart muscle is called a *myocardial infarct* (MI) or heart attack. Even though an area of ischemic heart muscle may be within a few millimeters of the left ventricular chamber, which is filled with oxygen-rich blood, oxygen cannot diffuse rapidly enough from the ventricular chamber to the ischemic region to sustain normal metabolism in the ischemic cardiac muscle. Only by reopening the thrombosed coronary artery can normal function be restored and an infarct avoided.

Cerebral vascular disease and coronary vascular disease are common in human medicine. Vascular disease is encountered less frequently in veterinary medicine. By contrast, cardiac

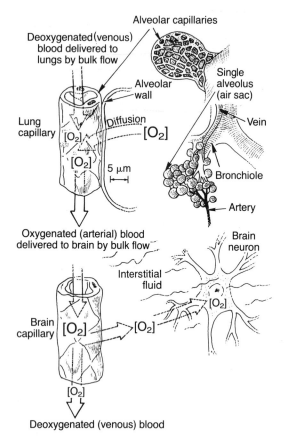

Figure 17–1. Oxygen is transported from the alveolar air sacs of the lungs (upper right) to all the tissues of the body by a combination of bulk flow and diffusion. Bulk flow is rapid; it can transport oxygen to all parts of the body within a few seconds. Diffusion can transport oxygen efficiently only over distances less than 100 μm.

disease (dysfunction of the heart muscle or valves, as distinguished from coronary vascular disease) is more common in veterinary medicine than in human medicine. Therefore, in the following chapters, cardiac physiology is emphasized more than vascular physiology. First, however, the general layout of the circulation is considered, and particular attention is paid to the hydrostatic pressure differences that drive bulk flow of blood through the circulation.

The Pulmonary and Systemic Circulations Are Arranged in Series, but the Various Organs Within the Systemic Circulation Are Arranged in Parallel

As shown in Figure 17–2, blood is pumped from the left ventricle into the aorta. The aorta divides and subdivides to form many arteries that deliver fresh, oxygenated blood to each organ of the body, except the lungs. The pattern of arterial branching that delivers blood of the same composition to each organ is called a *parallel* arrangement of blood vessels. After blood passes through the capillaries within individual organs, it enters veins. Small veins combine to form larger and larger veins, until the entire blood flow is delivered to the right atrium by way of the vena cava. The blood vessels between the aorta and the vena cava (including the blood vessels in all organs of the body except for the lungs) are collectively called the *systemic circulation*. Blood passes from the right atrium into the right ventricle, which pumps it into the pulmonary artery. The pulmonary artery branches into smaller and smaller arteries, which deliver blood to each lung capillary. Blood from lung capillaries is collected in pulmonary veins and brought to the left atrium. Blood then passes back into the left ventricle. The blood vessels of the lungs constitute the *pulmonary circulation*. The pulmonary circulation and the heart are collectively termed the *central circulation*. Note that the pulmonary circulation and the systemic circulation are arranged in *series;* that is, blood must pass through the pulmonary vessels between each passage through the systemic circuit.

In one pass through the systemic circulation, blood generally encounters only one capillary bed before being collected in veins and returned to the heart. There are three exceptions to this rule. The first is in the *splanchnic circulation* (blood supply of the digestive organs).

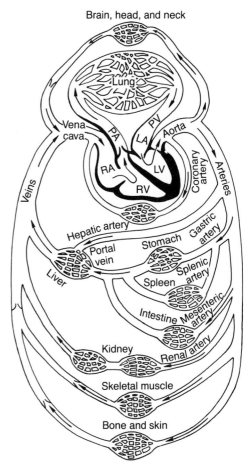

Figure 17–2. General layout of the cardiovascular system, showing that the systemic and pulmonary circulations are arranged in series and that the organs within the systemic circulation are arranged in parallel. *RA*, right atrium; *RV*, right ventricle; *LA*, left atrium; *LV*, left ventricle. (Adapted from Milnor WR: Cardiovascular Physiology. New York, Oxford University Press, 1990.)

As shown in Figure 17–2, blood that leaves the splenic, gastric, or mesenteric capillaries enters the *portal vein*. The portal vein carries splanchnic venous blood to the liver, where the blood passes through another set of capillaries before its return to the heart. This arrangement of two systemic capillary beds in series is called a *portal system*. The portal system in the splanchnic circulation allows nutrients that have been absorbed from the GI tract to be delivered directly to the liver. There the nutrients are transformed for storage or allowed to pass into the general circulation.

The kidneys contain the second example of a portal system (where blood traverses two capillary beds in series). As shown in Figure 17–2, blood entering a kidney passes first through the glomerular capillaries and then through the tubular capillaries. The kidneys utilize this portal system to adjust the amounts of water, electrolytes, and other solutes in the blood. The third portal system is found in the brain and is important in the control of hormone secretion by the pituitary gland. After traversing capillaries in the hypothalamus, blood enters portal vessels that carry it to the anterior pituitary gland (adenohypophysis) and to another set of capillaries. Substances that control the release of pituitary hormones are added to the blood as it traverses hypothalamic capillaries. When this blood reaches capillaries in the pituitary gland, these substances diffuse out of the blood stream and into the pituitary interstitial fluid, where they act to increase or decrease the secretion of specific hormones by pituitary cells. To summarize, the splanchnic, renal, and hypothamo-hypophyseal portal systems are the only major exceptions to the rule that blood encounters only one capillary bed in a single pass through the systemic circulation.

Cardiac Output Is the Volume of Blood Pumped Each Minute by the Left Ventricle

Typically, in a resting dog, about 1 minute is needed for blood to traverse the entire circulation (from the left ventricle back to the left ventricle). Because the pulmonary and systemic circulations are in parallel, the volume of blood pumped by the right heart each minute must equal the volume of blood pumped by the left heart each minute. The term *cardiac output* is used to refer to the volume of blood pumped per minute by either the left ventricle or the right ventricle. Among the common mammalian species encountered in veterinary medicine, cardiac output at rest is approximately 3 L/minute/m² of body surface area. Thus, in a large dog, cardiac output at rest is typically 2.5 L/minute. Note that the left and right ventricles together pump 5.0 L of blood/minute. In an animal at rest, blood entering the aorta is divided so that approximately 20% of it flows through the splanchnic circulation and 20% to the kidneys. Another 20% goes to the skeletal muscles. The brain receives about 15% of the cardiac output, and the coronary arteries carry about 3% of the cardiac output. The remainder goes to skin and bone.

The Perfusion Pressure for the Systemic Circulation Is Much Greater Than the Perfusion Pressure for the Pulmonary Circulation

When the left ventricle contracts and ejects blood into the aorta, the aortic pressure rises to a peak value called *systolic pressure* (typically 120 mmHg). Between ejections, blood continues to flow out of the aorta into the downstream arteries. This outflow causes aortic pressure to decrease. The minimum value of aortic pressure, just before the next ejection, is called *diastolic pressure* (typically 80 mmHg). The *mean* (average) value of the pulsatile pressure in the aorta is about 98 mmHg. The mean aortic pressure represents a potential energy for driving blood through the systemic circulation. As blood flows through the systemic circulation, this pressure energy is dissipated. The potential energy (blood pressure) remaining by the time the blood reaches the vena cava is only 3 mmHg. Therefore, the perfusion pressure for the systemic circuit is 98 mmHg minus 3 mmHg, or 95 mmHg.

The pressure in the pulmonary artery is typically 20 mmHg systolic and 8 mmHg diastolic, with a mean value of 13 mmHg. Pulmonary venous pressure is typically 5 mmHg, so the perfusion pressure for blood flow through the lungs is 8 mmHg (i.e., 13 mmHg–5 mmHg). Note that the perfusion pressure for the systemic circuit is much greater than the perfusion pressure for the lungs. Yet, the same volume of blood flows each minute through the systemic circulation and through the lungs. It takes a smaller perfusion pressure to push the cardiac output through the lungs than through the systemic circulation, because the resistance to blood flow is much lower in the pulmonary vessels than in the systemic vessels. Therefore, the systemic circulation is referred to as the high pressure, high resistance side of the circulation, and the pulmonary circuit is called the low pressure, low resistance side.

By convention, the hydrostatic pressures just mentioned are measured with reference to atmospheric pressure. That is, an arterial pressure of 98 mmHg means that the blood pressure is 98 mmHg higher than atmospheric pressure. Also, by convention, blood pressure is measured with reference to heart level. Pressure can be measured in an artery or vein at a level different from heart level, as long as a correction is made to account for the effect of gravity on the blood. Gravity increases the actual distending pressure in vessels lying below heart level and decreases the actual pressure in vessels above heart level.

Each Type of Blood Vessel Has Physical Properties Suited to Its Particular Function

In a resting animal, about 25% of the blood volume is in the central circulation and about 75% is in the systemic circulation (Table 17–1). Most of the blood in the systemic circulation is found in the veins. Only a small fraction is found in the arteries, arterioles, and capillaries. Therefore, the veins are known as the *blood reservoirs* of the circulation. The arteries are the *high pressure conduits* for delivery of blood to the capillaries. The arterioles are the *gates* of the systemic circulation; they constrict or dilate to control the blood flow to each capillary bed. Although only a small fraction of the systemic blood is found in capillaries, it is within these vessels that the important diffusional exchange takes place between the blood stream and the interstitial fluid.

Table 17–2 presents information about the size and number of the various types of vessels in the systemic circulation. As the aorta branches into smaller and smaller vessels, the diameter of the vessels becomes smaller, but the number of vessels increases. One aorta supplies blood to 45,000 terminal arteries, each of which gives rise to over 400 arterioles. Each arteriole typically branches into about 80 capillaries. The capillaries are so small in diameter that red blood cells have to deform to squeeze through them, and the red cells must pass through in single file. However, there are so many capillaries that the total cross-sectional area of the capillaries is much greater than the cross-sectional area of the preceding arteries and arterioles. Because capillary blood flow is spread out over such a large cross-sectional area, the flow velocity is low. Blood moves rapidly (about 13 cm/second) through the aorta. At this speed, blood is delivered from the heart to all parts of the body in less than 10 seconds. In each tissue, the velocity of blood flow decreases as the blood leaves arteries and enters arterioles and capillaries. The slow velocity of blood flow in capillaries causes blood to spend 1–5 seconds within a capillary, which allows time for diffusional exchange to take place between the capillary blood and the interstitial fluid. Blood from the capillaries is collected by venules and veins and is carried rapidly back to the heart. Figure 17–3 graphs the relationship between the total cross-sectional area and the velocity of flow within several types of vessels. This figure emphasizes the rapidity of bulk flow through large vessels and the relatively slow flow through the capillaries. Note that it is the *velocity* of blood flow that is lower in the capillaries. The same *volume* of blood flows each minute through an artery, the capillaries that it feeds, and the veins draining the capillaries.

In addition to having a large cross-sectional area and slow velocity of blood flow, capillaries have a large surface area. The total surface area of the wall of the aorta, for example, is about 200 cm^2, but the total surface area of the walls of all the capillaries is about 200,000 cm^2. This large surface area is important in promoting diffusional exchange.

Blood Is a Suspension of Cells in Liquid

As shown in Figure 17–4, blood can be separated into its cellular and liquid components by centrifugation. The liquid phase of blood is lighter than the cells and therefore ends up on the top of the centrifuge tube. The acellular or extracellular liquid in blood is called *plasma*. Water constitutes 93% of the plasma volume. Plasma also contains ions (*electrolytes*) in solution, mainly Na^+, K^+, Ca^{2+}, Mg^{2+}, Cl^-, HCO_3^-, HPO_4^{--} and SO_4^{--}. About 5–7% of the plasma volume is made up of protein molecules. Globulin, albumin, and fibrinogen are the primary *plasma proteins*. Globulin and albumin are important in the immune responses of the body. Fibrinogen is important in the process of blood clotting. Plasma contains small amounts of gases (O_2, CO_2, N_2) in solution. Of the 20 mL of O_2 carried in each 100 mL of blood, only 0.3 mL is carried in solution. Most of the O_2 in blood is carried in

Table 17–1
DISTRIBUTION OF BLOOD VOLUME IN THE CARDIOVASCULAR SYSTEM OF A NORMAL DOG

Between Pulmonary and Systemic Circuits	Percent
Pulmonary vessels and heart	25
Systemic vessels	75
	100

Within the Systemic Circuit	
Arteries and arterioles	15
Capillaries	5
Venules and veins	80
	100

Table 17–2
GEOMETRY OF SYSTEMIC CIRCULATION OF 30-KG DOG

Vessel	Number	Inside Diameter (mm)	Total Cross-Sectional Area (cm²)	Length (cm)	Velocity of Blood Flow (cm/second)	Mean Blood Pressure (mmHg)
Aorta	1	20.0	3.1	40.0	13.0	98
Small arteries	45,000	0.14	6.9	1.5	6.0	90
Arterioles	20,000,000	0.030	140.0	0.2	0.3	60
Capillaries	1,700,000,000	0.008	830.0	0.05	0.05	18
Venules	130,000,000	0.020	420.0	0.1	0.1	12
Small veins	73,000	0.27	42.0	1.5	1.0	6
Vena cava	1	24.0	4.5	34.0	9.0	3

Adapted from Milnor WR: Cardiovascular Physiology. New York, Oxford University Press, 1990.

chemical combination with hemoglobin (in the red blood cells). Likewise, only a small amount of the CO_2 in blood is carried in solution. More of it becomes hydrated to form HCO_3^-. However, most of the CO_2 in blood combines with

hemoglobin or plasma proteins to form carbamino compounds. The nutrient substances dissolved in plasma include glucose, amino acids, lipids, and some vitamins. The metabolic waste products include CO_2, urea, creatinine, uric acid, and bilirubin.

Normally, cells constitute about 40% of the blood volume. The fraction of cells in blood is called the *hematocrit*. The cells settle to the bottom in a tube of centrifuged blood. The cell component looks red because most of the blood cells are the *erythrocytes* or *red blood cells*. The red blood cells contain the protein *hemoglobin*, which functions as the primary carrier of oxygen and carbon dioxide in the blood. The *leukocytes* or *white blood cells* appear as a thin, white "buffy coat" on the top of the red blood cells; there are about 1000 times more red blood cells than white blood cells. The white blood cells are critical in the immune responses of the body. The cellular layer also

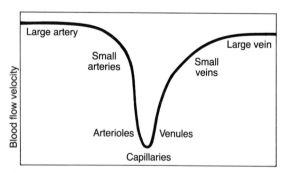

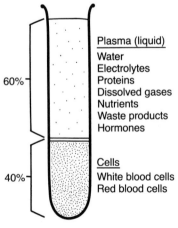

Figure 17–3. As the systemic arteries branch to form arterioles and capillaries, the total cross-sectional area of the vessels increases, so the forward velocity of blood flow decreases. As blood from the capillaries is collected into venules and veins, the total cross-sectional area is reduced, so the velocity of blood flow increases again. Therefore, blood moves quickly from the heart to the microvessels, where it stays for a few seconds, before moving rapidly back to the heart.

Figure 17–4. Blood can be separated into a liquid component (plasma) and a cellular component (mostly red blood cells) by centrifugation. The fraction of cells in blood is called the hematocrit.

contains *platelets,* which are specialized cells or cell fragments that are important in blood clotting.

Because most of the O_2 in blood is carried in chemical combination with the protein hemoglobin within red blood cells, the ability of blood to carry oxygen is determined by the amount of hemoglobin within each red blood cell times the number of red blood cells in the blood. Deviations from a normal hematocrit of 40% have critical consequences in terms of the ability of blood to carry oxygen. The hematocrit also affects the *viscosity* of blood as shown in Figure 17–5. Viscosity is a measure of resistance to flow. For example, honey is more viscous than water. Plasma, by itself, is about 1.5 times more viscous than water because of the presence of plasma protein molecules (albumin, globulin, fibrinogen). The presence of cells in normal blood (hematocrit of 40%) gives it a viscosity about two times greater than the viscosity of plasma. When hematocrit rises above 40%, viscosity increases rapidly. This condition is called *polycythemia,* which literally means "many cells in the blood." The blood of a patient with polycythemia can carry more than the normal 20 mL O_2/100 mL blood. However, the increased viscosity makes it hard for the heart to pump the blood. Therefore, polycythemia creates a heavy workload for the heart and can lead to heart failure if the heart is not healthy.

The opposite problem, in which hematocrit is too low, is called *anemia.* Anemia literally means "no blood," but in fact refers to a condition where there are abnormally few red blood cells in blood. Each 100 mL of blood of an anemic patient carries less than the normal 20 mL of oxygen. Therefore, cardiac output must be increased above normal in order to deliver the normal amount of oxygen each minute to the tissues. This need to increase cardiac output also poses an increased workload to the heart and can lead to the failure of a diseased heart. Thus, a hematocrit of about 40% represents a compromise that allows the blood to carry an adequate amount of oxygen without putting an undue workload on the heart.

Figure 17–6 provides an idea of the relative size and shape of the major constituents of blood. The plasma proteins are much larger than the ionic components of plasma. Red blood cells are many times larger than the plasma proteins.

CLINICAL CORRELATION

COLIC AND ENDOTOXIC SHOCK IN A HORSE SECONDARY TO STRONGYLE PARASITISM

HISTORY □ A 1-year-old standardbred is brought to your clinic by its new owner because the horse has been restless, rolling, kicking at its belly, and pawing the ground. The owner reports that the horse has had a poor appetite for several days and now refuses both hay and grain. The owner says he has wormed the horse recently, but the previous worming history is unknown.

CLINICAL EXAMINATION □ The horse is underweight and has a dull hair coat. It is obvious that the horse is in pain. Physical examination reveals an abnormally high temperature (103.5°F); fast, labored breathing (40 breaths/minute); and an elevated heart rate (80 beats/minute). All limbs feel cool to the touch. The mucous membranes are abnormally dark in color (indicating sluggish circulation). Abdominal auscultation is abnormal; no abdominal sounds are heard on either the left or right side. A rectal examination reveals several distended loops of bowel.

You perform abdominocentesis and withdraw some peritoneal fluid. Normally, peritoneal fluid is clear and straw-colored. The fluid from this

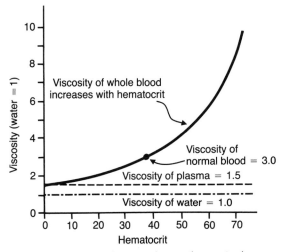

Figure 17–5. Plasma is more viscous than water because of the presence of plasma proteins. Blood is more viscous than plasma because of the presence of blood cells. Blood viscosity increases sharply when the fraction of cells (hematocrit) rises much above the normal value of 40%.

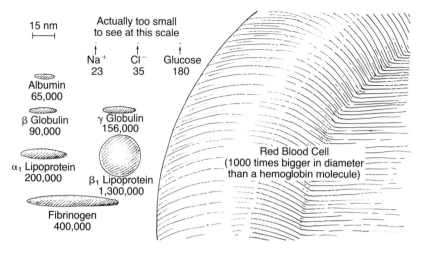

Figure 17-6. Relative size and shape of the major constituents of blood. The figure emphasizes that the plasma protein molecules are huge compared to molecules of glucose and the ionic electrolytes, and the blood cells (red and white) are huge compared to plasma protein molecules. Numbers under constituents are their molecular weights.

horse is darker than normal, and it has a turbid appearance. Measurements with a refractometer indicate that the peritoneal fluid contains five times more protein than normal. Microscopic examination of the fluid reveals the presence of four times the normal number of white blood cells, and the cells contain bacteria.

OUTCOME □ You tell the owner that the horse appears to have a badly damaged bowel and that the prognosis is grave. You inform him that surgical treatment is possible, but that expensive postoperative complications are likely, because infection appears to have spread into the peritoneum. After considering the options, the owner decides against surgery. You institute supportive therapy with intravenous (IV) fluids and analgesics.

The horse's condition deteriorates over the next 12 hours. Heart rate increases progressively to 100 beats/minute. The mucous membranes show evidence of declining blood flow (longer and longer capillary refill time). The horse begins to wheeze and becomes depressed. There are no bowel sounds. Despite the delivery of IV fluids, there is no output of urine. With the owner's consent, you euthanize the horse.

Necropsy examination indicates that this horse had thrombi (vascular obstructions) in several major branches of the mesenteric arteries, probably secondary to a severe infestation of blood worms (*Strongylus vulgaris*). Several areas of the intestine were necrotic. Gram negative bacteria were cultured in both the peritoneal fluid and the blood. The lungs were edematous, and fluid was found in the airways and thorax.

COMMENT □ *Strongylus vulgaris* in horses lodges in mesenteric arteries and decreases the blood flow to the intestine. Worming a severely infested horse can precipitate acute intestinal ischemia, because the worms break away from the walls of major arteries and drift into smaller arteries, which they occlude. Also, the dying worms release substances that trigger the formation of blood clots in the mesenteric arteries. Digestive processes become disrupted and may cease entirely. Intestinal ischemia and gaseous distention of the bowel cause severe pain. If ischemia persists, segments of the bowel become permanently damaged. The breakdown of the intestinal epithelium allows bacteria and bacterial products (endotoxins) to enter the peritoneum and blood. Bacteria and endotoxins cause the body to produce substances that depress the heart and disrupt the capillary endothelium, especially in the lungs. Pulmonary edema and heart failure lead to respiratory failure. Cardiovascular failure leads to renal failure. The progression becomes irreversible.

Bibliography

Cohn PF: Historical perspectives. *In* Cohn PF, Brown EJ Jr, Vlay SC (eds): Clinical Cardiovascular Physiology. Philadelphia, WB Saunders, 1985, p 3.

Haskin SC: Shock. *In* Fox PR (ed): Canine and Feline Cardiology. New York, Churchill Livingstone, 1988, p 229.

Milnor WR: The circulatory system. *In* Cardiovascular Physiology. New York, Oxford University Press, 1990, p 3.

Milnor WR: Normal state of the circulatory system. *In* Cardiovascular Physiology, New York, Oxford University Press, 1990, p 29.

Scher AM, Feigl EO: Introduction and physical principles. *In* Patton HD, Fuchs AF, Hille B, et al (eds): Textbook of Physiology, Vol 2, 21st ed. Philadelphia, WB Saunders, 1989, p 771.

Schmidt-Nielsen K: Blood. *In* Animal Physiology: Adaptation and Environment, 3rd ed. London, Cambridge University Press, 1983, p 70.

Schmidt-Nielsen K: Circulation. *In* Animal Physiology: Adaptation and Environment, 3rd ed. London, Cambridge University Press, 1983, p 97.

Wilson JA: Circulatory systems—nature and functions. *In* Principles of Animal Physiology, 2nd ed. New York, Macmillan Publishing, 1979, p 543.

PRACTICE QUESTIONS FOR CHAPTER 17

1. According to Table 17–2, how long does it take for blood to travel the length of a capillary?

    a. 0.05 second
    b. 0.1 second
    c. 1 second
    d. 10 seconds
    e. 20 seconds

2. In 1 minute, the amount of blood pumped by the left ventricle would equal

    a. the amount of blood that flowed through the coronary circulation.
    b. one half of the cardiac output.
    c. two times the cardiac output.
    d. the amount of blood that flowed through all organs of the systemic circulation except for coronary blood flow.
    e. the amount of blood that flowed through the lungs.

3. A transfusion of plasma would

    a. decrease the hematocrit of the recipient's blood.
    b. increase the viscosity of the recipient's blood.
    c. decrease the sodium concentration of the recipient's plasma.
    d. increase the number of cells in the recipient's blood.
    e. decrease the concentration of proteins in the recipient's plasma.

4. The walls of most capillaries have pores or clefts in them, which are approximately 4 nm in diameter (4×10^{-9} m). According to Figure 17–6,

    a. a capillary pore is approximately 20 times larger in diameter than a sodium ion.
    b. an albumin molecule is approximately 3.5 times longer than the diameter of a capillary pore.
    c. the diameter of a red blood cell is approximately 1880 times greater than the diameter of a capillary pore.
    d. a γ globulin molecule could just about squeeze through a capillary pore if it were lined up exactly right.
    e. All of the above

5. Which of the following sequences of capillary beds might a red blood cell encounter in a normal circulation?

    a. lungs . . . skin . . . lungs . . . brain
    b. coronary . . . kidney (glomerular) . . . kidney (tabular) . . . lungs
    c. spleen . . . liver . . . mesentery . . . lungs
    d. lungs . . . coronary . . . stomach . . . liver
    e. brain . . . lungs . . . liver . . . coronary

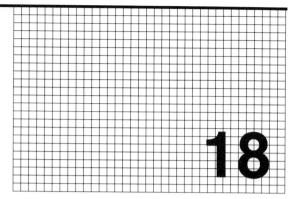

18

Electrical Activity of the Heart

1. Each heartbeat is initiated by an electrical action potential that spreads from cell to cell through cardiac muscle
2. Three features distinguish the initiation of muscle contraction in cardiac muscle from that in skeletal muscle
3. The long cardiac action potential results from prolonged changes in the permeability of cardiac cells to sodium, potassium, and calcium
4. A spontaneous decrease in potassium permeability accounts for the spontaneous depolarization of the pacemaker cells
5. Sympathetic and parasympathetic nerves act on cardiac pacemaker cells to increase or decrease heart rate
6. The specialized conduction system of the heart is responsible for originating, organizing, and synchronizing each heartbeat
7. Dysfunction in the specialized conducting system of the heart leads to abnormalities in cardiac rhythm (arrhythmias)
8. Cardiac tachyarrhythmias can result either from abnormal action potential formation (ectopic pacemaker) or from abnormal action potential conduction (re-entry)

Each Heartbeat Is Initiated by an Electrical Action Potential That Spreads from Cell to Cell Through Cardiac Muscle

The heart is a mechanical pump that propels blood through the blood vessels. As the heart muscle relaxes between beats, the heart fills with blood. With each contraction of the heart muscle, blood is ejected out of the left ventricle into the aorta and out of the right ventricle into the pulmonary artery. Each cardiac contraction (heartbeat) is initiated by an electrical action potential within the cardiac muscle cells. This chapter begins with a detailed de-scription of the properties of electrical action potentials in cardiac muscle cells. Next, there is a description of how the spread of these action potentials through a myocardium is synchronized and organized to make the contracting heart into an effective pump. Finally, several common electrical dysfunctions of the heart are discussed.

It is important to understand the electrical properties of single cardiac muscle cells, be-cause the heart functions electrically as if it were a single cell. The heart is said to form a *functional syncytium* (literally, "same cell"). Cardiac muscle cells are electrically linked to one another, unlike skeletal muscle cells, which are electrically isolated from one another. Therefore, action potentials spread from cell to cell throughout the heart.

The structural basis for the heart's ability to function as an electrical syncytium is evident under the light microscope (Fig. 18–1). Cardiac muscle appears as an array of fibers (individual cardiac muscle cells), which are arranged roughly parallel. The cardiac fibers are striated, just like skeletal muscle fibers. However, one difference between cardiac and skeletal muscle is that cardiac muscle cells are joined by *intercalated discs*. These discs contain *nexi*, or *gap junctions*, through which an action potential in one cardiac muscle cell can spread

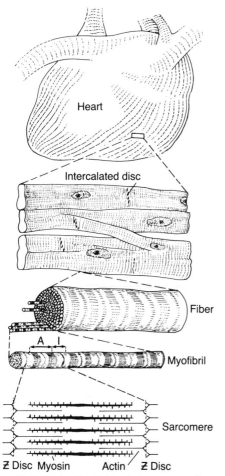

Figure 18–1. Under the light microscope, cardiac muscle fibers are seen to be joined by intercalated discs, which allow action potentials to spread from cell to cell. Cardiac muscle is striated, like skeletal muscle. With an electron microscope, the striations are seen to result from an orderly arrangement of actin and myosin filaments. These filaments are the structural and functional subunits of cardiac muscle, just as they are for skeletal muscle.

into the adjacent cardiac muscle cell. Skeletal muscle does not have intercalated discs or nexi. Action potentials in one skeletal muscle cell do not spread into neighboring muscle cells.

The striations of skeletal muscle and cardiac muscle have the same structural basis. Examining a single cardiac muscle cell under high magnification with the use of electron microscopy reveals that each striated fiber is made up of a few hundred myofibrils. Each *myofibril* has a repetitive pattern of light and dark bands. The various bands and lines within a myofibril are given letter designations (A-band, I-band, Z-disc). The alignment of these bands in adjacent myofibrils accounts for the striated appearance of the whole muscle fiber. Each repeating unit of myofibrillar bands is called a *sarcomere*. The word means "little muscle," because the sarcomere is both the anatomical and functional subunit of the cardiac muscle. A sarcomere extends from one Z-disc to the next, a distance of approximately 100 microns (μm). Each sarcomere is composed of an array of thick and thin filaments. The thin filaments are attached to the Z-discs, and they interdigitate with the thick filaments. The thin filaments are composed of *actin* molecules. The thick filaments are composed of *myosin* molecules. The myosin molecules have ends that protrude from the thick filament and form *cross-bridges* with the nearby thin filaments. A cycling or paddling of these cross-bridges pulls the thin filaments past the thick filaments. This sliding of thin filaments past thick filaments causes each sarcomere, and therefore the whole muscle cell, to contract. The molecular biochemistry of filament sliding and sarcomere shortening is described in Chapter 5.

Three Features Distinguish the Initiation of Muscle Contraction in Cardiac Muscle from that in Skeletal Muscle

The major differences between skeletal muscle and cardiac muscle are not in the biochemistry of contraction, but rather in the properties of the action potential that initiates the contraction. Table 18–1 shows the similarities and differences in the initiation of contraction in skeletal muscle and cardiac muscle. Normally a skeletal muscle cell contracts only in response to an action potential in the somatic motor neuron associated with the muscle cell. One action potential in a motor neuron causes

Table 18-1
SEQUENCE OF EVENTS IN INITIATION OF CONTRACTION OF SKELETAL MUSCLE AND CARDIAC MUSCLE

Skeletal Muscle	Cardiac Muscle
Action potential in somatic motor neuron	(NOTE: Action potentials in autonomic motor neurons are *not* needed to initiate heart beats; a completely denervated heart beats spontaneously)
Acetylcholine release	
Activation of muscarinic cholinergic receptors at motor end-plate	
Depolarization of muscle membrane (end-plate potential)	Spontaneous depolarizatioan of pacemaker cells (pacemaker potential)
Action potential forms in muscle cell but does not spread to other cells	Action potential forms in a pacemaker cell and spreads from cell to cell through whole heart
Tiny amount of Ca^{2+} enters cell through "fast Ca^{2+} channels"	Substantial amount of Ca^{2+} enters cell through "slow Ca^{2+} channels"
Ca^{2+} released from sarcoplasmic reticulum	Ca^{2+} released from sarcoplasmic reticulum
Ca^{2+} binds to troponin	Ca^{2+} binds to troponin
Actin-myosin cross-bridge cycling	Actin-myosin cross-bridge cycling
Muscle contracts ("twitch")	Heart contracts ("beat" or "systole")
Ca^{2+} taken up by sarcoplasmic reticulum	Ca^{2+} taken up by sarcoplasmic reticulum
Ca^{2+} that entered cell through fast Ca^{2+} channels pumped back into extracellular fluid	Ca^{2+} that entered cells through slow Ca^{2+} channels pumped back into extracellular fluid
Muscle relaxes	Heart relaxes (diastole)

one contractile twitch in the muscle cells that it innervates. A motor neuron action potential results in the release of acetylcholine. Acetylcholine activates cholinergic receptors on the skeletal muscle cell membrane at a specialized region called the *motor end-plate*. Acetylcholine depolarizes the membrane of the motor end-plate. When this depolarization brings the skeletal muscle membrane to threshold, an action potential forms in the muscle cell membrane. This action potential is propagated along the length of the skeletal muscle cell (see Chapter 4).

An action potential in skeletal muscle is primarily brought about by the influx of extracellular sodium ions across the cell membrane. However, there are also calcium ion channels within the muscle cell membrane, and these ion channels are opened during the action potential. Because calcium concentration is higher in the extracellular fluid than in the intracellular fluid, a small amount of calcium flows into a skeletal muscle cell during an action potential. The entire action potential in a skeletal muscle lasts only 1–2 ms, and the calcium ion channels open and close within this same length of time. Therefore, they are called *fast calcium channels*. The occurrence of an action potential somehow causes the release of calcium stores from the sarcoplasmic reticulum within the skeletal muscle cell. The amount of extracellular calcium that enters a skeletal muscle cell through fast calcium channels is tiny compared with the amount of calcium that an action potential releases from the sarcoplasmic reticulum. However, the entry of extracellular calcium may help initiate the release of calcium from the sarcoplasmic reticulum. The calcium ions freed from the sarcoplasmic reticulum bind to the protein troponin. This initiates the cycling of actin-myosin cross-bridges, which causes muscle contraction. The contraction initiated by a single action potential is very brief, because the free intracellular calcium is rapidly taken up by active transport into the sarcoplasmic reticulum, and the muscle relaxes.

The first major difference between the initiation of contraction in skeletal and cardiac muscle is that action potentials in motor neurons are not needed to initiate cardiac contractions. Instead, cardiac contractions are initiated by cardiac pacemaker cells, which spontaneously depolarize to threshold. The normal cardiac *pacemaker cells* are located in the right atrium, near the vena cava, at a site called the *sinoatrial (SA) node*.

When any one pacemaker cell depolarizes to threshold, an action potential forms in that cell. The action potential then spreads from cell to cell by way of the nexi in the intercalated discs. The ability of an action potential to spread from cell to cell is the second major difference between the initiation of contraction in cardiac muscle and skeletal muscle.

The third distinguishing feature of cardiac muscle contraction concerns the role of extracellular calcium. The cardiac action potential lasts 100–250 ms (100 times longer than the action potential in skeletal muscle). The prolonged action potential is brought about by prolonged changes in the permeability of the cardiac muscle membrane to potassium, sodium, and calcium ions. The ionic channels through which calcium ions cross the cell membrane are particularly important in prolonging the cardiac action potential. These channels are called *slow calcium channels*, because they stay open for 100–250 ms compared with 1–2 ms for the fast calcium channels in skeletal muscle. Because these calcium channels are open much longer, about 10 times more calcium enters a cardiac muscle cell than enters a skeletal muscle cell during an action potential. By itself, the extracellular calcium is insufficient to initiate a forceful contraction. However, the entry of extracellular calcium triggers the release of additional calcium from the sarcoplasmic reticulum of cardiac muscle cells. This process is called *calcium-triggered calcium release*. At the conclusion of a cardiac action potential, the slow calcium channels close. Most of the free, intracellular calcium is pumped back into the sarcoplasmic reticulum. In addition, the calcium that entered the cell through slow calcium channels is pumped back across the cell membrane into the extracellular fluid. Both of these processes involve active transport, because the calcium is being pumped against its electrochemical gradient. As the free intracellular calcium concentration is returned to its resting level, the cardiac muscle relaxes.

To summarize, the major differences between the initiation of contraction in cardiac and skeletal muscle are as follows:

1. the origin of muscle cell action potentials; action potentials are spontaneous in the case of cardiac muscle but are dependent on motor neuron action potentials in the case of skeletal muscle;
2. the spread of muscle cell action potentials; they spread from cell to cell in cardiac muscle but are confined within a single cell in skeletal muscle;
3. the role of extracellular calcium; it contributes directly to the initiation of actin-myosin cross-bridges cycling in cardiac muscle and also triggers the release of more calcium from the sarcoplasmic reticulum. In contraction of skeletal muscle, extracellular calcium plays only a trigger role.

Calcium channel blockers are drugs that bind to the slow calcium channels of cardiac muscle and decrease the entry of calcium into cardiac muscle cells during an action potential. Calcium channel blockers (e.g., verapamil and nifedapine) are used in clinical situations when a reduction in the forcefulness of cardiac contraction is desirable. One such situation is idiopathic hypertrophic subaortic stenosis (IHSS), in which excessively hypertrophied ventricular muscle bulges into the aortic opening during ventricular contraction. This obstruction reduces the volume of blood that is ejected from the ventricle into the aorta with each heartbeat. By decreasing the forcefulness of cardiac contractions, calcium channel blockers limit the degree of obstruction of the outflow. (They also reduce the progression of cardiac hypertrophy, for reasons that are described later.) Coronary artery disease is another situation in which a reduction in cardiac contractility might be desirable. In coronary artery disease, blood flow to the ventricular muscle becomes limited by atherosclerotic plaques in the coronary arteries. By reducing the forcefulness of cardiac contractions, calcium channel blockers reduce cardiac oxygen demand to a level that can be supplied by blood flow through the diseased coronary arteries.

The Long Cardiac Action Potential Results from Prolonged Changes in the Permeability of Cardiac Cells to Sodium, Potassium, and Calcium

Figure 18–2 shows an action potential in a typical ventricular muscle cell. As mentioned already, the cardiac action potentials last 100 times longer than action potentials in nerves or skeletal muscle fibers. However, the resting membrane potential (about -80 mV) is maintained by the same ionic conditions that account for the resting membrane potential of nerves and skeletal muscle fibers (see Chapter 3). That is, resting cardiac cells have a high permeability to potassium and a low permeability to sodium and calcium (Fig. 18–3). The upstroke of the action potential in cardiac muscle fibers is caused by a sudden increase in the permeability to sodium, just as it is in nerves and skeletal muscle fibers. The peak of the action potential is reached within a few milliseconds. Sodium permeability begins to decrease then, and the cardiac cell membrane potential begins to return toward its resting level. However, repolarization is interrupted, and there is a prolonged plateau of depolarization, which lasts over 100 ms. The plateau is brought about by three conditions that occur in cardiac muscle cells but not in nerves or skeletal muscle fibers:

1. potassium permeability decreases;
2. sodium permeability remains somewhat elevated rather than returning to its low resting condition;

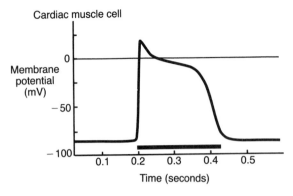

Cardiac muscle cell

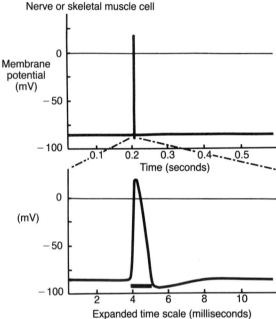

Nerve or skeletal muscle cell

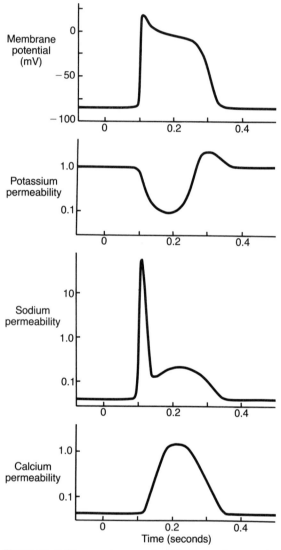

Figure 18–2. Action potentials in cardiac muscle cells (top trace) last 100 times longer than action potentials in nerve or skeletal muscle cells (lower traces). The prolonged phase of depolarization in cardiac muscle cells is called the *plateau of the action potential.* The dark bars under each action potential indicate the length of the absolute refractory period.

3. most important, calcium permeability increases.

It is during the plateau that calcium ions from the extracellular fluid flow into the cells through the slow calcium channels. The plateau ends when the cells' permeability to potassium increases. The resulting efflux of potassium makes the inside of the cells negative. Also, the sodium and calcium permeabilities return to their low resting levels, which decreases the influx of these positive ions. Therefore, the cells repolarize to a normal resting membrane potential.

The long duration of the cardiac action po-

tential creates a long refractory period. *Refractory period* (strictly, "absolute refractory period") is the time following the beginning of one action potential during which another action potential cannot be initiated. In nerves, skeletal muscle cells, and cardiac muscle cells, the refractory period lasts about as long as an action potential. Therefore, the refractory period in a nerve or skeletal muscle cell lasts

Figure 18–3. The membrane potential of a cardiac muscle cell (top trace) is determined by the relative permeabilities of the cell membrane to potassium, sodium, and calcium (three lower traces). At rest (left side of graphs), the cell is much more permeable to potassium than it is to sodium and calcium. A cardiac action potential (middle of graphs) is produced by a characteristic sequence of changes in the potassium, sodium, and calcium permeabilities. The action potential ends when the permeabilities return to their resting state (right side of graphs).

about 1 or 2 ms, but the refractory period in a cardiac muscle cell lasts 100–250 ms (see Fig. 18–2).

The importance of the long refractory period in cardiac muscle is that it guarantees a period of relaxation (and cardiac filling) between each cardiac contraction. As shown in Figure 18–4, each cardiac action potential results in a twitch-like contraction (beat) of the heart. Note that a cardiac action potential lasts nearly as long as a cardiac contraction; the contractile tension in the heart returns to almost zero by the time the action potential is over. If a second action potential occurred immediately after the first refractory period ended, the result would be a second, distinct cardiac contraction. Because of the long refractory period, the heart cannot sustain a continuous contraction. By contrast, the contractile twitch of a skeletal muscle fiber lasts much longer than the action potential itself. Several action potentials can occur during a single contractile twitch. Multiple action potentials cause muscle twitches that fuse together. The resulting contractile tension is greater than the tension that results from a single action potential. This phenomenon is called temporal summation. *Fusion* and

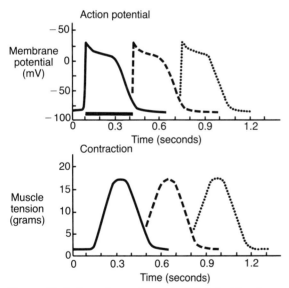

Figure 18–4. A cardiac action potential (left side of top graph) causes a cardiac contraction (left side of bottom graph). The heavy, horizontal bar under the action potential shows the duration of the absolute refractory period. The dashed lines in the top graph show the earliest possible occurrence of a second and third action potential (each one occurring right after the absolute refractory period for the preceding action potential). Because of the long refractory period, each contraction is almost over before the earliest possible next contraction can begin. This guarantees a period of cardiac relaxation between each contraction.

temporal summation are the mechanisms that permit graded and prolonged tension development in skeletal muscle. The long refractory period in cardiac muscle cells prevents the fusion and summation of cardiac contractions. Therefore, there is a guaranteed period of relaxation (and refilling) between each heartbeat.

A Spontaneous Decrease in Potassium Permeability Accounts for the Spontaneous Depolarization of Pacemaker Cells

The shape of the cardiac action potential varies from one region of the heart to another. The pattern discussed so far is found in the ventricular muscle cells. A somewhat different pattern is found in the pacemaker cells of the SA node. Figure 18–5 (top) shows the membrane potential in an SA node pacemaker cell during the initiation of one heartbeat. The most obvious difference between the action potential in an SA node cell and a ventricular cell is that the plateau phase of the SA node action potential is shorter. However, the most important difference is that the membrane potential of pacemaker cells does not stay at a stable resting level between action potentials. Instead, the membranes of pacemaker cells spontaneously depolarize until they reach the threshold voltage for initiation of an action potential. The spontaneous depolarization is called the *pacemaker potential*. Because the heart is a functional syncytium, only one SA node cell has to reach threshold and form an action potential in order to initiate an electrical depolarization that spreads across the whole heart. That is, the first pacemaker cell to reach threshold initiates a heartbeat.

The depolarization of pacemaker cells is the result of a spontaneous decrease in potassium permeability. As shown in Figure 18–3, the stable resting membrane potential of normal cardiac muscle cells results from constant levels of potassium, sodium, and calcium permeability. Depolarization toward threshold could be caused either by an increase in sodium or calcium permeability (which would increase the rate of entry of positive sodium or calcium ions) or by a decrease in potassium permeability (which would decrease the ease with which potassium ions leave the cell). In fact, it is the ratio between these permeabilities that primarily determines membrane potential. In a pacemaker cell, potassium permeability de-

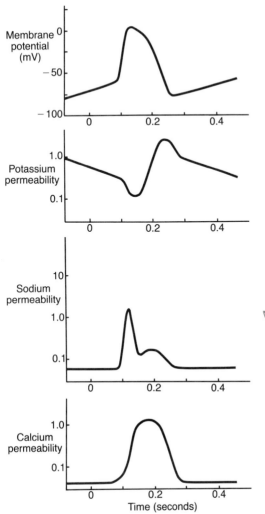

Figure 18–5. A pacemaker cell depolarizes spontaneously to threshold and initiates an action potential (top trace). The spontaneous depolarization (called the pacemaker potential) is the result of a spontaneous, progressive decrease in potassium permeability (second trace). Once threshold is reached, an action potential is produced by further changes in the potassium permeability together with changes in the sodium and calcium permeabilities (bottom two traces). Note that the sequence of permeability changes that cause the action potential is similar in pacemaker cells (this figure) and in nonpacemaker cells (Figure 18–3).

creases spontaneously, so the cell depolarizes toward threshold (see Fig. 18–5). As the membrane potential approaches threshold, there is also an increase in calcium permeability, which hastens the depolarization process. Once threshold for an action potential is reached, there is a sudden increase in sodium permeability, a further increase in calcium permeability, and a further decrease in potassium permeability. During the actual action potential, the changes in the permeabilities to po-

tassium, sodium, and calcium are similar in pacemaker cells and in regular cardiac cells.

Sympathetic and Parasympathetic Nerves Act on Cardiac Pacemaker Cells to Increase or Decrease Heart Rate

Figure 18–6 shows how the neurotransmitters norepinephrine and acetylcholine affect the pacemaker cells of the heart. Acetylcholine slows the spontaneous depolarization of pacemaker cells, because acetylcholine slows the spontaneous decrease in potassium permeability. Acetylcholine makes it take longer for the pacemaker cells to reach threshold, so there is a longer time between heartbeats. That is, the heart rate is slowed below its intrinsic or spontaneous rate. Norepinephrine has the opposite effect. Norepinephrine speeds up the spontaneous depolarization of pacemaker cells by speeding up the spontaneous decrease in their potassium permeability. Because the pacemaker cells reach threshold more quickly in the presence of norepinephrine, there is a shorter interval between heartbeats. That is, the heart rate is elevated above its intrinsic or spontaneous level. Parasympathetic neurons release acetylcholine at the SA node cells, so parasympathetic activity decreases the heart rate. Sympathetic neurons release norepinephrine at the SA node cells, so sympathetic nerve activity increases the heart rate.

Figure 18–7 indicates the way in which sympathetic and parasympathetic neurons interact in the control of the heart rate. In the absence of either sympathetic or parasympathetic action potentials, the heart beats at its intrinsic rate. For a large dog this rate is typically about 140 beats per minute. However, the heart rate is only 50–70 beats per minute during sleep, and about 90 beats per minute if the dog is quiet and awake. The only way these heart rates (below the intrinsic rate) can be achieved is by activation of parasympathetic neurons. Accordingly, the graph indicates that parasympathetic activity is high during sleep. The awake heart rate of 90 beats per minute is achieved by a somewhat smaller parasympathetic tone. Exercise or emotional arousal cause the heart rate to increase. The heart rate may rise as high as 250 beats per minute in a dog that is maximally exercising or badly frightened. Obviously, such heart rates are above the intrinsic rate. They are achieved by activation of the sympathetic nerves to the heart. By grading the level of sympathetic

Interval Between Heartbeats

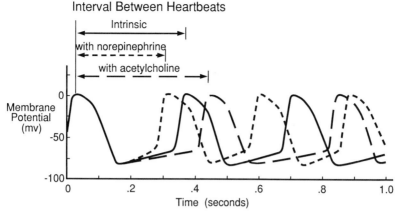

Time (seconds)

Figure 18–6. In the absence of neurohumoral influences, a pacemaker cell of the SA node will spontaneously depolarize to threshold and initiate a series of action potentials (solid line in graph). The interval between action potentials under these conditions determines the intrinsic or spontaneous heart rate. Acetylcholine decreases the rate of depolarization and therefore lengthens the interval between action potentials (long-dashed line). Norepinephrine increases the rate of depolarization and therefore shortens the interval between action potentials (short-dashed line).

tone, the heart rate can be adjusted to meet the demands of each behavioral situation. Sympathetic activity is maximal during periods of fear, fight, or flight.

Sympathetic and parasympathetic neurons to the heart are sometimes activated simultaneously. When both systems are activated, the resulting heart rate represents the outcome of a sort of tug-of-war between sympathetic action to increase the heart rate and parasympathetic action to decrease the heart rate. Typically, the sympathetic and parasympathetic systems are both partially activated when the heart rate is between about 90 beats per minute

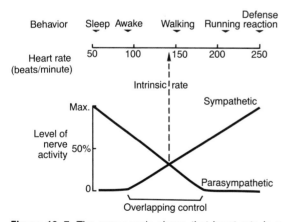

Figure 18–7. The upper scale shows that heart rate in a normal dog ranges from 50–250 beats per minute, depending on behavioral state. The graph shows that this wide range of heart rates is brought about by the interactions between parasympathetic nerve activity, which slows the heart below its intrinsic rate, and sympathetic nerve activity, which speeds the heart above its intrinsic rate.

and 175 beats per minute, with parasympathetic activity being predominant in the lower part of this range and sympathetic activity being predominant in the higher part of this range. When sympathetic activity and parasympathetic activity are equal, their effects cancel each other, and the heart rate is at its intrinsic or spontaneous level. Simultaneous activation of sympathetic and parasympathetic neurons appears to give the nervous system tight control over the heart rate under a wide variety of behavioral conditions.

The Specialized Conduction System of the Heart is Responsible for Originating, Organizing, and Synchronizing Each Heartbeat

When the SA node pacemaker cells initiate a normal heartbeat, both atria contract almost simultaneously. After that, there is a pause. Then, both ventricles contract almost simultaneously. After contracting, the whole heart relaxes and remains in a relaxed state until the next beat is initiated by the SA node pacemaker cells. The organization and synchronization of these cardiac events are brought about by the *specialized conducting system* of the heart, which consists of the *SA and atrioventricular (AV) nodes, AV bundle, bundle branches,* and *Purkinje's fibers* (Fig. 18–8).

The spontaneous depolarization to threshold of the SA node pacemaker cells has been described already. Other atrial cells do not exhibit pacemaker activity. That is, their membrane potential remains stable at a resting level

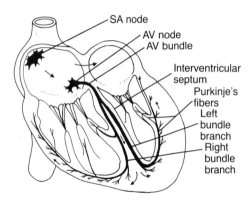

Figure 18–8. The specialized conduction system of the heart is responsible for the initiation and coordination of cardiac contractions.

(about −80 mV), unless they are depolarized to threshold by the occurrence of action potentials in neighboring cells. Thus, when a pacemaker cell in the SA node spontaneously depolarizes to threshold, the resulting action potential in that pacemaker cell spreads from cell to cell throughout both atria, and both atria contract.

The pause between atrial and ventricular contraction is brought about by the slow condition of action potentials through the AV node. Cells of the AV node are the only conducting path between the atria and ventricles. Elsewhere, the atria and ventricles are separated by a layer of connective tissue. Connective tissue cells neither form nor conduct action potentials. The AV node is composed of specialized cardiac muscle cells. AV node tissue conducts action potentials, but the velocity of propagation of the action potential is ten times slower through the AV node than through normal atrial tissue. Once an action potential passes through the AV node, it enters the *AV bundle* or *common bundle of His.* The bundle of His and the *bundle branches* are composed of specialized cardiac muscle cells that conduct action potentials rapidly, three times faster than atrial tissue. At the ventricular apex, the right and left bundle branches break up into a network of Purkinje's fibers, which carry the action potential rapidly along the inner walls of both ventricles. Thus, the slow conduction of action potentials through the AV node results in a delay between the atrial and ventricular contractions. However, once the action potential enters the ventricular bundles it is spread so rapidly through both ventricles that both ventricles contract almost simultaneously.

Figure 18–9 re-emphasizes the role of the specialized conduction system in organizing cardiac contractions. In this illustration, atrial excitation begins at time T=0, when one SA node cell reaches threshold. Within 0.1 seconds, the action potential initiated by this SA node cell spreads completely across the right and left atria, which leads to the almost simultaneous contraction of both atria. As the action potential spreads across the atria, it depolarizes cells of the AV node also, beginning at time T=0.04 seconds. While the atria are in a depolarized (excited) state, the action potential is also being propagated slowly from cell to cell through the AV node. After traversing the AV node, the action potential reaches the ventricular bundles, which carry it rapidly to the ventricular apex. The action potential arrives at the ventricular apex at time T=0.17 seconds. Note that it takes about 0.13 seconds (0.17 seconds minus 0.04 seconds) for the action potential to get through the AV node and bundles. That is, 0.13 seconds represent a typical delay between atrial depolarization and ventricular depolarization. Once the action potential has reached the ventricular apex, Purkinje's fibers spread it rapidly throughout both ventricles. Ventricular depolarization is complete by time T=0.22 seconds, and both ventricles contract. By this time the atria have repolarized to a resting state, and their refractory period is over. Therefore, atrial tissue is susceptible to a second action potential. However, the action potential that has spread throughout both ventricles cannot be propagated retrograde through the AV node and back into the atria; the AV node cells function as a one-way electrical gate. Therefore, following ventricular excitation and contraction, the whole heart relaxes and remains in a resting state until the next beat is originated by the SA node pacemaker cells.

Another important feature of the AV node is that the AV node cells can act as *auxiliary pacemakers.* As shown in Figure 18–10, the AV node cells spontaneously depolarize toward threshold, but much more slowly than the SA node cells. Therefore, under normal circumstances, the SA node cells reach threshold first and initiate a cardiac action potential. As this action potential spreads into the AV node, it encounters auxiliary pacemaker cells that are spontaneously depolarizing toward threshold. The spreading action potential depolarizes these pacemaker cells immediately to threshold, and they form an action potential. However, if the SA node is damaged and does not

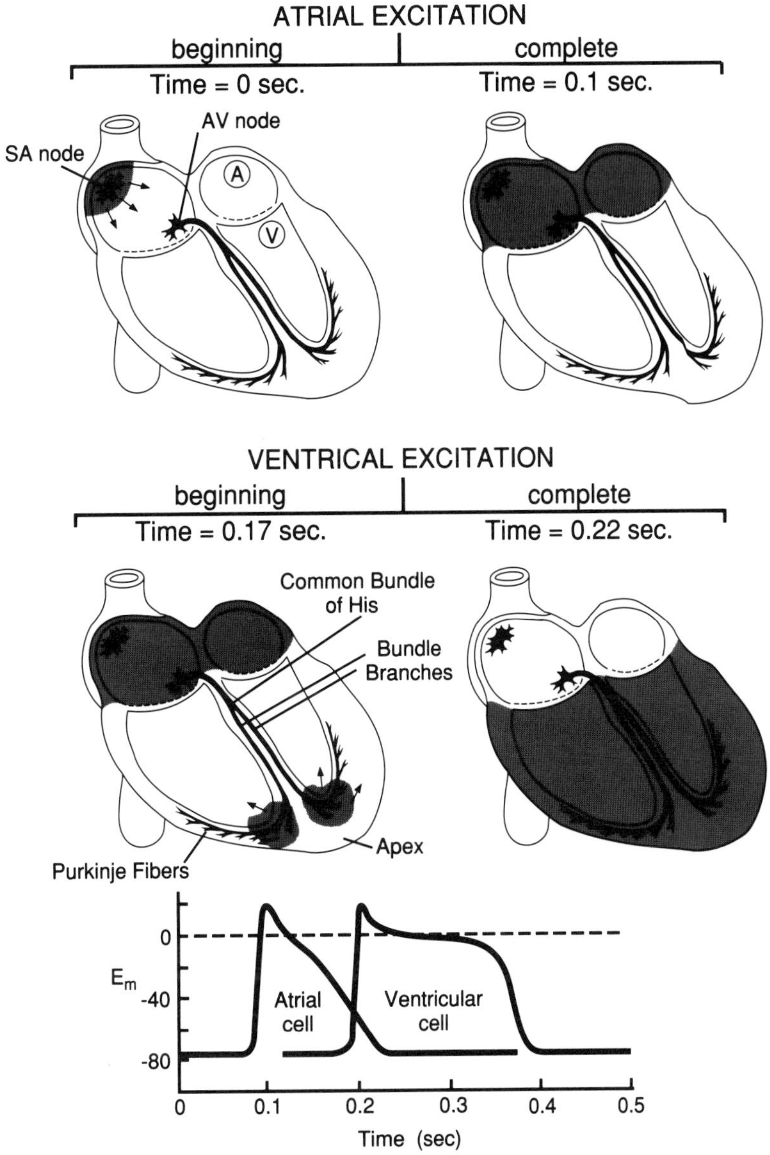

ATRIAL EXCITATION

| beginning | complete |
| Time = 0 sec. | Time = 0.1 sec. |

VENTRICAL EXCITATION

| beginning | complete |
| Time = 0.17 sec. | Time = 0.22 sec. |

Figure 18–9. The heart is pictured at four instants during the initiation of a normal contraction. In the upper-left drawing (time T = 0 seconds), a pacemaker cell in the SA node has just reached threshold, and an action potential has begun to spread outward across the atria. In the upper right (T = 0.1 seconds), the action potential has spread completely across both atria (all atrial cells are at the plateau of their action potentials). In the lower left drawing (T = 0.17 seconds), the action potential has passed down the bundle branches and has just reached the ventricular apex. A short time later (T = 0.22 seconds, lower right drawing), the action potential has just finished spreading across both ventricles (all ventricular cells are at the plateau of their action potentials). The graph shows the timing of action potentials in a left atrial cell and a left ventricular cell. These cells are at the locations labeled *A* and *V* in the upper left drawing. Their locations make these among the last cells to be depolarized as action potentials spread across the atria and ventricles.

depolarize to threshold, or if the cells at the beginning of the AV node are damaged and do not propagate atrial action potentials, then the AV node pacemaker cells reach threshold eventually and initiate ventricular contractions. The intrinsic or spontaneous ventricular rate resulting from AV node pacemakers is about 40 beats per minute in a resting dog, as compared with 140 beats per minute, which is the spontaneous rate of SA node pacemaker cells. Nevertheless, this ventricular rate is sufficient to sustain life if the SA node fails as a pacemaker or if the AV node fails to conduct atrial action potentials.

A final important feature of the AV node cells is that they have long refractory periods, even longer than the refractory period of normal atrial or ventricular tissue. The long refractory period of AV node cells helps protect the ventricles from being stimulated to contract at rates that are too rapid for efficient pumping. This protective function of the AV node is important in situations in which the atrial action potential frequency exceeds the rate at which ventricles could pump blood efficiently. This condition occurs during atrial flutter or atrial fibrillation, as explained later.

Table 18–2 summarizes the five important electrical characteristics of the AV node that have been discussed. Three of these charac-

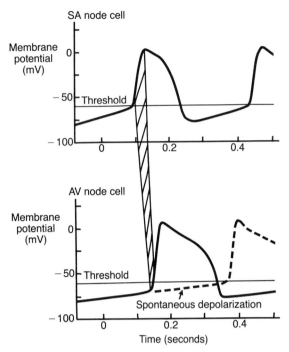

Figure 18–10. SA node cells and AV node cells both show pacemaker activity (spontaneous depolarization toward threshold). Normally, the SA node cells depolarize more quickly and reach threshold first (top graph). The resulting atrial action potential spreads into the AV node and depolarizes the AV node cells to threshold (solid line in bottom graph). However, if the SA node pacemaker cells were nonfunctional or if atrial action potentials were not conducted into the AV node, the AV node cells would eventually depolarize to threshold and initiate action potentials on their own (dashed line in bottom graph). In this way, the AV node cells serve as an auxiliary ventricular pacemaker.

teristics are influenced by the nervous system. As indicated in the table, parasympathetic activity decreases the conduction velocity of the AV node cells, lengthens their refractory period, and slows their auxiliary pacemaker activity. Sympathetic activation has the opposite effects. These sympathetic and parasympathetic effects bring about adjustments in AV node properties that are appropriate for different heart rates. When sympathetic activity is high and the SA node pacemakers are initiating heartbeats frequently, the whole process of cardiac contraction and relaxation must be sped up, including the delay between atrial and ventricular contractions. Thus, it is appropriate that sympathetic action also speeds the velocity of action potential conduction through the AV node. In addition, sympathetic activation shortens the AV node refractory period, which allows heartbeats to be conducted more frequently between the atria and the ventri-

cles. Finally, sympathetic activation enhances AV node auxiliary pacemaker activity, which speeds up the ventricular rate if the AV node is blocked. Conversely, when parasympathetic activation slows depolarization of the SA node pacemakers and decreases heart rate, then it makes sense for AV conduction velocity to be slowed, so there is a longer delay between atrial and ventricular contractions.

Dysfunction in the Specialized Conducting System of the Heart Leads to Abnormalities in Cardiac Rhythm (*Arrhythmias*)

Cardiac arrhythmias can result from problems in either action potential formation or action potential conduction. *Sick sinus syndrome* is an example of a problem with action potential formation. Patients with sick sinus syndrome have an abnormally slow heart rate at rest (*bradycardia*) and an insufficient increase in heart rate during exercise. As indicated by the name, this electrical dysfunction results from a sluggish depolarization of the SA node pacemaker cells. That is, the intrinsic sinus rate is very low. Even though the problem in sick sinus syndrome is intrinsic to the sinus itself, one treatment strategy is to administer a drug that blocks parasympathetic action on the heart (a cholinergic muscarinic antagonist,

Table 18–2
ELECTRICAL CHARACTERISTICS OF THE AV NODE

Characteristic	Sympathetic Effect	Parasympathetic Effect
Only conducting pathway between the atria and ventricles	—	—
Slow conduction velocity (Creates AV delay)	Increases velocity (Shorter AV delay)	Decreases velocity (Longer AV delay)
One-way conduction (atria to ventricles)	—	—
Spontaneous depolarization to threshold (acts as auxiliary pacemaker)	Faster depolarization	Slower depolarization
Long refractory period	Shortens refractory period	Lengthens refractory period

e.g., atropine). The logic behind this treatment is illustrated in Table 18–3. In a normal healthy dog, the intrinsic rate of the heart is 140 beats per minute. However, the heart rate at rest is about 90 beats per minute, because high parasympathetic tone slows the SA node pacemaker to a rate below its intrinsic rate. A drug that blocks parasympathetic effects on the heart returns the heart rate in the resting dog to 140 beats per minute. A dog with a sick sinus has a low intrinsic heart rate, perhaps 80 beats per minute. Parasympathetic tone makes the resting heart rate even lower, approximately 30 beats per minute. A drug that blocks parasympathetic effects restores the heart rate to its intrinsic level, 80 beats per minute. Therefore, a dog with sick sinus syndrome, treated with atropine, has a heart rate that closely matches the rate of a normal resting dog.

Another possible therapeutic approach is to increase the heart rate by administering a drug that mimics the action of sympathetic nerves. Specifically, a β-adrenergic agonist (e.g., isoproterenol) can be administered to activate the adrenergic receptors on the SA node cells that are normally activated by norepinephrine. Enough isoproterenol would be given to increase the resting rate from 30 beats per minute up to 80–90 beats per minute.

If drug treatment of sick sinus syndrome is ineffective, an alternative way to increase the heart rate is through the use of an artificial cardiac pacemaker. An artificial cardiac pacemaker is an electric stimulator that applies electrical shocks to the heart and depolarizes cardiac muscle to threshold. Shocks applied to the atria initiate atrial action potentials. If the AV node is functioning normally, these atrial action potentials are conducted to the ventricles, and the ventricles also contract.

Sick sinus syndrome exemplifies a dysfunction during action potential *formation*. AV node

block is a common electrical dysfunction of the heart during action potential *conduction*. If damage to the AV node prevents conduction of atrial action potentials to the ventricles, then the atria continue to beat at a rate determined by the SA node pacemaker cells. The ventricles continue to beat too, but at a much lower rate. When the AV node is blocked, ventricular contractions are initiated by AV node cells functioning as auxiliary pacemakers. Recall that the AV node pacemaker cells depolarize more slowly than the SA node pacemakers. In a resting dog with AV node block, the ventricles typically beat at 40 beats per minute, and these beats are completely desynchronized from the atrial contractions.

Three degrees of severity of AV node block are recognized. Complete block of the AV node, where no atrial action potentials are conducted to the ventricles, is called *third-degree AV node block*. If action potentials are conducted sporadically from the atria to the ventricles, so that the AV node transmits some atrial action potentials but not all of them, the condition is called *second-degree AV node block*. In a patient with second-degree block, some atrial contractions are followed by ventricular contractions and others are not. Strong parasympathetic activity can create or exaggerate second-degree AV node block, because parasympathetic activity increases the refractory period of the AV node cells. For example, in resting horses, parasympathetic activity is sometimes so strong, and the AV node refractory period is so long, that some atrial beats are not conducted to the ventricles. During exercise, these same horses do not show AV node block, because parasympathetic activity has been reduced, and sympathetic activity has been increased. Both of these changes shorten the refractory period of the AV node.

The mildest degree of AV node block is *first-degree block*. In first-degree block, every atrial action potential is transmitted to the ventricles, but the action potential is propagated even more slowly than normal through the AV node. Therefore, the delay between atrial contraction and ventricular contraction is abnormally long. Because the AV node conduction velocity can be slowed by parasympathetic activity and sped by sympathetic activity, the degree of nervous excitation of the heart can influence the severity of first-degree block.

AV node block can be caused by toxins, infections, ischemia, congenital heart defects, or cardiac fibrosis. Another common cause of AV node block is the inadvertent damage of

Table 18–3
TREATMENT OF SICK SINUS SYNDROME BY BLOCKING PARASYMPATHETIC EFFECTS ON HEART RATE WITH A CHOLINERGIC MUSCARINIC ANTAGONIST

Heart Rate	Normal Dog	Dog with Sick Sinus Syndrome
Intrinsic rate	140 bpm	80 bpm
Resting rate (with parasympathetic tone)	90 bpm	30 bpm
Rate after atropine	140 bpm	80 bpm

AV node tissue during the surgical repair of a ventricular septal defect. Second- or third-degree AV node block often involves the electrical phenomenon known as *decremental conduction.* Specific structural and electrical properties of the AV node cells cause the action potential to have a less rapid upstroke, a lower voltage amplitude, and a slower velocity of conduction in the AV node than in normal atrial or ventricular tissue. All these differences make conduction of the action potential from cell to cell less reliable in the AV node than in normal atrial or ventricular tissue. When the AV node cells are in an electrically depressed state, an atrial action potential may dissipate within the AV node and not be transmitted to the ventricles. This dying out of a cardiac action potential in a slowly conducting region is called *decremental conduction.*

AV node block must be treated if the resulting ventricular rate is too low to maintain adequate blood flow to the body. Drugs that block parasympathetic actions on the heart (cholinergic muscarinic antagonists such as atropine) might reduce the AV node refractory period and increase conduction velocity sufficiently to overcome a blocked state. Drugs that mimic the effect of sympathetic nerves by activating β-adrenergic receptors (e.g., isoproterenol) could have the same effect (refer to Table 18–2). If drug treatment fails to correct AV node block, then an electrical pacemaker may be implanted. In the case of AV node block, the pacemaker needs to be applied to the ventricles. Pacing the atria would not be beneficial, because atrial action potentials would not be transmitted to the ventricles.

Cardiac Tachyarrhythmias Can Result Either from Abnormal Action Potential Formation (Ectopic Pacemaker) or from Abnormal Action Potential Conduction (Re-entry)

Tachyarrhythmias are abnormalities in cardiac rhythm in which the atrial or ventricular rates, or both, are abnormally high. An isolated, occasional extra atrial or ventricular beat is called a *precontraction* or a *premature beat.* Precontractions often result from the presence in the atria or ventricles of an area of abnormal tissue that acts as a pacemaker by spontaneously depolarizing to threshold before the regular pacemaker does. Certain toxins, electrolyte imbalances, and ischemia can cause such *ectopic pacemaker* activity. Occasional pre-contractions are common in both animals and humans, and normally they have no clinical significance. If the precontractions become frequent or continuous, the condition is called *tachycardia,* which means "rapid heart."

Tachycardia refers to a heart rate that is more rapid than is appropriate for the behavioral circumstances (e.g., a heart rate of 160 beats per minute in a resting dog). Five common causes of tachycardia are cardiac infection, drug toxicity, electrolyte imbalances, myocardial ischemia, and myocardial infarction. The tachycardias are named for the site of the pacemaker where they originate. If the tachycardia originates from an ectopic pacemaker within the atria, it is called *atrial tachycardia.* Atrial tachycardia is common in some canine breeds, including boxers and wolfhounds. If the tachycardia appears to originate from the SA node pacemaker cells, the condition is called *sinus tachycardia. Junctional tachycardias* originate from ectopic pacemakers within the AV node or first part of the AV bundle. *Supraventricular tachycardia* is a general term that encompasses sinus tachycardia, atrial tachycardia, and junctional tachycardia. If the ectopic pacemaker causing the tachycardia is within the ventricles, the condition is called *ventricular tachycardia.* In this situation, the ventricles beat at a rapid rate, as dictated by the abnormal ventricular pacemaker, whereas the atria continue to beat at the rate dictated by the normal SA node pacemaker.

An extremely rapid atrial tachycardia is called *atrial flutter.* Atrial flutter does not lead to ventricular flutter because of the long refractory period of the AV node cells. The AV node transmits some but not all of the atrial depolarizations to the ventricle. In this way, the AV node protects the ventricles from beating at too rapid a rate, even though the atria are in flutter. If atrial contractions become so rapid that they lose synchrony, the condition is called *atrial fibrillation.* This is common in certain breeds of dogs, including Dobermans. Atrial fibrillation usually does not lead to ventricular fibrillation because of the protective, long refractory period of the AV node cells.

Synchronous ventricular contractions are essential for life. If the synchronization of the ventricular contractions is disrupted and the ventricles begin to fibrillate, ventricular pumping stops. In *ventricular fibrillation,* each tiny region of the ventricular wall contracts and relaxes at random in response to action potentials that spread randomly and continuously throughout the ventricles. The condition of ventricular fibrillation is synonymous with sudden cardiac death.

Whatever the underlying cause, tachycardia is thought to be triggered either by an ectopic pacemaker or by the phenomenon of re-entry. An *ectopic pacemaker* is an area of myocardial tissue (other than the SA node) that depolarizes spontaneously to threshold and initiates a spreading cardiac action potential. *Re-entry* occurs when an area of myocardium (other than the AV node) develops the twin properties of slow conduction of action potentials and an ability to conduct action potentials in only one direction. Figure 18–11 illustrates how an area of slow, one-way conduction can initiate tachycardia. If a normally originating action potential is conducted only in one direction through the abnormal area, and if the conduction is so slow that the normal tissue is past its refractory period by the time the action potential emerges from the abnormal region, the emerging action potential can trigger another action potential in the normal tissue. If this abnormally initiated action po-

tential spreads around the cardiac chamber and back into the abnormal region, a vicious cycle can develop. The action potential is once again propagated slowly through the abnormal region, and once again it emerges from the abnormal region after the normal tissue is past its refractory period. A second *re-entrant action potential* is formed in the heart. This movement of an action potential around and around a cardiac chamber is called a *circus movement*. The tachyrhythmia that results when an action potential from an abnormal area re-enters normal tissue is called a *re-entrant arrhythmia*. In effect, an area of slow, one-way conduction within the wall of a cardiac chamber functions as an ectopic pacemaker and initiates isolated precontractions, continuous tachycardia, or fibrillation.

In most cases, ventricular fibrillation can be reversed only by electrical *defibrillation*. In this process, a strong electrical current is passed briefly through the heart muscle. This current depolarizes all of the cardiac cells simultaneously and holds them for a moment in a

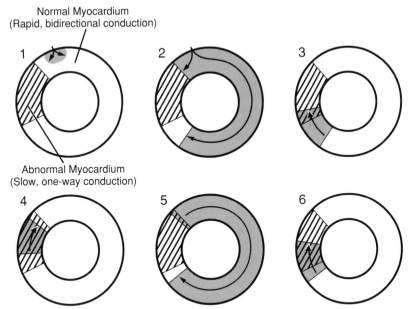

Figure 18–11. A cross section of a cardiac chamber (atrium or ventricle) is shown at six different moments in order to illustrate how reentrant arrhythmias occur. The abnormal region of the myocardium conducts action potentials slowly and only in one direction (upward in this example). *State 1:* An action potential is just entering this ring of tissue, and only the area shaded black is depolarized. *State 2:* The action potential is propagated rapidly in both directions through the normal cardiac tissue but is blocked from entering the abnormal myocardium in a counterclockwise direction. *State 3:* The clockwise-going action potential can enter the abnormal region. *State 4:* While the action potential is propagated slowly through the abnormal region, the normal cardiac tissue repolarizes to a resting state. *State 5:* The action potential emerges from the abnormal region into normal cardiac tissue and is propagated through the normal tissue for a second time. Meanwhile, the abnormal tissue repolarizes to a resting state. *State 6:* The action potential begins to move slowly through the abnormal region for a second time. Steps 4, 5, and 6 repeat themselves, so the abnormal region functions as an ectopic pacemaker.

depolarized state. When the current is turned off, it is hoped that all of the cardiac tissue will repolarize to a resting membrane potential simultaneously and that the normal pacemakers of the heart will then have a chance to initiate beats in an organized and synchronized manner once again.

Whereas ventricular fibrillation is generally lethal without electrical defibrillation, other tachycardias can be treated often by *antiarrhythmic drugs*. *Local anesthetics* (for example, lidocaine) are one category of antiarrhythmic drugs. They act by stabilizing the membrane potential of the cardiac muscle cells, particularly in cells that are tending to depolarize to threshold spontaneously. Local anesthetics partially block sodium channels in cardiac muscle cell membranes, and this counteracts membrane depolarization and action potential formation.

The *cardiac glycosides* (for example, digitalis) are another category of antiarrhythmic drugs. They slow conduction velocity through the AV node. They also increase the refractory period of AV node tissue and of ventricular cells. Cardiac glycosides act by inhibiting the sodium-potassium pump in the cell membranes.

Calcium channel blockers (e.g., verapamil) are a third category of antiarrhythmic drugs; they are especially effective for the treatment of supraventricular tachycardias. Verapamil appears to act by slowing conduction velocity through the AV node. Action potentials originated by ectopic atrial or AV node pacemakers tend to dissipate (through decremental conduction) in the slowly conducting and refractory tissue of the AV node and are not transmitted to the ventricular bundle branches.

β-*Adrenergic antagonist* drugs (for example, propranolol) are a fourth class of antirhythmics that also act by slowing conduction velocity and lengthening the refractory period of cardiac tissue. In addition, β blockers slow the spontaneous depolarization of pacemaker cells.

Electrical dysfunction of the heart has been discussed in order to illustrate that specific abnormalities in the specialized cardiac conduction system can result in specific and serious arrhythmias. Electrical dysfunction of the heart is encountered often in clinical practice, and it is often serious or even lethal in its consequences. Because electrical dysfunction is so important, the next chapter is devoted to an explanation of the *electrocardiogram (ECG)*,

which is the most commonly used technique for evaluating electrical dysfunction.

CLINICAL CORRELATION

THIRD-DEGREE ATRIOVENTRICULAR BLOCK

HISTORY □ A 5-year-old male English bulldog has fainted several times during the past 3 weeks. On each occasion he collapses, is apparently unconscious for a few seconds, and then slowly recovers. These episodes occur most often during exertion. In general, he tends to be less active than normal, but there are no other obvious signs of illness.

CLINICAL EXAMINATION □ The dog is moderately obese. There are no obvious neurological deficits. His mucous membranes appear normal; they are pink and the capillary refilling time is normal (1.5 seconds). Auscultation of the chest reveals a slow, regular heart rate of 45 beats per minute. The femoral pulse rate is also 45 per minute and strong. Thoracic radiography reveals a mildly enlarged heart, but the chest radiograph is otherwise within normal limits.

The ECG reveals a disparity between the atrial rate (atrial depolarizations occurring regularly 140 times per minute) and the ventricular rate (ventricular depolarizations occurring regularly 45 times per minute). There is no consistent time interval between the atrial and ventricular depolarizations.

COMMENT □ Voltage fluctuations are produced at the body surface by atrial and ventricular depolarizations (as explained in Chapter 19). An electrocardiograph detects these voltage changes and produces a graph of voltage as a function of time. The graph is called an electrocardiogram (ECG). The ECG of this dog shows a complete dissociation between atrial and ventricular depolarizations, and this provides definitive diagnostic evidence of complete (third-degree) AV node block. The dog's atria are depolarizing 140 times per minute in response to action potentials that are being initiated in the normal manner by pacemaker cells of the SA node. However, the atrial action potentials are not being transmitted through the AV node. Ventricular action potentials are being initiated, at the slow rate of 45 per minute, by auxilliary pacemaker cells that are located below the blocked region of the AV node.

The low ventricular rate in this dog allows a longer-than-normal time for ventricular filling between beats. Therefore, the volume of blood ejected with each beat (the stroke volume) is greater than normal. The increased stroke volume causes the femoral pulse to be very strong.

In a normal dog, heart rate is controlled by autonomic nerves acting on the SA node pacemaker cells. These nerves adjust the heart rate so that cardiac output is matched to the metabolic requirements of the body. In a dog with complete AV block, the ventricles do not respond to these autonomically mediated changes in atrial rate. Typically, the rate of ventricular contractions is abnormally low at rest and does not increase much during exercise. Therefore, cardiac output is less than normal at rest, and cardiac output does not increase enough during exertion to meet the increased metabolic needs of exercising skeletal muscle. The inadequate cardiac output results in a decrease in arterial blood pressure. In this bulldog, the decrease in arterial blood pressure during exertion causes brain blood flow to fall below the level needed to sustain consciousness. As a result, the dog faints.

TREATMENT □ Drug therapy for AV node block involves either blocking the effects of parasympathetic nerves on the AV node (with a muscarinic, cholinergic antagonist drug like atropine) or mimicking the effects of sympathetic activation (with cautious use of a β-adrenergic agonist drug like isoproterenol or dopamine). The rationale for these treatments is based on the following physiology. AV node block occurs because atrial action potentials die out in the AV node, a process called *decremental conduction.* The tendency for decremental conduction is increased by parasympathetic activation, because parasympathetic nerves act on AV node cells to increase their refractory period and to decrease the velocity with which action potentials spread from cell to cell. Therefore, blocking parasympathetic effects sometimes (but rather rarely) reverse AV node block. Sympathetic nerves decrease the refractory period of AV node cells and increase their conduction velocity. Therefore, sympathetic activation decreases the tendency for decremental conduction; a sympathomimetic drug (one that mimics the effects of sympathetic activation) has the same effect. In addition, sympathetic nerves act directly on the ventric-

ular auxiliary pacemaker cells to increase their rate. Therefore, even if a sympathomimetic drug does not unblock the AV node, it increases ventricular rate somewhat.

Many cases of third-degree AV block cannot be managed effectively with drugs, so an artificial ventricular pacemaker must be installed. A temporary pacemaker lead can be inserted into the right ventricle through the external jugular vein with only sedation and local anesthesia. This temporary pacemaker can be used to keep heart rate and cardiac output at a normal level during the induction of general anesthesia prior to surgical thoracotomy for the implantation of a permanent pacemaker on the ventricular epicardium.

Bibliography

Berne RM, Levy MN: Electrical activity of the heart. *In* Berne RM, Levy MN (eds): Cardiovascular Physiology. St. Louis, CV Mosby, 1986, p 5.

Giles WR: Intracellular electrical activity in the heart. *In* Patton HD, Fuchs AF, Hille B, et al (eds): Textbook of Physiology—Circulation, Respiration, Body Fluids, Metabolism, and Endocrinology, 21st ed. Philadelphia, WB Saunders, 1989, p 782.

Milnor WR: Properties of cardiac cells. *In* Cardiovascular Physiology. New York, Oxford University Press, 1990, p 62.

Noble D: The Initiation of the Heartbeat. New York, Oxford University Press, 1979.

PRACTICE QUESTIONS FOR CHAPTER 18

1. An increase in heart rate could result from

   a. an increase in sympathetic nerve activity to the heart.
   b. an abnormally rapid decrease in permeability of SA node cells to K^+ during diastole.
   c. an elevated body temperature.
   d. a decrease in parasympathetic nerve activity to the heart.
   e. All of the above

2. In which of the following arrhythmias will there be more atrial beats per minute than ventricular beats?

   a. Complete (third-degree) AV block
   b. Frequent premature ventricular contractions

   c. Sick sinus syndrome (sinus bradycardia)
   d. First-degree AV block
   e. Ventricular tachycardia

3. The normal pathway followed by a cardiac action potential is to begin in the SA node and then spread

   a. across the atria in the bundle of His.
   b. through the connective tissue layers that separate the atria and ventricles.
   c. across the atria and to the AV node.
   d. from the left atrium to the right atrium.
   e. from the left atrium to the left ventricle and from the right atrium to the right ventricle.

4. Which statement is true?

   a. The refractory period of cardiac muscle cells is much shorter than their mechanical contraction.
   b. The cardiac action potential is propagated from one cardiac cell to another through nexi or gap junctions.
   c. Purkinje's fibers are special nerves that spread the cardiac action potential rapidly through the ventricles.
   d. Ventricular muscle cells characteristically depolarize spontaneously to threshold.
   e. The permeability of ventricular muscle cells to Ca^{2+} is lower during the plateau of an action potential than it is at rest.

5. The pacemaker cells of the SA node characteristically

   a. exhibit pacemaker potentials instead of action potentials.
   b. increase their rate of spontaneous depolarization when acetylcholine is present.
   c. exhibit a spontaneous decrease in their permeability to K^+.
   d. have longer action potential plateaus than ventricular cells.
   e. depolarize to threshold as a result of the blockage of Ca^{2+} channels.

19

The Electrocardiogram

1. An electrocardiogram is simply a voltmeter that makes plots of voltage as a function of time
2. Atrial depolarization, ventricular depolarization, and ventricular repolarization cause characteristic voltage deflections in the electrocardiogram
3. Abnormal voltages in the electrocardiogram are indicative of cardiac structural or electrical abnormalities
4. Electrical dysfunctions in the heart cause abnormal patterns of electrocardiogram waves

An Electrocardiogram Is Simply a Voltmeter That Makes Plots of Voltage as a Function of Time

The *electrocardiogram (ECG)* is the most commonly used clinical tool for diagnosing electrical dysfunctions of the heart. In its most common application, two or more metal electrodes are applied to the skin surface, and the voltages recorded by the electrodes are beamed onto an oscilloscope screen or drawn onto a paper strip. How the heart produces detectable voltages at the body surface is extraordinarily complex. However, one can use elementary physical principles to develop an intuitive model of how the ECG works; this intuitive model is adequate for most clinical applications.

The development of this picture begins with the idea of an *electrical dipole* in a conductive medium (Fig. 19–1). A dipole is a pair of electrical charges (a plus charge and a minus charge) separated by a distance. A common flashlight battery is a good example of a dipole. A battery has a positive end (where excess

positive charges are) and a negative end (where excess negative charges are), and the two ends are separated by a distance. If such a dipole is placed within a conductive medium (for example, in a basin filled with sodium chloride solution), ionic currents flow through the solution. Positive ions flow in the solution from the positive end of the dipole toward the negative end, and vice versa. The flow of ions creates voltage differences within the salt solution. These voltage differences can be detected by placing the electrodes of a voltmeter at the perimeter of the salt solution. In Figure 19–1, an electrode placed at point A would measure a more positive voltage than an electrode placed at point B. There is a positive voltage at point A with respect to point B; equivalently, there is a positive voltage difference between point A and point B. Point C and point D are equally near the positive and negative ends of the dipole, so no voltage difference would exist between electrodes placed at points C and D.

In Figure 19–2, the battery in the basin of saline has been replaced with a single, elon-

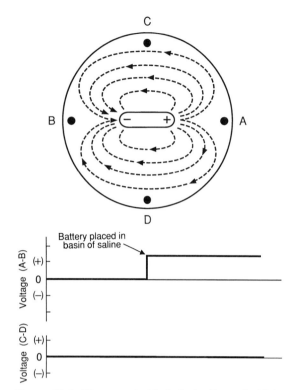

Figure 19–1. When an electrical dipole (like a flashlight battery) is placed into a conductive medium (like a basin of salt water), the flow of ionic currents creates voltage differences within the electrolyte solution. A simple voltmeter can be used to detect these voltage differences. In this example, point A will be positive with respect to point B (i.e., voltage A-B will be positive). No voltage difference will exist between point C and point D (i.e., voltage C-D will be zero).

gated cardiac muscle cell. The voltages detected at point A with respect to point B, and at point C with respect to point D, are plotted for five different conditions. In condition 1, the cell is at a resting membrane potential. The resting cell is charged negatively on the inside and positively on the outside, all around its perimeter. From the outside, the cell does not look like a dipole, because it is symmetrically charged around its perimeter. Therefore, the voltage difference between point A and point B would be zero. The voltage difference between point C and point D would also be zero.

In condition 2, an action potential has formed at the left end of the cell and is spreading toward the right end of the cell. That is, the left end of the cell is depolarized and is at the plateau of its action potential; the right end of the cell is still at a resting membrane potential. Under these conditions, the cell forms an electrical dipole, with the outside of the cell charged positively at the right end

and negatively at the left end. Therefore, a positive voltage would exist at point A with respect to point B. However, the voltage at point C with respect to point D would still be zero, because neither point is closer to the positive end of the cell than the negative end of the cell.

In condition 3, the entire cell is depolarized. That is, the entire cell is at the plateau of its action potential, so no voltage differences exist around the perimeter of the cell. Therefore, the recorded voltages are zero.

In condition 4, the cell is pictured as repolarizing; the left end of the cell has returned to a resting state and the right end of the cell is still at the plateau of its action potential. Under these conditions, the voltage at point A is negative with respect to point B, because the outside of the cell is charged negatively at its right end and positively at its left end. However, the voltage at point C with respect to point D is still zero.

In condition 5, the entire cell has returned to a resting state, so the voltage at point A with respect to point B is again zero. Note that points C and D "see the same electrical

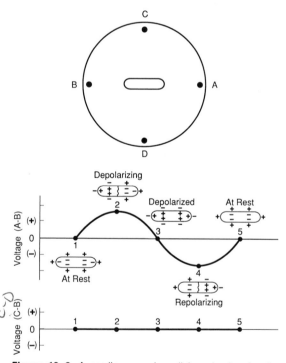

Figure 19–2. A cardiac muscle cell in a basin of saline would produce voltage differences between point A and point B during a phase of spreading depolarization or spreading repolarization but not when the whole cell is in a uniform state of polarization. No voltage difference is created between point C and point D.

view" throughout both the depolarization and repolarization of the cell, so the voltage at point C with respect to point D remains at zero. Also, note that if the repolarization (condition 4) had spread from right to left in the cell (instead of from left to right), the voltage at point A with respect to point B would remain positive.

Figure 19–3 takes the development of the ECG one step further by picturing the entire heart (rather than a single cardiac muscle cell) placed within the basin of saline. This is not a large conceptual step, because the heart is a functional syncytium and acts like one big cell. The graphs below the drawing show the voltages that would be detected by electrodes at the perimeter of the basin during atrial depolarization. The plots start at a time between

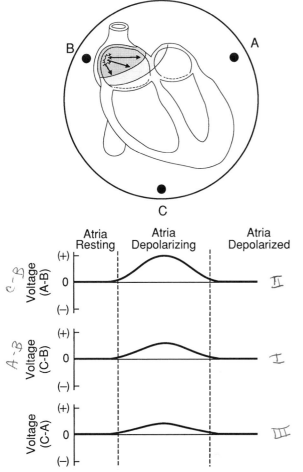

Figure 19–3. A resting heart, placed in a basin of saline, would not create voltage differences between electrodes A, B, and C. However, during depolarization of the atria, positive voltage differences would be created between points A and B, points C and B, and points C and A.

cardiac contractions, when the entire heart is at a resting membrane condition. Every cardiac cell is charged negatively on the inside of its membrane and positively on the outside. Therefore, the entire heart, viewed as one big cell, would carry a positive charge all the way around it, and there would be no voltage differences between any of the electrodes. When the cells in the sinoatrial (SA) node depolarize to threshold, they initiate an action potential that spreads outward from the SA node. As indicated by the arrows in the diagram, the action potential spreads downward in the right atrium and also across the right atrium toward the left atrium. During this atrial depolarization, the right atrial cells near the SA node become charged negatively on the outside, whereas the cells in the left atrium and the cells in the inferior part of the right atrium, which have not yet depolarized, remain positive on the outside. Therefore, the depolarizing atria create an electrical dipole that is angled downward and toward the left atrium. Because the left atrium is positive with respect to the right atrium, a voltage is created at point A that is positive with respect to point B. Because the inferior parts of the atria are positive with respect to the superior parts, the voltage at point C is also positive with respect to point B, as is the voltage difference between points C and A. These voltage differences are shown in the graphs. Once the atria are depolarized (that is, once every atrial cell is at the plateau of its action potential), the voltage differences in all leads return to zero.

Atrial Depolarization, Ventricular Depolarization, and Ventricular Repolarization Cause Characteristic Voltage Deflections in the Electrocardiogram

In Figure 19–4, the heart is pictured in its normal position in the thorax of a dog. The extracellular fluids of the body contain sodium chloride in solution, so the body can be imagined to be a substitute for the basin of saline that was shown in the previous figures. The positions of the left forelimb, right forelimb, and left hindlimb in Figure 19–4 correspond with points A, B, and C in Figure 19–3. Condition a in Figure 19–4 shows that atrial depolarization would cause a positive voltage in the left forelimb with respect to the right forelimb. This is simply a repetition of the idea that is illustrated in Figure 19–3, with the left

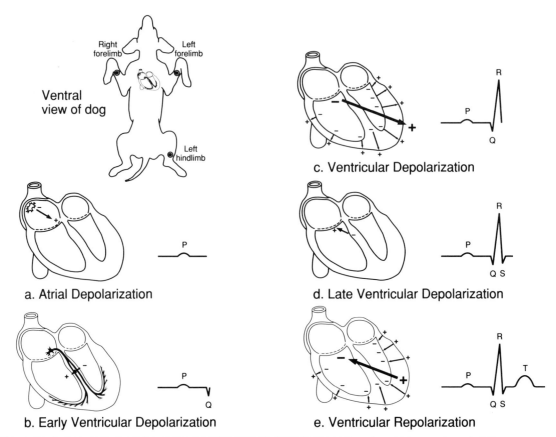

Figure 19–4. As a normal cardiac action potential spreads through the atria and ventricles, a characteristic sequence of voltage differences is created between the left forelimb (analogous to point A in Figure 19–3) and the right forelimb (analogous to point B in Figure 19–3). See text for a complete description.

forelimb being equivalent to point A and the right forelimb being equivalent to point B.

The deflection in the ECG trace during atrial depolarization is called the *P-wave*. At the end of atrial depolarization (that is, at the end of the P-wave) the ECG voltage returns to zero. At this moment during the actual cardiac cycle, the action potential is spreading through the atrioventricular (AV) node and the first part of the AV bundle. These tissues are so small that they generally do not create a detectable voltage difference at the body surface.

The next voltage differences that are detectable at the body surface are those associated with the depolarization of the ventricles. The first part of this event is usually a depolarization spreading from left to right across the interventricular septum, as shown in condition b. This first phase of ventricular depolarization usually causes a small voltage difference *(Q-wave)* between the left forelimb and the right forelimb, with the left forelimb being slightly negative with respect to the right.

The next event in ventricular depolarization usually causes a large, positive voltage at the left forelimb, with respect to the right, and this is shown in condition c. To understand why this *R-wave* is large and positive, recall that during ventricular depolarization, the left and right bundle branches bring the spreading action potential to the ventricular apex. From there, Purkinje's fibers carry the action potential rapidly up the inside walls of both ventricles. Then, the depolarization spreads outward through the walls of both ventricles, as pictured by the small arrows in the drawing of condition c. Each small arrow can be considered to be a dipole, with its positive end at the outside wall of the ventricle (because the inside surfaces of the ventricles depolarize before the outside surfaces). The *net* electrical effect of these action potentials spreading outward through the walls of both ventricles is a large electrical dipole pointed diagonally downward (caudad) and toward the dog's left.

The *net dipole* points toward the left for two

reasons. First, the cardiac axis is tilted toward the left (that is, the normal orientation in the heart is with the ventricular apex angled toward the left wall of the thorax). Second, the left ventricle is much more massive than the right ventricle, so the action potentials spreading outward in the wall of the left ventricle dominate electrically over the action potentials spreading outward in the wall of the right ventricle. The resulting large, positive R-wave is the predominant feature of a normal ECG. Abnormalities in the magnitude or polarity of the R-wave have great diagnostic significance, which is explained later.

After the cardiac action potential has spread outward through the walls of both ventricles, the voltage difference seen at the body surface returns to zero. Then, at the end of ventricular depolarization, there is sometimes a brief, small, negative voltage in the left forearm with respect to the right forearm, as shown in condition d. The physical basis of this small *S-wave* is obscure.

Altogether, the process of *ventricular depolarization* produces a pattern of voltages in the ECG called the *QRS-wave* (or *QRS-complex*). Condition e shows the electrical events during repolarization of the ventricles. Whereas the wave of *depolarization* spreads outward through the walls of both ventricles, the wave of *repolarization* usually spreads inward. That is, the outside surface of the ventricles is the last ventricular tissue to depolarize but the first to repolarize. Stated another way, cardiac muscle cells near the outside surfaces of the ventricles characteristically have shorter action potentials than do cells on the inside surfaces of the ventricles. The inward-going repolarization creates a net dipole with its negative end pointed upward (craniad) and toward the right. Therefore, *ventricular repolarization* creates a positive voltage in the left forelimb with respect to the right forelimb. The resulting positive-going wave in the ECG is called the *T-wave*.

The opposite directions of ventricular depolarization and repolarization make sense if one considers that depolarization leads to contraction in cardiac muscle and repolarization leads to relaxation. In order to create a contraction that pumps blood effectively, it is appropriate for the interior wall of both ventricles (the *subendocardium*) to begin contracting first. Then, the outer layer of the ventricles (the *subepicardium*) squeezes down on the already contracting interior layers. If the order were reversed, the exterior walls of the ven-

tricles would be contracting and squeezing on subendocardial muscle that is still relaxed and, therefore, not participating in pumping. Conversely, it is appropriate for ventricular relaxation to occur first in the outer layers and last in the inner layers. Thus, it makes sense that the outer layers of ventricular tissue are the last to depolarize and the first to repolarize.

To summarize, the P-wave is caused by atrial depolarization, the QRS-complex by ventricular depolarization, and the T-wave by ventricular repolarization. There is not a wave in the normal ECG that corresponds to atrial repolarization, because atrial repolarization does not proceed in an orderly enough pattern or direction to create a net electrical dipole. The pattern of ventricular repolarization varies from dog to dog, and it is not uncommon for the T-wave to be negative.

Because the predominant waves in an ECG correspond to specific electrical events in the heart, the time between these waves can be measured to determine the timing of events in the heart. Figure 19–5 identifies the important intervals and segments in the ECG. The *P-R interval* corresponds to the time between atrial depolarization and ventricular depolarization. This delay is introduced by slow conduction of the cardiac action potential through the AV node and is typically about 0.1 second. The duration of the *QRS-complex* corresponds to the time it takes for ventricular depolarization to occur, once the cardiac action potential emerges from the AV node and AV bundle. Typically, this is less than 0.1 second. The *Q-T interval* corresponds to the length of time that the ventricles remain depolarized (i.e., the length of the action potential in ventricular tissue). Typically, the Q-T interval is about 0.2 second. The time between successive P-waves *(P-P interval)* corresponds to the time between atrial contractions. The P-P interval can be used to calculate the number of atrial contractions per minute (the atrial rate), as illustrated in the figure. Likewise, the time between successive R-waves *(R-R interval)* corresponds to the time between ventricular contractions, so R-R interval can be used to calculate ventricular rate.

Figure 19–6 shows actual ECG records obtained from a normal dog. To obtain these recordings, electrodes were placed on the left forelimb, right forelimb, and left hindlimb. Electrodes on these limbs are usually envisioned as forming a triangle around the heart (just as electrodes at points A, B, and C form a triangle around the heart in Figure 19–3).

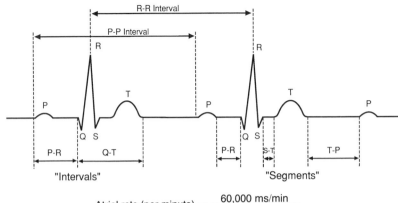

Figure 19–5. The time between various waves of the ECG corresponds to the timing of specific events in the heart. See text for a complete description. The equations show how atrial rate and ventricular rate can be calculated from the P-P and R-R intervals, respectively. Of course, in a normally functioning heart, atrial rate = ventricular rate = heart rate.

$$\text{Atrial rate (per minute)} = \frac{60{,}000 \text{ ms/min}}{\text{P-P Interval (in ms)}}$$

$$\text{Ventricular rate (per minute)} = \frac{60{,}000 \text{ ms/min}}{\text{R-R interval (in ms)}}$$

The various ECG traces in Figure 19–6 were obtained by interconnecting these electrodes in standardized combinations, as shown in the figure insert. These standardized interconnections were prescribed by Eintoven, inventor of the ECG. The voltage difference recorded between electrodes on the left forelimb and right forelimb is called *lead I* (first trace in figure). Note the presence of distinct P-, QRS-, and T-waves in this trace.

A similar pattern of voltage is measured typically between electrodes placed on the left hindlimb and right forelimb. This electrode configuration is called *lead II* (top middle trace in the figure). The *lead III* ECG (top right trace in the figure) shows the voltage difference

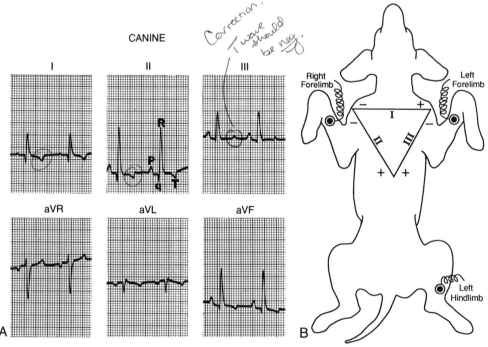

Figure 19–6. *(A)* ECG from a normal dog. *(B)* The usual convention for interconnecting the three limb electrodes to obtain lead I, lead II, and lead III ECGs. See text for additional explanation. (Reprinted with permission from Tilley LP: Essentials of Canine and Feline Electrocardiology: Interpretation and Treatment, 2nd ed. Philadelphia, Lea & Febiger, 1985.)

recorded between the left hindlimb and left forelimb. Leads I, II, and III provide different electrical views of the heart. Three additional views are provided by the *augmented unipolar limb leads* (aV_R, aV_L, and aV_F). Lead aV_R measures the voltage from the right forelimb electrode with respect to the average voltage from the other two limb electrodes. Similarly, aV_L and aV_F measure the voltages from the left forelimb and left hindlimb electrodes with respect to the average voltage from the other two electrodes. To make it easy to measure the intervals on an ECG, two standard chart speeds are used, whereby either five or ten major divisions equal one second. To make it easy to measure voltages on an ECG, a standard vertical calibration is used, whereby two major divisions equal 1 mV.

Leads I, II, and III are used routinely in veterinary electrocardiography. The augmented unipolar limb leads (aV_L, aV_R, and aV_F) are used less commonly. Occasionally, ECG electrodes are positioned at standardized sites on the thorax to aid in the evaluation of specific cardiac electrical dysfunctions. These *precordid (chest) leads* are used more commonly in human medicine than in veterinary medicine.

Abnormal Voltages in the Electrocardiogram Are Indicative of Cardiac Structural or Electrical Abnormalities

The ECG in Figure 19–7 was obtained from a dog with right ventricular hypertrophy. Note that the atrial and ventricular rates are about 100 beats per minute, and the sequence of waves in the ECG appears to be normal. That is, each heart beat begins with an upward-going P-wave, which is followed by a QRS-complex and a positive T-wave. However, the predominant polarity in the QRS-complex in lead I is negative instead of positive. Recall that the QRS-complex is caused by ventricular depolarization, and that its dominant feature is normally a large, positive R-wave. The R-wave is normally positive in lead I, because the cardiac axis is normally angled to the left side of the thorax and because the left ventricular wall is much more massive than the right ventricular wall. Therefore, reversal of this polarity suggests that the cardiac axis has shifted to the right, that the mass of the right ventricle has increased, or both. The abnormally high voltages of the QRS-complex in

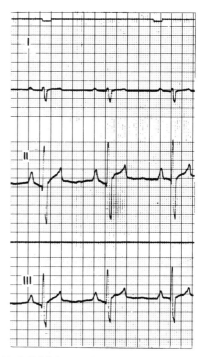

Figure 19–7. ECG from a dog with right ventricular hypertrophy. The paper speed is 50 mm/second, so 10 major grid divisions equals 1 second. The P-P and R-R intervals are both 0.6 seconds, so atrial and ventricular rates are both 100 per minute. The salient abnormalities are (1) predominantly negative QRS complexes in lead I and (2) large amplitude of QRS complexes in leads II and III. (From Ettinger SJ: Textbook of Veterinary Internal Medicine, 3rd ed. Philadelphia, WB Saunders, 1989, p 981.)

leads II and III are indicative also of ventricular hypertrophy. Right ventricular hypertrophy is a common consequence of cardiac defects that increase either the volume of blood that must be pumped by the right ventricle or the pressure that must be generated within the right ventricle during its contractions. Examples include pulmonic stenosis, patent ductus arteriosus, and ventricular septal defect (these are discussed in Chapter 20).

The ECG voltages are also sometimes abnormally low. One common cause of low voltage ECGs is an accumulation of fluid in the pericardium. This condition is called *cardiac tamponade*. In a sense, the pericardial fluid creates a short-circuit for ionic currents, so that less current flows outward toward the body surface. Therefore, the ECG voltages at the body surface are smaller than normal.

The ECG in Figure 19–8 looks normal in all respects except that there is an upward shift of the S-T segment compared with the rest of the ECG. An S-T segment shift is often indic-

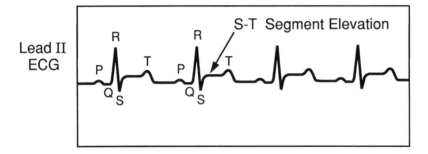

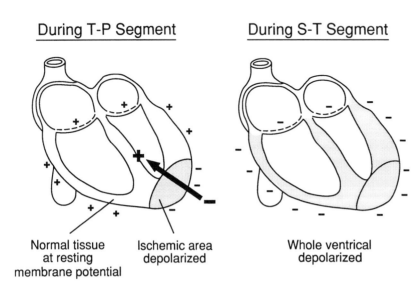

During T-P Segment

Normal tissue at resting membrane potential

Ischemic area depolarized

During S-T Segment

Whole ventrical depolarized

Figure 19–8. The voltage recorded during the S-T segment is elevated, compared to the baseline (T-P segment), in this lead II ECG from a dog with an inferior (caudal) ventricular infarct. The drawings show why an ischemic or infarcted area of ventricle creates a net electrical dipole in the resting ventricle (left) but not in the depolarized ventricle (right).

ative of an area of ischemic or infarcted ventricular tissue. As shown in the figure, the ischemic area does not maintain a normal resting membrane potential. Therefore, in between ventricular contractions (when ventricular cells are at rest), the ischemic area is depolarized compared with the normal tissue. This creates an electrical dipole within the resting ventricle. In the case shown here, the ischemic area is in the inferior (caudal) part of the ventricles, so a negative voltage is observed in lead II during ventricular rest (T-P segment). During the S-T segment, the entire ventricle, including the ischemic area, is depolarized, so there is not a strong dipole between the injured area and the normal area. Therefore, the ECG voltage during the S-T segment is close to a true zero level. However, the S-T segment is elevated compared to the more negative voltage during ventricular rest. *S-T segment elevation* (which is actually T-P segment depression) is indicative of an ischemic or infarcted area in the inferior (caudal) part of the ventricle. Ischemia or infarction in the anterior (cranial) ventricular area would cause *S-T segment depression*.

Making a diagnosis on the basis of abnormal ECG voltage alone is risky. Theoretically, if the structural and electrical properties of a particular heart are known, the appearance of the ECG can be predicted with certainty. However, the reverse situation is not strictly true. A given voltage abnormality in an ECG cannot be ascribed with certainty to a particular cardiac defect, because several defects may result in similar voltage abnormalities. However, in conjunction with other clinical data, ECG abnormalities are strongly indicative of specific structural or electrical abnormalities in the heart.

Electrical Dysfunctions in the Heart Cause Abnormal Patterns of Electrocardiogram Waves

Figure 19–9 shows an ECG from a dog with a premature ventricular contraction. This lead I strip begins with five normal beats (each QRS-complex is preceded by a P-wave and followed by a T-wave). The P-waves are evenly spaced, with a P-P interval of 0.5 second (heart

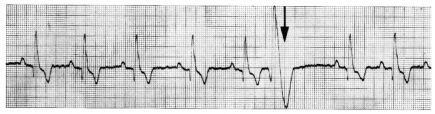

Figure 19–9. Lead I ECG of dog showing five normal beats followed by one premature ventricular beat. A sixth P-wave would be expected at the time marked by the arrow. This P-wave is obscured by the large voltages associated with the premature ventricular beat. Also, the refractory period associated with the premature beat prevented the sixth normal ventricular beat from occurring; this creates a long pause (called the *compensatory pause*) between the premature beat and the next regular beat. (From Ettinger SJ: Textbook of Veterinary Internal Medicine, 3rd ed. Philadelphia, WB Saunders, 1989.)

rate = 120 beats per minute). After five normal beats, a large voltage complex of abnormal shape occurs without a preceding P-wave. This is indicative of a premature ventricular depolarization, because electrical activity in the atria could not possibly produce such large voltage deflections. The positive polarity of the large premature R-wave in this lead I ECG indicates that the ventricular depolarization spreads predominantly from right to left in the ventricles. The abnormal shape and long duration of the premature QRS complex indicate that the premature action potential did not spread across the ventricles by way of the rapidly conducting bundle branches. Instead, the ventricular depolarization must have spread through more slowly conducting pathways. That is, the ectopic site that originated these beats was not within the AV bundle or in the normal bundle branches. The abnormally large T-wave associated with the premature beat further emphasizes the abnormal

pattern of spread of the premature action potential across the ventricles.

Had the premature beat originated from an ectopic pacemaker within the AV bundle or bundle branches, the pattern of ventricular depolarization and the pattern of ventricular repolarization would have been normal in appearance. That is, the QRS-complex and the T-wave of the premature beat would have looked like the other QRS- and T-waves. They would simply have occurred earlier than expected and would not be preceded by a P-wave. Note that in the case of a premature atrial contraction, the QRS-complex and T-wave would be expected to have a normal size and shape, because normal ventricular pathways would be involved in ventricular depolarization and repolarization.

The ECGs in Figure 19–10 show additional examples of cardiac electrical dysfunction. The ECG in Figure 19–10A was recorded from a resting dog. The R-waves are spaced regularly

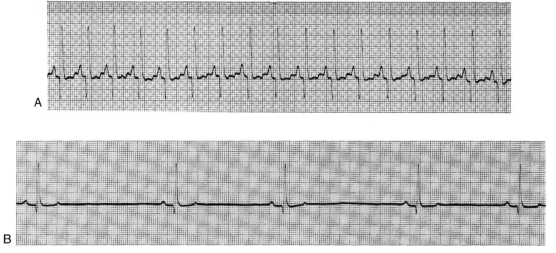

Figure 19–10. Sinus tachycardia *(A)* and sinus bradycardia *(B)* are evident in these otherwise normal ECGs from two resting dogs. (From Ettinger SJ: Textbook of Veterinary Internal Medicine, 3rd ed. Philadelphia, WB Saunders, 1989.)

and indicate a ventricular rate of 235 beats per minute. This is fast for a resting dog. However, the pattern of ECG waves appears to be normal. That is, each QRS-complex is preceded by a clear, positive P-wave and is followed by a positive T-wave (which overlaps the next P-wave). Therefore, the most likely diagnosis is *sinus tachycardia* (rapid heart rate initiated by SA node pacemakers). Figure 19–10B shows the opposite extreme. The pattern of ECG waves is normal, but the heart rate is only 55 beats per minute. The diagnosis is *sinus bradycardia* (the SA node is the pacemaker, but its rate is slow).

The ECG provides an easy way to diagnose AV node block. The ECG in Figure 19–11A looks normal, except that there is an abnormally long P-R interval, suggesting an abnormally long delay in the propagation of the action potential through the AV node and AV bundle. This would be indicative of *first-degree AV block*. In Figure 19–11B, the P-wave spacing indicates an atrial rate of 123 beats per minute.

Four of the P-waves are followed by QRS-complexes and large, negative T-waves, but the other seven P-waves are not followed by QRS-complexes. The ECG indicates that some, but not all, atrial depolarizations are transmitted through the AV node. Therefore, the condition is second-degree AV block. Second-degree AV block is not life-threatening unless there are so many missed ventricular beats that cardiac output falls to dangerously low levels.

Figure 19–11C shows an example of third-degree (complete) AV node block. Two large QRS-complexes are visible, followed by negative T-waves. (The S-T segments are depressed.) The R-R interval is about 2.9 seconds, indicating that the ventricular rate is only 21 beats per minute. The QRS-complexes are not preceded by P-waves. Small, positive P-waves are present, indicating an atrial rate of 142 beats per minute, but there is no synchronization between the P-waves and the QRS-complexes. Apparently, atrial action po-

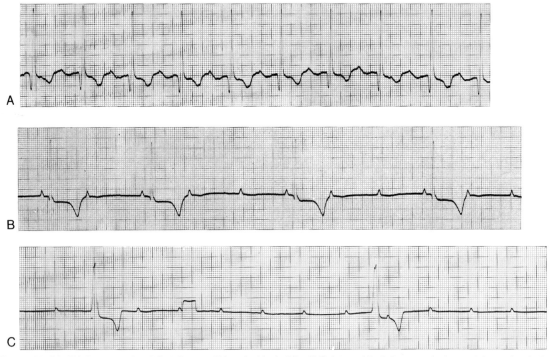

Figure 19–11. *(A)* An example of first-degree AV node block. The P-R interval is 0.2 seconds (normal for a dog is less than 0.14 seconds). The heart rate is 120 beats per minute. Each QRS complex is preceded by a positive P-wave and followed by a negative T-wave. *(B)* An example of second-degree AV node block. The small, positive deflections are P-waves. The broad, negative deflections are T-waves, which follow the faintly visible QRS complexes. Where P-waves are followed by QRS complexes, the P-R interval is normal. However, only every second or third P-wave is followed by a QRS complex. That is, there are two or three atrial beats for every ventricular beat. *(C)* An example of third-degree (complete) AV node block. The positive P-waves are regularly spaced (two of them are obscured by the large ventricular complexes). The rectangular deflection one third of the way through the record is a voltage calibration signal. (From Ettinger SJ: Textbook of Veterinary Internal Medicine, 3rd ed. Philadelphia, WB Saunders, 1989.)

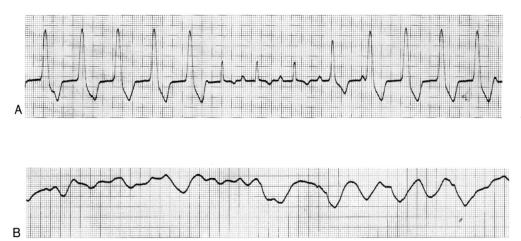

Figure 19–12. *(A)* An example of ventricular tachycardia, which reverts briefly to a sinus rhythm. The ventricular rate is about 165 beats per minute. This pattern would be typical for a dog with an ectopic ventricular pacemaker running at almost the same rate as the SA node pacemaker; some ventricular beats would be initiated by the ectopic pacemaker and others would be initiated in the normal way through the AV node. *(B)* An example of ventricular fibrillation. Whether the atria are fibrillating is not apparent; the random voltage fluctuations generated by the fibrillating ventricles would obscure any P-waves that might be present. (From Ettinger SJ: Textbook of Veterinary Internal Medicine, 3rd ed. Philadelphia, WB Saunders, 1989.)

tentials are being blocked at the AV node. The ventricles are beating slowly in response to an auxiliary pacemaker in the AV node or in the bundle of His.

Figure 19–12 shows an ECG record of a dog that is drifting in and out of ventricular tachycardia. The first five waves are abnormally shaped ventricular complexes, indicative of an ectopic ventricular pacemaker located outside of the normal ventricular conduction system. No P-waves are observed. Then, there are three normal-appearing QRS-T sequences, with preceding P-waves, suggesting that a normal rhythm is being established. However,

the ectopic ventricular pacemaker regains control, and ventricular tachycardia returns.

Ventricular tachycardia degenerates frequently into ventricular fibrillation. Figure 19–12B shows an ECG indicative of ventricular fibrillation. The record shows irregular voltage fluctuations with no discernible pattern. The atria may or may not be fibrillating. It is possible that regularly occurring P-waves are present but are obscured by the random electrical activity in the ventricles. However, ventricular fibrillation stops the heart from pumping blood, whether or not the atria continue to contract in a synchronized fashion.

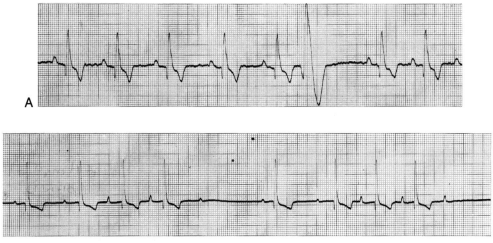

Figure 19–13. Lead I ECG records from two dogs. *A* is the basis for Practice Question #4. *B* is the basis for Practice Question #5. (From Ettinger SJ: Textbook of Veterinary Internal Medicine, 3rd ed. Philadelphia, WB Saunders, 1989.)

Very sophisticated techniques are available for the analysis of ECGs, and these are widely used in human medicine and in many veterinary clinics. The purpose in this section is to introduce only enough complexity to illustrate the usefulness of the ECG in the diagnosis of cardiac abnormalities. In addition, this discussion of the ECG is also intended to reinforce the student's understanding of electrical dysfunction of the heart.

CLINICAL CORRELATION

DILATIVE CARDIOMYOPATHY WITH PAROXYSMAL ATRIAL TACHYCARDIA

HISTORY ☐ The owner of a 5-year-old male Saint Bernard brings the dog to you because of a distended abdomen, weakness, coughing, and difficulty breathing. The owner believes these signs developed gradually over a period of several weeks; however, there were occasional episodes when the dog suddenly seemed weak and listless.

CLINICAL EXAMINATION ☐ Palpation reveals that the dog has muscle wasting and a fluid-filled abdomen. The jugular veins are distended. The arterial pulse is rapid and irregular. There are frequent pulse deficits (missing beats). Thoracic radiography reveals an enlarged heart and an accumulation of fluid near the lung hilus.

You record the dog's ECG for several minutes. The ECG shows that P-waves usually occur at a rate of 160–170 per minute; each P-wave is followed by a QRS-T complex. However, the ECG also shows frequent episodes when there are 210–230 P-waves per minute. During these episodes, most P-waves are followed by QRS-T complexes, but others are not. As a result, the QRS-T complexes occur irregularly, and there are only about 180 of them per minute.

Echocardiography reveals severe dilation of all four cardiac chambers, particularly the atria. The ventricular contractions are weak.

COMMENT ☐ The ECG indicates that this dog has atrial tachycardia. One cannot tell from the information presented whether the atrial pacemaker is located in the SA node or somewhere else in the atria. It is likely that one atrial pacemaker area is initiating depolarizations at

a rate of 160–170 per minute and that another atrial area intermittently pre-empts the first pacemaker by initiating depolarizations at the more rapid rate of 210–230 per minute. When the atrial rate is 160–170 per minute, the AV node transmits every atrial action potential to the ventricles, so the ventricles also contract 160–170 times per minute. However, when the atrial rate is 210–230 per minute, some of the atrial action potentials arrive at the AV node when the nodal cells are still refractory from the preceding action potential. These atrial action potentials are not transmitted into the ventricles. As a result, there are only about 180 ventricular contractions per minute. This is a case where a second-degree AV node block, created by the relatively long refractory period of AV node cells, is beneficial, because it prevents the ventricles from beating too rapidly. As the frequency of ventricular contractions increases, the time available between contractions for ventricular refilling becomes shorter and shorter. As a result, the volume of blood pumped with each beat (stroke volume) decreases, and so does cardiac output. At ventricular rates above 180 per minute, the cardiac output could fall to such a low level that the dog would collapse.

This dog's primary problem is probably a chronic, progressive weakening of his heart muscle *(cardiomyopathy)*. All the clinical signs, including atrial tachycardia, can be attributed to a primary cardiomyopathy. Dilative cardiomyopathy is common in giant-breed dogs, especially males, and often (as in this case) there is no discernible cause. Even though the cause of the cardiomyopathy could not be determined from the evidence available in this case, the sequence of dysfunctions that resulted from the cardiomyopathy can be inferred with near certainty.

Ventricular weakness (heart failure) caused cardiac output to fall below normal, especially during exercise. The dog's body attempted to compensate for the heart failure by increasing blood volume, which increased both venous and atrial pressures far above normal. The elevated atrial pressure had the beneficial effect of "supercharging" the ventricles with an extra volume of blood before each contraction, which partially returns stroke volume toward normal. However, the excessive volume and pressure of blood in the veins caused pulmonary edema (which led to coughing and difficulty breathing) and systemic edema (which led to abdominal distension). Also, distension of the atria made the atrial cells more excitable electrically. This resulted in the formation of ectopic pacemakers and the onset of atrial tachycardia. The tachycardia limited ventricular refilling time, which brought about a further compromise in cardiac output. A serious vicious cycle began in which decreased cardiac output caused further venous congestion and atrial distension, which aggravated the arrhythmia, and so forth. The prognosis is poor without treatment.

This case of heart failure provides a good preview for the next several chapters, which deal in detail with the physiological mechanisms of cardiac and vascular control in both normal and heart failure states.

TREATMENT □ A diuretic drug (e.g., furosemide) is administered to promote an increase in urine formation. The goal is to reduce blood volume and venous and atrial pressures. This reduces the signs resulting from congestion and edema. Sometimes the paroxysmal atrial tachycardia resolves following diuretic-induced reductions in atrial size. If not, antiarrhythmic drugs (e.g., quinidine, a cardiac glycoside) can be used to try to reduce the electrical excitability of atrial tissue.

Bibliography

Berne RM, Levy MN: Electrical activity of the heart. *In* Berne RM, Levy MN (eds): Cardiovascular Physiology. St. Louis, CV Mosby, 1986, p 5.

Ettinger SJ: Cardiac arrhythmias. *In* Ettinger SJ (ed): Textbook of Veterinary Internal Medicine—Diseases of the Dog and Cat, Vol 1, 3rd ed. Philadelphia, WB Saunders, 1989, p 76.

Hilwig RW: CArdiac arrhythmias. *In* Robinson NE (ed): Current Therapy in Equine Medicine. Philadelphia, WB Saunders, 1987, p 154.

Katz AM: Physiology of the Heart. New York, Raven Press, 1977.

Miller MS, Tilley LP: Electrocardiography. *In* Fox PR (ed): Canine and Feline Cardiology. New York, Churchill Livingstone, 1988, p 43.

Milnor WR: The electrical activity of the heart. *In* Cardiovascular Physiology. New York, Oxford University Press, 1990, p 140.

Noble D: The Initiation of the Heartbeat, 2nd ed. Clarendon Press, 1979.

Scher AM: The electrocardiogram. *In* Patton HD, Fuchs AF, Hille B, et al (eds): Textbook of Physiology—Circulation, Respiration, Body Fluids, Metabolism, and Endocrinology, 21st ed. Philadelphia, WB Saunders, 1989, p 796.

PRACTICE QUESTIONS FOR CHAPTER 19

1. In which of the following arrhythmias will the ECG characteristically show the *same number* of P-waves and QRS-complexes?

   a. Complete (third-degree) AV block
   b. First-degree AV block
   c. Ventricular tachycardia
   d. Atrial flutter
   e. All of the above

2. The time required for the conduction of the cardiac action potential through the AV node would be approximately equal to the

   a. R-R interval.
   b. P-R interval.
   c. S-T interval.
   d. P-P interval.
   e. Q-T interval.

3. The T-wave in a normal ECG represents

   a. atrial depolarization.
   b. atrial repolarization.
   c. the pacemaker potential.
   d. ventricular depolarization.
   e. ventricular repolarization.

4. The ECG in Figure 19–13A indicates

   a. sinus arrhythmia.
   b. right ventricular hypertrophy.
   c. S-T segment elevation.
   d. premature ventricular contraction.
   e. atrial fibrillation.

5. The ECG in Figure 19–13B indicates

   a. second-degree AV block.
   b. third-degree AV block.
   c. sinus bradycardia.
   d. ventricular tachycardia.
   e. ST segment elevation.

20

The Heart as a Pump

1. Each heartbeat is made up of ventricular systole and diastole
2. Cardiac output equals heart rate times stroke volume
3. Up to a point, increases in end-diastolic volume cause increases in stroke volume
4. Ventricular contractility is the major factor that affects ventricular end-systolic volume
5. Increasing heart rate does not increase cardiac output substantially unless stroke volume is maintained
6. Murmurs are abnormal heart sounds caused by turbulent flow through cardiac defects
7. Cardiac defects increase the heart's workload because they require one or both ventricles to pump extra blood at an elevated pressure
8. The pathology associated with cardiac defects is a direct result of the abnormal pressures, volumes, and workloads created in the cardiac chambers

Each Heartbeat Is Made Up of Ventricular Systole and Diastole

The heart is a pump, or rather it is two pumps that work together. Each of these pumps (ventricles) works in a cycle, first filling with blood and then emptying. In each *cardiac cycle* (heartbeat) the left ventricle takes a volume of blood from the pulmonary veins and left atrium and ejects it into the aorta. The right ventricle takes a similar volume of blood from the systemic veins and right atrium and ejects it into the pulmonary artery.

The events of a single cardiac cycle are shown in Figure 20–1. Because cardiac contractions are triggered by electrical depolarizations, a normal electrocardiogram (ECG) trace is presented at the top of this figure. Ventricular contraction is initiated by ventricular depolarization, which is indicated by the QRS-complex. The period of ventricular con-

traction, during which blood is ejected from the ventricles, is called *ventricular systole*. Each systole is followed by *ventricular diastole*, during which the ventricles relax and refill with blood prior to the next ventricular systole.

Ventricles do not empty completely during systole. As shown in the graph of ventricular volume, about 60 mL of this blood is contained in each ventricle of a large dog at the end of diastole. This is called the *end-diastolic volume*. During systole, about 30 mL of this blood is ejected from each ventricle, but 30 mL remains. This is called the *end-systolic volume*. The volume of blood ejected from one ventricle in one beat is called the *stroke volume*. Stroke volume equals end-diastolic volume minus end-systolic volume.

As shown in Figure 20–1, left ventricular pressure is low at the beginning of ventricular systole, but it increases rapidly. There is a

4.P.

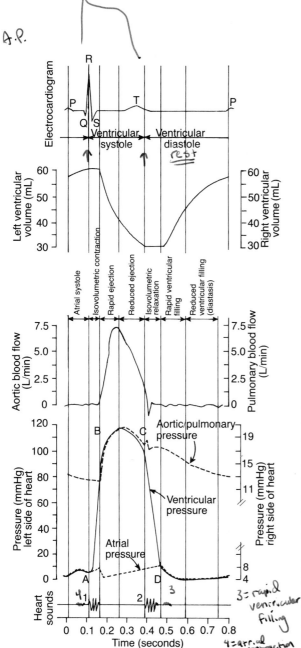

Figure 20–1. The events and terminology associated with one cardiac cycle (heartbeat) in a normal dog. The vertical scales on the left side of the graphs are for the left side of the heart. The vertical scales on the right side of the graphs are for the right side of the heart. *Point A:* closure of mitral valve. *Point B:* opening of aortic valve. *Point C:* closure of aortic valve. *Point D:* opening of mitral valve. See text for details.

momentary backflow of blood from the left ventricle to the left atrium, which closes the left atrioventricular (AV) valve (the *mitral valve*). However, there is no ejection of blood from the left ventricle into the aorta, because the aortic valve remains closed until left ventricular pressure exceeds aortic pressure.

Therefore, there is no change in ventricular volume during this first phase of systole, which is called *isovolumetric contraction*.

When left ventricular pressure rises above aortic pressure, the aortic valve does open, and there is a *rapid ejection* of blood into the aorta. This is followed by a phase of *reduced ejection* of blood, as ventricular pressure and, therefore, aortic pressure pass their peak (*systolic*) values and begin to decrease. (During the period of reduced ejection, ventricular pressure actually falls below aortic pressure, but ejection continues for a few moments, because the blood flowing out of the ventricle is carried along by the momentum imparted to it during rapid ejection.) As ventricular pressure continues to decrease, ejection comes to an end. There is a momentary backflow of blood from the aorta into the left ventricle, which closes the aortic valve. The end of ejection and the closure of the aortic valve demarcate the end of ventricular systole and the beginning of ventricular diastole.

During the first phase of ventricular diastole, the ventricular muscle relaxes, and left ventricular pressure declines from a value near aortic pressure to a value near left atrial pressure. However, no filling of the ventricle occurs, because the mitral valve remains closed until left ventricular pressure drops below left atrial pressure. This first phase of ventricular diastole is called *isovolumetric relaxation*, because there is neither filling nor emptying of the ventricle.

When left ventricular pressure does fall below left atrial pressure, the mitral valve swings open, and ventricular filling commences. First, there is a period of *rapid ventricular filling*, which is followed by a phase of *reduced ventricular filling (diastasis)*. Diastasis is followed by *atrial systole*, during which the atrial muscle contracts. Ventricular volume is nearly at its end-diastolic level even before atrial systole. In a dog at rest, 80–90% of ventricular filling typically occurs prior to atrial systole. Atrial systole simply "tops up" the almost full ventricles. An important clinical consequence of this fact is that dogs can function well at rest even if their atria are in fibrillation and not contracting. During exercise, atrial contractions make a greater contribution to ventricular filling, because the rapid heart rate in exercise leaves a shorter time for diastolic filling. Therefore, animals with atrial fibrillation typically exhibit exercise intolerance.

At the end of atrial systole, the atria begin to relax. Left atrial pressure drops slightly.

There is a momentary backflow of blood from the left ventricle to the left atrium, and the mitral valve closes. The ventricles begin to contract, and another ventricular systole begins. Therefore, the closure of the mitral valve marks the beginning of left ventricular systole.

The preceding paragraphs discussed pressure changes in the left atrium, left ventricle, and aorta. However, all the events of ventricular systole and diastole occur on both sides of the heart. Therefore, all the statements made earlier also hold true for the right side of the heart. Simply substitute "right" for "left," "pulmonary artery" for "aorta," "pulmonic valve" for "aortic valve," and "tricuspid valve" for "mitral valve." The only important difference between the left and right sides of the heart is that the right side of the heart reaches a systolic pressure of only about 20 mmHg, whereas the left side of the heart reaches 120 mmHg. For this reason, there are different scales on the pressure axes for the left and right sides.

The timing of the two major heart sounds is also shown on Figure 20–1. The first heart sound is associated with the closure of the AV valves (the mitral valve on the left side of the heart and the tricuspid valve on the right side of the heart). It is not the actual closure of the valves that makes the heart sound. Rather it is the reverberation created in the blood and in the cardiac walls when the valves close. The valve leaflets are light; they do not have enough mass to create much sound. However, the momentary backflow of blood from the ventricles to the atria at the end of ventricular diastole causes the AV valves to close quickly. The backflow of blood is brought suddenly to a stop. A sound is created that is analogous to the "water hammer" sometimes heard when a water faucet is suddenly closed.

The second heart sound is associated with the closure of the aortic valve on the left side of the heart and the pulmonic valve on the right side of the heart. It is usually briefer, sharper, and higher-pitched than the first heart sound. Again, it is not the valve leaflets closing that make the sound, but rather the reverberations produced when the momentary backflow of blood into the ventricles is brought to a sudden stop by closure of the valves. The closure of the aortic and pulmonic valves is normally coincident. However, under certain circumstances, the two valves close at slightly different times. The second heart sound is heard as two distinct sounds, a condition called a *split heart sound*.

Note that the AV valves close at the beginning of ventricular systole, and the aortic and pulmonic valves close at the end of ventricular systole. Therefore, ventricular systole can be defined also as that part of the cardiac cycle between the first heart sound and the second heart sound.

Cardiac Output Equals Heart Rate Times Stroke Volume

All of the events diagrammed in Figure 20–1 occur during each heartbeat, and each heartbeat results in the ejection of one stroke volume of blood into the pulmonary artery and aorta. The number of heartbeats per minute is called the heart rate. Therefore, the total volume of blood pumped by each ventricle in 1 minute is equal to stroke volume times heart rate. Cardiac output can be increased only if heart rate increases, stroke volume increases, or both. Therefore, to understand how the body controls cardiac output one must understand how the body controls heart rate and stroke volume. Figure 20–2 summarizes the factors that affect heart rate and stroke volume. These factors are described in detail in the following three sections.

Up to a Point, Increases in End-Diastolic Volume Cause Increases in Stroke Volume

Because stroke volume equals end-diastolic volume minus end-systolic volume, stroke volume can be increased only by increasing end-diastolic volume (that is, filling the ventricles fuller during diastole) or by decreasing end-systolic volume (that is, emptying the ventricles more completely during systole).

The relationship between end-diastolic ventricular volume and stroke volume is plotted in Figure 20–3A. Increases in end-diastolic volume lead to increases in stroke volume. The detailed physiological mechanisms underlying this relationship are complex. Basically, however, a greater ventricular filling during diastole places the ventricle in a more favorable geometry for ejection of blood during the next systole. Also, stretching the ventricular muscle fibers during diastole causes a greater amount of Ca^{2+} to be released from the sarcoplasmic reticulum during the subsequent systolic contraction. Under resting conditions in a normal animal, ventricular filling is only part of the way up this *ventricular function curve*. Therefore, increases or decreases from

Figure 20–2. The control of cardiac output. Solid arrows show direct or primary effects. Dashed arrows indicate influences that tend to reduce the primary effect. For example, a decrease in systolic duration would partially offset a decrease in diastolic filling time. The relationships shown here are described in detail in the text.

↑Cardiac Output

↑ Stroke Volume   ↑ Heart Rate

↑ End-Diastolic Volume   ↓ End-Systolic Volume

↑ Ventricular Compliance   ↑ Preload   ↑ Contractility ◄— ↑Sympathetic Activity   ↓ Parasympathetic Activity

↑ Venous or Atrial Pressure   ↓ Systolic Duration

↓ Diastolic Filling Time

-----► negative feedback

normal ventricular end-diastolic volume result in roughly proportional increases or decreases in stroke volume.

End-diastolic ventricular volume is determined by ventricular preload and ventricular compliance. *Preload* is the distending pressure within a ventricle at the end of diastole (ventricular end-diastolic pressure). Normal values of preload are 3 mmHg for the right ventricle and 5 mmHg for the left ventricle. Ventricular preload is determined by the atrial pressure at the end of diastole. Because there are no valves

between the veins and the atria, atrial pressure is equivalent to the pressure within the nearby veins. Thus, pulmonary venous pressure, left atrial pressure, and left ventricular end-diastolic pressure are all essentially equivalent measures of left ventricular preload. Similarly, right ventricular end-diastolic pressure, right atrial pressure, and vena cava pressure are all essentially equivalent measures of right ventricular preload. Right ventricular preload is measured in the clinic by way of a catheter that is introduced into a peripheral vein (e.g.,

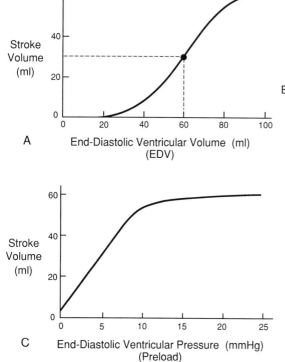

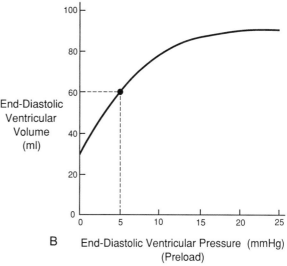

Figure 20–3. (A) Increases in end-diastolic ventricular volume cause increases in stroke volume. The data are for the left ventricle of a large dog. The dashed lines indicate the normal values. (B) Up to a point, increases in end-diastolic ventricular pressure (preload) cause increases in end-diastolic ventricular volume. The data are for the left ventricle of a large dog. (C) The combined relationships of A and B show that, up to a point, increases in ventricular preload cause increases in stroke volume.

jugular vein) and advanced into the thoracic vena cava or right atrium. Such a catheter is called a *central venous catheter,* and the pressure measured at its tip is called *central venous pressure.* Left ventricular preload is more difficult to measure clinically, because there is no easy way to place a catheter tip into the left atrium or pulmonary veins.

Figure 20–3B shows the relationship between end-diastolic ventricular volume and end-diastolic ventricular pressure (preload) for a normal left ventricle. The ventricle has a natural volume of 30 mL in a relaxed, non-pressurized state (i.e., when preload equals 0). Increases in preload distend and fill the ventricle. A preload of 5 mmHg brings about the normal left ventricular end-diastolic volume of 60 mL. However, an elastic limit is reached when ventricular volume approaches 90 mL. Further increases in preload do not cause much additional ventricular filling.

Because increases in end-diastolic ventricular volume cause stroke volume to increase (Fig. 20–3A), and because increases in ventricular preload are associated with increases in end-diastolic volume (Fig. 20–3B), increases in ventricular preload must cause increases in stroke volume. This relationship is shown in Figure 20–3C. The relationships between ventricular preload, end-diastolic volume, and stroke volume were first studied in detail by Starling. The idea that an increase in preload (or end-diastolic volume) causes stroke volume to increase is called *Starling's law of the heart.* The Starling mechanism plays a critical role in moment-to-moment adjustments of cardiac stroke volume. For example, if the right ventricle begins to pump an increased stroke volume, the additional pulmonary blood flow results in an increase in pulmonary venous flow and an increase in pulmonary venous pressure. The increased pulmonary venous pressure increases left atrial pressure, which increases left ventricular preload, which increases the filling of the left ventricle during diastole. The increase in left ventricular end-diastolic volume results in a greater stroke volume from the left ventricle. Thus, an increase in right ventricular stroke volume quickly results in a corresponding increase in left ventricular stroke volume. The reverse is also true. Obviously, this sequence has the potential for developing into a vicious circle, with runaway increases in stroke volume. Other control mechanisms prevent this from happening, and these are discussed later (Chapter 24). The point is that the Starling

mechanism keeps the stroke volumes of the left and right ventricles balanced. If this equality is not maintained (and one ventricle pumps more blood than the other for several minutes), a large part of the body's blood volume accumulates either in the lungs or in the systemic circulation.

Because of its role in regulating stroke volume, Starling's law of the heart is also referred to as *heterometric autoregulation.* The name implies a self-control (autoregulation) of cardiac output as a result of different (hetero) initial volumes (metric); that is, heterometric refers to different end-diastolic volumes.

Hemorrhage is one situation in which a change in preload alters stroke volume. The rapid loss of a substantial amount of blood from the systemic circulation results in a decreased venous pressure at the right side of the heart and, therefore, a decreased right atrial pressure. Right atrial pressure is the preload for the right ventricle, and a decrease in right atrial pressure results in decreases in right ventricular end-diastolic volume and, therefore, in right ventricular stroke volume. This quickly results in a corresponding decrease in left ventricular stroke volume. The resulting decrease in cardiac output causes systemic arterial pressure to drop. The consequences could be life-threatening if arterial pressure decreased so much that adequate blood flow to the brain, heart, and other critical organs was not maintained.

End-diastolic ventricular volume is determined not only by preload, but also by *ventricular compliance.* Compliance measures the ease with which the ventricular walls stretch to accommodate incoming blood during diastole. A compliant ventricle is one that yields easily to preload pressure and readily fills with blood during diastole. More rigorously, compliance is defined as change in volume divided by change in pressure. Ventricular compliance therefore corresponds to the slope of a ventricular volume-pressure curve like the one shown in Figure 20–3B. The figure shows that a normal ventricle is quite compliant over the range of volumes near normal end-diastolic ventricular volume. That is, small changes in preload result in substantial changes in end-ventricular volume. However, at preloads above about 10 mmHg, the ventricle becomes less compliant (stiffer). Inelastic connective tissue in the ventricular walls limits further increases in ventricular volume.

With advancing age or as a result of certain cardiac diseases, the ventricular walls become

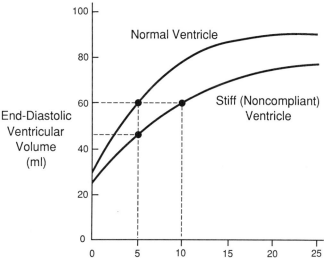

Figure 20–4. A stiff, noncompliant ventricle requires a higher filling pressure (preload) in order to reach a normal degree of filling (end-diastolic volume).

stiff and noncompliant even at normal preloads. Figure 20–4 shows a comparison of volume-pressure curves for a normal ventricle and for a noncompliant ventricle. For any given increase in ventricular preload, there is a smaller increase in ventricular volume in the noncompliant ventricle. Larger than normal preloads are required to obtain normal end-diastolic ventricular volumes in a ventricle with decreased compliance.

Preload and compliance are the two factors that most directly affect end-diastolic ventric-

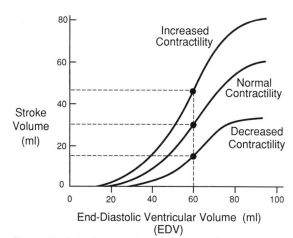

Figure 20–5. An increased cardiac contractility is identifiable graphically as a leftward and upward shift of the ventricular function curve. An increase in contractility means that there will be a larger stroke volume for any given end-diastolic volume. Conversely, a decrease in contractility (rightward and downward shift) means that there will be a smaller stroke volume for any given end-diastolic volume.

ular volume. Heart rate is an additional factor that exerts an important, but indirect, influence on ventricular filling. At normal resting heart rates, there is ample time for ventricular filling during diastole. As mentioned earlier, ventricular filling is nearly complete in a resting dog even before atrial systole occurs. However, as heart rate increases above resting levels, the period available for diastolic filling is reduced to shorter and shorter times. Typically, at heart rates above 150 to 180 beats per minute, the time available for diastolic filling is too short for normal filling to take place, even though atrial pressure, atrial systolic contraction, and ventricular compliance are normal. This limitation on ventricular filling would dramatically reduce stroke volume when heart rate is high, if not for an additional, compensating influence that is discussed later in the chapter.

Ventricular Contractility Is the Major Factor That Affects Ventricular End-Systolic Volume

An increase in *ventricular contractility* results in a more complete emptying of the ventricle during systole and, therefore, a decreased end-systolic volume. Contractility can be defined as the pumping ability of a ventricle. An increase in contractility can bring about an increase in stroke volume without a change in end-diastolic volume. As shown in Figure 20–5, increased contractility results in an increased stroke volume for any given end-diastolic volume. For example, at a normal end-diastolic volume of 60 mL, end-systolic volume is 30 mL, so the stroke volume is 30 mL. An increased contractility with no change in end-diastolic volume results in more systolic emptying; if end-systolic volume is reduced to 15 mL, stroke volume increases to 45 mL.

Cardiac contractility can be increased by sympathetic nerve activity through the action of the neurotransmitter norepinephrine. Norepinephrine activates β-adrenergic receptors on ventricular muscle cells. As a result of this activation, increased amounts of intracellular calcium are made available at the initiation of contraction. Therefore, the contraction is more forceful. Other β-adrenergic agonist drugs (e.g., epinephrine and isoproterenol) mimic this action of norepinephrine on the heart and also increase cardiac contractility. The cardiac glycosides are another class of drugs that increases cardiac contractility by making more calcium available. The most common example is the drug digitalis.

If stroke volume is observed to be below normal for any given end-diastolic volume, there must have been less than normal ventricular emptying during systole. That is, there must have been an increase in end-systolic volume, and the most likely reason is that cardiac contractility has decreased. This is shown in Figure 20–5. A decreased sympathetic activity decreases cardiac contractility, as does β-adrenergic antagonist drugs, which block β-adrenergic receptors on ventricular muscle cells. Propranolol is the β antagonist used most commonly in the clinic to decrease cardiac contractility. Propranolol blocks the effects of sympathetic nerves on the heart and thereby decreases the amount of calcium available to initiate ventricular contraction. Like β antagonists, calcium channel–blocking drugs also decrease cardiac contractility by making less calcium available for activation of the contractile proteins. Barbiturates depress cardiac contractility too, and this must be kept in mind when administering barbiturates for anaesthesia or analgesia. A decrease in cardiac contractility decreases stroke volume and, therefore, cardiac output. Blood pressure may fall to dangerously low levels.

A decreased cardiac contractility is also the hallmark of the general clinical condition called *heart failure*. Although there are many kinds of heart failure, they share the symptom of a decreased pumping ability of the ventricle. Heart failure can result from coronary artery disease, cardiac hypoxia, myocarditis, diseases of the cardiac valves, toxic reactions, or electrolyte imbalances.

Although ventricular contractility is usually the predominant factor affecting ventricular end-systolic volume, the effect of arterial blood pressure must be considered also. Substantial increases in arterial blood pressure impair ventricular ejection. End-systolic volume increases, and stroke volume decreases, because left ventricular pressure during systole must exceed aortic pressure before the aortic valve opens and ejection of blood from the ventricle occurs. Aortic pressure is called the *cardiac afterload*. It is the pressure against which the ventricle must pump in order to eject blood. The higher the afterload, the more difficult it is for the ventricle to eject blood. Therefore, a high afterload causes less complete ventricular emptying; end-systolic volume increases. This effect is minor for a normal heart and within the normal range of arterial pressure. However, end-systolic volume becomes much more strongly influenced by afterload if a heart is in failure.

Increasing Heart Rate Does Not Increase Cardiac Output Substantially Unless Stroke Volume Is Maintained

Because cardiac output is equal to stroke volume times heart rate, one might expect that cardiac output would be proportional to heart rate. That is, if stroke volume did not change, doubling heart rate would double cardiac output (see dashed line in Figure 20–6). However, if one experimentally increases heart rate above its normal level with an electrical pacemaker, cardiac output increases to a point, but not in proportion to the increase in heart rate. As mentioned earlier, when heart rate is increased, diastolic filling time is reduced. The resulting reduction in end-diastolic volume reduces stroke volume, so cardiac output does not increase in proportion to heart rate (see lower line in Figure 20–6). In fact, at heart rates above 180–200 beats per minute, stroke volume falls so much that cardiac output actually decreases with further increases in heart rate. This problem was encountered when early versions of artificial cardiac pacemakers malfunctioned in ways that caused high ventricular rates. Decreases in stroke volume at high heart rates are also encountered in certain cardiac arrhythmias. In *paroxysmal atrial tachycardia* (PAT), for example, a rapid heart rate is

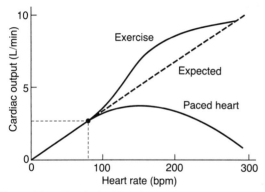

Figure 20–6. The dashed line shows that increases in heart rate would cause proportional increases in cardiac output if stroke volume did not change. However, if the heart is paced to higher and higher rates, the increase in cardiac output is less than expected, because stroke volume decreases (lower line). When a dog increases its own heart rate through sympathetic activation (e.g., during exercise), cardiac output increases more than expected because stroke volume increases (upper line).

originated by an ectopic atrial pacemaker. The tachycardia occurs typically in bursts or paroxysms. The rapid heart rate limits diastolic filling so much that cardiac output falls below normal. Blood pressure can fall so low that the patient becomes weak or faints.

In contrast to cardiac pacing, which does not cause a large increase in cardiac output, increases in heart rate in the normal course of daily activity are accompanied by substantial increases in cardiac output. An example is the increase in cardiac output that normally accompanies exercise. As shown in Figure 20–6 (upper curve), the actual increase in cardiac output during progressively more intense exercise is even greater than would be expected on the basis of the increase in heart rate. The reason that cardiac output increases so much during exercise is that stroke volume increases also. During exercise, increases in heart rate are brought about by increases in sympathetic activity. This sympathetic activation also increases cardiac contractility, so the ventricles empty more completely with each beat. In addition, sympathetic activation shortens the duration of systole. That is, under sympathetic action, the heart not only contracts more frequently (increased rate) and more forcefully (increased contractility), it contracts and relaxes more quickly. This shortening of systole helps to preserve diastolic filling time.

As shown in Figure 20–7, when the heart rate is 60 beats per minute, each beat takes 1 second. This 1 second must be composed of one systole and one diastole. Typically, systole

lasts about one third of the beat, or one third of a second. If the heart rate is increased to 120 beats per minute, each beat lasts only one half of a second. If systole remains at one third of a second, there is only one sixth of a second left for diastolic filling. However, if the increase in heart rate occurs because of an increase in sympathetic activity, systole becomes shorter, and this helps to preserve diastolic filling time. Although diastole is shorter under these conditions than at rest, it is longer than it would have been if systole were not shortened. Thus, we say that sympathetic activation helps to preserve diastolic filling time by shortening systole. Because sympathetic activation increases both heart rate and stroke volume, it can create large increases in cardiac output.

Parasympathetic nerves have little effect on ventricular contractility or systolic duration. However, a reduction in parasympathetic activity is an additional factor that increases heart rate during exercise. (Because parasympathetic activation decreases heart rate, decreases in parasympathetic activity allow heart rate to increase.) The overall effect of sympathetic and parasympathetic actions during the transition from rest to exercise is to bring about a four- or fivefold increase above normal in cardiac output. These changes are summarized in Table 20–1.

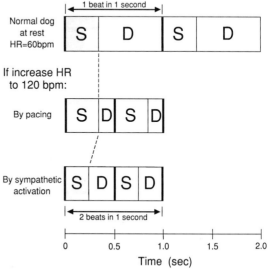

Figure 20–7. If heart rate is increased from 60 beats per minute (top) to 120 beats per minute by an artificial pacemaker, the duration of systole remains the same, and diastolic duration (filling time) is greatly reduced (middle). If the same increase in heart rate is brought about by sympathetic activation, systole becomes shorter, which helps to preserve diastolic filling time (bottom).

Table 20–1
TYPICAL CARDIAC CHANGES DURING VIGOROUS EXERCISE IN A LARGE DOG

	Rest	Exercise
Ventricular end-diastolic volume (mL)	60	55
Ventricular end-systolic volume (mL)	30	15
Stroke volume (mL)	30	40
Heart rate (beats/minute)	80	240
Cardiac output (L/minute)	2.4	9.6

The control of cardiac output is summarized in Figure 20–2. Cardiac output is determined by stroke volume and heart rate. Stroke volume is determined by end-diastolic volume and end-systolic volume. End-diastolic volume depends on preload, ventricular compliance, and diastolic filling time. End-systolic volume depends on contractility and arterial pressure or afterload (not shown in figure). Diastolic filling time is decreased when heart rate is high. Heart rate is increased by sympathetic activation and parasympathetic withdrawal. Sympathetic activation also increases contractility and shortens systolic duration (which helps to preserve diastolic filling time).

Murmurs Are Abnormal Heart Sounds Caused by Turbulent Flow Through Cardiac Defects

Cardiac murmurs are abnormal heart sounds, and they often indicate the presence of cardiac abnormalities. Murmurs can take the form of abnormalities in the first or second heart sound, or they can be additional, abnormal heart sounds. Figure 20–1 indicates that the first heart sound is associated with the closure of the AV valves at the beginning of ventricular systole. The second heart sound is associated with the closure of the aortic and pulmonic valves at the end of ventricular systole. Occasionally, faint third and fourth normal heart sounds are audible with the stethoscope. By comparison, clinically important murmurs are much louder. Often, murmurs are even louder than the normal first and second heart sounds.

Murmurs are caused by turbulent flow through cardiac defects. The underlying physical principle is that *laminar or smooth flow* of blood through the heart and blood vessels is quiet, whereas *turbulent flow* is noisy. An analogy is that a river does not make any sound as it flows smoothly through a broad, relatively flat channel. If the same river enters a channel that is restricted or drops steeply, then a rapid or cataract forms. The flow becomes turbulent, and the turbulent flow makes noise. The same volume of river water passes through the flat area and down the rapids, but the flow is turbulent and noisy only in the area of the rapids. The flow of blood through the heart and blood vessels is normally smooth, and therefore quiet, during all parts of the cardiac cycle, except two. The first moment of turbulent flow occurs at the beginning of ventricular contraction, upon closure of the AV valves. It is not the closure of the valves themselves that creates the first heart sound, but rather the turbulence and vibration caused as flowing blood comes to a sudden stop. The second moment of turbulent flow normally occurs at the end of ventricular systole, when the aortic and pulmonic valves close. As they close, the backward-flowing blood comes to a sudden stop, which again creates a moment of turbulence and vibration in the valve leaflets and in the walls of the aorta and pulmonary arteries. This vibration is heard as the second heart sound.

Table 20–2 lists cardiac valve defects that cause additional sites of turbulent flow and, therefore, murmurs. The table also indicates the timing of the murmurs relative to the cardiac cycle. Some murmurs occur during ventricular systole; these are *systolic murmurs*. Some murmurs occur during ventricular diastole; these are *diastolic murmurs*. *Continuous murmurs* occur during both systole and diastole. The timing of each murmur is easy to remember if you keep in mind two basic

Table 20–2
CARDIAC VALVE DEFECTS AND THE MURMURS THEY CAUSE

Site of Defect	Systolic Murmur	Diastolic Murmur
AV valves	Incompetence (insufficiency)	Stenosis
Aortic/pulmonic valves	Stenosis	Incompetence (insufficiency)

principles: murmurs are caused by turbulent blood flow, and blood flows in response to pressure differences. That is, turbulent (noisy) flow through a cardiac defect occurs only if there is a substantial pressure difference from one side of the defect to the other.

Figure 20–8 indicates how these principles can be used to account for systolic murmurs. The numbers in the figure indicate the maximum pressures that normally exist in each cardiac chamber during ventricular systole. Note, for example, that the pressure in the left ventricle is normally much higher than the pressure in the left atrium during ventricular systole. The mitral valve is normally closed during ventricular systole, so no blood flows backward from the ventricle to the left atrium. However, if the mitral valve fails to close completely during ventricular systole, the large pressure difference between the left ventricle and the left atrium causes a rapid, backward flow of blood through the partially closed valve. This turbulent backflow creates a murmur that is heard during systole. A mitral valve that fails to close completely is said to

be *insufficient* or *incompetent*. The backflow across the valve is called *regurgitation*. Mitral regurgitation is present in one out of twelve dogs over 5 years of age.

Blood flows through a *ventricular septal defect (VSD)* from the left ventricle to the right ventricle during ventricular systole, because systolic pressure is much higher in the left ventricle than in the right ventricle. Typically, the flow of blood through a VSD is turbulent, and a systolic murmur is created.

Systolic turbulence is created also if the aortic valve does not open widely. Blood ejected from the ventricle accelerates to a high velocity as it squeezes through the restricted aortic opening, and turbulence occurs. A valve that fails to open widely is called a *stenotic valve*, and therefore the defect of *aortic stenosis* produces a systolic murmur. Pulmonic stenosis also causes a systolic murmur. Aortic and pulmonic stenosis are common congenital defects in dogs.

A *patent ductus arteriosus (PDA)* (a persistence after birth of the opening between the aorta and the pulmonary artery; see Chapter 49) produces a murmur during systole, because the pressure in the aorta is much higher than the pressure in the pulmonary artery. Blood flows from the aorta into the pulmonary artery, and turbulence occurs. However, the murmur of PDA is not restricted to systole, because aortic pressure remains higher than pulmonary artery pressure throughout diastole. Therefore, the murmur of PDA is heard in both systole and diastole. It is a *continuous murmur*. It is also called a *machinery murmur*, because it characteristically sounds like the rumble of machinery. PDA is common in dogs, especially in females. Occasionally, animals exhibit open pathways for blood flow between peripheral arteries and peripheral veins. These are called *arterial-venous fistulae*. Arterial-venous fistulae carry flow (and create turbulence) during both systole and diastole and, therefore, create a continuous murmur. The murmur of an arterial-venous fistula is most audible at the body surface close to the point of the fistula. The murmur of a patent ductus is characteristically heard best at a specific point on the thorax. The site from which a murmur can be heard best is often indicative of the particular type of defect that causes the murmur.

Figure 20–9 depicts the minimum pressures that normally exist in the various cardiac chambers during ventricular diastole. These pressures form the basis for understanding

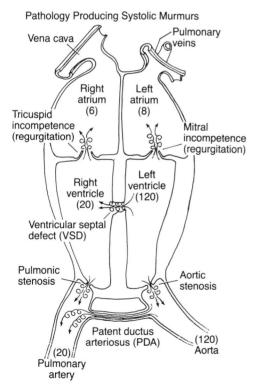

Figure 20–8. Schematic view of the heart showing cardiac defects that cause systolic murmurs. The numbers in parentheses indicate normal maximum pressure (mmHg) during ventricular systole. The swirled arrows indicate the sites of turbulent (noisy) flow.

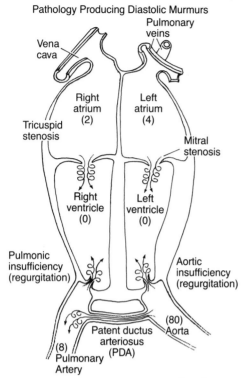

Pathology Producing Diastolic Murmurs

Figure 20–9. Cardiac defects that cause diastolic murmurs. The numbers in parentheses indicate normal minimum pressures (mmHg) during ventricular diastole. The swirled arrows indicate the sites of turbulent (noisy) flow.

be produced also by defects on the right side of the heart. Pulmonic regurgitation produces a diastolic murmur, but it is relatively rare. Tricuspid stenosis is uncommon, at least as a congenital defect. However, the presence of heartworms in the right side of the heart sometimes creates a stenosis at the tricuspid valve, and a diastolic murmur occurs.

The presence of cardiac murmurs (and the defects that cause them) is not clinically important if these defects do not cause pathological changes in the body. But cardiac defects typically lead to three different pathological consequences: (1) an abnormally high or low blood flow to one region of the body; (2) abnormally high or low blood pressures in a particular region of the body; and (3) *cardiac hypertrophy* (enlargement of cardiac muscle).

It is not difficult to understand why cardiac defects lead to abnormal blood flows or abnormal blood pressures. For example, a ventricular septal defect leads to an abnormally high blood flow through the pulmonary circulation. Mitral stenosis leads to an abnormally high left atrial pressure. It may be more difficult to see why cardiac defects lead to cardiac hypertrophy. The underlying principle is that cardiac defects lead to an increase in the workload of one or more cardiac chambers, and an increase in workload of the cardiac muscle leads to hypertrophy. An understanding of cardiac energetics (see next section) is needed to develop this concept more fully.

Cardiac Defects Increase the Heart's Workload Because They Require One or Both Ventricles to Pump Extra Blood at an Elevated Pressure

Cardiac hypertrophy resulting from the increase in cardiac muscle workload takes weeks to develop. It is analogous to the fact that an increase in skeletal muscle workload (physical conditioning) leads to skeletal muscle hypertrophy. To develop this analogy more fully, recall that a skeletal muscle does work by exerting a force while shortening. The mechanical work done by a skeletal muscle is equal to the force developed by the contracting muscle, times the distance moved during one contraction, times the number of contractions. Therefore, the mechanical work done by a skeletal muscle can be increased by increasing the forcefulness of contraction, the distance moved, or the number of contractions. In weightlifting conditioning, the emphasis is on

why certain cardiac defects commonly produce diastolic murmurs. First consider *mitral stenosis*. A normal mitral valve opens widely during ventricular diastole and creates a low resistance pathway for blood flow. The resistance of an open mitral valve is normally so low that left atrial pressure is only 1–2 mmHg higher than ventricular pressure during ventricular filling. However, if the mitral valve fails to open widely, ventricular filling must occur through a stenotic (restricted) mitral valve. This creates turbulent flow and a diastolic murmur. Mitral stenosis is a common murmur in humans who develop calcification of the mitral valve as a result of rheumatic heart disease.

During diastole, the normal aortic valve is shut tightly, and no blood flows backward from the aorta into the left ventricle. If the aortic valve does not close tightly, blood flows backward (regurgitates) from the aorta to the left ventricle during diastole. Therefore, *aortic regurgitation* produces a diastolic murmur. The defect is called *aortic incompetence* or *aortic insufficiency*. Aortic regurgitation is common in horses but not in dogs. Diastolic murmurs can performing a few forceful contractions of skeletal muscle. Weightlifting leads to an increase in muscle workload and, therefore, a muscular hypertrophy. Conditioning that involves repetitive, low-force contractions of skeletal muscle (such as running or swimming) primarily emphasizes the distance and duration components of skeletal muscle work. "Distance work" also leads to hypertrophy. However, a common observation in skeletal muscle conditioning is that weight work causes more hypertrophy than distance work.

The function of the heart is to pump blood, and the *mechanical (external) work* performed by any pump is equal to the pressure generated by the pump, times the volume of fluid that is pumped in one pump stroke, times the number of pump strokes. Therefore, the work done by the left ventricle in one cardiac cycle, called the *stroke work,* is equal to the pressure produced, times the stroke volume. In 1 minute, the work done by the left ventricle is equal to the pressure created, times the stroke volume, times the heart rate. The pressure produced by the left ventricle can be approximated by the average pressure in the aorta. Therefore, the *minute work* done by the left ventricle is equal to the average aortic pressure, times the stroke volume, times the heart rate.

In our analogy with skeletal muscle, the average aortic pressure is analogous to the force developed by the contracting muscle, stroke volume is analogous to the distance moved during one contraction, and heart rate is analogous to the number of contractions. Obviously, the external work done by the left ventricle could be increased by increasing the pressure that the left ventricle develops during systolic ejection of blood into the aorta, by increasing the amount of blood pumped by the left ventricle in one beat, or by increasing heart rate. Notice that a 50% increase in ventricular work can result from a 50% increase in left ventricular pressure, a 50% increase in left ventricular stroke volume, or a 50% increase in heart rate. Clinically, any of these changes results, over a period of weeks, in left ventricular hypertrophy. However, a common clinical observation is that an increase in ventricular pressure causes a much more pronounced hypertrophy than does an increase in stroke volume or heart rate. This clinical observation is summarized by the statement that "pressure work is harder for the heart (and causes more hypertrophy) than volume work." Note the analogy between this observation and the observation that weight work causes more skeletal muscle hypertrophy than distance work. The basis for this difference is that weight work in skeletal muscle and pressure work in the heart involve the generation of a great deal of *internal, wasted work,* which appears as heat. This greatly increases the *total work* (external work plus internal work) being done by the skeletal or cardiac muscle.

Under normal conditions, about 85% of the metabolic energy consumed by the heart appears as heat and only 15% appears as external work. A physicist would say that the heart has a thermodynamic efficiency of about 15%. However, the cardiac efficiency depends on the kind of work being done by the ventricles. The heart becomes less efficient when external work is increased by increasing pressure. Conversely, the heart becomes more efficient when the external work is increased by increasing the volume of blood pumped. Thus, an increase in pressure and an increase in volume may cause the same increase in external work, but an increase in pressure causes a much greater increase in the heat produced by the heart than does an increase in volume. It is the total energy consumption of the heart, not just the external work, that is the primary stimulus for ventricular hypertrophy. Again, an increase in pressure work causes greater cardiac hypertrophy than does an increase in volume work.

The dominant role of pressure in determining total ventricular energy consumption is evident from a comparison of the work done by the left and right ventricles. The stroke volume and heart rate are equivalent for the left and the right ventricles, but the left ventricle develops about five times more pressure during systole than the right ventricle. Therefore, the external work done by the left ventricle is roughly five times greater than the external work done by the right ventricle. The total metabolic energy consumption of the left ventricle is much more than five times greater than the energy consumption of the right ventricle, because the extra external work performed by the left ventricle is in the form of greater pressure. As a result, almost all of the energy consumed by the heart is consumed by the left ventricle. Therefore, almost all of the coronary blood flow is delivered to the left ventricular muscle, and almost all of the oxygen consumed by the heart is consumed by the left ventricle. Because of the high amount of pressure work done by the left ventricle compared with the right ventricle, the left ventricle develops much heavier and thicker muscular walls than the right ventricle.

A clinical observation from human medicine provides a further illustration of how an increase in ventricular pressure work leads to ventricular hypertrophy. About 20% of the adult human population has hypertension. In most of these patients, arterial blood pressure is elevated because of an increased resistance to blood flow in the systemic arterioles. Cardiac output is generally normal in hypertensive patients, but an elevated ventricular pressure is required to force this cardiac output through the constricted systemic arterioles. This increases the pressure work done by the left ventricle in hypertensive patients and results in a pronounced left ventricular hypertrophy.

Up to a point, left ventricular hypertrophy is an appropriate and beneficial adaptation to the increased workload imposed on the left ventricular muscle. However, excessive hypertrophy is deleterious for two reasons. First, the enlarged ventricular muscle restricts the opening of the aortic valve. Aortic stenosis, in turn, necessitates an even greater systolic pressure within the left ventricle, which leads to more hypertrophy, in a vicious circle. Second, if the coronary circulation cannot provide enough blood flow to meet the increased metabolic demands of the hypertrophic ventricle, hypoxia, ischemia, and acidosis may develop. Inadequate coronary blood flow becomes especially likely if the coronary vessels have become constricted because of atherosclerosis. The combination of hypertension and coronary artery disease is a common and especially serious problem in human medicine. The hypertensive patient with coronary artery disease may have adequate blood flow to the hypertrophic ventricles during rest, but the increase in blood flow may be insufficient during exercise. As a result, hypertensive patients with coronary artery disease characteristically experience cardiac ischemia (and myocardial infarction) or cardiac arrhythmias (and sudden death) during periods of exercise.

The Pathology Associated with Cardiac Defects Is a Direct Result of the Abnormal Pressures, Volumes, and Workloads Created in the Cardiac Chambers

Figure 20–10 summarizes pathological consequences associated with some common mur-

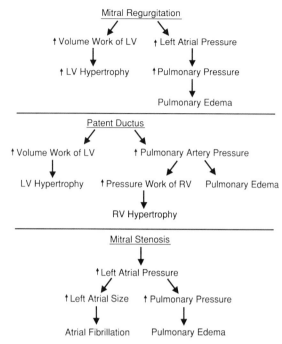

Figure 20–10. The pathological consequences of several common cardiac defects.

murs. First consider mitral regurgitation. With each contraction of the left ventricle, a normal volume of blood is ejected into the aorta, and an additional volume of blood is ejected backward into the left atrium. As a result, there is an increase in the volume work performed by the left ventricle. This increase of left ventricular external work also brings about a moderate increase in the total heat produced by the left ventricle. Therefore, mild to moderate left ventricular hypertrophy develops. Also in a heart with mitral regurgitation, the left atrium continues to receive a normal volume of blood each minute through the pulmonary circulation, and additionally receives blood that flows backward from the left ventricle with each beat. Therefore, the left atrium becomes distended, and left atrial pressure increases. Blood also backs up, or dams up, in the pulmonary blood vessels, which increases the pressure there. Elevated pressures in the pulmonary blood vessels cause water and electrolytes to be filtered out of the blood stream and into the pulmonary interstitial spaces. The accumulation of water in the lung tissue causes a "water-logging" or swelling that is called *pulmonary edema*. Clinically, when left atrial pressures rise above 20–25 mmHg, pulmonary edema becomes so severe that there is a substantial reduction in the ability of the lungs to transfer oxygen and carbon dioxide into and out of the blood stream. The result is respiratory distress.

The clinical consequences of mitral regurgitation are usually more noticeable during exercise than during rest. One reason is that, despite the regurgitation, the left ventricle can usually adapt enough through hypertrophy and increases in heart rate to maintain a normal cardiac output into the aorta (and therefore into the systemic circulation) at rest. Also, despite some pulmonary edema, the exchange of oxygen and carbon dioxide is sufficient to meet the animal's needs during rest. During exercise, however, the output of the left ventricle into the systemic circulation must increase to several times normal if it is to supply adequate blood to exercising skeletal muscle. Also, the rate of exchange of oxygen and carbon dioxide in the lungs must increase to several times normal. Despite the hypertrophy, the left ventricle may not be able to maintain adequate blood flow to the systemic circulation during exercise if mitral regurgitation is serious. Again, the lungs may not be able to exchange enough carbon dioxide and oxygen to support the metabolism of the exercising animal if the pulmonary edema is serious.

Consider next the pathology associated with aortic stenosis (not shown in Figure 20–10). In order to eject a normal volume of blood with each beat through a stenotic aortic valve, the left ventricle must develop an abnormally high systolic pressure. This increases the pressure work of the left ventricle, which leads to a pronounced left ventricular hypertrophy. The left ventricular hypertrophy has the desirable effect of increasing the contractility of the left ventricular muscle so that it can generate the increased pressure required to maintain a normal cardiac output. However, the hypertrophy has two undesirable side effects. The first is that the coronary blood vessels may be unable to deliver the increased amounts of blood required by the enlarged left ventricular muscle fibers. If coronary blood flow is inadequate for the level of work being performed by the cardiac muscle, hypoxia and acidosis may develop, which can lead to ventricular arrhythmias. The second problem with ventricular hypertrophy is that, as the left ventricular muscle enlarges, the ventricular muscle begins to impinge on the aortic outflow pathway, which further hampers the ability of the ventricle to eject blood. In a sense, the ventricular

muscle that is hypertrophying "gets in its own way" or becomes "muscle bound." Limitations in coronary blood flow and geometric restrictions in aortic outflow are much more likely to be noticeable during exercise than at rest. Therefore, a patient with aortic stenosis may be able to function normally at rest but may exhibit exercise intolerance. That is, the patient may have limited ability to exercise and may exhibit ventricular arrhythmias during exercise.

Typically PDA results in both left and right ventricular hypertrophy (see Fig. 20–10). In a typical patient with a patent ductus, the left ventricle pumps a normal volume of blood per minute to the systemic circulation and also pumps two to three times that volume of blood per minute through the patent ductus. As a result, the volume work done by the left ventricle is above normal, and this leads to left ventricular hypertrophy. The blood flowing through the patent ductus enters the pulmonary artery, so pulmonary arterial pressure increases above normal. This, in turn, increases the pressure work that must be done by the right ventricle. The right ventricle receives a normal volume of blood back from the systemic circulation each minute, and the right ventricle has to generate an elevated systolic pressure in order to eject this blood into the high-pressure pulmonary artery. The increased pressure work for the right ventricle is a powerful stimulus for hypertrophy, so a pronounced right ventricular hypertrophy develops.

In a patient with PDA, the pulmonary artery and the pulmonary blood vessels must carry not only the normal volume of blood (represented by the output of the right ventricle), but also the blood that is pumped through the patent ductus. Therefore, pulmonary blood flow is typically three or four times normal in a patient with a patent ductus. The resulting increases in pulmonary vascular pressure can lead to pulmonary edema. A surgical repair of a patent ductus in a young animal leads to a rapid reversal of all of these pathological changes.

The preceding examples make predictable the pathological consequences of a ventricular septal defect. These consequences include increased volume work of the left ventricle, moderate left ventricular hypertrophy, increased volume and pressure work of the right ventricle, pronounced right ventricular hypertrophy, increased blood flow through the lungs, possible pulmonary edema, and possible exercise intolerance. It should also be clear why pulmonary stenosis leads to increased pressure work for the right ventricle and pronounced right ventricular hypertrophy (see Clinical Correlation, below).

Figure 20–10 summarizes pathological consequences associated with the diastolic murmur of mitral stenosis. Left atrial pressure must increase above normal in order to force a normal volume of blood through the stenotic mitral valve and into the left ventricle during each ventricular diastole. The elevated left atrial pressure distends the left atrium, which makes it susceptible to fibrillation. There also may be some hypertrophy of the atrial muscle. However, the atrium continues to function mainly as a reservoir to collect and hold blood during ventricular systole rather than as a pumping chamber to force blood into the ventricle during its diastole. The increase in left atrial pressure also causes blood to back up and accumulate in the pulmonary blood vessels, which can cause pulmonary edema. One might suppose that the back-up of blood in the pulmonary vessels would eventually increase the pressure in the pulmonary artery also, and thereby increase the pressure work of the right ventricle. That is, one might predict that mitral stenosis would lead to right ventricular hypertrophy. This prediction is a logical one, but in practice, animals with elevated left atrial pressures usually die from the effects of pulmonary edema before right ventricular pressures have had a chance to become high enough to induce right ventricular hypertrophy. Therefore, mitral stenosis does not generally lead to hypertrophy of either ventricle.

The defect of aortic regurgitation is associated classically with left ventricular hypertrophy. The hypertrophy occurs because, with each systole, the left ventricle has to eject a normal stroke volume of blood into the systemic circuit, plus an additional volume of blood that simply regurgitates back from the aorta into the left ventricle during diastole. Thus, the volume work of the left ventricle is increased above normal, and left ventricular pressures may rise. Both of these stimulate left ventricular hypertrophy. In severe cases of aortic regurgitation, diastolic ventricular pressures become elevated, because the left ventricle receives blood both from the left atrium and from the aorta during diastole. Left atrial pressure increases, and pulmonary edema develops.

The foregoing consideration of the pathol-

ogy associated with cardiac defects is important for two reasons. First, these defects and their consequences are commonly encountered in the clinic. Second, this discussion illustrates how the symptoms and consequences of disease states can be understood and predicted in a rational way, based on an understanding of basic principles of cardiac physiology.

CLINICAL CORRELATION

PULMONIC STENOSIS

HISTORY □ A 6-month-old female schnauzer is referred to your clinic because of a heart murmur that was detected during a routine health care visit. The puppy is fairly active but is slightly smaller than her female littermates. She also tires more quickly than her littermates when they play together.

CLINICAL EXAMINATION □ All physical parameters are normal except for a systolic heart murmur that can be heard best over the left third to fourth intercostal space. Femoral pulses are normal, and the jugular veins are not distended. Electrocardiography reveals that the dog is in normal sinus rhythm with a heart rate of 118 beats per minute. The P-R interval is normal. However, the major QRS-deflection is negative in leads I and AvF. Also, deep S-waves are noted in leads II and III, and the QRS-complexes are slightly prolonged, owing to the wide S-waves. Thoracic radiographs show right ventricular enlargement; the right border of the cardiac silhouette is more rounded than normal and closer than normal to the right thoracic wall.

A catheter is inserted into the jugular vein, and the following pressures are measured as the catheter is advanced through the right heart and into the pulmonary artery:

Central venous pressure (mean right atrial pressure) = 6 mmHg

Right ventricular systolic pressure = 56 mmHg

Pulmonary artery systolic pressure = 16 mmHg

The jugular catheter is withdrawn until the catheter tip is in the right ventricle. Then, additional radiographs are taken while a radiopaque dye is injected through the catheter. These radiographs reveal that the right ventricular outflow tract is narrowed just below the pulmonic valve, and that the pulmonic valve does not open widely during ventricular systole.

COMMENT □ The young age of this dog and the absence of other signs of illness suggest that the murmur results from a congenital cardiac abnormality. Murmurs are graded on a scale of 1 through 6, with 6 being the most severe. This dog's murmur is grade 4. A systolic murmur can result from aortic or pulmonic stenosis, mitral or tricuspid incompetence, or a ventricular septal defect (see Fig. 20–8). On the basis of the location from which this murmur can be heard best, aortic or pulmonic stenosis is the most likely cause. All the additional clinical evidence supports a diagnosis of pulmonic stenosis.

The ECGs indicate that cardiac action potentials are initiated and spread through the heart in the normal way. However, the abnormalities observed in the polarity and shape of the QRS-complex are indicative of right ventricular hypertrophy. The thoracic radiographs support this diagnosis. Pulmonic stenosis leads to right ventricular hypertrophy, because the right ventricle must generate much higher pressures than normal during systole in order to eject blood through the narrow outflow tract. Right ventricular systolic pressure is 56 mmHg in this dog, compared with a normal pressure of 20 mmHg.

Normally, the pulmonic valve opens widely during systole, and ventricular systolic pressure equals pulmonary artery systolic pressure. In this dog, there is a difference of 40 mmHg between right ventricular systolic pressure and the systolic pressure in the pulmonary artery just beyond the pulmonic valve. This difference indicates a moderate pulmonic obstruction. The degree of obstruction can be evaluated visually from the radiographs taken during dye injection.

Right ventricular hypertrophy is one of two adaptive responses that helps this dog maintain a nearly normal right ventricular stroke volume, despite the pulmonic stenosis. The other adaptive response is that mean right atrial pressure is higher than normal (6 mmHg instead of 3 mmHg). Right atrial pressure is elevated, because blood backs up or dams up in areas upstream from the stenosis (i.e., in the right ventricle, right atrium, and vena cava). The elevated atrial pressure is adaptive, because it increases right ventricular preload, which increases end-diastolic volume, which (by Starling's law of the heart) helps keep right ventricular stroke volume at a normal level, despite the stenosis. Right atrial pressure is not high enough in this dog to cause abdominal ascites or systemic edema. However, both these signs are seen occasionally in dogs with severe pulmonic stenosis, because excessively elevated right atrial pressure leads to marked increases in capillary hydrostatic pressure (upstream from the right atrium).

The combined effects of right ventricular hypertrophy and elevated right ventricular preload allow this dog's heart to pump a nearly normal stroke volume during rest. However, the pulmonic obstruction limits the increase in stroke volume that can occur during exercise. The resulting limitation in cardiac output accounts for this dog's lack of stamina during exercise. Over a prolonged period, such a limitation in cardiac output can also stunt growth.

TREATMENT □ Theoretically, the best treatment for pulmonic stenosis is to remove the obstruction surgically. A valve dilator can be used or an artificial conduit can be installed across the stenotic valve. Although the most seriously affected dogs require surgical treatment, many dogs with pulmonic stenosis can lead sedentary lives without any treatment.

Some clinicians believe that the adverse effects of pulmonic stenosis can be minimized by administration of β-adrenergic antagonists (e.g., propranolol) or calcium channel blockers (e.g., verapamil). Although the mechanism and efficacy of these drugs remain unclear, there is speculation that these drugs act by limiting ventricular contractility, which limits the work of the heart. Because an increase in cardiac work is the stimulus for hypertrophy, a drug that limits the increase in work also limits the hypertrophy. Although moderate hypertrophy can be adaptive (as explained earlier), excessive hypertrophy is detrimental for two reasons. First, the enlarged ventricular muscle can crowd the pulmonic outflow tract, making the stenosis even worse. Second, the coronary circulation may be unable to deliver the increased amounts of blood flow required by the massive ventricular muscle.

Bibliography

Berne RM, Levy MN: The cardiac pump. *In* Berne RM, Levy MN (eds): Cardiovascular Physiology. St. Louis, CV Mosby, 1986, p 50.

Brown CM: Acquired disorders of cardiac blood flow. *In*

Robinson NE (ed): Current Therapy in Equine Medicine. Philadelphia, WB Saunders, 1987, p 164.

Button C: Congenital disorders of cardiac blood flow. *In* Robinson NE (ed): Current Therapy in Equine Medicine. Philadelphia, WB Saunders, 1987, p 167.

Cohen PF: Cardiac pumping action and its regulation. *In* Cohen PF, Brown EJ Jr, Vlay SC (eds): Clinical Cardiovascular Physiology. Philadelphia, WB Saunders, 1985, p 61.

Huntsman LL, Feigl EO: Cardiac mechanics. *In* Patton HD, Fuchs AF, Hille B, et al (eds): Textbook of Physiology, Vol 2. Philadelphia, WB Saunders, 1989, p 820.

Katz AM: Physiology of the Heart. New York, Raven Press, 1977.

Knight DH: Pathophysiology of heart failure. *In* Ettinger SJ (ed): Textbook of Veterinary Internal Medicine. Philadelphia, WB Saunders, 1989, p 899.

Milnor WR: The heart as a pump. *In* Milnor WR (ed): Cardiovascular Physiology. New York, Oxford University Press, 1990, p 111.

Olivier NB: Congenital heart disease in dogs. *In* Fox RR (ed): Canine and Feline Cardiology. New York, Churchill Livingstone, 1988, p 357.

Scher AM: Events of the cardiac cycle: Measurements of pressure, flow, and volume. *In* Patton HD, Fuchs AF, Hille B, et al (eds): Textbook of Physiology, Vol 2. Philadelphia, WB Saunders, 1989, p 834.

PRACTICE QUESTIONS FOR CHAPTER 20

1. In the normal cardiac cycle,

   a. ventricular systole and ventricular ejection begin at the same time.
   b. the second heart sound coincides with the end of ventricular ejection.
   c. the highest left ventricular pressure is reached just as the aortic valve closes.
   d. aortic pressure is highest at the beginning of ventricular systole.
   e. atrial systole occurs during rapid ventricular ejection.

2. Figure 20–11 shows a plot of the changes in pressure and volume that occur in the left ventricle during one cardiac cycle. Which of the following is true?

   a. Point D marks the beginning of isovolumetric relaxation.
   b. Point B marks the closure of the aortic valve.
   c. Point C marks the opening of the mitral valve.
   d. Point A marks the beginning of isovolumetric contraction.
   e. Point D marks the beginning of ventricular systole.

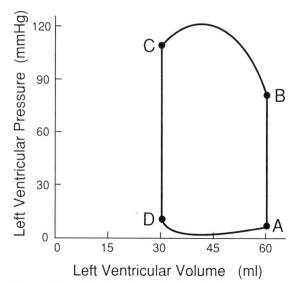

Figure 20–11. The closed loop depicts the changes in left ventricular pressure and volume that occur during one cardiac cycle. This graph is the basis for Practice Question #2. The first step in understanding the figure is to determine whether the normal sequence of events proceeds clockwise or counterclockwise around the loop. To make this distinction, recall that the ventricles fill when ventricular pressure is low and empty when ventricular pressure is high. Next, identify the phases of the cardiac cycle that correspond with each limb of the loop. Finally, determine what happens to the mitral and aortic valves at each corner of the loop. Hint: *A, B, C,* and *D* in this figure match with the similarly labeled events in Figure 20–1.

3. Which statement is true for a normal heart?

   a. Sympathetic activation causes end-systolic ventricular volume to increase.
   b. An increase in ventricular preload causes end-diastolic ventricular volume to decrease.

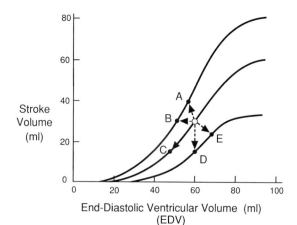

Figure 20–12. This graph of three ventricular function curves is the basis for Practice Question #4.

c. An increase in ventricular contractility causes systolic duration to increase.

d. An increase in ventricular contractility causes the external work of the heart to decrease.

e. Pacing the heart at a high rate causes stroke volume to decrease.

4. Starting at the open circle in Figure 20–12, which point would be reached after contractility decreased and preload increased?

a. Point A
b. Point B
c. Point C
d. Point D
e. Point E

5. You examine a 7-year-old poodle and find evidence of a systolic murmur (no diastolic murmur), pulmonary edema (rapid respiration, cough), left ventricular hypertrophy (no right ventricular hypertrophy), and exercise intolerance. The most likely explanation for the symptoms is

a. mitral regurgitation.
b. mitral stenosis.
c. aortic regurgitation.
d. pulmonary stenosis.
e. ventricular septal defect.

21

The Systemic and Pulmonary Circulations

1. Blood pressure represents a potential energy that propels blood through the circulation
2. *Resistance* is defined as the pressure difference driving flow through a tube or set of tubes, divided by the resulting flow
3. The net resistance of the systemic circulation is called the total peripheral resistance
4. The pulmonary circulation offers much less resistance to blood flow than the systemic circulation does
5. Arterial pressures are measured in terms of their systolic, diastolic, and mean levels
6. Pulse pressure increases when stroke volume increases, heart rate decreases, aortic compliance decreases, or total peripheral resistance increases

Blood Pressure Represents a Potential Energy That Propels Blood Through the Circulation

It is useful to divide the cardiovascular system into the *central circulation* and the *systemic circulation.* The central circulation is composed of the right side of the heart, the pulmonary circuit, and the left side of the heart. Blood enters the central circulation from the vena cava and leaves the central circulation through the aorta. The systemic circulation has the aorta as its inlet point and the vena cava as its outlet point. In a normal resting animal, approximately 25% of the blood volume resides in the central circulation and about 75% in the systemic circulation. Most of the blood in the systemic vessels is in the systemic veins.

Figure 21–1 shows the normal pressure profile in the systemic circulation. The blood pressure is highest in the aorta (typically, 98 mmHg) and lowest in the vena cava (3 mmHg). It is this pressure difference that forces blood to flow through the systemic vessels. Blood pressure can be thought of as the potential energy available to move blood; the decrease in pressure in the sequential segments of the systemic circuit represents the amount of this potential energy that is "used up" in moving blood through each segment. The pressure that is used up is actually converted to heat, which is generated through friction as the blood is pushed through the vessels. Blood pressure decreases only about 3 mmHg as blood moves through the aorta and large arteries, which means that little pressure energy is used up in moving blood through the aorta and major arteries, because these vessels offer little resistance to blood flow. The greatest pressure decrease (and the greatest expenditure of energy) occurs in forc-

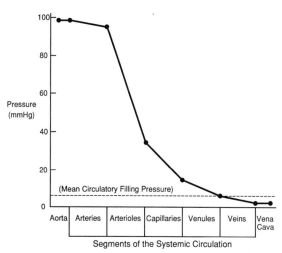

Figure 21–1. The graph shows the blood pressures (hydrostatic pressures) that typically exist in the systemic circulation of a dog at rest. The actual blood pressure in the aorta and arteries is pulsatile; the values plotted here are the average (mean) values of those pulsatile pressures. *Mean circulatory filling pressure* is the pressure that would exist if the heart were stopped (see text for fuller description). All pressures are measured with reference to atmospheric pressure.

ing blood to flow through arterioles. That is, the arterioles provide a greater resistance to blood flow than any other segment of the systemic circulation. Although the capillaries and the venules also offer a substantial resistance to blood flow, the resistance (and therefore the pressure decrease) is not as great in these vessels as in the arterioles. The large veins and the vena cava are low-resistance vessels, so little pressure energy is expended in driving the blood flow through these vessels.

It is the pumping of blood by the heart that maintains the pressure difference between the aorta and the vena cava. If the heart stops, blood continues to flow for a few moments from the aorta toward the vena cava. This removal of blood from the aorta causes pressure to decrease in the aorta. Addition of blood to the vena cava increases the pressure there. Soon, there is no pressure difference between the aorta and the vena cava. Blood flow in the systemic circuit ceases, and the pressure everywhere in the systemic circulation is the same. Experimentally, it has been demonstrated that this eventual, average pressure is about 7 mmHg. This pressure, in a static circulation, is called the *mean circulatory filling pressure*. Mean circulatory filling pressure is above zero, because there is a fullness to the circulation. That is, even if the heart stops,

blood still distends the vessels that contain it. If a transfusion of blood is given to an animal with the heart stopped, the vessels become more distended, and the mean circulating filling pressure rises above 7 mmHg. Conversely, if blood is removed from an animal with the heart stopped, the pressure everywhere falls to a level below 7 mmHg.

Consider what happens if the heart is restarted in an animal after the pressure has equalized everywhere at 7 mmHg. With each heartbeat, the heart takes blood out of the vena cava and moves it into the aorta. The volume of blood in the vena cava decreases, and vena caval pressure drops below 7 mmHg. The volume of blood in the aorta increases, and aortic pressure rises above 7 mmHg. The vena caval pressure drops about 4 mmHg (from 7 to 3), and the aortic pressure rises about 91 mmHg (from 7 to 98). It is important to understand why the pressure decreases only a little in the vena cava and why it increases so much in the aorta, even though the volume of blood removed from the vena cava with each heartbeat is the same as the volume of blood added to the aorta. The reason is that the veins are much more compliant than the arteries. That is, one can add or remove blood from veins without changing the venous pressure very much, whereas adding or removing blood from arteries changes the arterial pressure a great deal.

A compliant vessel readily distends when pressure or volume is added. A compliant vessel is one that yields under hydrostatic pressure. By definition, *compliance* is the change in the volume within a vessel or a chamber divided by the associated change in pressure. Figure 21–2 shows curves depicting the relationship between volume and pressure in veins (which have a high compliance) and arteries (which have a low compliance). Compliance corresponds to the slope of a line on a volume-versus-pressure graph. This graph shows that, at a pressure of 7 mmHg, the veins contain a greater volume of blood than the arteries, because the veins are more compliant than the arteries. When the heart removes some blood from the veins, the pressure in the veins decreases from 7 mmHg to 3 mmHg. When that same volume of blood is added to the less compliant arteries, the arterial pressure rises from 7 mmHg to 98 mmHg. The pressure increase in the arteries is about 20 times greater than the pressure decrease in the veins. That is, the arteries are about 20 times less compliant than the veins.

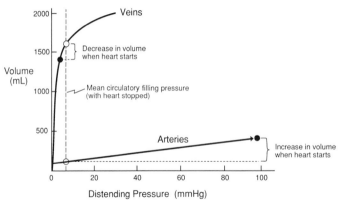

Figure 21–2. Veins are more compliant (distensible) than arteries, so they hold a greater volume of blood for a given distending pressure. For example, if the heart were stopped and the pressure throughout the systemic circulation were 7 mmHg (typical value for mean circulating filling pressure), the veins would contain about 1600 ml of blood and the arteries only 125 ml (open circles on graphs). Restarting the heart would cause a decrease in venous volume and an equivalent increase in arterial volume (closed circles). However, because the veins are so much more compliant than the arteries, the decrease in venous pressure when the heart starts would be much smaller than the increase in arterial pressure.

The difference in compliance between arteries and veins is appropriate, considering the fundamentally different function of these two types of vessels. The veins comprise the body's major blood reservoir, so it is appropriate that they can accept or give up a large volume of blood without much of a change in pressure. The arteries function as a temporary storage site for the pressure energy created when the heart ejects blood. A high arterial pressure is necessary to force blood to flow through the systemic tissues. The large arteries must be tough, relatively noncompliant vessels so they can hold and maintain a pressure high enough to drive blood through the systemic circulation both during and between cardiac ejections.

Maintaining a normal blood flow through the systemic tissues requires a high arterial pressure primarily because the arterioles offer such a large resistance to blood flow. In addition to being the site of the greatest resistance to blood flow in the systemic circulation, the arterioles are the site of adjustable resistance in the systemic circulation. By changing their resistance to blood flow, the arterioles in a particular organ can adjust the amount of blood delivered to that organ. The concept of arteriolar resistance and its adjustment is important to an understanding of cardiovascular physiology.

Resistance Is Defined As the Pressure Difference Driving Flow Through a Tube or Set of Tubes, Divided by the Resulting Flow

The pressure difference (Δ pressure) used in calculating the resistance of a tube or set of tubes is the pressure at the inlet, minus the pressure at the outlet. Figure 21–3 shows a typical relationship between flow and driving pressure for two simple tubes. The smaller tube has higher resistance, and the larger tube has lower resistance. For a given pressure difference, flow is higher in the tube that has lower resistance.

The definition of resistance is

$$\text{resistance} = \frac{\Delta \text{ pressure}}{\text{flow}}$$

In the example shown in Figure 21–3, a pressure difference of 60 mmHg caused a flow of 1600 mL/minute through the large tube. Thus, the resistance of the large tube was 37.5 mmHg/L/minute. The same driving pressure (60 mmHg) caused a flow of only 100 mL/minute through the small tube. The resistance of the small tube was 600 mmHg/L/minute. The resistance of the small tube was 16 times greater than the resistance of the large tube.

The French physician Poiseuille demonstrated over 100 years ago that radius is the primary determinant of the resistance of a tube. He demonstrated that the resistance of a tube can be predicted from the following equation.

$$\text{resistance} = \frac{8 \eta l}{\pi r^4}$$

The resistance of a tube varies inversely with the fourth power of the radius, so that doubling the radius (r) of the tube decreases its resistance by a factor of 16 (2^4). Also, resistance is proportional to the length (l) of the tube. This makes intuitive sense; it is harder to force fluid through a long tube than through a short tube of the same radius. The final important determinant of resistance is the viscosity (η) of the fluid. The higher the viscosity of the fluid, the higher the resistance to its flow through a tube. For example, honey is more viscous than water, so a tube would offer a higher resistance to the flow of honey than to the flow of water.

As noted earlier (see Fig. 21–1), the pressure difference driving blood through the arterioles is greater than the pressure difference driving blood through the capillaries. Therefore, it was concluded that the arterioles offer *more* resistance to blood flow than do the capillaries. This may seem paradoxical, because radius is the main determinant of resistance. Capillaries have a *smaller* radius than arterioles, so why

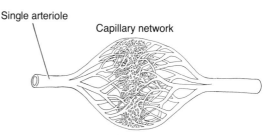

Resistance of arteriole is less than resistance of capillary

Figure 21–4. Arterioles are larger in diameter than capillaries. Therefore, the resistance of a single arteriole is less than the resistance of a single capillary. However, each arteriole typically supplies blood to a network of capillaries, and the resistance of a capillary network is less than the resistance of the arteriole that supplies it.

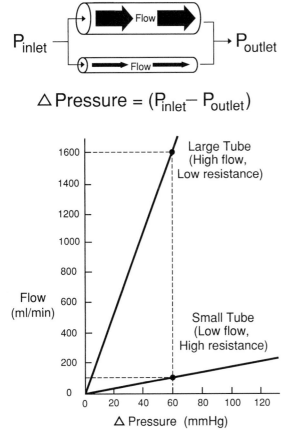

$$\triangle Pressure = (P_{inlet} - P_{outlet})$$

Figure 21–3. Flow through a tube is determined by resistance and perfusion pressure (the pressure difference between the inlet and outlet). Large tubes have a much lower resistance than small tubes, so they carry a much greater flow for any given perfusion pressure (as shown by the closed circles).

do they have a *lower* resistance? The explanation for this apparent paradox is illustrated in Figure 21–4. It is true that each capillary has a smaller diameter and therefore a greater resistance than each arteriole. However, each arteriole in the body distributes blood to many capillaries, and the *net* resistance of all of those capillaries is less than the resistance of the single arteriole that delivers blood to them. To re-emphasize, it is only because each arteriole delivers blood to so many capillaries that the net resistance of the capillaries is less than the resistance of the arteriole.

By varying their resistance, the arterioles control how much blood flows to an organ or to a region within an organ. The arterioles change their resistance by contracting or relaxing the smooth muscle within their walls. Contraction of the arteriolar smooth muscle decreases the radius of arterioles, which substantially increases resistance to blood flow. Relaxation of the smooth muscle increases the radius of the vessels, and this vasodilation substantially reduces the resistance to blood flow. Figure 21–5 shows that small changes in the radius of arterioles in an organ can substantially alter the blood flow to the organ. In this example, arterial pressure is 93 mmHg, and venous pressure is 3 mmHg. Brain blood flow is initially 90 mL/minute (0.090 L/minute). Therefore, the resistance of the brain blood vessels to blood flow is 1000 mmHg/L/minute, as shown in the calculations. Most of

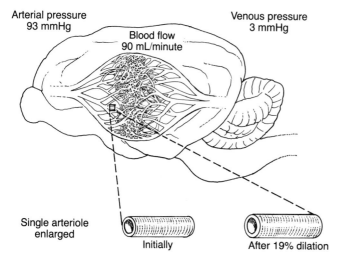

Arterial pressure
93 mmHg

Venous pressure
3 mmHg

Blood flow
90 mL/minute

Figure 21–5. Example to illustrate how a small arteriolar dilation could substantially increase blood flow to the brain. Further discussion in text.

Single arteriole enlarged

Initially

After 19% dilation

Initially,

$$\text{Resistance} = \frac{\Delta \text{Pressure}}{\text{Blood Flow}} = \frac{(93 - 3)\ \text{mmHg}}{90\ \text{mL/minute}} = 1000\ \text{mmHg/L/minute}$$

After dilation of arterioles, resistance = 500 mmHg/L/minute

$$\text{Blood Flow} = \frac{\Delta \text{Pressure}}{\text{Resistance}} = \frac{(93 - 3)\ \text{mmHg}}{500\ \text{mmHg/L/minute}} = 180\ \text{mL/minute}$$

this resistance is provided by the brain arterioles. If the arteriolar smooth muscle relaxed slightly, so that the radius of the arterioles increased by 19%, the arteriolar resistance would be cut in half. To understand why such a small change in radius causes such a large change in resistance, recall that resistance varies inversely as the fourth power of the radius. The resistance would then be 500 mmHg/L/minute. As calculated in Figure 21–5, the brain blood flow would then double to 180 mL/minute. This example illustrates how a small change in arteriolar radius brings about a large change in the blood flow.

The Net Resistance of the Systemic Circulation Is Called the Total Peripheral Resistance

Like any other resistance, total peripheral resistance (TPR) is defined as a pressure difference (perfusion pressure) divided by a flow. In calculating the resistance of the systemic circulation, the perfusion pressure is the pressure in the aorta minus the pressure in the vena cava. The flow is the total amount of blood flowing through the systemic circuit, which is equal to the cardiac output. For a typical dog at rest, mean aortic pressure is 98 mmHg, mean vena caval pressure is 3 mmHg,

and cardiac output is 2.5 L/minute. Under these conditions, TPR is 38 mmHg/L/minute. A TPR of 38 mmHg/L/minute means that it takes a driving pressure of 38 mmHg to force 1 L/minute of blood through the systemic circuit.

Because the pressure in the vena cava is usually close to zero, this pressure is sometimes ignored in calculating TPR. The resulting, simplified equation states that TPR is approximately equal to aortic pressure divided by cardiac output. Usually this equation is rearranged to form the statement that mean aortic blood pressure is equal to cardiac output times TPR ($\underline{BP = CO \times TPR}$). Thus, if aortic pressure is increased, it must be because cardiac output increased, TPR increased, or both. For example, as mentioned earlier, human hypertension is characterized by an excessive constriction of the systemic arterioles, which increases TPR above normal. Cardiac output is typically close to normal in human hypertension. In other situations, TPR and cardiac output change in opposite directions. For example, in the transition from rest to exercise in dogs, TPR decreases to as low as one fifth of its normal value, because the arterioles in the working skeletal muscle dilate in order to increase skeletal muscle blood flow. Cardiac output increases during exercise, and may be five times normal during heavy exercise. The result is that aortic pressure is hardly changed. As a final example, hemorrhage characteristically reduces cardiac output (because cardiac preload decreases). However, compensating reflexes (discussed later) increase TPR by constricting the arterioles in the kidneys, splanchnic circulation, and resting skeletal muscle. The result is that aortic blood pressure decreases only a small amount. This maintenance of aortic pressure is essential to provide adequate blood flow to the brain, heart, and any exercising skeletal muscle.

The Pulmonary Circulation Offers Much Less Resistance to Blood Flow Than the Systemic Circulation Does

Like any other resistance, pulmonary resistance is calculated as a pressure difference (perfusion pressure) divided by a flow. The perfusion pressure forcing blood through the pulmonary circuit is the pressure in the pulmonary artery minus the pressure in the pulmonary veins. The flow that traverses the pulmonary circuit is equal to the cardiac output. For a typical dog at rest, mean pulmonary arterial pressure is 13 mmHg, mean pulmonary venous pressure is 5 mmHg, and cardiac output is 2.5 L/minute. Thus, pulmonary resistance is 3.2 mmHg/L/minute. Note that this is only about one twelfth of the resistance of the systemic circulation.

Pulmonary blood vessels dilate and pulmonary resistance decreases during exercise. The reason is that, as exercise begins, cardiac output increases. Cardiac output may increase to five times its resting value during vigorous exercise. Therefore, pulmonary blood flow also is five times higher than normal. This raises pulmonary artery pressure. Pulmonary blood vessels are compliant, and the increase in pulmonary arterial pressure distends the pulmonary vessels. Because resistance is inversely proportional to the fourth power of vessel radius (Poiseuille's equation, mentioned earlier), a small increase in the radius of the pulmonary vessels greatly decreases their resistance.

The distension of pulmonary blood vessels during exercise is advantageous, because it lowers pulmonary resistance, which allows pulmonary flow to increase greatly without necessitating a large increase in pulmonary arterial pressure. However, in other circumstances, the distensibility of the pulmonary vessels can lead to adverse consequences. An

example is the effect of gravity on pulmonary blood flow. Gravity pulls downward on the blood within lung blood vessels, which increases the distending pressure in vessels low in the lungs compared with vessels higher up (Fig. 21–6). The distended vessels have a lower resistance to blood flow, so more of the pulmonary blood flow traverses the lower (dependent) regions of a lung than the higher regions. Gravity also affects the airways of the lungs. For reasons explained later (Chapter 44), the effect of gravity on the airways causes more air to be delivered to the dependent regions of the lungs than to the higher regions. However, gravity has a greater effect on blood flow than on air delivery, so there is a tendency for blood flow to be excessive (relative to air delivery) in the dependent region of a lung. Any such imbalance between air delivery and blood flow is called a ventilation-perfusion mismatch. This inherent problem is most severe in large animals, where the large size of the lungs leads to substantial gravitational effects.

Hypoxic vasoconstriction is an important mech-

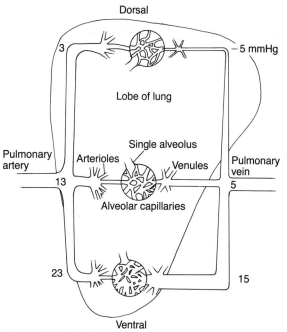

Figure 21–6. Gravity pulls downward on the blood within the lungs, which increases the pressure within blood vessels low in the lungs (see numbers in the figure). The pressure outside of the blood vessels (intrapleural pressure) is not affected much by gravity (because air is so much lighter than blood). Therefore, the low-lying blood vessels are distended, which decreases their resistance to blood flow. As a result, more blood flows through the lower parts of the lungs than through the upper parts.

anism that helps offset ventilation-perfusion mismatches in the lungs, whether these mismatches result from gravitational effects or from any other cause. The pulmonary blood vessels are sensitive to the local concentration of oxygen (measured as oxygen partial pressure, P_{O_2}). A low P_{O_2} *(hypoxia)* causes pulmonary vessels to constrict. Hypoxic vasoconstriction takes place in any region of the lung where ventilation (the delivery of fresh air and oxygen) is reduced relative to blood flow. The vasoconstriction increases the resistance of blood vessels in that lung region, and thereby reduces blood flow (perfusion). In this way, hypoxic vasoconstriction brings about a better match between ventilation and perfusion.

Like many compensatory mechanisms, hypoxic vasoconstriction can sometimes have undesirable consequences. For example, consider what happens if ventilation becomes depressed throughout both lungs. This occurs acutely during an allergic constriction of the airways *(asthma)* or chronically as the result of long-term pulmonary disease that obstructs the airways *(chronic obstructive pulmonary disease,* common in horses). The depressed ventilation causes hypoxia throughout the lungs. The hypoxia causes pulmonary vasoconstriction, which increases pulmonary vascular resistance. The increased resistance necessitates a substantial increase in pulmonary arterial pressure in order to maintain pulmonary blood flow. The condition of elevated pulmonary arterial pressure is called *pulmonary hypertension.* Pulmonary hypertension greatly increases the workload of the right ventricle. In extreme cases, it leads to right ventricular failure (see Clinical Correlation in Chapter 44).

Arterial Pressures Are Measured in Terms of Their Systolic, Diastolic, and Mean Levels

The pressures in the aorta and pulmonary artery are not constant but pulsatile, as shown in Figure 21–7 (femoral artery pressure, also shown in Figure 21–7, will be discussed later). With each cardiac ejection, the aorta and pulmonary artery become distended with blood, which causes the aortic and pulmonary artery pressures to increase to peak values, called *systolic pressures.* In between cardiac ejections (that is, during ventricular diastole), blood continues to flow out of the aorta and pulmonary artery into the systemic and pulmonary circulations, respectively. As the volume

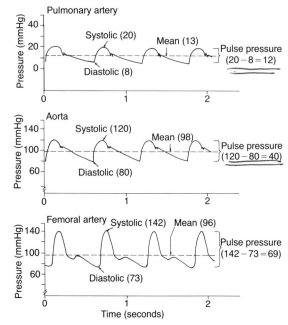

Figure 21–7. Blood pressure in the large arteries is pulsatile. The pressure patterns typical of the pulmonary artery, aorta, and femoral artery are shown.

of blood in these large arteries decreases, the arteries become less distended, so arterial pressure decreases. Pressure continues to decrease until the next cardiac ejection begins. The minimum pressure reached before each new ejection is called the *diastolic pressure.* Figure 21–7 shows the characteristic patterns of the pressure pulsations for the aorta and pulmonary artery, and indicates typical values for systolic and diastolic pressures.

The amplitude of the pressure pulsations in an artery is called the *pulse pressure.* Specifically,

aortic pulse pressure =
(aortic systolic pressure) −
(aortic diastolic pressure)

pulmonary artery pulse pressure =
(pulmonary artery systolic pressure) −
(pulmonary artery diastolic pressure)

Typical values for pulse pressure are indicated in Figure 21–7. Note how much lower the systolic, diastolic, and pulse pressures are in the pulmonary artery than in the aorta. These differences illustrate why the pulmonary circulation is called the low-pressure circulation and the systemic circulation is called the high-pressure circulation.

It is important to distinguish systolic pressure, diastolic pressure, and pulse pressure from each other and to distinguish all of them from *mean pressure*. Mean aortic pressure is the average pressure in the aorta over the course of one or more complete cardiac cycles. Likewise, mean pulmonary artery pressure is the average pressure in that vessel. Obviously, the mean pressure in an artery is somewhere between the systolic (maximum) and diastolic (minimum) pressure levels. However, because the pressure patterns in arteries are asymmetrical, the mean pressure is not necessarily midway between the systolic and diastolic pressures (see Fig. 21–7).

A popular rule is that mean pressure is about one third of the way up from diastolic toward systolic pressure. That is, mean arterial pressure = diastolic pressure + ⅓ (pulse pressure). Figure 21–7 reveals that this is *not* a valid approximation for determining mean pressure in the aorta. However, the approximation is a good one for pressures measured in the femoral artery or in most other major arteries distal to the aorta. The reason that the rule applies in the distal arteries but not in the aorta is that the pattern of the arterial pressure pulsations changes as the pulses move out away from the heart. The pressure pulses become narrower and more sharply peaked. This pronounced asymmetry of the pressure pulses causes the mean level in distal arteries to be much closer to the diastolic pressure than to the systolic pressure (see Fig. 21–7).

For complex reasons, the pulse pressure typically *increases* as blood flows from the aorta into the distal arteries. However, the mean pressure *decreases* in accordance with the principle of conservation of energy. Mean arterial pressure is a measure of the potential energy in the blood stream, and this potential energy is used up (converted into heat by friction) as blood flows from the aorta through the systemic circulation. As stated earlier, most of the resistance to blood flow is found in the arterioles and capillaries. Therefore, the largest decrements in *mean pressure* occur in these segments of the systemic circulation (see Fig. 21–1). The aorta and large arteries offer only a small resistance to blood flow. Therefore, mean arterial pressure is only slightly lower downstream in the femoral artery than it is upstream in the aorta. This difference in pressure is typically only 1–3 mmHg (see Fig. 21–7). In summary, compared with pressure in the aorta, the systolic pressure in the femoral artery is typically greater, the diastolic pressure lower, and the pulse pressure higher. The mean pressure is necessarily lower.

Mean pressures are the pressures that must be used in calculating vascular resistance from the equation

$$resistance = perfusion\ pressure/blood\ flow.$$

In calculating total peripheral resistance, the perfusion pressure is *mean* aortic pressure minus *mean* vena cava (or right atrial) pressure. In calculating pulmonary resistance, the perfusion pressure is *mean* pulmonary arterial pressure minus *mean* pulmonary vein (or left atrial) pressure. Therefore, the concept of mean pressure has tremendous fundamental and theoretical importance.

The only way to measure mean vascular pressures is by inserting a needle or catheter into the vessel of interest. The first direct measurement of mean arterial blood pressure was carried out by Stephen Hales, an English clergyman. In about 1730, Hales inserted a tube (catheter) into the femoral artery of a conscious horse and found that blood rose in the tube to a height of more than 8 feet. An 8-foot column of blood represents a pressure above 180 mmHg, almost twice the mean arterial pressure expected in a normal resting animal. The high pressure undoubtedly reflected the physical and emotional distress of the horse, which was restrained upside down during the episode. Nowadays, arterial catheterization is common in human medicine (e.g., in cardiac catheterization laboratories) but not in veterinary medicine. However, the lesson that physical or emotional distress can dramatically increase blood pressure is as relevant today as it was in Hales' time.

In human medicine, systolic and diastolic arterial pressures can be measured quite accurately with a blood pressure cuff and stethoscope. A blood pressure cuff is not as easy or accurate to use on veterinary species, so systolic and diastolic arterial pressures are seldom directly measured in veterinary medicine. However, the pulse is commonly palpated by placing the fingertips over a major artery, such as the femoral artery. Palpating an artery allows one to get some idea of the pulse pressure by sensing the magnitude of the pulsations felt in the artery. A low pulse pressure is referred to as a "thready" or weak pulse. A high pulse pressure may be called a "bounding" or strong pulse.

Pulse Pressure Increases When Stroke Volume Increases, Heart Rate Decreases, Aortic Compliance Decreases, or Total Peripheral Resistance Increases

An increase in stroke volume tends to increase pulse pressure. Because cardiac ejections create the pulsations in arterial pressure, it should not be surprising that larger ejections create bigger pulsations (Fig. 21–8A). The graph shows that an increase in stroke volume also increases mean pressure, because an in-

creased stroke volume increases cardiac output.

A second factor that tends to increase pulse pressure is a decrease in heart rate. In between cardiac ejections, blood continues to run out of the aorta and through the systemic circulation, and aortic pressure decreases. It falls to a minimum (diastolic) level before being boosted again by the next cardiac ejection. When heart rate decreases, there is a longer time between beats (ejections) and a longer time for blood to run out of the aorta and into

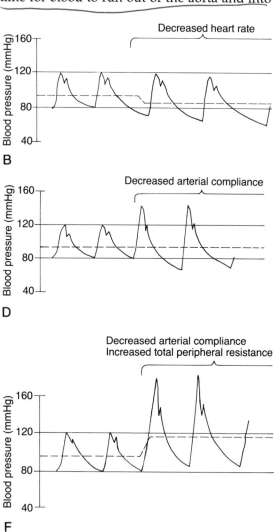

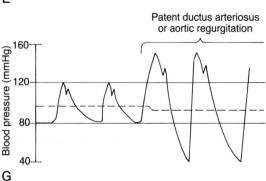

Figure 21–8. Various conditions that increase arterial pulse pressure are compared with regard to their effects on systolic pressure, diastolic pressure, and mean pressure (see text for fuller description).

the systemic circulation. Therefore, blood pressure in the aorta falls to a lower level before the next cardiac ejection, and pulse pressure is increased (Fig. 21–8B). Note that a decrease in heart rate also decreases mean arterial pressure, because a decreased heart rate results in a decreased cardiac output, which decreases mean arterial pressure.

Figure 21–8C diagrams the effect of a simultaneous increase in stroke volume and a decrease in heart rate. In this example, cardiac output, which is stroke volume times heart rate, remains unchanged. Therefore, mean arterial pressure remains unchanged. However, pulse pressure is markedly increased as a result of the combined effects of an increase in stroke volume and a decrease in heart rate. Aerobic conditioning in humans, and in some animals, leads to an increase in stroke volume and a decrease in heart rate at rest. Therefore, mean arterial pressure in a well-trained athlete is typically normal, but pulse pressure is greater than normal. Palpation of the arteries of an athlete at rest reveals a strong, slow pulse.

A decrease in arterial compliance is the third factor that tends to increase pulse pressure (Fig. 21–8D). With each ventricular systole, the heart ejects blood into the aorta and large arteries, which distends these vessels. The stiffer the walls of the large arteries, the greater the increase in pressure required to distend them.

Arterial stiffening increases systolic pressure, because arterial pressure rises higher with each cardiac ejection. Arterial stiffening also decreases diastolic arterial pressure, because pressure falls more as blood leaves the stiffer arteries in between cardiac ejections. In general, neither cardiac output nor TPR is affected by arterial stiffening. Therefore, *mean arterial pressure*, the product of cardiac output and TPR, is unchanged. The major arteries tend to become stiffer as a result of the normal aging process, particularly in humans, and this accounts for the increase in pulse pressure that is typical in older persons.

As shown in Figure 21–8E, an increase in TPR is the fourth factor that commonly increases pulse pressure. In actuality, TPR does not affect pulse pressure directly, but acts through a stiffening of the arteries. The mechanism is as follows: (1) an increase in TPR (arteriolar constriction) causes blood to back up or accumulate in the large arteries; (2) mean arterial pressure increases; (3) the arteries become more distended than normal; (4) disten-

sion forces the larger arteries toward their elastic limit, so distended arteries are stiffer than arteries under normal pressurization (Fig. 21–9). This stiffening of the arteries causes pulse pressure to increase. Note that an increase in TPR increases both pulse pressure and mean arterial pressure. As mentioned earlier, TPR is elevated in human hypertension. Therefore, mean arterial pressure and pulse pressure are both typically elevated. Whereas a normal arterial pulse pressure is 40 mmHg (120 systolic minus 80 diastolic), a severely hypertensive person might have a pulse pressure of 80 mmHg (190 systolic minus 110 diastolic). The increase in pulse pressure in hypertensive persons is often accentuated by a simultaneous aging process, which further decreases the compliance of the arteries. The combination of decreased arterial compliance and increased TPR increases pulse pressure dramatically (see Fig. 21–8F). An older, severely hypertensive person might have a pulse pressure of 110 mmHg (200 systolic minus 90 diastolic).

In summary, pulse pressure tends to be increased by increased stroke volume, decreased heart rate, decreased arterial compliance, or increased TPR.

Some of the cardiac defects that produce murmurs also cause characteristic changes in pulse pressure. For example, a patient with patent ductus arteriosus (PDA) has a large left

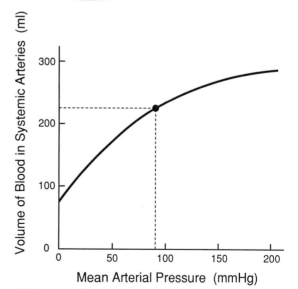

Figure 21–9. This volume-pressure relationship shows that normal systemic arteries become stiffer (less compliant) when they are distended by arterial pressure above normal. (Recall that compliance is equal to the slope of a volume-pressure relationship.)

ventricular stroke volume. Typically, aortic systolic pressure is elevated but diastolic pressure is much lower than normal because, between cardiac ejections, blood runs from the aorta out into the systemic circuit and also through the open ductus. A similar characteristic increase in pulse pressure is caused by aortic regurgitation (see Fig. 21–8G). In aortic regurgitation, more blood than normal leaves the aorta during diastole, part of it going through the systemic circuit and part of it returning through the incompetent aortic valves and into the left ventricle.

CLINICAL CORRELATION

CANINE HEARTWORM DISEASE WITH PULMONARY EMBOLISM

HISTORY □ You examine a 6-year-old male beagle who has been used as a hunting companion by his owner for several years. The owner reports that the dog tires more easily than usual and has developed a cough that is worse when exercising. You had treated this dog when he was 3 years old for a laceration, and your records indicate that the dog was otherwise in excellent health at that time. The owner acknowledges that the dog has not been given any immunizations or heartworm prophylactic medication for the past 2 years.

CLINICAL EXAMINATION □ On physical examination of the dog, you note the cough reported by the owner and an apparent modest accumulation of fluid in the abdominal cavity (ascites). You also note a systolic murmur, heard loudest over the left third to fourth intercostal spaces. The chest radiograph and ECG show evidence of right ventricular hypertrophy. In addition, the pulmonary vessels are more prominent than normal on the radiograph, and they are tortuous. You take a blood sample and centrifuge it. You pipette a bit of the buffy coat onto a glass slide and examine it microscopically. You find the microfilaria of *Dirofilaria immitus.* You diagnose canine heartworm parasitism.

COMMENT □ Adult heartworms develop from microfilaria, which are transmitted by mosquitoes from the blood stream of infected dogs to the blood stream of noninfected dogs. The adult worms, which grow to a length of 10–20 cm,

cling to the walls of the pulmonary artery and its major branches. Heartworm infestation typically causes pulmonary arterial vessels to become enlarged and tortuous (twisted). In heavily infested dogs, adult worms also reside in the right ventricle and right ventricular outflow tract, where they cause pulmonary stenosis. The resulting turbulence during right ventricular ejection accounts for the murmur heard in this dog. The pulmonic stenosis and the increased pulmonary resistance created by the worms also lead to right ventricular hypertrophy, exercise intolerance, and ascites (review Clinical Correlation in Chapter 20).

TREATMENT □ You advise the owner that the dog should be treated with an arsenic-containing medication that kills adult worms over a period of several days. However, you also warn the owner that the treatment of severely infested dogs is risky. Dead adult worms break away from the right ventricle and pulmonary artery and lodge in smaller pulmonary vessels. These vascular occlusions (emboli) restrict pulmonary blood flow and reduce cardiac output. Therefore, it is necessary to keep the dog in a quiet, unstressed state for 8–10 days after beginning treatment. In addition to restricting pulmonary blood flow, the emboli are also likely to cause inflammation and blood clots in the lungs. Pulmonary edema is expected. Also, pulmonary blood vessels may break down, allowing blood to enter the airways of the lungs. Respiratory failure is possible. Anti-inflammatory and antithrombotic drugs (aspirin initially, plus prednisolone after 4–5 days) is given to reduce these complications.

With the owner's consent, you keep the dog at your clinic for 2 days (to allow it to become accustomed to the surroundings) and then begin treatment. Over the next week, the dog becomes even more lethargic than before and begins to cough up blood. The dog has a low-grade fever (102–103° F), and his ascites becomes worse. However, his systolic murmur begins to fade. After 1 week, all the clinical signs have improved markedly. The dog is sent home for a prolonged period of recuperation. The long-term prognosis is good.

Bibliography

Berne RM, Levy MN: The arterial system. *In* Berne RM, Levy MN (eds): Cardiovascular Physiology. St. Louis, CV Mosby, 1986, p 124.

Brown EJ Jr, Cohen PF: The systemic circulation. *In* Cohen PF, Brown EJ Jr, Vlay SC (eds): Clinical Cardiovascular Physiology. Philadelphia, WB Saunders, 1985, p 129.

Butler J: The circulation of the lung. *In* Patton HD, Fuchs AF, Hille B, et al (eds): Textbook of Physiology, Vol 2. Philadelphia, WB Saunders, 1989, p 961.

Feigl EO: The arterial system. *In* Patton HD, Fuchs AF, Hille B, et al (eds): Textbook of Physiology, Vol 2. Philadelphia, WB Saunders, 1989, p 849.

Milnor WR: Principles of hemodynamics. *In* Milnor WR (ed): Cardiovascular Physiology. New York, Oxford University Press, 1990, p 171.

Milnor WR: Pulmonary circulation. *In* Milnor WR (ed): Cardiovascular Physiology. New York, Oxford University Press, 1990, p 357.

PRACTICE QUESTIONS FOR CHAPTER 21

1. If aortic compliance is decreased while heart rate cardiac output and TPR remain unchanged,

   a. pulse pressure is unchanged.
   b. pulse pressure is increased.
   c. pulse pressure is decreased.
   d. One cannot know the effect on pulse pressure because stroke volume may have changed.

2. Mean aortic pressure increases if

   a. stroke volume increases from 30 mL to 40 mL, and heart rate decreases from 100 beats/minute to 60 beats/minute.
   b. arterial compliance decreases.
   c. heart rate decreases.
   d. arterioles throughout the body dilate.
   e. TPR increases.

3. The following measurements are made on a dog:

heart rate	80 beats/minute
stroke volume	30 mL
mean aortic pressure	96 mmHg
mean pulmonary artery pressure	30 mmHg
left atrial pressure	5 mmHg
right atrial pressure	12 mmHg

TPR (taking into account both arterial and atrial pressures) is

   a. 10.42 mmHg/L/minute.
   b. 12.50 mmHg/L/minute.
   c. 35.00 mmHg/L/minute.
   d. 37.92 mmHg/L/minute.
   e. 40.00 mmHg/L/minute.

4. A change from breathing normal air (21% O_2 and 0% CO_2) to breathing a gas mixture of 10% O_2 and 5% CO_2 causes pulmonary blood vessels to _____ and pulmonary resistance to _____.

   a. constrict .... increase
   b. constrict .... decrease
   c. dilate .... increase
   d. dilate .... decrease
   e. remain unchanged .... remain unchanged

5. An abdominal aorta is studied during autopsy. It is 15 cm long and 1.1 cm in diameter. If one also knows the viscosity of blood, this information can be used to estimate the aorta's

   a. resistance to blood flow.
   b. velocity of blood flow.
   c. compliance.
   d. blood pressure.
   e. permeability.

22

Capillaries and Fluid Exchange

1. Capillaries, the smallest blood vessels, are the site for the exchange of water and solutes between the blood stream and the interstitial fluid
2. Lipid-soluble substances diffuse readily through capillary walls, whereas lipid-insoluble substances must pass through capillary pores
3. Fick's law of diffusion is a simple, mathematical accounting of the physical factors that affect the rate of diffusion
4. Water moves across capillary walls both by diffusion (osmosis) and by bulk flow
5. Several common physiological changes alter the normal balance of Starling's forces and increase the filtration of water out of capillaries
6. Edema is a clinically noticeable excess of interstitial fluid

Capillaries, the Smallest Blood Vessels, Are the Site for the Exchange of Water and Solutes Between the Blood Stream and the Interstitial Fluid

Because of their small size, the capillaries are sometimes called the *microcirculation*. They are also called the *exchange vessels*, because the exchange of water and solutes between the blood stream and the interstitial fluid takes place across the walls of the capillaries. Each type of blood vessel in the body is structurally suited for its primary function, and the walls of the capillaries are especially well adapted for their exchange function.

Figure 22–1 shows the contrasting features of the walls of the various types of blood vessels. The distinguishing feature of the walls of the aorta and large arteries is the presence of a large amount of elastic material along with the smooth muscle. These vessels are called

the *elastic vessels;* elasticity is necessary because the aorta and large arteries must distend with each pulsatile ejection of blood from the heart. The small arteries, and particularly the arterioles, have relatively thick walls with less elastic tissue and a predominance of smooth muscle, so they are called the *muscular vessels.* The muscle enables these vessels to constrict or dilate, which varies their resistance to blood flow. The muscular vessels vary the total peripheral resistance (TPR) and also direct blood flow to particular organs or to particular regions within an organ. The capillaries are the smallest vessels, being about 8 μm in diameter and less than 0.5 mm long. Capillaries are so small that red blood cells (8 μm in diameter) must squeeze through in single file. Capillary walls consist of a single layer of endothelial cells. The small diameter and the thinness of the vessel wall permit the blood within the

Figure 22–1. Each type of blood vessel in the systemic circulation is specifically suited to its particular function by its size, wall thickness, and wall composition. The vessels are shown in cross section in this scale drawing (the arteriole, capillary, and venule are magnified 250 times to make them visible). Also shown are the relative proportions of the three most important types of tissue found in blood vessel walls.

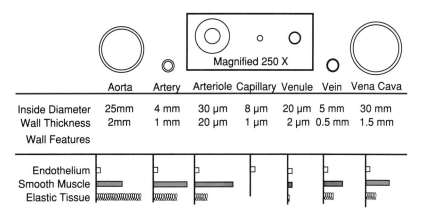

	Aorta	Artery	Arteriole	Capillary	Venule	Vein	Vena Cava
Inside Diameter	25mm	4 mm	30 µm	8 µm	20 µm	5 mm	30 mm
Wall Thickness	2mm	1 mm	20 µm	1 µm	2 µm	0.5 mm	1.5 mm
Wall Features							
Endothelium							
Smooth Muscle							
Elastic Tissue							

capillaries to pass close to the interstitial fluid outside the capillaries. The venules and veins are larger than the capillaries, and they have thicker walls. Venules and veins have both elastic tissue and smooth muscle in their walls. However, the walls of veins are not as thick or as muscular as the walls of the arteries or arterioles. The primary role of the veins is to serve as *reservoir vessels*. The veins are very compliant. In addition, it is normal for many veins in the body to be in a state of partial collapse. Therefore, substantial changes in venous blood volume can occur without much change in venous pressure.

Capillaries form a network (see Fig. 17–3). In most tissues, the capillary network is so dense that each cell of the tissue is within 100 µm of a capillary. However, not all the capillaries of a tissue carry blood all the time. In most tissues, a periodic constriction of each arteriole reduces or even stops blood flow for a short time in some capillaries. Also, in some tissues (e.g., intestinal circulation) there are tiny sphincter muscles at points where capillaries branch off from arterioles. Contraction of these *precapillary sphincters* can also decrease or stop the flow of blood in individual capillaries. When the metabolic rate of a tissue increases (and therefore its need for blood flow increases), the arterioles and precapillary sphincters dilate. As a result, capillaries already carrying blood carry an increased amount, and capillaries previously shut off open up so that they begin to carry blood. In this way, the flow of blood through the capillaries of a rapidly metabolizing tissue can be increased. Also, when blood begins to flow through capillaries that were previously shut, the distance between each cell of the tissue and the nearest capillary carrying bulk flow of blood is effectively decreased, and this speeds up diffusional exchange.

Lipid-Soluble Substances Diffuse Readily Through Capillary Walls, Whereas Lipid-Insoluble Substances Must Pass Through Capillary Pores

The rate of diffusional exchange between capillary blood and the surrounding interstitial fluid depends both on the features of the capillary wall and also on the properties of the substance being exchanged. In most tissues, *water-filled pores* or *clefts* lie between the endothelial cells that form capillary walls (Fig. 22–2). These pores provide a channel through which water and water-soluble (lipid-insoluble) substances can move from the capillary lumen to the interstitial space or vice versa. Lipid-insoluble substances that pass through these water-filled pores include the plasma electrolytes, glucose, and amino acids. By contrast, lipid-soluble substances in blood, such as dissolved oxygen and carbon dioxide, fatty acids, ethanol, and lipid-soluble hormones, can diffuse through both the water-filled pores and the endothelial cells of the capillary wall. That is, a lipid-soluble substance like oxygen can diffuse right through the cell membranes and cytoplasm of the capillary endothelial cells. Because the area of the pores typically constitutes only about 1% of the total wall surface area of a capillary, lipid-insoluble substances are restricted to a much smaller surface area for exchange between the capillary fluid and the surrounding interstitial fluid compared to lipid-soluble substances. As a result, the rate of diffusional exchange is much slower for lipid-insoluble substances than for lipid-soluble substances.

The characteristics of the capillary pores vary from tissue to tissue. Two extremes are found in the liver and brain. The capillary pores or clefts in the liver are so large that even plasma proteins like albumin and globulin can pass through them. This is an appro-

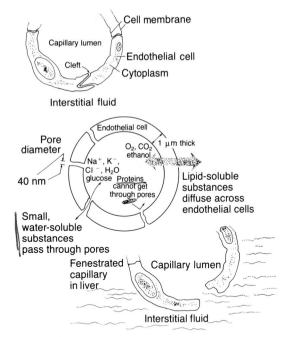

Figure 22–2. Most capillaries have pores or clefts between endothelial cells (top diagram). Water and lipid-insoluble compounds move between the capillary plasma and the interstitial fluid through these water-filled channels (center diagram). The size of the capillary pores varies greatly from tissue to tissue, the largest capillary pores being found in the liver (bottom diagram).

priate feature for the liver capillaries, because the plasma proteins are produced in the liver. The large clefts permit the newly synthesized protein molecules to enter the blood stream. The large pores in liver capillaries are appropriate also for the role of the liver in detoxification. Some toxins that become bound to plasma proteins are removed from the blood stream by the liver and chemically changed into less toxic substances. Because of their large pores, capillaries in the liver are called *fenestrated capillaries* ("capillaries with windows") (see Fig. 22–2, bottom). The other extreme in pore size is represented by the capillaries of the brain. The pores of brain capillaries are so small that only water molecules and electrolyte molecules can pass through them. Glucose, amino acid molecules, and plasma proteins cannot pass through these tiny pores. The tight barrier provided between the blood stream and the brain tissue by the small pores is called the *blood-brain barrier* (see Chapter 14). The neurons of the brain use glucose as their primary metabolic substrate, so glucose has to be able to pass from the blood stream into the brain tissue.

For this purpose, the membranes of the endothelial cells of brain capillaries are equipped with special proteins that carry glucose across the capillary wall. This carrier-mediated process by which glucose moves from the blood stream into the brain tissue is called *facilitated diffusion.*

Fick's Law of Diffusion Is a Simple Mathematical Accounting of the Physical Factors That Affect the Rate of Diffusion

Most of the factors that affect the rate of diffusional exchange between capillary blood and interstitial fluid have already been mentioned. These factors include the size of the capillary pores and the properties of the diffusing substance (i.e., lipid-soluble versus lipid-insoluble). Fick incorporated the factors that affect the rate of diffusion into an equation called *Fick's law of diffusion*. Figure 22–3 shows how Fick's law applies to the diffusional exchange between capillary fluid and interstitial fluid. The rate of diffusion of any substance (S) depends, first of all, on the *concentration difference* of the substance between the capillary fluid and the interstitial fluid. Diffusion is driven by a concentration difference, and diffusion always proceeds from the area of higher concentration toward the area of lower concentration. Next, the rate of diffusion is determined by the *area available for diffusion*. For lipid-soluble substances, this area is equivalent to the total surface area of the capillaries. For lipid-insoluble substances, this area is much smaller, being equal to the area of the capillary pores or clefts.

The term Δx in the equation represents the *distance* over which diffusion must occur. In most tissues, Δx represents the distance from a cell of the tissue to the nearest capillary that is carrying bulk flow of blood. The greater the distance from a tissue cell to a capillary, the slower the rate of diffusional exchange of substances between that cell and the capillary blood. Therefore, Δx appears in the denominator in the equation.

The term *D* in the equation is a *diffusion coefficient*. The value of *D* increases with temperature, because diffusion is dependent upon the random Brownian motion of particles in solution, and the amount of that motion increases with temperature. *D is different for different substances.* For example, the diffusion coefficient for carbon dioxide is about 20

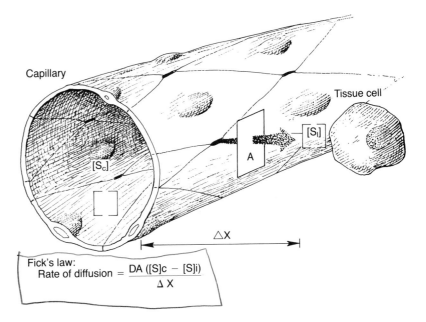

Figure 22–3. The factors affecting the rate of diffusion of a substance, S, from the capillary plasma to the interstitial fluid next to a tissue cell are $[S_c] - [S_i]$, the concentration difference between the capillary plasma and interstitial fluid; A, the area available for diffusion; Δx, the distance involved; and D, the diffusion coefficient.

Capillary

Tissue cell

$[S_i]$

A

$[S_c]$

ΔX

Fick's law:
$$\text{Rate of diffusion} = \frac{DA\,([S]c - [S]i)}{\Delta X}$$

times greater than the diffusion coefficient for oxygen. As a result, carbon dioxide diffuses much more rapidly than oxygen does for a given concentration difference, area, and diffusion distance. This difference is inconsequential under normal physiological conditions. However, in certain disease states, the diffusion of oxygen and carbon dioxide between the blood stream and tissues becomes limited by an inadequate area for diffusion or by an excessive diffusion distance. Because oxygen has a lower diffusion coefficient than carbon dioxide, the delivery of oxygen to the metabolizing cells of a tissue generally becomes inadequate before the removal of carbon dioxide from the cells becomes inadequate. That is, when physiological diffusion limitations exist, body tissues generally exhibit *hypoxia* (low oxygen) before they exhibit *hypercapnia* (elevated carbon dioxide).

Several of the factors affecting the rate of diffusion are physiologically adjustable. For example, in skeletal muscle at rest, the arterioles are constricted, and blood flow through capillaries is low. In fact, at any one moment, blood flows through only about one quarter of the skeletal muscle capillaries. The rest carry no flow. Nevertheless, this low blood flow is adequate to deliver oxygen and nutrients to the resting skeletal muscle cells and to remove the small amounts of carbon dioxide being produced by those resting muscle cells. During exercise, the skeletal muscle arterioles dilate. Capillaries already carrying blood carry a

larger flow, and capillaries previously not carrying blood begin to carry it. These changes act in three ways to speed the delivery of oxygen and metabolic substrates to the exercising muscle cells and to facilitate the removal of carbon dioxide and other metabolic waste products. First, when more capillaries carry blood, the area available for diffusion (A in Fick's diffusion equation) is increased. Second, because more capillaries carry blood, the distance between each exercising skeletal muscle cell and the nearest open capillary (Δx in the diffusion equation) is decreased. Third, the concentration difference for oxygen between the capillary blood and the interstitial fluid (the driving force for diffusion) is greatly increased. The driving force for diffusion is increased for two reasons. First, the greater blood flow brings more oxygenated blood into the tissue, which increases the concentration of oxygen in capillary blood. Second, the rapid utilization of oxygen by the exercising skeletal muscle cells decreases the concentration of oxygen within the skeletal muscle cells and in the surrounding interstitial fluid.

The same factors that increase the rate of oxygen diffusion also increase the rate at which carbon dioxide and other metabolic products are removed from the cells and into the blood stream. In the case of carbon dioxide and other metabolic products, the concentration is highest in the cells and lowest in the capillary plasma, so diffusional movement is from the cells toward the blood stream.

Water Moves Across Capillary Walls Both by Diffusion (Osmosis) and by Bulk Flow

The exchange of water between the capillary plasma and the interstitial fluid merits special consideration for two reasons. First, the forces governing its movement are more complicated than the forces affecting solute movement. Second, the control of water movement has special clinical implications; when an excessive amount of water accumulates in the interstitial space, the condition is called *edema.*

As the preceding discussion has emphasized, solutes such as oxygen, carbon dioxide, glucose, electrolytes, and fatty acids move between the capillary plasma and the interstitial fluid by diffusion. The driving force for the diffusion of a particular solute is the concentration difference of that solute between the capillary plasma and the interstitial fluid. Water also moves by diffusion, through the capillary pores, from the side of the capillary where the water concentration is highest to the side where the water concentration is lowest. However, this diffusional movement of water is more commonly described as a movement from an area of low total solute concentration toward an area of high total solute concentration. This tendency of water to move down its concentration gradient by diffusion is called *osmosis*. The physical prerequisites for osmosis are (1) the presence of a *semipermeable membrane* (a membrane that is permeable to water but not to specific solutes), and (2) a difference in the total concentration of impermeable solutes on the two sides of the membrane.

The capillary wall constitutes a semipermeable membrane. It is permeable to water but not to certain solutes. Specifically, the capillary walls in most organs are impermeable to the plasma proteins. (Albumin and globulin molecules are just slightly too large to pass through the pores in most capillaries.) Normally the concentration of plasma proteins is 7 g/dL within the capillary plasma and only 0.2 g/dL in the interstitial fluid. The higher protein concentration within the capillaries creates a tendency for water molecules to move by osmosis from the interstitial fluid into the capillary blood plasma. Movement of water in this direction is called *reabsorption*.

The tendency for water to move by diffusion is quantified by osmotic pressure. By definition, the *osmotic pressure* of a solution is equal to the hydrostatic pressure that would be required to stop the diffusion of water into the solution across a semipermeable membrane. The *osmotic pressure of capillary plasma,* generated by the plasma proteins, is also called *plasma oncotic pressure or colloid osmotic pressure*. (The term colloid is used, because the plasma proteins are not in a true solution but rather in a colloidal suspension.) The normal oncotic pressure of capillary plasma is 25 mmHg. That is, the entry of water into the capillaries because of the osmotic attraction of the plasma proteins could be stopped by a hydrostatic pressure in the capillaries of 25 mmHg.

The concentration of plasma proteins in the interstitial fluid is much lower than in the capillary plasma; the oncotic pressure of interstitial fluid is normally only 1 mmHg. Therefore, the net oncotic pressure acting on water, calculated by subtracting the oncotic pressure of interstitial fluid from the oncotic pressure of capillary blood, is 25 mmHg − 1 mmHg = 24 mmHg, favoring reabsorption. Note that it is only the plasma protein molecules that generate an osmotic pressure acting on water. The other solutes in the blood and in the interstitial fluid (oxygen, carbon dioxide, glucose, electrolytes) can pass across the capillary wall. Therefore, the total concentration of these solutes is almost exactly equal in the capillary plasma and in the interstitial fluid, and they do not generate an osmotic pressure difference between the capillary plasma and the interstitial fluid.

In addition to being affected by diffusional (osmotic) forces, the movement of water across the capillary wall is affected also by hydrostatic forces. Hydrostatic pressure differences between the capillary plasma and the interstitial fluid cause water to move by bulk flow through the capillary pores. The hydrostatic pressure within the capillaries (capillary blood pressure) is normally about 18 mmHg (see Fig. 21–1). Interstitial fluid hydrostatic pressure is normally about −7 mmHg. (The negative sign means that interstitial fluid pressure is normally *less* than atmospheric pressure.) The negative interstitial fluid pressure (−7 mmHg), together with the positive capillary hydrostatic pressure (18 mmHg), creates a *hydrostatic pressure difference* of 25 mmHg that tends to force water out of the capillaries and into the interstitial spaces. Movement of water out of capillaries and into the interstitial space is called *filtration.*

The tendency for this hydrostatic pressure difference to filter water out of capillaries is nearly balanced by the tendency for the oncotic pressures to reabsorb interstitial water back into the capillaries. However, the balance is rarely perfect. Usually the hydrostatic pressure difference (favoring filtration) slightly exceeds the oncotic pressure difference (favoring reabsorption), so there is a small net filtration of water out of the capillaries. This water would simply accumulate in the interstitial spaces and cause swelling there, were it not for the lymph vessels, which collect excess interstitial fluid and return it to the blood stream through the subclavian vein (Fig. 22–4).

Note that the hydrostatic pressures mentioned earlier are measured with reference to atmospheric pressure. To say that interstitial pressure is negative does not imply that a vacuum exists, but only that the interstitial pressure is slightly below atmospheric pressure. If the interstitial spaces of the body were always pressurized more than atmospheric pressure, then all parts of the body would bulge outward. The subatmospheric interstitial fluid pressure probably accounts for the ability of some body surfaces to assume a concave shape (e.g., the axillary space or the orbits of the eyes).

The origin of the negative interstitial fluid pressure is easy to understand. If interstitial fluid hydrostatic pressure were not negative, then the oncotic pressure difference (favoring reabsorption) would predominate over the hydrostatic pressure difference (favoring filtration). Water would be reabsorbed from the interstitial space. However, this process would shrink the interstitial space, so the hydrostatic pressure there would decrease. Reabsorption would continue until the tendency for water to be reabsorbed (by osmotic action) became balanced by the tendency for water to be filtered in response to the increasing hydrostatic pressure difference between capillary blood and interstitial fluid. Typically, the osmotic and hydrostatic influences come into an approximate balance when enough water has been reabsorbed from the interstitial space to lower the interstitial fluid hydrostatic pressure a few millimeters below atmospheric pressure.

The following equation expresses mathematically the interaction between osmotic pressures and hydrostatic pressures in determining the net force (net pressure) acting on water. Nominal values for each pressure are also listed.

net pressure $= [(P_c - P_i) - (\pi_c - \pi_i)]$
where $P_c =$ capillary hydrostatic pressure

$P_i =$ interstitial fluid hydrostatic pressure
$\pi_c =$ capillary plasma oncotic pressure
$\pi_i =$ interstitial fluid oncotic pressure

Nominal values:

$P_c = 18$ mmHg
$P_i = -7$ mmHg
$\pi_c = 25$ mmHg
$\pi_i = 1$ mmHg

Solving the equation, using nominal values:

net pressure $= [(18 \text{ mmHg}) - (-7 \text{ mmHg})]$
$- [(25 \text{ mmHg}) - (1 \text{ mmHg})] =$
$+1$ mmHg

The positive sign for net pressure indicates that the net pressure favors filtration. The small magnitude of the net pressure (1 mmHg) indicates that the hydrostatic and osmotic forces affecting water are nearly in balance (i.e., there is only a slight tendency for filtration). The quantitative analysis of how osmotic and hydrostatic pressures affect water movement across capillary walls was first derived by Starling (the same scientist for whom Starling's law of the heart is named). Therefore, the interaction of osmotic and hydrostatic pressure is referred to as "the balance of Starling forces." Starling realized that the actual rate of water movement across capillary walls is affected both by the magnitude of the imbalance between hydrostatic and osmotic forces and by the permeability of the capillary wall to water. These ideas are expressed in the following equation, which indicates that the movement of water is equal to the permeability of the capillary wall (given as the filtration coefficient, K_f) times the net difference between hydrostatic and oncotic pressures.

transcapillary water flux $=$
$K_f [(P_c - P_i) - (\pi_c - \pi_i)]$

Examination of this equation reveals that the tendency for filtration of water out of capillaries can be enhanced by (1) increasing the hydrostatic difference between capillary blood and interstitial fluid, (2) decreasing the osmotic tendency for water to be reabsorbed, or (3) increasing the permeability of the capillary to water (i.e., increasing the filtration coefficient).

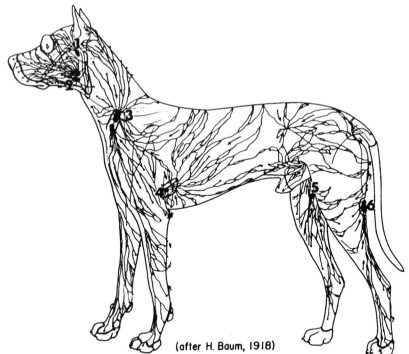

(after H. Baum, 1918)

Figure 22–4. The lymphatic vessels collect excess interstitial fluid from tissues throughout the body and carry it to the subclavian vein (not shown), where the lymph enters the blood stream. Lymph moves through lymph vessels by bulk flow, and the driving force for this flow is the pressure difference between the interstitial fluid hydrostatic pressure and the subclavian vein pressure. Valves in the lymph vessels prevent a reverse flow of lymph. The numbers identify the major lymph nodes. (From Getty R: Sisson and Grossman's The Anatomy of the Domestic Animal, Vol 2. Philadelphia, WB Saunders, 1975, p 1653.)

Several Common Physiological Changes Alter the Normal Balance of Starling's Forces and Increase the Filtration of Water Out of Capillaries

An increase in capillary hydrostatic pressure (P_c) favors filtration of water. Capillary hydrostatic pressure can be increased by an increase in arterial blood pressure or by a decrease in arteriolar resistance. An increase in arterial pressure causes more pressure to be transmitted down through the arterioles and into the capillaries. Likewise, a decrease in arteriolar resistance (e.g., a dilation of the arterioles) allows a greater portion of the arterial pressure to be transmitted into the capillaries. Capillary hydrostatic pressure can be increased also by a backing up (damming up) of venous blood. An increase in central venous pressure causes blood to accumulate in the capillaries and raises capillary pressure. An obstruction to venous outflow (e.g., too tight a dressing on a limb) also causes blood to back up in the capillaries, and this also increases capillary hydrostatic pressure.

Whereas several factors commonly affect capillary hydrostatic pressure, the only important determinant of interstitial fluid hydrostatic pressure is the volume of fluid present in the interstitial space. An accumulation of interstitial fluid increases interstitial hydrostatic pressure. Removal of interstitial fluid decreases the pressure. As stated earlier, interstitial fluid hydrostatic pressure is usually subatmospheric (e.g., -7 mmHg). When interstitial fluid hydrostatic pressure rises above atmospheric pressure, the accumulation of interstitial fluid becomes clinically noticeable as a swelling or *edema.*

The osmotic forces exerted on water depend on the concentrations of proteins in the capillary plasma and in the interstitial fluid. The normal plasma protein concentration is 7 g/dL of plasma, which results in a plasma oncotic pressure of 25 mmHg. Any alteration in the concentration of proteins in the capillary plasma alters the plasma oncotic pressure. Similarly, changes in the interstitial protein concentration alter interstitial fluid oncotic pressure. Under normal circumstances, protein molecules are slightly too large to pass through the capillary pores or clefts. Under abnormal circumstances (e.g., during tissue inflammation), the clefts may widen enough to allow plasma proteins to move from the capillary blood into the interstitial fluid.

Under normal circumstances, the main route for the delivery of plasma proteins into the interstitial fluid is by the process of *pinocytosis.* The first step in pinocytosis is called *endocyto-*

sis. This process involves the invagination of the capillary endothelial cell membrane to form an intracellular vesicle that contains plasma, including plasma proteins. The next step in pinocytosis is the migration of these vesicles across the capillary endothelial cell from the side facing the blood stream to the side facing the interstitial fluid. The final step in pinocytosis involves *exocytosis,* in which the vesicles containing plasma fuse with the outer membrane of the capillary endothelial cells; the vesicles discharge their contents into the interstitial space. An increase in pinocytotic activity increases the delivery of plasma proteins into the interstitial space and increases interstitial fluid oncotic pressure.

Plasma proteins get removed from the interstitial space through the lymph vessels. The lymphatic vessels carry the interstitial fluid, and any plasma proteins contained in it, to the thorax, where the fluid enters the subclavian vein.

The role of lymphatic flow in preventing the accumulation of excessive interstitial fluid is especially important in the lungs. Lung capillaries are more permeable to plasma proteins than are most capillaries in the systemic circulation. As a result, the concentration of proteins in lung interstitial fluid is almost as high as the concentration in the capillary blood. That is, the oncotic pressure of interstitial fluid in the lungs is normally about 18 mmHg, compared with 25 mmHg for capillary blood. Capillary hydrostatic pressure in the lung is generally about 12 mmHg. This value is lower than capillary hydrostatic pressure for systemic capillaries, because pulmonary arterial pressure is so much lower than systemic arterial pressure. Interstitial hydrostatic pressure in the lungs is generally about −5 mmHg (the same as intrapleural pressure). The following equation shows the summation of these Starling forces for lung capillaries:

$$
\begin{aligned}
\text{net pressure} &= [(P_c - P_i) - (\pi_c - \pi_i)] \\
&= [(12 \text{ mmHg}) - (-5 \text{ mmHg})] \\
&\quad - [(25 \text{ mmHg}) - (18 \text{ mmHg})] \\
&= +10 \text{ mmHg}
\end{aligned}
$$

A net pressure of +10 mmHg indicates that there is a substantial net tendency for filtration of fluid out of the capillaries and into the lung interstitial spaces. The lung interstitial spaces would fill rapidly with water, and pulmonary edema would develop, if not for the well-developed system of lymph vessels in the

lung. These vessels continuously remove interstitial fluid and prevent its excessive accumulation.

Edema Is a Clinically Noticeable Excess of Interstitial Fluid

Edema is a common clinical problem. One common cause is increased venous pressure. Increased venous pressure can result from the application of too tight a dressing on the extremity of an animal. The resulting constriction of the veins impedes the outflow of venous blood from the limb. Blood backs up in the limb veins, which increases venous pressure. Blood then backs up in the capillaries and increases capillary hydrostatic pressure.

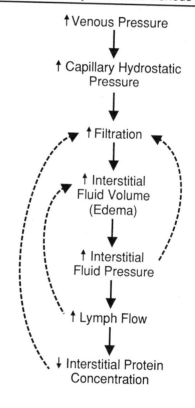

Edema Caused by Increased Venous Pressure

↑Venous Pressure

↑ Capillary Hydrostatic Pressure

↑ Filtration

↑ Interstitial Fluid Volume (Edema)

↑ Interstitial Fluid Pressure

↑ Lymph Flow

↓ Interstitial Protein Concentration

- - - - ▶ negative feedback

Figure 22–5. An increase in venous pressure leads to an increase in interstitial fluid volume (edema). The dashed lines indicate the effects of the three safety factors against edema. First, an increase in interstitial fluid hydrostatic pressure reduces the rate of filtration back toward normal. Second, an increase in lymph flow reduces interstitial fluid volume back toward normal. Third, a decrease in interstitial fluid protein concentration reduces the rate of filtration back toward normal.

As shown in Figure 22–5, this increase in capillary hydrostatic pressure leads to an excessive filtration of capillary fluid into the interstitial space. When this accumulation becomes clinically noticeable, the patient is said to exhibit edema.

Three factors (safety factors) limit the degree of edema. All three safety factors depend on the fact that an increased interstitial fluid volume leads to an increase in interstitial fluid hydrostatic pressure. The first safety factor is that this increased interstitial fluid pressure acts directly to oppose or limit filtration. Interstitial fluid pressure does not have to rise above capillary hydrostatic pressure to limit edema. Any increase in interstitial fluid pressure (e.g., from a normal value of -7 mmHg to $+2$ mmHg) helps to change the net balance of the Starling forces in the direction of reducing excessive filtration.

The increased interstitial fluid pressure also promotes lymph flow. Lymph flow removes edema fluid from the tissue and, therefore, helps limit the degree of edema. Increased lymph flow is the second safety factor against edema.

The third safety factor is an indirect consequence of increased lymph flow. Recall that interstitial fluid normally has a small amount of plasma protein present in it, primarily as the result of pinocytosis. This protein exerts a small but significant oncotic pressure that reduces the osmotic reabsorption of water. When filtration becomes excessive and edema forms, the newly filtered fluid (delivered to the interstitial space through the capillary pores or clefts) is almost entirely free of proteins. As lymph carries away interstitial fluid under these circumstances, the proteins originally present in the interstitial fluid are carried away by the lymph, while fluid relatively free of proteins is being added to the interstitial space by the increased filtration. Therefore, interstitial protein concentration and interstitial fluid oncotic pressures decrease, and this helps reduce filtration.

To summarize, venous obstruction causes capillary hydrostatic pressure to change in a direction that increases filtration. Edema occurs. Then, three safety factors come into play to limit the degree of edema. A new steady-state condition is eventually reached, wherein interstitial fluid is removed by lymph vessels as fast as it is filtered.

Another common clinical situation that leads to an increased venous pressure (and therefore edema) is heart failure. If the right ventricle fails (that is, if the right ventricular contractility decreases), blood backs up or pools in the right atrium and the vena cava. This increase in venous and atrial pressures is beneficial in one respect; it helps promote diastolic filling of the failing ventricle. The resulting increase in diastolic ventricular volume helps restore the stroke volume of the ailing right ventricle back toward its normal level (recall Starling's law of the heart). Although the increased venous pressure is beneficial in terms of restoring stroke volume toward normal, the increased venous pressure often leads to excessive capillary filtration and edema in the systemic organs. Systemic edema is therefore a common complication of right heart failure. In humans with heart failure, the edema is often most noticeable in the lower extremities, particularly if the patient remains standing or seated for a long time. In animals with heart failure, systemic edema is often most noticeable in the abdomen. Excess interstitial fluid in the abdominal organs tends to ooze out into the peritoneal space and accumulate there. Excessive fluid in the peritoneum is called *ascites*. Marked ascites is common in patients with right heart failure.

Failure of the left ventricle leads to increased left atrial pressure and increased pulmonary venous pressure. The result is an increase in capillary filtration in the lungs, which leads to an increase in the amount of interstitial fluid in the lung tissue, or *pulmonary edema*. In extreme cases, some of the excess interstitial fluid oozes into the alveolar and bronchial air spaces of the lungs, so that frank fluid is found in the airways. Such a patient typically coughs up a frothy fluid.

A decreased plasma protein concentration also leads to edema, because it reduces the capillary plasma oncotic pressure (Fig. 22–6). One common cause of decreased plasma protein concentration is a decrease in the rate of plasma protein production by the liver. This occurs in malnutrition and leads to the clinical syndrome of *kwashiorkor*. Victims of kwashiorkor typically look emaciated, except that their abdomens are grossly distended by ascites (edema fluid in the peritoneum). Another cause of abnormally low plasma protein concentration is an increase in the rate of loss of proteins from the body. Protein loss occurs in kidney disease. For example, in *nephrotic syndrome*, the kidney glomerular capillaries become permeable to plasma proteins. Plasma proteins leave the blood stream and enter the urinary tubules (nephrons) of the kidney. A chronic loss of proteins in the urine reduces plasma protein concentration. Hence, the presence of plasma proteins in the urine is an alarming clinical sign.

Another common cause for the loss of plasma proteins from the body is severe burns. The capillaries of burned skin become permeable to both fluid and proteins. Substantial amounts of plasma can leave the body through these damaged capillaries. The presence of plasma proteins in the fluid weeping from a burn site accounts for the typical yellow color of that fluid. If the water and electrolytes lost through burns are replaced (by intravenous administration of saline or Ringer's solution, or by ingestion of salt and water) and if the plasma proteins are not replaced, plasma protein concentration decreases.

Whether it results from decreased production or increased loss, a decrease in plasma protein concentration leads to a decrease in plasma colloid osmotic pressure. This alters the balance of Starling forces in a direction that favors excessive filtration of fluid from the capillaries. Interstitial fluid accumulates, and edema is noticed. However, the same

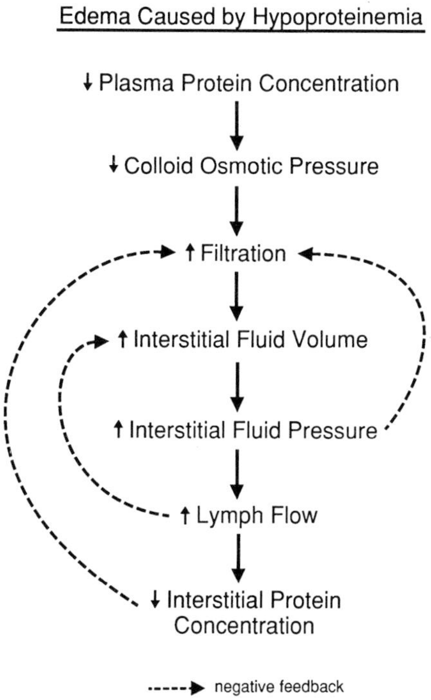

Edema Caused by Hypoproteinemia

↓ Plasma Protein Concentration

↓ Colloid Osmotic Pressure

↑ Filtration

↑ Interstitial Fluid Volume

↑ Interstitial Fluid Pressure

↑ Lymph Flow

↓ Interstitial Protein Concentration

- - - -▶ negative feedback

Figure 22–6. A decrease in plasma protein concentration leads to edema, but three safety factors limit the degree of the edema, just as in Figure 22–5.

Edema Caused by Lymphatic Obstruction

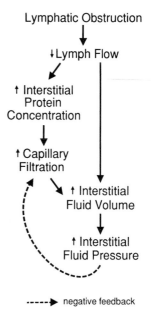

- - - -▶ negative feedback

Figure 22–7. Lymphatic obstruction leads to edema. Lymphedema is clinically troublesome because only one of the normal three safety factors is operative to limit the degree of edema.

three safety factors that limited edema in the case of increased venous pressure (see Fig. 22–5) also operate in the case of decreased plasma protein concentration (Fig. 22–6). Overall, a decreased plasma protein concentration causes excessive filtration and edema, but the degree of edema is limited by the three safety factors: (1) an increased interstitial fluid pressure, (2) an increased lymph flow, and (3) a decreased interstitial protein concentration.

Edema can also result from lymphatic obstruction. Clinically, this situation is called *lymphedema*. Common causes of lymphedema are inflammatory diseases and cancers that obstruct the lymphatic vessels. Also, in certain parasitic diseases, microfilaria lodge in the lymph nodes and obstruct lymph flow. Filarial parasites cause the pronounced edema seen in cases of *elephantiasis*. Lymphedema also occurs as a secondary consequence of surgical procedures that damage lymph nodes. A common example of this in human medicine is the edema of the arm that follows radical mastectomy. The removal of axillary lymph nodes during radical mastectomy creates scar tissue that impairs lymphatic drainage from the arm.

Figure 22–7 traces the causes of edema following lymphatic obstruction and shows why lymphedema is clinically so troublesome.

Lymphatic obstruction decreases lymph flow. Interstitial fluid accumulates instead of being removed, and edema results. The accumulation of edema fluid raises interstitial fluid pressure, which acts as a safety factor to limit the excess capillary filtration. However, the second and third safety factors discussed earlier are absent in the case of lymphedema, because these safety factors depend on an increase in lymph flow. In lymphedema a decreased lymph flow is the causative problem, so there cannot be an increased lymph flow (second safety factor) to compensate for the edema. When lymph flow decreases, interstitial proteins accumulate instead of being carried away by the lymph. Therefore, the third safety factor against edema (decreased interstitial fluid oncotic pressure) is also absent in lymphedema.

Edema is a common result of physical injury or allergic reactions to antigen challenges. Physical trauma, like a scratch or a cut on the skin, results in a local bump or swelling. A similar swelling is observed when the skin reacts to some irritating agent or antigen challenge. An allergic swelling can also occur in bronchial tissue during an asthmatic reaction. The edema of asthma can be life-threatening, because it limits air flow to the lungs. As shown in Figure 22–8, an injury or antigen challenge leads to the release of the chemical *histamine* from the tissue cells. Histamine has two effects that cause edema. First, histamine increases the permeability of capillaries to proteins. As proteins leave the blood stream and accumulate in the interstitial space of the damaged tissue, they increase the interstitial fluid oncotic pressure, which promotes filtration of fluid. Secondly, histamine promotes filtration by acting on arteriolar smooth muscle to relax it. The arterioles dilate, and the resulting decrease in arteriolar resistance allows more of the arterial blood pressure to impinge on the capillaries. The resulting increase in the capillary hydrostatic pressure promotes filtration. Although histamine promotes excess filtration and edema through two mechanisms, all three safety factors against edema are intact and act to limit the degree of edema.

Other situations also cause edema, but these examples cover some of the most common causes of clinical edema and reinforce an understanding of the interplay of the osmotic and hydrostatic forces that act on water to govern its filtration out of capillaries or reabsorption into capillaries.

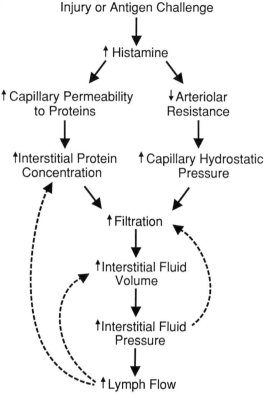

Edema Caused by Injury or Allergic Reaction

Figure 22–8. Histamine mediates the changes that lead to edema in response to a physical injury or antigen challenge. The normal three safety factors against edema are intact and help to limit the degree of edema. Treatment with an antihistamine (drug that blocks histamine receptors on arterioles and capillaries) also helps to reduce edema in these cases.

CLINICAL CORRELATION

ACUTE PROTEIN-LOSING ENTEROPATHY IN A HORSE

HISTORY □ You are called to a home a few miles from your clinic by parents who are concerned about their daughter's 4-year-old quarter horse. They report that the horse is listless and has had diarrhea for 2 days.

CLINICAL EXAMINATION □ You arrive at the client's home to find that the horse is stabled in a small barn with no access to pasture. Poor-quality grass hay is stacked in the barn. On physical examination, you find the horse to be somewhat emaciated, with dry mucous membranes, a foul-smelling diarrhea, and a fast heart rate (tachycardia). When you pinch up a section of his skin, it falls back to the normal position slowly, which indicates dehydration.

You take a blood sample and then begin an intravenous (IV) administration of polyionic fluid (lactated Ringer's). You tell the clients that you will return later. Analysis of the blood sample indicates a hematocrit of 55% (normal range 35–45%) and a plasma protein concentration of 4.5 g/dL (normal range 5.9–7.8 g/dL). You become concerned that your administration of fluids, without replacement of plasma proteins, will exaggerate the horse's hypoproteinemia. Therefore, you arrange to obtain plasma from a donor horse, and you return to examine the horse. You find the horse is still listless. Edema is now evident along the ventral abdomen and in the limbs.

COMMENT ☐ Acute enteropathy (intestinal disorder) often causes diarrhea. The loss of water and solutes leads to dehydration. Prior to treatment, blood volume and interstitial fluid volume are both reduced. Hematocrit (fraction of cells in blood) is typically elevated, because fluid is removed from the blood stream but blood cells are not. In some forms of enteropathy (called protein-losing enteropathy), the capillaries in the intestine become leaky to plasma proteins. Albumin, in particular, moves from the blood stream into the intestinal lumen and is eliminated in the feces.

This horse has a severe shortage of plasma proteins. The shortage of plasma proteins probably resulted from a combination of poor nutrition (which depresses the liver's production of plasma proteins) and the protein-losing enteropathy. The deficit of plasma proteins in this horse is even more severe than one might suspect on the basis of the plasma protein concentration of 4.5 g/dL, because this value is the net result of two opposing processes. The loss of protein in the diarrhea lowers plasma protein concentration, but the dehydration raises plasma protein concentration.

The administration of IV fluids added water and electrolytes to the circulating blood volume, but the plasma proteins remaining in the blood stream were further diluted. As a result, plasma oncotic pressure decreased, and this led to excess filtration of water out of capillaries and into the interstitial space. The result was edema, especially in the dependent regions of the body (ventral abdomen and legs). Restoration of a normal plasma protein concentration would reverse the edema.

TREATMENT ☐ The enteropathy in cases such as this one is often self-limiting. Therefore, the aim of treatment should be to remedy the dehydration, the electrolyte loss, and the plasma protein deficit. IV administration of both polyionic fluids and plasma is usually effective.

Bibliography

Berne RM, Levy MN: The microcirculation and lymphatics. *In* Berne RM, Levy MN (eds): Cardiovascular Physiology. St. Louis, CV Mosby, 1986, p 136.
Bolton GR, Ettinger SJ: Peripheral edema. *In* Ettinger SJ (ed): Textbook of Veterinary Internal Medicine. Philadelphia, WB Saunders, 1989, p 41.
Cunningham SL: The physiology of body fluids. *In* Patton HD, Fuchs AF, Hille B, et al (eds): Textbook of Physiology, Vol 2. Philadelphia, WB Saunders, 1989, p 1098.
Milnor WR: Capillary and lymphatic systems. *In* Milnor WR (ed): Cardiovascular Physiology. New York, Oxford University Press, 1990, p 327.
Renkin EM: Microcirculation and exchange. *In* Patton HD, Fuchs AF, Hille B, et al (eds): Textbook of Physiology, Vol 2. Philadelphia, WB Saunders, 1989, p 860.
Ware WA, Bonagura JD: Pulmonary edema. *In* Fox RR (ed): Canine and Feline Cardiology. New York, Churchill Livingstone, 1988, p 205.

PRACTICE QUESTIONS FOR CHAPTER 22

1. Which of the following will NOT cause pulmonary edema?

   a. Increased capillary permeability to protein
   b. Blockage of pulmonary lymph vessels
   c. Increased left atrial pressure
   d. Constriction of pulmonary arterioles
   e. Left heart failure

2. A patient with a form of protein-losing kidney disease has a plasma colloid osmotic pressure of 10 mmHg. The patient has edema but is not getting any worse. Blood pressure and heart rate are normal. Which of the following is probably preventing further edema?

   a. Increased interstitial fluid hydrostatic pressure
   b. Increased capillary hydrostatic pressure
   c. Decreased lymph flow
   d. Increased plasma sodium ion concentration
   e. Increased interstitial fluid oncotic pressure

3. The following parameters were measured in the microcirculation of a skeletal muscle:

P_c (capillary hydrostatic pressure) = 34 mmHg

P_i (interstitial fluid hydrostatic pressure) = 10 mmHg

π_c (capillary plasma oncotic pressure) = 24 mmHg

π_i (interstitial fluid oncotic pressure) = 1 mmHg

Which of the following is true?

a. These conditions would favor filtration.
b. These conditions would favor reabsorption.
c. These conditions would favor neither filtration nor reabsorption.
d. One cannot say what these conditions favor because the concentration of plasma protein is not specified.

4. During a 30-minute hemorrhage, the mean arterial pressure of a horse decreases from 90 to 75 mmHg. Heart rate increases from 40 to 90 beats per minute. The skin has become cold. After the hemorrhage you take a blood sample and measure the hematocrit, which is 28%. You can conclude that

a. capillary hydrostatic pressure is increased.
b. interstitial fluid volume is decreased.
c. interstitial fluid pressure is increased.
d. capillary colloid osmotic pressure is increased.
e. arteriolar resistance has decreased.

5. The rate of diffusion of glucose molecules from capillary blood to interstitial fluid is most directly affected by

a. the voltage difference between capillary blood and interstitial fluid.
b. the interstitial fluid hydrostatic pressure.
c. the size and number of capillary pores.
d. the amount of oxygen in the blood.
e. the hematocrit.

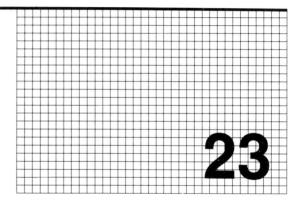

23

Local Control of Blood Flow

1. The amount of blood flowing through a tissue is affected by intrinsic and extrinsic control mechanisms
2. Metabolic control of blood flow is a local mechanism that matches the blood flow of a tissue to its metabolic rate
3. Autoregulation is a relative constancy of blood flow in an organ despite changes in perfusion pressure
4. Mechanical compression can reduce blood flow to a tissue

The Amount of Blood Flowing Through a Tissue Is Affected by Intrinsic and Extrinsic Control Mechanisms

The blood flow in every tissue of the body is affected by both intrinsic and extrinsic control mechanisms. *Extrinsic control mechanisms* act from outside a tissue, through nerves or hormones, to alter blood flow. *Intrinsic control* is exerted by local mechanisms within a tissue. For example, histamine is released from the cells of most tissues in response to injury or during allergic reactions. Histamine acts locally on the arteriolar smooth muscle to relax it. Dilation of the arterioles decreases arteriolar resistance and, therefore, increases the blood flow to the tissue. A second example of intrinsic control is the arteriolar dilation and increased blood flow during exercise in skeletal muscle. This example also illustrates the general phenomenon of metabolic control of blood flow: tissues tend to increase their blood flow whenever their metabolic rate increases.

Although the blood flow in all tissues is affected by both intrinsic and extrinsic mechanisms, intrinsic mechanisms predominate in the control of blood flow in the coronary vessels, brain, and working skeletal muscle. By contrast, extrinsic mechanisms predominate in the control of blood flow to the kidneys, splanchnic organs, and resting skeletal muscle. Skin is an example of a tissue in which both intrinsic and extrinsic control mechanisms have an important influence. In general, local (intrinsic) control dominates extrinsic control in the so-called critical tissues—those that must have enough blood to meet their metabolic needs on a second-by-second basis in order to maintain the animal's survival. Extrinsic control dominates intrinsic control in tissues that can withstand temporary reductions in blood flow (and metabolism) in order to make extra blood available for the critical tissues.

By definition, vascular resistance of a tissue

is equal to the *perfusion pressure* (arterial pressure minus venous pressure) divided by the blood flow. Rearranging this equation shows that the blood flow through a tissue is always equal to the perfusion pressure divided by the resistance of the blood vessels in the tissue. Local control mechanisms cannot alter perfusion pressure directly (because they cannot change the body's arterial pressure or venous pressure), but they can alter the resistance of the blood vessels in a tissue. Recall that most of the resistance to blood flow in a tissue is in the arterioles. Local control of blood flow usually involves dilation or constriction of arterioles to change the resistance to blood flow through the tissue.

Metabolic Control of Blood Flow Is a Local Mechanism That Matches the Blood Flow of a Tissue to Its Metabolic Rate

Metabolic control of blood flow is the most important local control mechanism. For example, metabolic control accounts for the 40-fold increase in blood flow in skeletal muscle during exercise (from 2.5 mL/minute/100 g during rest to 100 mL/minute/100 g during maximal exercise). The functional significance of metabolic control of blood flow is that it matches the blood flow in a tissue to the metabolic rate of the tissue. An increase in tissue blood flow in response to increased metabolic rate is called *active hyperemia* ("hyper" means elevated, "emia" refers to blood, and the word "active" implies an increased metabolic rate).

Metabolic control of blood flow works via chemical changes in the tissue. When the metabolic rate of a tissue increases, its consumption of oxygen increases, and there is an increased rate of production of metabolic products, including carbon dioxide, adenosine, and lactic acid. Also, some potassium moves from the intracellular fluid to the interstitial fluid. Therefore, as a tissue's metabolism increases, the interstitial concentration of oxygen decreases, and the interstitial concentrations of metabolic products and potassium increase. All of these changes have the same effect on arteriolar smooth muscle: they relax it. As a result, there is an arteriolar dilation and a decreased arteriolar resistance to blood flow. More blood flows through the tissue. Low levels of oxygen and high concentrations of metabolic products and potassium also cause

the precapillary sphincters to relax, so that more of the capillaries of the tissue open to blood flow. As explained in Chapter 22, the opening of more capillaries decreases the diffusion distance between fresh, oxygenated blood and the metabolizing cells of the tissue. Opening more capillaries also increases the total capillary surface area for diffusional exchange. The net result of the increased blood flow, the decreased diffusion distance, and the increased total capillary surface area is a more rapid removal of metabolic products from the tissue and a more rapid delivery of oxygen and other metabolic substrates to the tissue.

Metabolic control of blood flow involves negative feedback. The accumulation of metabolic products and the lack of oxygen initiate a vasodilation and increase blood flow, which removes the accumulating metabolic products and delivers additional oxygen. A new balance is reached when the increased blood flow closely matches the increased metabolic needs of the tissue. The major features of metabolic control of blood flow are diagrammed in Figure 23–1.

Reactive hyperemia is a temporary increase above normal in the flow of blood to a tissue following a period when blood flow was restricted. As the name implies, hyperemia (increased flow) is a response (reaction) to a period of inadequate blood flow. Mechanical compression of blood vessels is one of the most common causes of restricted blood flow in a tissue.

Reactive hyperemia after mechanical compression is easy to demonstrate in nonpigmented epithelial tissue. Press a finger against nonpigmented skin hard enough to occlude blood flow. Maintain the pressure for about 1 minute and then release. The previously compressed area of skin looks darker (redder) for a short time, because the arterioles there have dilated, and blood flow is greater than normal when the compression is released.

The same metabolic control mechanisms that account for active hyperemia also explains reactive hyperemia. During the period of restricted blood flow, metabolism continues in the compressed area, so metabolic products accumulate, and the local concentration of oxygen decreases. These metabolic effects cause dilation of the arterioles and a decrease in arteriolar resistance. When the mechanical obstruction to flow is removed, flow increases above normal until the "oxygen debt" is repaid and the excess metabolic products have been

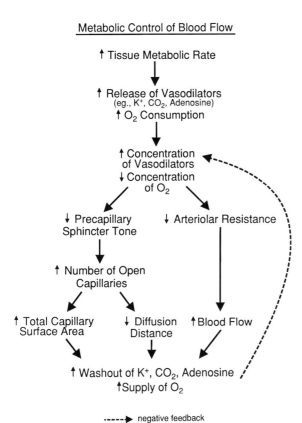

Metabolic Control of Blood Flow

Figure 23–1. Metabolic control of blood flow is a local (intrinsic) mechanism that acts within a tissue to match blood flow to metabolic rate. As a tissue becomes more active metabolically, this mechanism increases blood flow and thereby regulates the concentration of oxygen and metabolic products in the tissue.

removed from the compressed tissue. Active and reactive hyperemia are compared in Figure 23–2.

Autoregulation Is a Relative Constancy of Blood Flow in an Organ Despite Changes in Perfusion Pressure

Metabolic control mechanisms probably account also for the phenomenon known as *blood flow autoregulation*. Autoregulation is an intrinsic control mechanism that is evident in denervated organs and organs in which local control of blood flow is predominant over neural and humoral control (i.e., in coronary circulation, brain, and working skeletal muscle).

Figure 23–3 summarizes an experiment that demonstrates autoregulation in the brain. The top and middle graphs in the figure indicate that blood flow to the brain is 100 mL/minute in an animal whose perfusion pressure (arte-

rial pressure minus venous pressure) is 100 mmHg. This initial condition is also plotted as point A in the bottom graph. The top and middle graphs next show the effect on the brain's blood flow when perfusion pressure is increased suddenly to 140 mmHg. The increase in perfusion pressure causes an instant increase in the brain's blood flow to 140 mL/minute. However, the middle graph shows that the brain's blood flow does not remain at this elevated level, but begins to return toward its initial level over the next 20–30 seconds. Eventually, blood flow reaches a stable level of about 110 mL/minute. This stable response is plotted on the bottom graph as point B. The rest of the bottom graph was obtained in a similar way. That is, perfusion pressure was set artificially to various levels, ranging from 40 mmHg to 220 mmHg, and the resulting steady state levels of blood flow were plotted. Notice that over a considerable range of perfusion pressure (from about 60 to 190 mmHg), there is relatively little change in blood flow to the brain. That is, brain blood flow is autoregulated. The range of perfusion pressures over which flow stays relatively constant is called the *autoregulatory range*. Note that autoregulation fails at very high and very low perfusion pressures. Extremely high pressures result in marked increases of blood flow, and extremely low pressures result in marked decreases of blood flow. Nevertheless, over a considerable range of perfusion pressure, autoregulation keeps blood flow relatively constant.

Figure 23–4 shows that the metabolic control mechanisms previously described can account also for the phenomenon of autoregulation. If the metabolic rate of an organ does not change, but perfusion pressure is increased above normal, the increased pressure forces additional blood through the organ. The additional blood flow accelerates the removal of metabolic products from the interstitial fluid and increases the rate of oxygen delivery to the interstitial fluid. Therefore, the concentration of vasodilating metabolic products in the interstitial fluid decreases, and the concentration of oxygen in the interstitial fluid increases. These changes cause the arterioles of the tissue to constrict, which increases the resistance to blood flow through the tissue. Therefore, blood flow decreases back toward its initial level, despite a continuing elevated perfusion pressure.

To summarize, metabolic control mechanisms can account for active hyperemia (the

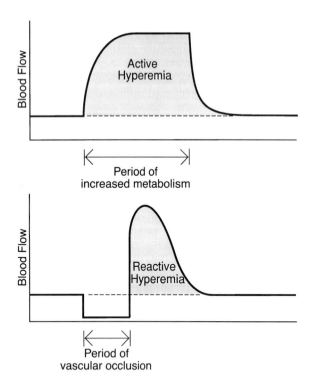

Figure **23–2.** Both active and reactive hyperemia involve increases above normal in blood flow, and both are brought about by mechanisms for the local, metabolic control of blood flow.

increase in blood flow in an organ in response to an increased metabolic rate in the absence of any blood pressure change). The same metabolic mechanisms can account also for reactive hyperemia (the increase in blood flow above normal in an organ following a period of flow restriction). In addition, the same metabolic mechanisms can account for autoregulation (the relative constancy of blood flow in an organ when there has been no change in metabolic rate, but blood pressure has either increased or decreased). There are other theories about the mechanism of autoregulation, and the student may encounter discussions of these in other texts under the headings of the *myogenic hypothesis* and the *tissue pressure hypothesis*. However, metabolic control is the most likely explanation for autoregulation of blood flow in the body's critical tissues (brain, coronary vessels, and exercising skeletal muscle).

Mechanical Compression Can Reduce Blood Flow to a Tissue

The final mechanism to be considered under the category of local or intrinsic control of blood flow is the effect of mechanical compression. Mechanical compression can reduce

blood flow in a tissue by literally squeezing down on the blood vessels. The example of mechanical pressure decreasing skin blood flow has already been mentioned. Long-term mechanical pressure on the skin must be avoided, because a prolonged period of subnormal blood flow (ischemia) leads to irreversible tissue damage and cell death (infarction). Pressure sores (e.g., bedsores) are an example. Three other specific instances of mechanical compression will be mentioned because of their clinical importance.

Figure 23–5 diagrams the effect of mechanical compression on coronary blood flow. The top tracing shows the changes in arterial (aortic) blood pressure during one whole cardiac cycle and part of another one. The periods of ventricular systole and ventricular diastole are labeled at the bottom of the figure. One would expect that left coronary blood flow would be highest during ventricular systole (when the aortic pressure is highest), and lowest during diastole (when the aortic pressure is lowest). However, the tracings of left coronary blood flow indicate that blood flow is actually depressed during systole and much higher during diastole. Flow even reverses and flows in a backward (negative) direction for a brief period near the beginning of systole. The fact

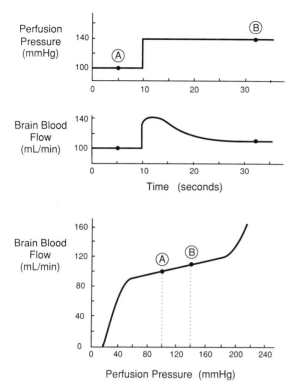

Figure 23–3. The experiment summarized here demonstrates autoregulation of brain blood flow. Perfusion pressure was artificially set to various levels (top graph), and the resulting steady-state values of blood flow were measured (middle graph) and plotted on a graph of brain blood flow versus perfusion pressure (bottom graph).

that coronary blood flow is much lower during systole, even though the perfusion pressure is higher, implies that coronary resistance must be substantially higher during systole than during diastole.

Coronary resistance is high during systole because the contracting ventricular muscle squeezes down on the coronary blood vessels, which increases their resistance to blood flow. The coronary vessels are not constricted in this way during diastole, because the ventricular muscle is relaxed. Therefore, coronary vascular resistance decreases dramatically during diastole, and blood flow increases. The bottom trace in Figure 23–5 indicates that mechanical compression does not have much influence on right coronary blood flow. That is, the magnitude of right coronary blood flow follows closely the changes in arterial pressure (being highest during systole and lowest during diastole). The reason that right coronary flow is not restricted by mechanical compression during systole is that the right ventricle contracts with much less force than the left ventricle.

The right ventricle does not develop enough compressive force to constrict its own blood vessels.

The reduction in left coronary flow by mechanical compression has great clinical importance. Most of the blood that is needed to support left ventricular metabolism must be delivered during ventricular diastole. In a resting animal with a low heart rate, there is adequate time during diastole for the coronary vessels to supply the amount of blood needed by the ventricular tissue. During exercise, heart rate and cardiac contractility increase. Left ventricular metabolism increases greatly, and the ventricular tissue needs more blood than normal. Also, during exercise the dura-

Mechanism of Autoregulation

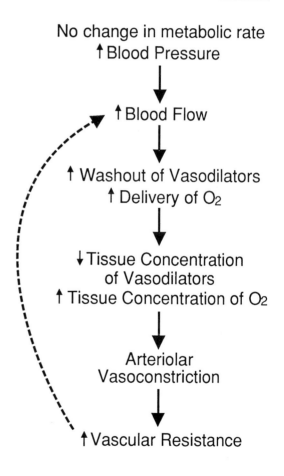

Figure 23–4. The same metabolic mechanism that is responsible for active hyperemia and reactive hyperemia can also account for autoregulation.

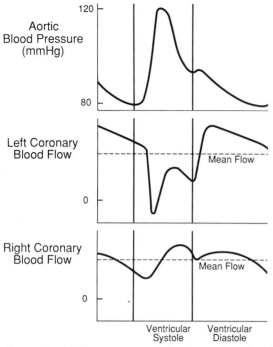

Figure 23–5. Left coronary blood flow is greatly reduced during ventricular systole by mechanical compression of left ventricular blood vessels. Right coronary flow is less affected by mechanical compression.

tion of diastole is greatly reduced, so there is less than normal time to deliver more than normal flow. Nevertheless, normal, healthy coronary vessels have a low enough resistance during diastole to supply the needed blood, even during maximal exercise. However, in coronary artery disease, where coronary vessels are restricted in diameter because of atherosclerosis, there is insufficient blood flow during diastole to supply the needs of the vigorously pumping ventricle. Therefore, ventricular ischemia develops during exercise in patients with coronary artery disease. The ischemic areas of the ventricle fail to contract normally. Ischemia can also cause arrhythmias or even ventricular fibrillation (sudden death).

Mechanical compression caused by muscle contraction also can restrict blood flow through skeletal muscles. The blood vessels that supply blood to skeletal muscle become compressed during strenuous, sustained contractions of the muscle. The compression reduces blood flow and can create ischemic conditions in the exercising muscle. Ischemia decreases the strength of muscular contractions. Ischemia also activates sensory nerve endings in the muscle, which cause the sensations of pain that are experienced during

sustained, forceful muscle contractions. Activation of the muscle ischemia receptors also triggers a reflex increase in arterial pressure. The high arterial pressure is advantageous, because it partially overcomes the effects of mechanical compression on blood flow. That is, a high arterial pressure helps to keep skeletal muscle blood vessels open despite the compressive effects of muscle contraction.

In the pulmonary vessels, where arterial pressure is much less than in systemic vessels, mechanical compression can more easily reduce blood flow. Figure 23–6 diagrams a situation commonly encountered in veterinary medicine in which mechanical compression impedes pulmonary blood flow. The diagram shows pulmonary vessels passing through a region of the lung. Panel A depicts normal conditions in which the pulmonary vessels are not compressed. The arterial pressure is 13 mmHg, and the venous pressure is 5 mmHg. The pressure in the alveolar air spaces of the lung is near zero (that is, near atmospheric pressure). This situation is normal, because alveolar pressures typically vary between −1 mmHg (during inspiration) and +1 mmHg (during expiration).

Panel B of this figure depicts a situation in which abnormally high alveolar pressure compresses pulmonary blood vessels. This would happen if this patient had a tracheal tube inserted into the airway and if the tracheal tube was attached to a source of elevated pressure. An elevated pressure could be generated by a mechanical respirator or by an anesthetist's squeezing the bag on an anesthesia machine that is attached to the tracheal tube. In an intubated patient, pressures generated in the tracheal tube are transmitted to the alveoli. An increase in alveolar pressure also increases the external, compressing pressures applied around the pulmonary blood vessels. Alveolar pressures in excess of 10–15 mmHg compress pulmonary blood vessels to a significant extent and raise the resistance to blood flow through the lungs. Therefore, pulmonary blood flow decreases. Two things happen as a result. First, less blood reaches the left atrium and left ventricle, which causes left ventricular stroke volume and aortic blood pressure to decrease. Second, blood ejected by the right ventricle dams up in the pulmonary arteries. This causes pulmonary arterial pressure to increase. An elevated pulmonary arterial pressure helps force blood through the compressed vessels. However, the increased pulmonary artery pressure also places an in-

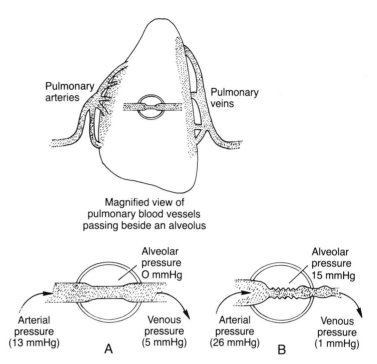

Figure 23–6. When alveolar pressure increases from 0 mmHg (A) to 15 mmHg (B), the pulmonary blood vessels are compressed. The resulting increase in pulmonary vascular resistance causes pulmonary arterial pressure to increase and venous pressure to decrease.

creased workload on the right ventricle. If the alveolar pressure is not excessively high, the right ventricle is able to generate sufficient pulmonary arterial pressure to restore pulmonary blood flow to normal. However, extremely high alveolar pressures restrict pulmonary blood flow, because the right ventricle is unable to raise pulmonary arterial pressure high enough to sustain flow. Under these conditions the patient can develop systemic hypotension and ischemia, with potentially fatal consequences. The veterinary clinician must remember this whenever a patient is intubated and attached to a mechanical respiratory device.

CLINICAL CORRELATION

PATENT DUCTUS ARTERIOSUS

HISTORY □ A 3-month-old female Welsh corgi is brought to your clinic by its owner, who has noticed a "rumbling noise" in the dog's chest. The dog is smaller than her littermates and a little less playful. The dog coughs occasionally, but the cough does not produce fluid.

CLINICAL EXAMINATION □ The dog appears to be in good health except for an occa-

sional cough. The mucous membranes are pink, and capillary refill time is normal (1.5 seconds). However, when you place your hand on the anterior left chest, you feel an abnormal vibration (*thrill*) with each heartbeat. With a stethoscope, you can auscultate a cardiac murmur that is loudest during systole but continues throughout both systole and diastole. The murmur is heard most loudly at the ventral third intercostal space on the left side. Expiratory sounds are slightly louder than normal. The pulse rate is 152 beats per minute, which you consider to be above normal for a dog of this size and age.

The electrocardiogram (ECG) indicates that the dog has sinus tachycardia; the atrial and ventricular rates are both 152 beats per minute. The R-waves are abnormally large in leads II and III (2.5 and 3.5 mV, respectively). The QRS-complex in lead I shows a large negative deflection followed immediately by an equally large positive deflection.

Thoracic radiographs show a generalized enlargement of the heart. The initial portion of the pulmonary artery is also substantially larger than normal, and the pulmonary blood vessels appear generally to be more prominent than normal.

COMMENT □ A murmur in a young, otherwise healthy dog is most likely the result of a congenital cardiac abnormality. A continuous murmur can occur only if there is a defect that causes turbulent flow throughout both diastole and systole. The loudness of the murmur indicates that there is a large flow through the defect. Because flow can occur only when there is a pressure gradient, the defect in this dog must be located where a substantial pressure gradient is present during both systole and diastole. No single intracardiac defect meets these criteria. That is, a stenotic or regurgitant valve produces either a systolic murmur or a diastolic murmur, but not both. A valve that is both stenotic and regurgitant produces two murmurs, one in systole and one in diastole. However, in such a case, there are moments during the cardiac cycle when no pressure gradient exists across the valve, so there are moments of silence between the systolic murmur and the diastolic murmur.

The only common cardiac defect that causes turbulent flow throughout both systole and diastole is a patent ductus arteriosus (PDA). This vessel is normal in the fetus but should close shortly after birth. The flow is continuous, because aortic pressure is higher than pulmonary artery pressure throughout the cardiac cycle. The murmur of PDA is usually heard best in the left third intercostal space. All the other clinical signs in this dog are also consistent with the diagnosis of PDA. The prominence of the pulmonary vessels on the radiographs indicates that pressure is abnormally high in the pulmonary artery and its branches. In a dog with a PDA, a large volume of blood flows from the aorta into the pulmonary artery, and this increases both pulmonary arterial pressure and pulmonary flow.

The radiographs and ECGs indicate that this dog has both right and left ventricular hypertrophy. The large R-waves in leads II and III indicate left ventricular hypertrophy, and the large negative deflection during the QRS in lead I indicates that the right ventricle is hypertrophic, too. The left ventricle becomes hypertrophic in a dog with PDA because it is called on to pump three to five times the normal cardiac output. (It pumps a normal volume to the organs of the systemic circulation and two to four times that much through the PDA.) The flow through the PDA is large, because the PDA offers little resistance to flow. The demand on the left ventricle to pump so much blood (increased volume work) leads to left ventricular hypertrophy. The volume of blood pumped by the right ventricle is nearly normal; it only has to pump the blood that returns through the vena cava

from the systemic organs. However, the right ventricle has to develop much higher systolic pressures than normal in order to eject this blood into the pulmonary artery, because pulmonary artery pressure is much higher than normal, as explained earlier. This increase in pressure work leads to right ventricular hypertrophy.

Because the PDA carries so much blood away from the aorta, dogs with PDA tend to have an abnormally low aortic pressure. Diastolic pressure is particularly reduced because of the rapid outflow of blood from the aorta during ventricular diastole. Therefore, PDA is typically associated with low mean aortic pressure but elevated pulse pressure.

Two mechanisms work together to keep blood flow to the systemic organs nearly normal despite the fact that a large fraction of cardiac output is "lost" through the PDA. First, reflex mechanisms (which are discussed in detail in Chapter 24) increase sympathetic activity to the heart, which increases heart rate and contractility above normal. These sympathetic effects keep left ventricular output (and aortic pressure) high enough to supply blood to both the systemic organs and the PDA. Second, metabolic control mechanisms cause the systemic organs to vasodilate, which keeps their blood flow nearly normal despite the subnormal aortic pressure.

Although the compensatory mechanisms just described allow a dog with a PDA to maintain a nearly normal blood flow to the systemic organs at rest, the heart cannot increase its output enough to supply the blood flow needed by the muscles during exercise. Therefore, a dog with a PDA appears less playful and energetic than its normal littermates. Over a period of months, the inability of the heart to supply the blood flow needed by metabolically active tissues causes a stunting of growth. Without treatment, the long-term prognosis is poor.

TREATMENT ☐ You show the dog's owner a diagram of the fetal circulation and explain that the ductus arteriosus normally closes and seals itself within 1–6 weeks after birth. However, the ductus fails to close spontaneously in about 1 out of every 700 newborns (the condition is four times more common in female pups). To treat the condition, the ductus is tied shut. An open-chest surgery is required, and most dogs treated before the age of 6 months lead completely normal lives. However, you advise the owner that PDA is hereditary, and that this puppy should probably not be used for breeding.

The owner elects to have the dog treated. The surgery is successful. The murmur and cough disappear immediately. Within 1 week, the dog is noticeably more energetic than before. By the time she is 6 months old, the dog has "grown into" her enlarged heart, and all physical findings are within normal limits.

Bibliography

Feigl EO: Coronary circulation. *In* Patton HD, Fuchs AF, Hille B, et al (eds): Textbook of Physiology, Vol 2. Philadelphia, WB Saunders, 1989, p 933.

Johnson JM: Circulation to skeletal muscle. *In* Patton HD, Fuchs AF, Hille B, et al (eds): Textbook of Physiology, Vol 2. Philadelphia, WB Saunders, 1989, p 887.

Milnor WR: Regional circulation to skeletal muscle. *In* Milnor WR (ed): Cardiovascular Physiology. New York, Oxford University Press, 1990, p 387.

Stephenson RB: The splanchnic circulation. *In* Patton HD, Fuchs AF, Hille B, et al (eds): Textbook of Physiology. Philadelphia, WB Saunders, 1989, p 911.

Stephenson RB: The renal circulation. *In* Patton HD, Fuchs AF, Hille B, et al (eds): Textbook of Physiology, Vol 2. Philadelphia, WB Saunders, 1989, p 924.

Suter PF: Peripheral vascular disease. *In* Ettinger SJ (ed): Textbook of Veterinary Internal Medicine. Philadelphia, WB Saunders, 1989, p 118.

PRACTICE QUESTIONS FOR CHAPTER 23

1. The increase in coronary blood flow during exercise is

    a. called Starling's law of the heart.
    b. caused by sympathetic activation of α-adrenergic receptors.
    c. caused by compression of the coronary blood vessels during systole.
    d. closely matched to the metabolic requirements of the heart.
    e. called reactive hyperemia.

2. A dog with an arterial blood pressure of 120/80 has a cerebral blood flow (CBF) of 100 mL/minute. When blood pressure is increased to 130/100, CBF increases to 105 mL/minute. This is an example of

    a. active hyperemia.
    b. autoregulation.
    c. reactive hyperemia.
    d. the blood-brain barrier.
    e. hypoxic vasoconstriction.

3. Local control of blood flow through an organ

    a. usually dominates over neurohumoral control.
    b. usually is subservient to neurohumoral control.
    c. can either dominate or be subservient to neurohumoral control, depending upon the organ.
    d. is always balanced by neurohumoral control.

4. In response to an increase in perfusion pressure, the arterioles of an autoregulating organ _____ and the vascular resistance of the organ _____.

    a. constrict .... increases
    b. constrict .... decreases
    c. dilate .... increases
    d. dilate .... decreases

5. When a young dog with a patent ductus arteriosus (PDA) begins to exercise,

    a. arterioles in the exercising skeletal muscle constrict.
    b. oxygen concentration in the skeletal muscle interstitial fluid decreases.
    c. left ventricular output decreases.
    d. right ventricular output decreases.
    e. mean arterial pressure increases to very high levels.

24

Neural and Hormonal Control of Blood Pressure and Blood Volume

1. Neurohumoral mechanisms regulate blood pressure and blood volume in order to ensure adequate blood flow for all body organs
2. The autonomic nervous system affects the cardiovascular system through the release of the neurotransmitters norepinephrine or acetylcholine
3. The arterial baroreceptor reflex regulates arterial blood pressure
4. The atrial volume receptor reflex regulates blood volume and helps to stabilize blood pressure
5. The cardiovascular state of conscious subjects is determined by an ongoing and ever-changing mixture of reflex effects and psychogenic responses

Neurohumoral Mechanisms Regulate Blood Pressure and Blood Volume in Order to Ensure Adequate Blood Flow for All Body Organs

The influences of the nervous system and hormones on the cardiovascular system are referred to collectively as the *neurohumoral* mechanisms of cardiovascular control. The neurohumoral mechanisms are also called *extrinsic control mechanisms,* because they act on organs from the outside. In review, the mechanisms of cardiovascular control that act locally, within individual tissues, are referred to

as *intrinsic control mechanisms.* The local or intrinsic mechanisms predominate in the control of blood flow to the critical organs, which include the heart (i.e., coronary blood flow), brain, and working skeletal muscle. In contrast, neurohumoral or extrinsic control mechanisms predominate in the control of blood flow to the noncritical organs, which include the kidneys, the splanchnic organs, and resting skeletal muscle.

Neurohumoral mechanisms also have strong effects on the heart; they act to alter heart rate and stroke volume. Note that cardiac muscle is under neurohumoral control,

Table 24–1
RECEPTORS INVOLVED IN NEUROHUMORAL CONTROL OF THE CARDIOVASCULAR SYSTEM

Receptor Type	Where Found	Effect of Receptor Activation	Function	Normal Activator
Alpha-adrenergic	Arterioles (all organs)	Constrict	Decrease blood flow to organ Increase total peripheral resistance	Norepinephrine from sympathetic neurons
	Veins (abdominal organs)	Constrict	Displace blood toward heart	Norepinephrine from sympathetic neurons
Beta-adrenergic	Heart SA node AV node Ventricles Ventricles	Increases heart rate Speeds AV conduction Increases contractility Shortens systole	Increases cardiac output	Norepinephrine from sympathetic neurons
	Arterioles (coronary)	Dilate	Increase coronary blood flow	Circulating epinephrine
	Arterioles (skeletal muscle)	Dilate	Increase muscle blood flow	Circulating epinephrine
Muscarinic cholinergic	Heart SA node AV node	Decreases heart rate Slows AV conduction	Decreases cardiac output	Acetylcholine from parasympathetic neurons
	Arterioles (coronary)	Dilate	Increase coronary blood flow	Acetylcholine from parasympathetic neurons
	Arterioles (genitals)	Dilate	Cause erection	Acetylcholine from parasympathetic neurons
	Arterioles (skeletal muscle)	Dilate	Increase muscle blood flow	Acetylcholine from sympathetic neurons
	Arterioles (most other organs)	Dilate	Function unknown	No normal activator known

whereas the coronary blood vessels are primarily under local control. When neurohumoral mechanisms increase heart rate or cardiac contractility, cardiac metabolic rate must also increase. The increased metabolism causes local metabolic control mechanisms to increase coronary blood flow.

The overall function of the neurohumoral control mechanisms is to control blood pressure and blood volume in such a way that adequate blood flow can be delivered to all organs of the body, or at least to the critical organs. In order to provide adequate blood flow for the critical organs, neurohumoral mechanisms may temporarily reduce the blood flow to noncritical organs below a normal or ideal level.

There are many important neurohumoral control mechanisms, but four are emphasized in the following presentation. Two of them are cardiovascular reflexes, which include the baroreceptor reflex and the atrial volume receptor reflex. The other two neurohumoral mechanisms are examples of psychogenic influences on the cardiovascular system. These are the defense alarm reaction and vasovagal syncope. Each of these mechanisms includes both neural and hormonal components. The neural components are emphasized in this chapter.

The Autonomic Nervous System Affects the Cardiovascular System Through the Release of the Neurotransmitters Norepinephrine or Acetylcholine

Table 24–1 summarizes the most important neural influences on the cardiovascular system. The neurotransmitters, either norepinephrine or acetylcholine, act on receptor sites on the membranes of cardiac muscle cells or on the smooth muscle cells of blood vessels.

Norepinephrine is released from most postganglionic sympathetic neurons. It activates *adrenergic receptors*. There are two major subtypes, α-*adrenergic receptors* and β-*adrenergic receptors*. Adrenergic receptors can be activated also by *epinephrine*. Epinephrine is released along with norepinephrine from the adrenal medulla in response to strong sympathetic activation. These substances are released directly into the blood stream, and they circulate to all organs in the body.

Acetylcholine is released from all parasympathetic postganglionic neurons and from certain postganglionic sympathetic neurons. Acetylcholine activates cholinergic receptors. There are two major subtypes, *muscarinic cholinergic receptors* and *nicotinic cholinergic receptors.* Cardiac muscle and vascular smooth muscle have muscarinic cholinergic receptors.

Alpha-adrenergic receptors are located on the membranes of the smooth muscle cells of the arterioles in all organs of the body. Alpha receptors are also found on the smooth muscle of the abdominal veins. The α-adrenergic receptors on arterioles and abdominal veins are innervated by postganglionic sympathetic neurons. Activation of the α-adrenergic receptors leads to constriction of the arterioles or the veins.

Arteriolar vasoconstriction in an organ increases the resistance and decreases the blood flow through that organ. If one or more major body organs are vasoconstricted, then the total peripheral resistance (TPR) increases. TPR (along with cardiac output) determines arterial blood pressure, so widespread α-adrenergic vasoconstriction in the body leads to an increase in arterial blood pressure. The increase in arterial pressure increases blood flow to the nonvasoconstricted organs. In this way, the sympathetic nervous system can use *vasoconstriction* in some organs to direct blood flow to other, nonvasoconstricted organs.

The major role of veins is to act as reservoirs for blood. *Venoconstriction* displaces blood toward the central circulation, which increases central venous pressure, ventricular preload, and stroke volume. Venoconstriction in the abdominal organs is particularly important in controlling central blood volume and, therefore, central venous pressure. The veins, whether constricted or dilated, offer little resistance to blood flow compared to the arterioles. Therefore, α-adrenergic venoconstriction causes only a small increase in the resistance to blood flow through an organ.

Sympathetic control on the heart is exerted through the β-adrenergic receptors that are found on every cardiac muscle cell. Beta receptors are activated by norepinephrine or epinephrine. Activation of β receptors increases heart rate, speeds up conduction through the atrioventricular (AV) node, increases ventricular contractility, and decreases the duration of ventricular systole. The last two of these effects increase stroke volume.

The overall effect is an increase in cardiac output.

Beta-adrenergic receptors are found on the arterioles also, particularly in the coronary circulation and in skeletal muscles. Activation of arteriolar β-adrenergic receptors causes relaxation of the vascular smooth muscle and dilation of the arterioles. However, these β-adrenergic receptors are not innervated by the sympathetic nervous system, so they are not activated directly by sympathetic nerves. Instead, these β-adrenergic receptors appear to respond to circulating epinephrine and norepinephrine, which are released by the adrenal medulla. The adrenal medulla releases epinephrine and norepinephrine in situations involving trauma, fear, or anxiety. Dilation of arterioles in the coronary circulation and in skeletal muscles is appropriate in such "fight or flight" situations, because the dilation results in an anticipatory increase in blood flow to the heart and skeletal muscle. Note that β-adrenergic vasodilation can overpower α-adrenergic vasoconstriction in the heart and skeletal muscle.

Cholinergic muscarinic receptors respond to the neurotransmitter acetylcholine. These receptors are located, most importantly, in the cardiac muscle cells. Cholinergic muscarinic receptors are particularly concentrated in the cells of the sinoatrial (SA) node and the AV node. The SA and AV nodes are innervated by postganglionic parasympathetic neurons. Activation of cholinergic muscarinic receptors at the SA node slows the spontaneous depolarization of pacemaker cells and decreases heart rate. This brings about a decrease in cardiac output. Activation of cholinergic muscarinic receptors in the AV node slows AV conduction, which creates a longer delay between atrial contractions and ventricular contractions. A prolonged AV delay is an appropriate accompaniment to a decreased heart rate.

Cholinergic muscarinic receptors are found also on the arterioles in most organs. Activation of these receptors causes the arterioles to dilate. However, these cholinergic muscarinic receptors are only innervated in three tissues. In the coronary circulation and in the external genitalia, parasympathetic neurons activate the cholinergic muscarinic receptors on arterioles. The vasodilatory effect is minor in the arterioles of the heart, and the function of this innervation is not well understood. In the genital organs, parasympathetic vasodilation results in erection. In cats and dogs, postganglionic sympathetic neurons that release acetylcholine (rather than norepinephrine) as a neurotransmitter innervate the cholinergic muscarinic receptors of skeletal muscle blood vessels. These *sympathetic-cholinergic neurons* appear to be activated specifically in anticipation of muscular exercise and during the defense-alarm reaction. The resulting vasodilation increases blood flow through the skeletal muscle just before, and during the initiation of, exercise. However, the cholinergic muscarinic receptors in skeletal muscle arterioles appear not to be innervated in other species, including most primates. An anticipatory vasodilation of skeletal muscle arterioles can be brought about in primates by activation of β-adrenergic receptors by epinephrine and norepinephrine that are released from the adrenal medulla, as mentioned earlier. To summarize, although arterioles throughout the body are dilated by acetylcholine, only the arterioles of the heart, external genitalia, and (in some species) skeletal muscle are innervated by acetylcholine-releasing autonomic neurons. The functional significance of muscarinic receptors on arterioles in other organs is unclear, because no neurons (either sympathetic or parasympathetic) appear to innervate them.

Of all the autonomic influences on the cardiovascular system just mentioned, three stand out as most important. The first is α-adrenergic vasoconstriction, brought about by the sympathetic nervous system in the arterioles of all body organs. The second is β-adrenergic excitation of cardiac muscle, brought about by the sympathetic nervous system and resulting in increased heart rate and stroke volume. The third is the cholinergic muscarinic effect on the heart, which decreases heart rate.

The Arterial Baroreceptor Reflex Regulates Arterial Blood Pressure

Blood pressure is monitored by pressure-sensitive nerve endings known as baroreceptors. The baroreceptors send afferent impulses to the central nervous system (CNS), which reflexly alters cardiac output or TPR to keep blood pressure at a normal level.

The *arterial baroreceptor reflex* is initiated by activation of specialized nerve endings that are embedded in the walls of the carotid arteries and aortic arch. These nerve endings are sensitive to stretch or distention of the arterial

wall. In effect, they sense arterial pressure, because blood pressure is the natural force that distends these arteries. Therefore, these nerve endings are called *baroreceptors* ("pressure sensors"), even though the actual physical factor being sensed is not pressure but rather the stretch or distortion of the nerve ending.

Baroreceptors (Fig. 24–1) are concentrated at the origin of each internal carotid artery in enlarged parts of the arteries, called the *carotid sinuses*. Similar nerve endings are found in the wall of the aortic arch, especially at the origin of its major branches. With every beat of the heart, neural impulses (action potentials) are initiated by the baroreceptors. The frequency of impulses is proportional to the arterial blood pressure. The afferent neurons from the aortic arch baroreceptors run in the vagus nerves. In some species the aortic baroreceptor afferents form a distinct bundle within the vagal nerve sheath, called the *aortic depressor nerve*. The stretch receptors in the carotid sinuses have their afferents in the carotid sinus nerves (Hering's nerves), which join into the glossopharyngeal (IX cranial) nerves. By way of these afferent neurons, the brain receives continuous information about the arterial blood pressure.

Figure 24–2 summarizes the effect of different arterial blood pressures on the sensory afferent nerve activity of arterial baroreceptors. The top trace depicts the pulsatile arterial pressure on three successive heartbeats. The mean level of arterial pressure is shown by the dashed line. The next trace below shows the pattern of action potentials that would be seen typically in a baroreceptor afferent neuron when the mean arterial pressure is lower than normal, in this case 50 mmHg. Note that there are only one or two action potentials with each heartbeat. These action potentials occur during the rapid upstroke of the pressure wave, because the baroreceptors are sensitive to rate of change of pressure. If the mean arterial pressure is at a higher level, perhaps 75 mmHg, more action potentials are formed during each heartbeat, but the action potentials still tend to occur during the rapid pressure increase at the beginning of each beat. As mean arterial pressure increases to 100 mmHg and beyond, there are more and more action potentials with each beat. However, the action potentials still occur as a cluster or burst during the upstroke of the pressure pulse. If mean arterial pressure reaches an extremely high level, like 200

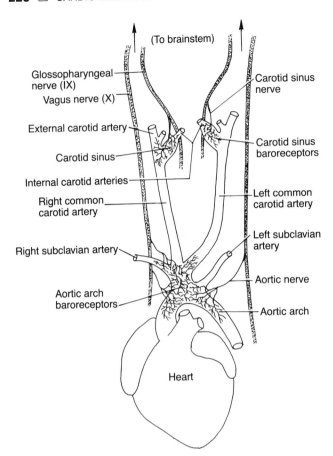

(To brainstem)

Glossopharyngeal nerve (IX)

Vagus nerve (X)

External carotid artery

Carotid sinus

Internal carotid arteries

Right common carotid artery

Right subclavian artery

Aortic arch baroreceptors

Heart

Carotid sinus nerve

Carotid sinus baroreceptors

Left common carotid artery

Left subclavian artery

Aortic nerve

Aortic arch

Figure 24–1. Arterial baroreceptors are located in the walls of the carotid sinuses and in the walls of the aortic arch and its major branches.

mmHg, the action potential activity in the baroreceptors becomes continuous (occurs during both systole and diastole). Thus, the arterial baroreceptors signal increases in pressure by increasing their action potential frequency. Because the baroreceptors are active when arterial pressure is normal (mean pressure near 100 mmHg), they can also signal a decrease in arterial pressure by decreasing their action potential frequency.

The reflex consequences of a decrease in afferent baroreceptor activity are summarized in Figure 24–3. The brain responds to a decrease in the afferent activity from the baroreceptors by increasing sympathetic activity. Sympathetic activity is increased to the arterioles of all organs, but particularly to the arterioles of noncritical organs (kidney, splanchnic organs, and resting skeletal muscle). Sympathetic activation causes vasoconstriction of these arterioles, which increases the resistance to blood flow through these organs and, therefore, increases TPR. The increase in peripheral resistance helps restore arterial blood pressure back toward its normal level. Sympathetic activity to the heart is increased also. This results

in increased contractility and decreased systolic duration, which combine to increase stroke volume and therefore cardiac output. Sympathetic activation also increases heart rate, which further increases cardiac output. The increase in cardiac output helps to restore blood pressure toward normal. The sympathetically driven increase in heart rate is augmented by a simultaneous reduction in parasympathetic activity to the SA node. Thus, the baroreceptor reflex uses reciprocal changes in sympathetic and parasympathetic activity to control heart rate.

To correctly understand the function of the baroreceptor reflex, it is important to recognize that the reflex does not *reverse* disturbances in blood pressure, but only minimizes them. Also, it is important to distinguish between cause and effect when thinking about the baroreflex. For example, what *causes* blood pressure to decrease *below normal* is a decrease *below normal* in cardiac output, TPR, or both. *There is no other way to lower blood pressure.* In a case where TPR falls below normal and *causes* blood pressure to decrease below normal, the *compensatory response* of the baroreceptor reflex

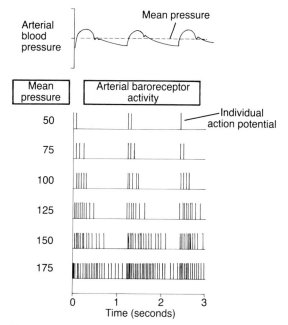

Figure 24–2. Each arterial pressure pulse causes action potentials to be generated in baroreceptor afferent neurons. The number of action potentials generated per heart beat increases dramatically with increases in mean arterial pressure.

is (1) to minimize the decrease in peripheral resistance by initiating a sympathetic vasoconstriction in the noncritical organs, and (2) to increase cardiac output above normal through increased sympathetic (and decreased parasympathetic) activation of the heart. After compensation by the baroreceptor reflex, peripheral resistance is still *below* normal (but not as far below normal as in the uncompensated state), and cardiac output is *above* normal. Blood pressure is still *below* normal, but not as far below normal as in the uncompensated state.

All of the reflex responses just illustrated for a decrease in arterial blood pressure occur in reverse in response to an increase in arterial blood pressure above its normal level. Hence, the baroreceptor reflex acts to combat either decreases in blood pressure or increases in blood pressure. As a regulator of arterial blood pressure, the baroreflex is both powerful and rapid. It can initiate compensations for changes in blood pressure within 1 second. A hemorrhage that would decrease blood pressure only 10 mmHg with intact baroreflexes, would cause a 40–50 mmHg decrease in blood pressure if there were no baroreflex. The bar-

oreflex also acts to maintain blood pressure close to normal during changes in posture or activity. In a dog without baroreflexes, changes in posture are accompanied by large, uncontrolled variations in blood pressure, as shown in Figure 24–4. By minimizing fluctuations in blood pressure, the baroreflex functions to assure an adequate blood flow to the critical organs.

Although the baroreceptor reflex is essential for the moment-to-moment stability of blood pressure, it does not appear to be the major mechanism responsible for setting the long-term level of arterial blood pressure, because baroreceptors adapt slowly or *reset* to the prevailing level of arterial pressure. That is, the baroreceptors come to accept whatever the prevailing blood pressure is as if it were the normal pressure. Baroreceptor resetting causes the baroreflex to "lose track of" normal blood pressure. For example, in an animal or human who has been hypertensive for a few days or weeks, the baroreflex functions to regulate blood pressure at the elevated level rather than to restore blood pressure toward its normal level. The baroreflex can become reset also in a downward direction during a period of sustained hypotension. For example, in chronic heart failure, where arterial pressure may be below normal for a period of days or weeks, the baroreflex appears to regulate blood pressure at a depressed level rather than to push it back toward its normal level. In summary, the baroreflex responds quickly and powerfully to counteract sudden changes in blood pressure, but it has little influence on the chronic level of blood pressure over a period of days or weeks.

The Atrial Volume Receptor Reflex Regulates Blood Volume and Helps to Stabilize Blood Pressure

Blood volume is monitored by specialized nerve endings in the cardiac atria. These atrial volume receptors send afferent impulses to the CNS, which responds reflexly to restore blood volume to normal.

The *atrial volume receptor reflex* is initiated by specialized sensory nerve endings that are located in the walls of the left and right atria. These nerve endings are activated by stretch. These stretch receptors are called *volume receptors,* because it is the volume of blood in each atrium that determines how much the atrial wall will be stretched. For example, a decrease

Baroreceptor Reflex

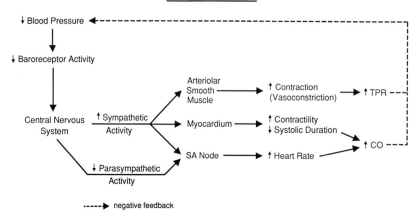

Figure 24–3. The arterial barore-ceptor reflex responds to de-creases in blood pressure (upper left) by changing cardiac output, total peripheral resistance, or both (far right). These reflex effects off-set the initial fall in blood pressure (dashed line).

in the body's total blood volume (e.g., a hem-orrhage) results in a decrease in the amount of blood in the major veins of the body and in the atria. If atrial volume decreases, atrial pressure decreases, and so does the stretch on the atrial walls. This decreases the frequency of action potentials generated in atrial stretch receptors. Conversely, increases in blood vol-ume result in increased atrial stretch and an increased frequency of action potentials gen-erated by the atrial stretch receptors. There-fore, these atrial stretch receptors are sensitive detectors of atrial blood volume and, indi-rectly, total blood volume.

Figure 24–5 summarizes the reflex effects of a change in the activity of the atrial volume receptors. If blood volume decreases, the re-sult is a decrease in the afferent activity from the atrial volume receptors. The CNS responds reflexly to this decreased afferent activity by increasing sympathetic efferent activity to the heart and systemic organs and decreasing parasympathetic efferent activity to the heart. The target organs for these changes in sym-pathetic and parasympathetic activity are the

same for the atrial volume receptor reflex as for the baroreceptor reflex. That is, a decrease in blood volume leads reflexly to arteriolar vasoconstriction, an increase in cardiac con-tractility, a decrease in systolic duration, and an increase in heart rate.

All of these changes help combat the de-crease in arterial blood pressure that would otherwise result from a decreased blood vol-ume. In this way, the atrial volume receptor reflex augments the baroreceptor reflex as a regulator of blood pressure. The volume re-ceptor reflex also acts in three additional ways to help restore the lost blood volume. First, the reflex acts through the hypothalamus to increase the sensation of thirst. If water is available, the animal drinks. This provides the fluid necessary to increase blood volume back toward normal. Second, the atrial volume re-ceptor reflex acts via the hypothalamus and pituitary gland to increase the release of *anti-diuretic hormone* (ADH). ADH is synthesized in the hypothalamus, but it is transported to the posterior pituitary gland for storage and release. ADH acts on the kidneys to decrease urine flow.* The third effect of the atrial vol-ume receptor reflex on blood volume is to increase the release of the hormone *renin* from the kidneys. Renin acts to increase the pro-duction of the hormone *angiotensin II*, which acts to increase production of the hormone *aldosterone*, which acts to decrease the amount of sodium and chloride excreted by the kid-neys. That is, activation of the renin-angioten-sin-aldosterone system causes the body to conserve available sodium chloride (NaCl). The combination of decreased sodium excre-tion (by actions of renin) and decreased urine

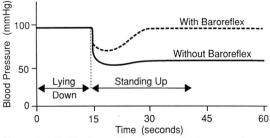

Figure 24–4. The baroreflex is essential for normal, mo-ment-to-moment stability of blood pressure. Dogs in which baroreflexes are eliminated exhibit much larger decreases in blood pressure in response to postural changes than do dogs with intact baroreflexes.

---

*ADH is also called arginine vasopressin (AVP).

Atrial Volume Receptor Reflex

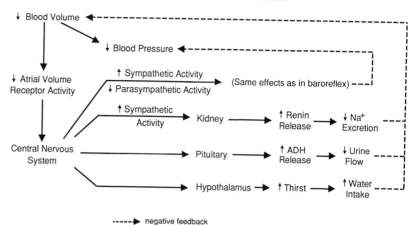

Figure 24-5. The atrial volume receptor reflex responds to a decrease in blood volume by decreasing sodium and water loss in the urine and by increasing oral water intake. The reflex also helps support blood pressure by increasing cardiac output and total peripheral resistance (similar to baroreflex).

flow (by actions of ADH) results in the conservation of body fluid. The conservation of body fluid, combined with an increased water intake, eventually restores blood volume back toward normal.

The Cardiovascular State of Conscious Subjects Is Determined by an Ongoing and Ever-Changing Mixture of Reflex Effects and Psychogenic Responses

The baroreceptor reflex and the atrial volume receptor reflex are just two of several important cardiovascular reflexes. They are primarily responsible for the regulation of blood pressure and blood volume, and they serve also to illustrate several properties common to all cardiovascular reflexes. First, these reflexes originate from stimuli to peripheral sensory receptors. Second, the reflexes occur at a subconscious level through neural pathways that primarily involve cardiovascular centers in the brainstem and midbrain. Third, cardiovascular reflexes persist in unconscious and anesthetized subjects, although the strength and character of the reflexes is altered by anesthesia. Finally, the reflexes use sympathetic and parasympathetic neurons as well as hormonal responses to bring about cardiovascular changes.

In conscious subjects, neurohumoral control of the cardiovascular system involves both cardiovascular reflexes and psychogenic effects. Psychogenic responses originate from conscious perceptions or emotional reactions. They are eliminated by unconsciousness or general anesthesia. They involve neural pathways of the midbrain and forebrain, including

the limbic system and cerebral cortex. Psychogenic responses are often triggered by sensory stimuli. For example, the sights, sounds, and smells of a veterinary clinic may trigger perceptions and emotions that cause increases in heart rate and blood pressure both in animal patients and their human companions. Psychogenic responses can occur also without any obvious sensory triggers. For example, anxiety about a future event can increase heart rate and blood pressure, at least in human beings. Cardiovascular reflexes and psychogenic reactions utilize the same sympathetic and parasympathetic neurons and some of the same hormonal responses to bring about cardiovascular changes.

Two important psychogenic responses are the defense-alarm reaction and vasovagal syncope (the "playing dead reaction"). The *defense-alarm reaction* is also called the *fear, fight, or flight response.* The defense-alarm reaction is an emotional response to threatening situations, physical injury, or trauma. This reaction involves increased sympathetic activity and decreased parasympathetic activity. Sometimes the sympathetic activation is strong enough to cause release of epinephrine and norepinephrine from the adrenal medulla. The cardiovascular responses during a defense-alarm reaction include an increased heart rate, increased stroke volume, vasoconstriction (in the kidneys, splanchnic organs, resting skeletal muscle, and skin), vasodilation (in coronary vessels and in working skeletal muscle), and increased blood pressure. The cardiovascular responses during the defense reaction are enhanced also by other circulating hormones, including ADH, angiotensin II, and adrenocorticotropic hormone (ACTH). The elevated

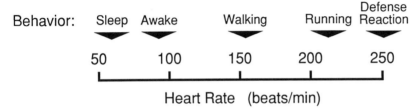

Figure 24–6. The defense-alarm reaction is simply the extreme of a continuum of emotional and physical arousal. The cardiovascular system (heart rate, for example) responds sensitively to every change along this arousal scale.

blood pressure helps to assure adequate blood flow for the exercising skeletal muscles, the heart, and the brain. The baroreceptor reflex is reset by the CNS during a defense alarm reaction, so that it regulates blood pressure at an elevated level rather than acting to oppose the increased pressure. This is analogous to resetting the cruise control on a car so that it regulates speed at an elevated level rather than acting to oppose an increased speed.

During a defense-alarm reaction, sympathetic activity is maximal, and parasympathetic activity is minimal. However, it is important to realize that this reaction is simply the extreme form of a continuum of states of emotional arousal. Sleep is at the opposite end of this cardiovascular and emotional continuum. In quiet rest or sleep, sympathetic activity is minimal, and parasympathetic activity is maximal. Animals and humans experience increases and decreases in emotional arousal from moment to moment during ordinary and extraordinary daily activities. Cardiovascular variables, such as heart rate and blood pressure, are sensitive to these changes in emotional state (Fig. 24–6). For example, it may be entirely normal for a large dog to have a heart rate of 130 beats per minute in a clinic if the dog is frightened in that setting. Another important point for the clinician to remember is that emotional responses are subjective.

Situations that severely agitate one animal may only cause a mild alerting response in another animal. The clinician must evaluate heart rate, blood pressure, and other cardiovascular signs with respect to the patient's emotional state.

Vasovagal syncope is another psychogenic response that may be encountered in the veterinary clinic. This response is also called the "playing dead reaction" or "playing opossum." In response to certain threatening or emotional situations, some humans and animals experience a psychogenic decrease in blood pressure and may faint. In many ways this response is the opposite of the defense-alarm reaction. As shown in Figure 24–7 vasovagal syncope involves a decrease in sympathetic activity and an increase in parasympathetic activity. These neural changes bring about a vasodilation of the noncritical organs and a decrease in TPR. Heart rate and cardiac output also decrease, so there is a large drop in arterial blood pressure. If blood pressure falls so low that there is inadequate cerebral blood flow, then *syncope (fainting)* results. The name vasovagal syncope denotes *vaso*-dilation, *vagal* (parasympathetic) activation, and *syncope* (fainting). It is not clear why some animals respond to a threatening situation with a defense-alarm reaction, whereas others exhibit vasovagal syncope. It is also unclear what the survival value of "playing dead" is, although

Vasovagal Syncope

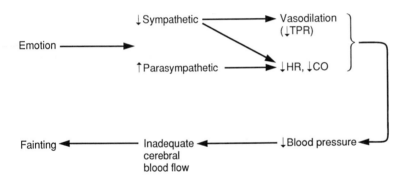

Figure 24–7. Vasovagal syncope (playing dead reaction) is an emotional response that involves decreases in sympathetic activity and increases in parasympathetic activity.

this response seems to have served opossums well over several million years.

CLINICAL CORRELATION

INTRAOPERATIVE HEMORRHAGE

HISTORY □ Four hours following abdominal surgery for a splenic sarcoma, a 30 kg, 9-year-old Labrador retriever is severely depressed and recumbant. An abnormally large amount of hemorrhage occurred during the surgical removal of the spleen, because the dog suffered from a hereditary blood-clotting defect (von Willebrand's disease).

CLINICAL EXAMINATION □ The dog's gums are pale, and his capillary refilling time is abnormally prolonged (3 seconds). His extremities are cool to the touch. The femoral pulse is rapid and weak. An electrocardiogram (ECG) indicates sinus tachycardia at a rate of 185 beats per minute. The hematocrit (packed cell volume) is 38%, and the plasma protein concentration is 5.6 g/dL; both these values are below normal. A jugular catheter is inserted, and central venous pressure is measured and found to be −1 mmHg (normal 0–3 mmHg). Despite being given 600 mL of lactated Ringer's solution intravenously (IV) during surgery, the dog has not produced any urine.

The dog's abdomen is tapped (abdominocentesis), and 100 mL of bloody fluid is removed.

COMMENT □ This case illustrates the clinical signs typical of hemorrhage. Most of the blood in a dog is in the systemic veins, so most of the blood missing after hemorrhage is missing from the veins. The result is an abnormally low central venous pressure, as observed in this dog. The decreased central venous pressure leads to a decreased ventricular preload and a decreased ventricular end-diastolic volume. This decreases stroke volume (Starling's law of the heart), cardiac output, and arterial blood pressure. Inadequate cardiac output and blood pressure lead to behavioral depression.

Neurohumoral compensations for the hemorrhage are initiated by the atrial volume receptor reflex and the arterial baroreceptor reflex. Heart rate is increased by the combination of increased sympathetic activation and decreased parasympathetic activation. The combination of high heart rate and low stroke vol-ume accounts for the rapid, but weak, femoral pulse. Sympathetic activity also causes vasoconstriction in the mucous membranes, skeletal muscle, splanchnic organs, and kidneys. The reduced blood flow in these tissues accounts for the gums being pale and showing slow refilling of capillaries, for the limbs being cool, and for the kidneys not producing urine. Urine formation by the kidneys is also being depressed by the combined hormonal effects of ADH and the renin-angiotensin-aldosterone system.

Hemorrhage, *per se,* does not reduce either hematocrit or plasma protein concentration, because whole blood is being lost. However, two factors caused hematocrit and plasma protein concentration to decrease in this dog. First, the fluid given IV during surgery (lactated Ringer's) did not contain either red blood cells or plasma proteins, so the cells and proteins remaining in the blood stream were diluted. Second, the hemorrhage reduced not only venous and arterial pressures, but also capillary hydrostatic pressure, and this changed the balance of hydrostatic and oncotic forces across the capillary walls in favor of reabsorption. The interstitial fluid that was reabsorbed into the blood stream contained no red blood cells and almost no plasma proteins. This caused a further dilution of the cells and proteins in the blood.

TREATMENT □ Therapy for this case involves measures to stop ongoing blood loss and restoration of the lost blood volume. In this dog, the hemorrhage is predominantly seepage from small intra-abdominal vessels as a result of the coagulation defect. Transfusions of fresh blood or plasma, or concentrated preparations of clotting proteins, promote clotting, limit subsequent hemorrhage, and expand the intravascular fluid volume. Additional crystalloid solutions (like lactated Ringer's) can be infused in this dog also, because the hematocrit and plasma protein concentration are not dangerously low. If crystalloid solutions are administered, the hematocrit and plasma protein concentration should be monitored closely to avoid the hypoxia that results from too much dilution of the red blood cells, or the edema that results from too much dilution of the plasma proteins.

Bibliography

Berne RM, Levy MN: Interplay of central and peripheral factors in the control of circulation. *In* Berne RM, Levy

MN (eds): Cardiovascular Physiology. St. Louis, CV Mosby, 1986, p 235.

Berne RM, Levy MN: The peripheral circulation and its control. *In* Berne RM, Levy MN (eds): Cardiovascular Physiology. St. Louis, CV Mosby, 1986, p 153.

Milnor WR: Autonomic and peripheral control mechanisms. *In* Milnor WR (ed): Cardiovascular Physiology. New York, Oxford University Press, 1990, p 249.

Milnor WR: The cardiovascular control system. *In* Milnor WR (ed): Cardiovascular Physiology. New York, Oxford University Press, 1990, p 219.

Scher AM: Cardiovascular control. *In* Patton HD, Fuchs AF, Hille B, et al (eds): Textbook of Physiology. Philadelphia, WB Saunders, 1989, p 972.

PRACTICE QUESTIONS FOR CHAPTER 24

1. The dilation of arterioles that occurs during steady state exercise in active skeletal muscle could be eliminated by

    a. pharmacological blockade of all autonomic ganglia.
    b. complete surgical removal of sympathetic innervation of the skeletal muscles.
    c. the administration of a cholinergic muscarinic-blocking agent.
    d. the administration of a β-receptor blocking agent.
    e. None of the above

2. A drug is injected IV into a dog and causes a transient increase in mean arterial pressure and a transient decrease in heart rate. The baroreceptor nerves are cut, and the drug is injected again and now causes a greater increase in blood pressure but no change in heart rate. Which choice is most likely to explain the results caused by the first injection of the drug?

    a. It caused activation of muscarinic cholinergic receptors of arterioles.
    b. It caused a reflex slowing of the heart.
    c. It caused β-receptor activation of the pacemaker cells of the atrium.
    d. It blocked α receptors of peripheral arterioles.
    e. It decreased the activity of arterial baroreceptors.

3. A dog has suffered a hemorrhage. Heart rate is increased above normal, and the skin is cold. The mucous membranes are pale. In this situation (as compared to normal)

    a. the baroreceptor nerves are firing at a higher rate.
    b. the sympathetic nerves to the heart are firing at a decreased rate.
    c. the sympathetic nerves to the blood vessels of the skin and mucous membranes are firing at an increased rate.
    d. the parasympathetic fibers to the blood vessels are firing at an increased rate.
    e. the release of renin by the kidney is decreased.

4. Vasovagal syncope

    a. involves decreased blood pressure and heart rate.
    b. involves increased sympathetic activity.
    c. involves a decrease in cardiac parasympathetic activity.
    d. prepares an animal for fight or flight.
    e. involves constriction of splanchnic arterioles.

5. Blood (250 mL) is taken from a vein of a dog. Mean arterial pressure does not decrease. Nevertheless, it is likely that

    a. stimulation of atrial stretch receptors has decreased.
    b. stroke volume has increased.
    c. stimulation of aortic arch baroreceptors has increased.
    d. TPR has decreased.
    e. secretion of ADH by the pituitary has decreased.

25

Integrated Cardiovascular Responses

1. Heart failure is compensated by both Starling's mechanism and the arterial baroreflex
2. Serious complications secondary to heart failure include edema, kidney failure, septic shock, and decompensation
3. The immediate cardiovascular effects of hemorrhage are minimized by compensations initiated by the atrial volume receptor reflex and the arterial baroreceptor reflex
4. The blood volume lost in hemorrhage is restored by a combination of capillary fluid shifts, and hormonal and behavioral responses
5. The initiation of exercise involves an interplay of local and neural changes to increase cardiac output and deliver increased flow to exercising muscle

In the preceding sections the various elements of cardiovascular function and control are described. However, an understanding of these individual elements is not sufficient to provide a basis for diagnosing and treating cardiovascular abnormalities. Instead, the interaction of these elements in normal and abnormal function must be understood. In addition, a discussion of integrated cardiovascular responses serves as a review and summary of the most important ideas presented previously. Three situations are considered to illustrate the integrated function of the cardiovascular system: first, the response to heart failure; second, the response to hemorrhage; and third, the response to exercise.

Heart Failure Is Compensated by Both Starling's Mechanism and the Arterial Baroreflex

Clinically, there are many kinds and causes of heart failure, but they share the basic underlying characteristic of decreased cardiac contractility. If the decrease in contractility affects both sides of the heart, the condition is called *bilateral heart failure*. In other circumstances, failure may be restricted primarily to either the left ventricle or to the right ventricle. A helpful way to envision the consequences of heart failure and the compensations for heart failure is to plot ventricular function curves for the failing ventricle, as shown in Figure 25–1. The curve labeled "normal" indicates the relation between stroke volume and preload for a normal animal. The curve labeled "initially severe failure" shows that a ventricle in failure has a depressed contractility, and therefore, a smaller stroke volume for any given preload. If a normal heart suddenly goes into severe failure, stroke volume decreases from its normal value (shown by point #1) to the low value (shown by point #2). For purposes of illustration, imagine that these curves define the function of the left ventricle, and that the left ventricle is the one that fails. A decrease in left ventricular stroke volume causes a decrease in left ventricular output (cardiac output), which results in a decrease in mean arterial blood pressure. If this fall in blood pressure is not compensated, there may be inadequate perfusion of the critical organs. Death may result. However, several mechanisms act to compensate for heart failure.

One compensation for heart failure is Starling's mechanism. If the left ventricle suddenly decreases its stroke volume, blood backs up (dams up or accumulates) in the left atrium and pulmonary veins, because the right ventricle, at least for a short time, maintains a higher stroke volume than does the failing left ventricle. Some of the excess blood pumped by the right ventricle accumulates in the left atrium, so left atrial pressure increases. The increase in left atrial pressure creates an increase in left ventricle preload, which leads to an increase in left ventricular end-diastolic

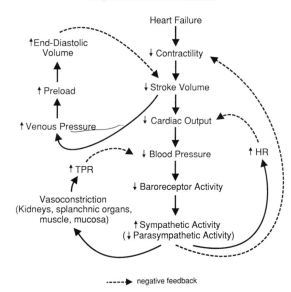

Compensation for Heart Failure

----▶ negative feedback

Figure 25–2. The consequences and compensations for heart failure. The changes described here include those presented graphically in Figure 25–1.

volume and (by Starling's mechanism) an increase in stroke volume. That is, instead of remaining at the point on the graph labeled point #2, the left ventricle moves to the right along the curve of initially severe failure, to point #3, with a higher preload and a somewhat higher stroke volume. This sequence of events, whereby an increase in preload helps offset the fall in stroke volume, is diagrammed in the upper-left loop of Figure 25–2. Note that this compensation does not return stroke volume to its normal value, but only brings it to a level somewhat higher than it would have been otherwise.

Another compensatory mechanism for heart failure involves the arterial baroreflex. Because stroke volume remains below normal, even after Starling's compensation, left ventricular output and arterial blood pressure remain below normal also. This results in a baroreceptor activity that is below normal. The central nervous system (CNS) responds reflexly by increasing sympathetic efferent activity to the heart and blood vessels, and by decreasing parasympathetic activity to the heart. The sympathetic effect on the heart increases ventricular contractility. Contractility is not restored to normal, but is brought to a higher level than would exist in the absence of reflex compensation. Graphically, the effect of the baroreflex on ventricular contractility corresponds to a transition to a ventricular function

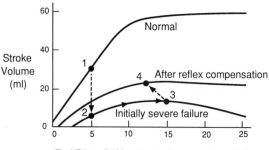

Figure 25–1. Ventricular function curves depicting the consequences and compensations for heart failure in terms of changes in preload and stroke volume. Details are given in the text.

curve that is intermediate between the normal curve and the curve of initially severe failure (point #4 in Fig. 25–1). Note that the increase in contractility also brings stroke volume back toward (but not reaching) its normal level. Sympathetic actions on the heart also increase the heart rate and decrease the systolic duration, and these changes help to restore cardiac output back toward normal despite a depressed stroke volume. Finally, sympathetic activation causes vasoconstriction in the noncritical organs, which increases the total peripheral resistance (TPR). This also helps to return blood pressure toward its normal level. The net effect of the compensations by way of Starling's mechanism and the baroreflex is that blood pressure can be maintained near its normal level despite a severe ventricular failure. These reflex effects are summarized also in Figure 25–2.

Serious Complications Secondary to Heart Failure Include Edema, Kidney Failure, Septic Shock, and Decompensation

Even though Starling's mechanism and the baroreflex can compensate for severe heart failure, there are important, secondary complications that often develop. These complications make heart failure a serious clinical problem, even in cases where arterial pressure is maintained near normal. The first of these complications is edema.

It was already noted that blood backs up or dams up in the veins and the atrium behind the failing ventricle. In the case of left ventricular failure, left atrial pressure increases, and so does pressure in the pulmonary veins and pulmonary capillaries. The increase in pulmonary capillary hydrostatic pressure leads to an increase in the filtration of capillary fluid into the lung's interstitial spaces. As fluid accumulates in the interstitial space, pulmonary edema develops. These events are summarized in the center of Figure 25–3. Excess interstitial fluid in the lungs slows the transfer of oxygen from the lung alveoli into the lung capillaries and can result in systemic hypoxia. In extreme cases, pulmonary edema results in the actual accumulation of fluid in the intrapleural space (*pleural effusion*) or in the alveolar air spaces, and this causes a further reduction in lung function. The resulting systemic hypoxia can lead to death.

In a case of right ventricular failure, the increase in venous pressure occurs in the systemic circulation. Therefore, the resulting edema occurs in the systemic organs, particularly in dependent extremities and in the abdomen. The edema is limited by the three safety factors previously discussed (see Fig. 22–5). These safety factors are all consequences of the fact that edema leads to an increase in interstitial pressure. Increased interstitial fluid pressure reduces the rate of filtration back toward normal and also increases lymph flow above normal. The increased lymph flow removes some of the edema fluid from the interstitial space. Also, the combination of filtration and increased lymph flow decreases interstitial fluid protein concentration. Therefore, interstitial fluid oncotic pressure decreases, which further reduces excess filtration.

An additional complication in severe heart failure is inadequate perfusion of the noncritical organs. When the baroreceptor reflex responds to an abnormally low arterial pressure in heart failure, it brings about arteriolar vasoconstriction, primarily in the kidneys, splanchnic organs, and resting skeletal muscle. In severe failure, the skin and mucous membranes may be vasoconstricted also. These organs have been referred to as noncritical in the sense that they can function temporarily with less than normal blood flow. Vasoconstriction in these organs permits the available cardiac output to be routed to the critical organs (brain, heart, and working skeletal muscle). However, a persistent vasoconstriction leads to prolonged tissue hypoxia, and organ function eventually fails.

Kidney failure, secondary to renal vasoconstriction, is a frequent complication to heart failure. The vasoconstricted kidney cannot form urine in a normal fashion and, therefore, cannot rid the body of excess salt and water or of nitrogenous or acidic waste products. Furthermore, after a prolonged period of intense vasoconstriction, the kidney tissue becomes irreversibly damaged. Uremia, acidosis, and salt and water retention may persist even if cardiac output and blood pressure can be restored toward normal. For this reason, renal failure is often the terminal event in chronic heart failure.

The mucosa of the gastrointestinal (GI) tract are also susceptible to damage secondary to prolonged, intense vasoconstriction. Normally, the intestinal mucosa creates a barrier between the intestinal lumen and the blood stream. Prolonged intestinal vasoconstriction

Complications Secondary to Heart Failure

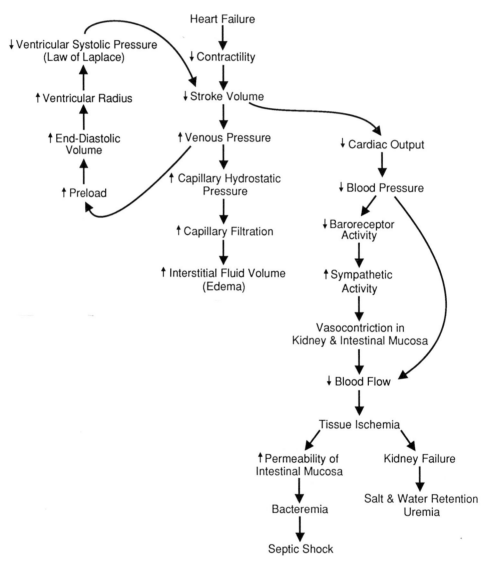

Figure 25–3. Four life-threatening complications secondary to heart failure are edema, kidney failure, septic shock, and decompensation. See text for details.

damages the mucosa, which allows bacteria and bacterial toxins to pass into the blood stream or the peritoneum. The resulting bacteremia or peritonitis can lead to septic shock and death. The adverse effects of heart failure on the kidneys and intestine are summarized in Figure 25–3, lower right.

The fourth common complication secondary to heart failure (in addition to edema, kidney failure, and septic shock) is cardiac decompensation. Although difficult to understand, cardiac decompensation is important, because it is the terminal event in many cases of severe cardiac failure. Cardiac decompensation is triggered by a mechanism that competes with Starling's mechanism. In the previous discussions of Starling's mechanism, an inherent limitation to increasing stroke volume by increasing preload has been overlooked. This limitation derives from the physical principle known as the *Law of Laplace*. Laplace pointed out that there is an unavoidable increase in the wall tension of a chamber whenever the fluid pressure within the chamber increases. Wall tension also increases when the radius of the chamber increases (even if fluid pressure is constant). This relationship is expressed mathematically as

$$T = P \cdot r$$
$$T = \text{wall tension}$$
$$P = \text{fluid pressure within the chamber}$$
$$r = \text{chamber radius}$$

The law of Laplace applies to the contracting ventricle as follows. In order to eject blood into the aorta, a contracting ventricle must develop a pressure higher than aortic pressure. If the radius of a ventricle increases, a greater wall tension is required to raise ventricular pressure above aortic pressure. A healthy ventricle can generate this increased wall tension; a failing ventricle may not.

An increase in end-diastolic ventricular volume has four effects, three that are favorable for increasing stroke volume and one that is unfavorable. The first favorable effect is that there is more blood in the ventricle at the end of diastole, and therefore more blood to eject in the following systole. The second favorable effect is that a greater diastolic distension of the ventricle places the cardiac muscle fibers in a more advantageous geometry for contraction. That is, there is a greater ability of the ventricular muscle to squeeze down on the contained fluid, without the muscle getting in its own way. The third favorable effect is that

a greater stretch of ventricular muscle fibers during diastole somehow causes more Ca^{2+} to be released from the sarcoplasmic reticulum during the subsequent systolic contraction. This increases the force of contraction. The fourth, unfavorable, effect of an increase in diastolic ventricular volume is that the greater radius of the ventricle at the end of diastole requires the muscle fibers in the wall of the ventricle to develop a greater tension in order to raise ventricular pressure high enough to eject blood (law of Laplace).

The ventricular function curve of a normal ventricle slopes upward, which indicates that the three advantageous effects of increasing ventricular diastolic volume are dominant over the fourth, unfavorable consequence of increasing diastolic volume. In the failing ventricle, the advantageous effects of greater ventricular filling are weaker, because the ventricular muscle fibers have a limited ability to increase their contractual force with increased ventricular end-diastolic volume. However, the limitation imposed by the law of Laplace is just as strong in the failing heart as in the normal heart. Thus, as the failing heart is distended beyond its normal diastolic volume, the failing ventricular muscle is stretched to a better geometry for contraction, but it cannot develop enough additional force of contraction to generate a ventricular pressure adequate for ejection during systole. As a result, there is little increase in stroke volume as preload increases. More importantly, with excessive preload there can actually be a *decreased* stroke volume for further increases in preload (right end of bottom curve in Fig. 25–1). This condition involves a vicious cycle, where an *increase* in preload results in a *decrease* in stroke volume, which results in an additional backing up of blood in the atrium behind the failing ventricle, which results in a further *increase* in ventricular preload, which results in yet a further *decrease* in stroke volume (upper left loop of Fig. 25–3). A patient exhibiting this vicious cycle of events is said to be in *decompensated heart failure*. This situation leads to death within a few hours, unless substantial clinical intervention takes place.

Four major complications secondary to heart failure have been presented (edema, kidney failure, septic shock, and decompensation). Each complication has been illustrated to be potentially life-threatening. Therefore, careful clinical diagnosis and treatment of heart failure is imperative, even in cases where compensatory mechanisms have maintained blood pressure near its normal level. In evaluating the severity of heart failure and the extent of compensation, it is clinically useful to group the symptoms of heart failure into two categories. The first category is referred to as the symptoms of *backward heart failure.* These include the changes in the circulation *upstream* from the failing ventricle, namely increased atrial pressure, increased venous pressure, excessive capillary filtration, edema, and the functional changes secondary to edema (such as respiratory failure). The heading of *forward heart failure* includes the consequences of heart failure *downstream* from the failing ventricle. These include decreased cardiac output, decreased arterial blood pressure, excessive vasoconstriction of the kidneys, splanchnic organs, or mucous membranes, and failure of normal function in any of these organs secondary to prolonged, excessive vasoconstriction.

Exercise intolerance is an additional, common symptom of heart failure. In many patients, the compensations for heart failure (by Starling's mechanism and reflexes) are able to maintain blood pressure and cardiac output near a normal level during rest or during mild physical activity. However, when the animal with heart failure attempts more vigorous muscular exercise, the heart is unable to provide the increased cardiac output required to deliver the necessary blood flow to the exercising skeletal muscle. Therefore, the patient with heart failure typically exhibits weakness

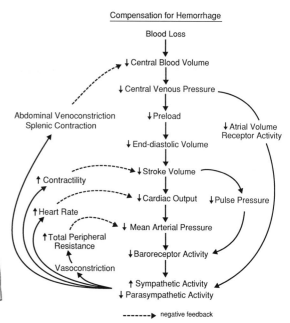

Figure 25–5. The effects of hemorrhage and the immediate compensations brought about by the arterial baroreflex and by the atrial volume receptor reflex. The changes described here include those presented graphically in Figure 25–4.

and an inability to exercise normally. In a normal animal, the ability of the heart to increase cardiac output during exercise depends on sympathetically mediated increases in stroke volume and heart rate. However, in a patient with heart failure, the ability of sympathetic activation to increase cardiac output is utilized simply to maintain a normal cardiac output in the resting state. Therefore, the patient's attempt to exercise is not accompanied by an effective further increase in sympathetic activity.

The Immediate Cardiovascular Effects of Hemorrhage Are Minimized by Compensations Initiated by the Atrial Volume Receptor Reflex and the Arterial Baroreceptor Reflex

The cardiovascular responses to hemorrhage are summarized graphically in Figure 25–4 and verbally in Figure 25–5. The curve labeled "Normal" in Figure 25–4 shows that the maintenance of a normal stroke volume is dependent on the maintenance of a normal level of ventricular preload. When hemorrhage occurs, blood is lost from the whole cardiovascular system and, particularly, from the veins, which are the blood reservoirs of the body. Central venous volume decreases, as does

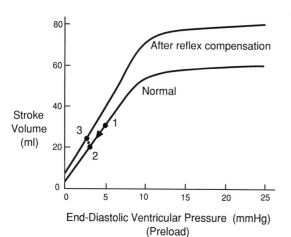

Fizgure 25–4. The direct effect of hemorrhage is to decrease ventricular preload, which decreases stroke volume (going from point #1 to point #2). Stroke volume is restored *toward normal* by a reflex increase in sympathetic activity, which increases ventricular contractility *above normal* (going from point #2 to point #3).

central venous pressure and atrial pressure. The decrease in atrial pressure causes decreases in ventricular preload and end-diastolic volume. In the absence of any compensations, the stroke volume decreases from point #1 in Figure 25–4 to point #2. Note that the normal ventricular function curve is rather steep to the left of the normal operating point (point #1). Therefore, a 40% hemorrhage results in approximately 40% reductions in central venous pressure, left atrial pressure, ventricular preload, ventricular end-diastolic volume, and stroke volume. If there were no compensation, there would be 40% reductions also in cardiac output and mean arterial pressure. Mean arterial pressure would be inadequate then to provide the blood flow necessary for normal function of the brain and the coronary circulation. The animal would die. However, a normal animal can compensate for hemorrhage and can withstand a 40% hemorrhage, without death, and with only a 5–10% decrease in mean arterial pressure.

The immediate compensations for hemorrhage are initiated by the arterial baroreflex and by the atrial volume receptor reflex. The decrease in mean arterial pressure causes a decrease in the activity of arterial baroreceptors. The baroreflex acts through the CNS to increase sympathetic activity and decrease parasympathetic activity. The increased sympathetic activity acts on the heart to increase cardiac contractility. This helps restore stroke volume back toward normal, despite a persistent, subnormal preload and end-diastolic volume. The effect of this sympathetic compensation for hemorrhage is diagrammed in Figure 25–4 as point #3. Note that stroke volume is not returned to normal. After compensation for a 40% hemorrhage, stroke volume may remain 25% below normal.

Additional compensations occur that help restore blood pressure closer to normal. First, heart rate increases above normal, which brings cardiac output back to within about 20% of its normal level, despite the persistent low stroke volume. In addition, sympathetic vasoconstriction in the noncritical organs raises TPR above normal, resulting in a mean arterial pressure that remains within 5 or 10% of its normal level, despite a 20% drop in cardiac output. The reader may wish to review the compensations described thus far by locating them on Figure 25–5.

The perceptive reader may wonder why baroreflex compensatory actions continue if mean arterial pressure is returned most of the way toward normal. Compensatory baroreflex responses are sustained because baroreceptors are responsive to changes in pulse pressure as well as to changes in mean arterial pressure, and pulse pressure remains low. There are two reasons for the subnormal pulse pressure: (1) the persistent decrease in stroke volume, and (2) the increase above normal in heart rate. Thus, even if the mean arterial pressure were returned completely to normal following a hemorrhage, arterial baroreceptor action potential frequency would remain below normal, because of the persistent, subnormal pulse pressure.

The atrial volume receptor reflex also sustains an increased sympathetic activity following hemorrhage. As shown in Figure 25–5, hemorrhage leads to a persistent decrease in central venous pressure and atrial pressure. Therefore, the activity of the atrial volume receptors is decreased below normal. The CNS responds to this decreased afferent activity from atrial volume receptors by elevating sympathetic efferent activity and decreasing cardiac parasympathetic efferent activity. Thus, the atrial volume receptor reflex and the arterial baroreflex work synergistically to compensate for hemorrhage.

In extreme hemorrhage, the reflex increases in sympathetic activity affect not only the heart and resistance vessels, but also the veins. The abdominal veins, in particular, are constricted when sympathetic activation is intense. Sympathetic venoconstriction displaces blood from the abdominal veins and moves it toward the central circulation, which helps to increase central venous pressure back toward normal. As a result, atrial pressure (cardiac ventricular preload) is higher than it would otherwise be (see Fig. 25–5). In addition, a substantial volume of blood can be moved from the spleen into the central circulation in those species that have large spleens (e.g., dogs and horses). Sympathetic activation constricts both the blood vessels within the spleen and the muscular capsule around the spleen. The blood that is sequestered in the spleen is expelled into the veins. In the dog and the horse, splenic contraction can mobilize a volume of blood equal to 10% of the total blood volume. An additional, adaptive feature of the blood sequestered in the spleen is that it has a higher than normal hematocrit. The mobilization of these sequestered red blood cells helps to offset the fall in hematocrit that is a normal consequence of interstitial fluid reabsorption following hemorrhage.

The arterial baroreceptor reflex and the atrial volume receptor reflex act within a few seconds to restore *blood pressure* toward its normal level after a hemorrhage. Other compensations come into play in the minutes and hours following hemorrhage to restore the lost fluid volume.

The Blood Volume Lost in Hemorrhage Is Restored by a Combination of Capillary Fluid Shifts and Hormonal and Behavioral Responses

Hemorrhage causes both venous and arterial pressures to fall below normal, so capillary hydrostatic pressure also falls below normal throughout the body. This alters the balance of hydrostatic and oncotic pressures acting on water in a direction that favors reabsorption of interstitial fluid back into the capillaries (Fig. 25–6). The volume of interstitial fluid that can be reabsorbed by this process in 1 hour is approximately 10% of the volume lost in the hemorrhage. However, the rate of reabsorption of interstitial fluid becomes limited after 3–4 hours, because as interstitial fluid is reabsorbed, there is a decrease in interstitial fluid

hydrostatic pressure (it becomes even more negative than normal), and this opposes further reabsorption. Also, as interstitial fluid is reabsorbed, the interstitial fluid protein concentration increases (the interstitial proteins are not reabsorbed); the resulting increase in interstitial fluid oncotic pressure also limits the amount of interstitial fluid that can be reabsorbed. In spite of these limits, the reabsorption of interstitial fluid is an important compensation for hemorrhage in the first few hours.

A complication that results from the reabsorption of interstitial fluid following hemorrhage is that the reabsorbed fluid contains no plasma proteins or blood cells. Therefore, the proteins and cells that are in the blood stream are diluted as interstitial fluid is reabsorbed. The concentration of plasma proteins in blood decreases, as does the hematocrit (fraction of cells in blood). For this reason, a decreasing hematocrit over a period of a few hours in an otherwise normal patient is presumptive evidence that a recent hemorrhage has occurred.

The restoration of blood volume following hemorrhage also involves hormonal and behavioral responses. As already mentioned, hemorrhage leads to a decrease in the action potential frequency of both the arterial baroreceptors and the atrial volume receptors. The immediate reflex effects on sympathetic and parasympathetic activity have been described already (Fig. 25–5). In addition, the arterial baroreceptors and the atrial volume receptors also have important hormonal effects. The increase in sympathetic activity increases renin secretion from the kidneys. Renin leads to increases in the hormones angiotensin II and aldosterone. Angiotensin is a potent vasoconstrictor (helps sustain blood pressure), and aldosterone acts on the kidneys to decrease sodium excretion. The arterial baroreflex and the atrial volume receptor reflex also act through the hypothalamus to increase the secretion of antidiuretic hormone (ADH) from the pituitary gland. ADH circulates to the kidneys where it reduces urine formation. Through the combined actions of the renin-angiotensin-aldosterone system and ADH, both sodium excretion and water excretion are decreased. Note that these actions *conserve* the available blood volume following hemorrhage, but they do not restore it to normal. The actual restoration of blood volume following hemorrhage requires an increased fluid intake. The baroreceptor reflex and the atrial volume receptor reflex act through the hypothalamus to

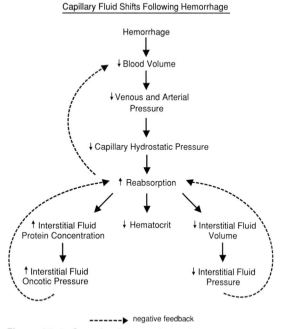

Capillary Fluid Shifts Following Hemorrhage

Hemorrhage
↓
↓ Blood Volume
↓
↓ Venous and Arterial Pressure
↓
↓ Capillary Hydrostatic Pressure
↓
↑ Reabsorption

↑ Interstitial Fluid Protein Concentration   ↓ Hematocrit   ↓ Interstitial Fluid Volume

↑ Interstitial Fluid Oncotic Pressure   ↓ Interstitial Fluid Pressure

------▶ negative feedback

Figure 25–6. Over the first 3–4 hours following a hemorrhage, interstitial fluid is reabsorbed into the blood stream, which helps compensate for the lost blood volume. A complication is that hematocrit decreases. Reabsorption is stopped eventually by decreases in interstitial fluid hydrostatic pressure and increases in interstitial fluid oncotic pressure.

Fluid Volume Replacement Following Hemorrhage

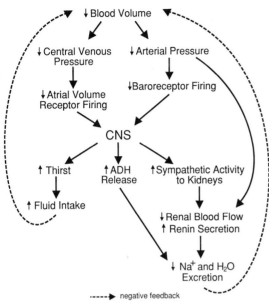

Figure 25–7. The humoral responses following hemorrhage result in a conservation of body fluid and electrolytes. The actual restoration of the fluid lost in a hemorrhage requires an increased fluid intake.

increase the sensation of thirst. If water is available, there is an increase in fluid intake until the lost blood volume is restored to normal. This may take 1–2 days. The hormonal and behavioral effects of hemorrhage are summarized in Figure 25–7.

The final compensation for hemorrhage involves the restoration of the lost plasma proteins and blood cells. The plasma proteins are synthesized by the liver, and the blood cells are produced by the bone marrow. The time required may be several days to a week or so.

The preceding discussion has focused on the effects of severe hemorrhage. All of the same compensations, except for constriction of the veins and spleen, occur to a milder degree following mild hemorrhage. For example, when a human donates blood, 0.5 L (about 10% of the blood volume) is removed. All of the compensations just described are evident following this 10% hemorrhage.

In humans and in some large animals, the transition from a supine to a standing posture elicits many of the same cardiovascular responses as with hemorrhage. The reason for this can be understood if one considers the effect of gravity on the blood contained within the body's blood vessels. In a standing subject, gravity increases the distending pressure in

the vessels of the legs. The gravitational effect does not result in much accumulation of blood in the arteries, arterioles and capillaries, because these vessels are not distensible (they have low compliance). However, the veins of the legs are compliant, and the increased venous hydrostatic pressure generated by gravity results in a distention of the leg veins. The distention of the leg veins slows the return of blood from the legs to the central circulation. Therefore, in an upright human there is a decrease in central blood volume and central venous pressure, just as there would be following hemorrhage. Thus, upright posture causes decreased cardiac filling, decreased stroke volume, decreased cardiac output, and so on. In a normal human, the assumption of an upright posture is equivalent to a 10% hemorrhage. All of the compensations for hemorrhage that have been described also occur in response to upright posture. The gravitational effect of standing is negligible in small animals. In large animals, such as cattle and horses, the pooling of blood in leg veins is minimized by the relatively small size of veins in the extremities.

The Initiation of Exercise Involves an Interplay of Local and Neural Changes to Increase Cardiac Output and Deliver Increased Flow to Exercising Muscle

A normal dog at rest has a cardiac output of about 2.5 L per minute. During maximal exercise, cardiac output rises to reach levels of 10–15 L per minute. TPR decreases by a factor of 5–6. The mechanisms that bring about these dramatic alterations are summarized in Figure 25–8. As skeletal muscle begins to exercise, metabolic products accumulate in the muscle tissue, and the local oxygen concentration decreases. The metabolic products and hypoxia both cause dilation of the arterioles within the exercising muscle. This vasodilation is a local response, not dependent on nerves or hormones. This metabolic control mechanism results in an increased blood flow to the exercising muscle. The increased blood flow delivers more oxygen and removes some of the accumulated metabolic vasodilating products. In this way, muscle blood flow is matched to metabolic rate.

Metabolic control of blood flow can succeed only if arterial blood pressure is maintained at a level sufficient to provide the additional blood flow to the exercising skeletal muscle.

However, when a substantial portion of the body's skeletal muscle is involved in exercise, the metabolic vasodilation causes a large decrease in TPR. This decrease in TPR would cause a large decrease in arterial blood pressure if not for three compensating neural mechanisms: the arterial baroreflex, the exercise reflex, and central command.

A decrease in blood pressure causes a decrease in baroreceptor action potential frequency, which acts through the CNS to increase sympathetic activity and decrease parasympathetic activity. Another mechanism that drives sympathetic and parasympathetic responses in exercise is the *exercise reflex*. The exercise reflex is initiated by specialized nerve endings within muscles and joints. An increase in muscular work and in the movement of the body joints somehow results in an increased frequency of action potentials in these muscle and joint receptors. The increased afferent activity results reflexly in an increased sympathetic and decreased parasympathetic efferent drive. Although the exact mechanism for excitation of these muscle and joint receptors is not completely understood, it is clear that the reflex effect of these muscle and joint receptors is necessary to keep blood pressure from falling during exercise. Finally, blood pressure is supported during exercise by a psychogenic effect called *central command*. Even prior to the initiation of exercise, the CNS acts to increase sympathetic activity and decrease parasympathetic activity. These autonomic effects cause vasoconstriction in nonworking muscle and in the kidneys, splanchnic organs, and skin. This vasoconstriction helps to offset the fall in TPR caused by the vasodilation in working skeletal muscle. Nevertheless, even after compensatory vasoconstriction of noncritical organs, peripheral resistance in a maximally exercising animal may be only one sixth of normal. Arterial pressure is maintained at a near-normal level during exercise by an increase in cardiac output to five or six times normal. The increase in sympathetic activity and decrease in parasympathetic activity brought about by the baroreflex, exercise reflex, and central command are the major causes of the increased cardiac output (see Fig. 25–8).

Two non-neural mechanisms also help to increase the cardiac output during exercise. The first of these is the *muscle pump* (Fig. 25–9). When skeletal muscles contract, they tend to squeeze down on the blood vessels contained within them. One effect of this, already

mentioned, is the tendency for a muscle to restrict its own blood flow during a sustained contraction. However, if the contractions are rhythmic, each contraction causes blood to be expelled out of the muscle veins and toward the central circulation. There is minimal backflow of blood from the central circulation back into the veins during muscular relaxation, because the veins have one-way valves within them. Thus, the pumping action of muscle, which massages the veins, displaces venous blood toward the central circulation and increases central venous pressure. In this way, the muscle pump increases ventricular preload above the level that would otherwise exist.

The second nonneural mechanism that helps to increase cardiac output during exercise is the *respiratory pump*. Vigorous exercise involves an increase in both the rate and depth of respiration. With each inspiration, a subatmospheric pressure is generated within the thorax. This negative pressure "pulls" outward on the airways of the lungs to expand them. It also pulls outward on the central veins and the heart and distends them. In this

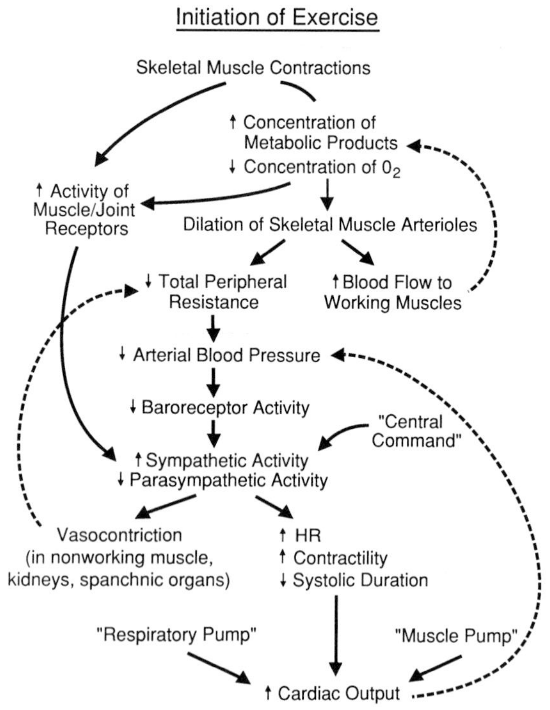

Initiation of Exercise

Figure 25–8. The initiation of exercise involves a complex interplay of local mechanisms and reflexes that increases blood flow in exercising muscle, decreases blood flow in the noncritical organs, increases cardiac output, and maintains arterial blood pressure.

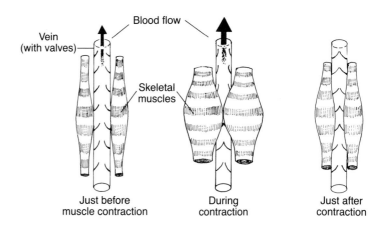

Figure 25–9. During dynamic exercise, the rhythmic contractions of skeletal muscles squeeze venous blood out of the muscle and back toward the central circulation. This so-called muscle pump helps increase central venous pressure in an exercising animal.

Blood flow

Vein
(with valves)

Skeletal
muscles

Just before
muscle contraction

During
contraction

Just after
contraction

way, the negative intrathoracic pressure during inspiration helps draw blood from the abdominal veins into the central veins and the atria. In addition, the diaphragm muscle moves caudally during inspiration and compresses the abdominal organs. This increases intra-abdominal pressure and squeezes blood out of the abdominal veins and back toward the central veins. This respiratory pumping action helps to increase venous return, central venous volume, and ventricular preload during exercise. The combined effect of sympathetic and parasympathetic responses, the muscle pump, and the respiratory pump is that cardiac output can increase to six times the resting level during severe exercise.

Note that the success of the mechanisms that increase cardiac output during exercise depends on an ability of the heart to respond normally both to increased sympathetic drive and to increases in preload. As mentioned earlier, a failing heart has an attenuated response to an increase in preload. Also, during heart failure, the autonomic mechanisms available to increase cardiac contractility and heart rate are invoked simply to maintain a normal cardiac output in the resting stage. Therefore, the autonomic nervous system in a patient with heart failure has a limited ability to bring about further increases in cardiac output during the initiation of exercise. For this reason, patients with heart failure typically exhibit exercise intolerance.

Maximal exercise ability in normal humans and animals appears to be limited by cardiac output. That is, the respiratory system can oxygenate as much blood as the heart can deliver to the lungs, and skeletal muscle can take up and metabolize as much oxygen as the heart can deliver to it. But, when cardiac output has reached a maximal level, oxygen transport from the lungs to the skeletal muscle is maximized also. This sets the upper limit to the level of exercise that can be sustained.

CLINICAL CORRELATION

EXERCISE INTOLERANCE SECONDARY TO CONGESTIVE HEART FAILURE

HISTORY ☐ An 8-year-old female Great Dane has been diagnosed previously with idiopathic dilative cardiomyopathy. Severe, generalized cardiac enlargement is evident on thoracic radiographs. The dog is losing weight and is unable to complete daily walks with her owners.

CLINICAL EXAMINATION ☐ Femoral pulses are weak but regular at 140 beats per minute. The mucous membranes are pale, and the capillary refilling time is prolonged. Respiration is rapid at 45 breaths per minute. The abdomen is distended, and the abdominal organs are difficult to palpate. The electrocardiogram (ECG) shows sinus tachycardia with broad, high voltage QRS-complexes. Thoracic radiography reveals a greatly enlarged heart and moderate pulmonary edema.

Additional diagnostic tests are conducted to help assess the degree of complications secondary to the heart failure. Percent saturation of hemoglobin in arterial blood is 78% (normal 95–100%); the difference in oxygen content between arterial and venous blood is 8.5 mL O_2/dL blood (normal 4–6 mL); serum creatinine concentration is 3 mg/dL (normal is less than 1 mg/dL); urine specific gravity equals 1.036 (high normal); and central venous pressure is 14 mmHg (normal 0–3 mmHg).

When persuaded to exercise, the dog appeared to become tired after walking less than one block. Her legs began to tremble, and then she collapsed. Her pulse rate was 180 beats per minute, and her mucous membranes were dark and cyanotic (blue).

COMMENT □ Chronic heart failure secondary to cardiomyopathy is common in large dogs over 4 years of age. Often, the cardiomyopathy is idiopathic (of unknown cause). The case presented here is fairly typical of advanced heart failure. All of the clinical findings are either direct consequences of the heart failure or consequences of the body's attempts to compensate for the heart failure (see Figs. 25–1, 2, and 3). In brief, ventricular failure (decreased contractility) leads to decreased stroke volume, cardiac output, and blood pressure. Compensations for the heart failure involve reflex decreases in parasympathetic activity, increases in sympathetic activity, and increases in the release of ADH and renin. Heart rate is increased, which helps raise cardiac output back toward normal. Pulse pressure, judged by palpating the femoral pulse, is reduced (because heart rate is high and stroke volume is low). The mucosa, splanchnic organs, kidneys, and resting skeletal muscle are vasoconstricted, which helps support arterial pressure and reserves the available cardiac output for the heart and brain. The vasoconstriction is evident in the pale color and slow refilling of the mucous membranes. Renal vasoconstriction reduces the rate of urine formation. Urinary loss of salt and water is further reduced by the actions of ADH and renin. The urine that is formed has a high solute concentration (high specific gravity). Metabolic products (e.g., creatinine) that are normally eliminated by the kidneys accumulate in the blood. Salt and water retention increases blood volume above normal. Most of the excess blood volume is in the veins, so venous and atrial pressures are above normal. The elevated atrial pressure (preload) also increases ventricular end-diastolic volume above normal, which helps the failing heart to pump a larger stroke volume than it otherwise would. However, the excessive volume and pressure of blood in the veins also causes systemic edema (distended abdomen) and pulmonary edema (visible on the radiograph). Pulmonary edema impairs the ability of the lungs to oxygenate blood. Therefore, the hemoglobin saturation and the oxygen content of arterial blood are both below normal in this dog. The tissues of the body respond to the low rate of oxygen delivery by unloading as much oxygen as they can from the blood as it flows through the tissue. This makes the arteriovenous difference in oxygen content greater than normal. The general inadequacy of cardiovascular transport leads to metabolic stresses on the dog's tissues, and weight loss occurs.

Despite many compensatory mechanisms, this dog is unable to deliver a normal amount of well-oxygenated blood to the body tissues, even at rest. When the dog tries to exercise, cardiac output increases little. Therefore, when exercise-induced vasodilation occurs in the exercising muscles, TPR and blood pressure would both fall dramatically. There is a further decrease in blood flow in the tissues of the systemic circulation that were already vasoconstricted (e.g., the mucous membranes), and these tissues become hypoxic and cyanotic. Inadequate blood flow in the exercising skeletal muscles leads to hypoxia and acidosis, and the dog collapses.

TREATMENT □ The ideal treatment strategy for this dog is to improve the contractile performance of the myocardium. Theoretically, one could use β-adrenergic agonists or cardiac glycosides to increase cardiac contractility. However, the currently available drugs are either ineffective or only mildly effective in dogs with severe, chronic heart failure. Therefore, treatment should emphasize symptomatic therapy, with the goals of controlling pulmonary congestion and improving cardiac output. Diuretics or venodilators reduce venous pressures and are usually effective in controlling signs of congestion, but they create the risk of exacerbating the low cardiac output. Arteriolar vasodilators can augment the output of a failing heart by reducing the afterload (arterial pressure) against which the heart must eject blood. An appropriate, initial treatment for this dog includes a diuretic (furosemide) and a cardiac glycoside (digitalis). If digitalis fails to improve cardiac contractility in this advanced case of cardiomyopathy, an arteriolar vasodilator (prazosin) or a mixed vasodilator-venodilator (captopril) can be added to the furosemide regimen.

Bibliography

Cohn PF: Pathophysiology of cardiovascular disease states. *In* Cohn PF, Brown EJ Jr, Vlay SC (eds): Clinical Cardiovascular Physiology. Philadelphia, WB Saunders, 1985, p 203.
Hamlin RL: Pathophysiology of heart failure. *In* Fox PR

(ed): Canine and Feline Cardiology. New York, Churchill Livingstone, 1988, p 159.

Kittleson MD: Management of heart failure: Concepts,
therapeutic strategies, and drug pharmacology. *In* Fox
PR (ed): Canine and Feline Cardiology. New York,
Churchill Livingstone, 1988, p 171.

Littlejohn A: Exercise-related cardiovascular problems. *In*
Robinson NE (ed): Current Therapy in Equine Medicine.
Philadelphia, WB Saunders, 1987, p 176.

Sisson D: The clinical evaluation of cardiac function. *In*
Ettinger SJ (ed): Textbook of Veterinary Internal Medicine, Vol 1, 3rd ed. Philadelphia, WB Saunders, 1989,
p 923.

Sparks HV, Rooke TW: Integrated cardiovascular responses. *In* Essentials of Cardiovascular Physiology.
Minneapolis, University of Minnesota Press, 1987, pp
177–189.

PRACTICE QUESTIONS FOR CHAPTER 25

1. During experimental trials on a new, artificial aortic valve, a dog is anesthetized and
   placed on cardiac bypass for 1 hour. (That
   is, a heart-lung machine is substituted for
   the dog's own heart and lungs.) After successful installation of the artificial valve, the
   dog is taken off bypass, and his normal
   circulation is restored. Ten minutes later,
   the dog's central venous pressure is 40
   mmHg, mean arterial pressure 90 mmHg,
   and heart rate 130 beats/minute. His cardiac
   output is not measured, but the surgeon
   suspects that it is too low, and that therefore, the patient's tissues are not being
   adequately supplied with blood.

   Which of the following measures would
   you select to improve the patient's condition?

   a. Transfusion with 500 mL of whole blood
   b. Administration of isoproterenol (a selec-
      tive β-adrenergic agonist)
   c. Increasing the heart rate by electrical
      pacing
   d. Administration of norepinephrine (an α-
      and β-adrenergic agonist)
   e. Administration of a β-adrenergic block-
      ing agent, such as propranolol

2. One of the nerves leading to a dog's heart
   is stimulated for 1 minute while left atrial
   pressure, heart rate, and left ventricular
   output are measured (Fig. 25–10). During
   this stimulation,

   a. venous return to the left atrium tran-
      siently exceeds left ventricular output.

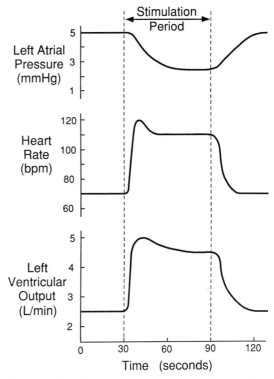

Figure 25–10. The cardiovascular data for Practice Question #2.

   b. the increase in left ventricular output at
      the beginning of stimulation can be ex-
      plained by Starling's law of the heart.
   c. stroke volume is lower after 15 seconds
      of stimulation than prior to stimulation.
   d. the effects of stimulation are the same
      as those caused by sympathetic activa-
      tion.
   e. the progressive decline in left ventricular
      output during the stimulation is proba-
      bly caused by a progressive increase in
      ventricular end-diastolic volume.

3. One hour after a severe hemorrhage, a
   dog's arterial pulse pressure, mean pressure, and hematocrit are all below normal.

   Which of the following statements is true?

   a. His diminished pulse pressure reflects
      decreased aortic compliance
   b. His diminished mean pressure probably
      results from decreased TPR
   c. His diminished hematocrit probably re-
      sults from reabsorption of interstitial
      fluid into the blood stream
   d. Under these conditions, the action po-
      tential frequency of the arterial baro-
      receptors is greater than normal

e. Under these conditions, sympathetic activity is probably less than normal

4. When a sheep is held in a vertical, head-up position, arterial pressure decreases because

   a. the baroreceptor reflex causes an increase in TPR.
   b. valves in the leg veins promote the return of blood to the heart.

c. the respiratory pump sucks blood into the thorax.
d. central blood volume is increased.
e. right atrial pressure is decreased.

5. During exercise

   a. TPR is decreased.
   b. cardiac output is increased.
   c. stroke volume is increased.
   d. blood pressure is nearly normal.
   e. All of the above.

THOMAS HERDT

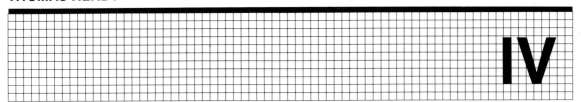

GASTROINTESTINAL PHYSIOLOGY/ METABOLISM

26

Regulation of Gastrointestinal Function

1. The intrinsic gastrointestinal nervous system lies in planes between the muscular and mucosal layers of the gut wall
2. The intrinsic nervous system contains receptors, sensory neurons, interneurons, and motor neurons
3. The gut also receives extrinsic innervation from the autonomic nervous system
4. The gastrointestinal system has an intrinsic endocrine system
5. Regulatory peptides exert a tropic effect on gastrointestinal epithelial cells
6. Regulatory peptides may originate from neurons, as well as from endocrine cells

The gastrointestinal (GI) system is regulated at two levels. One level of control is applied by the extrinsic central nervous and endocrine systems and is exerted in a manner similar to that for other organ systems. The second level of control is unique to the GI system and is exerted by intrinsic nervous and endocrine components located within the gut. This *intrinsic* level of control allows the gut to autonomously regulate its functions based on local conditions, such as the amount and type of food contained in the lumen. Control of the gut by the central nervous system (CNS) is mainly secondary; the CNS applies an influence on the intrinsic systems, which then directly regulate gut function (Fig. 26–1).

The Intrinsic Gastrointestinal Nervous System Lies in Planes Between the Muscular and Mucosal Layers of the Gut Wall

The intrinsic GI nervous system is extensive and highly sophisticated, containing about as many neurons as the spinal cord. The elements of the GI nervous system lie within the gut wall, and a brief review of GI anatomy may be helpful before discussing the intrinsic nervous system. The GI wall, from the esophagus to the rectum, is composed of two layers of muscle: a spongy *submucosa* composed of connective tissue and vascular elements, and a one cell–thick mucosal layer that lines the

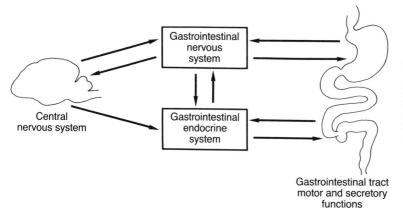

Figure 26–1. Gut function is under direct regulation by the intrinsic GI nervous system and the GI endocrine system. Most CNS influence on the gut is mediated through indirect effects on the GI endocrine and intrinsic nervous systems.

gut lumen. The outer layer of muscle has its fibers oriented parallel to the long axis of the gut and is called the *longitudinal* layer. The fibers of inner muscle are oriented circumferentially around the gut and are referred to as the *circular* layer. The submucosa is composed of loosely woven connective tissue and an extensive network of blood and lymph vessels. The submucosa is located between the circular muscle and mucosa (Fig. 26–2).

The intrinsic nervous system consists of cell bodies and their associated neurons. The cell bodies are arranged into two systems of ganglia: the *myenteric* (Auerbach's) plexus and the *submucosal* (Meissner's) plexus. (See Chapter 12 for a more general discussion of ganglia.) The myenteric plexus consists of ganglia located between the circular and longitudinal muscle layers. The submucosal plexus has its ganglia in the submucosal layer. Axons from

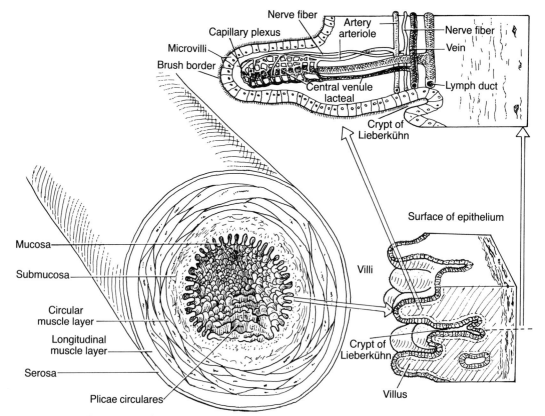

Figure 26–2. Schematic illustration of the cross-sectional anatomy of the gut wall.

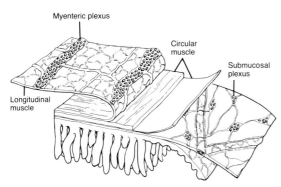

Figure 26–3. Schematic illustration of the organization of the GI intrinsic nervous system. Note the arborizations of nerve fibers that run between the individual ganglia of the myenteric and submucosal plexus.

the cell bodies project in rich networks near the ganglia. A thick net of neurons runs in the plane between the circular and longitudinal muscle layers, connecting the ganglia of the myenteric plexus. Individual neurons leave the neuronal network to innervate structures within the gut wall and to intercommunicate between the myenteric and submucosal plexuses (Fig. 26–3).

The Intrinsic Nervous System Contains Receptors, Sensory Neurons, Interneurons, and Motor Neurons

The plexuses of the intrinsic nervous system contain sensory (afferent) neurons, interneu-

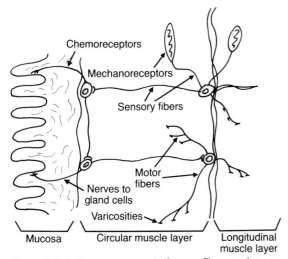

Figure 26–4. The arrangement of nerve fibers and receptors within the intrinsic GI nervous system. Varicosities release neuroregulatory substances in the vicinity of muscle fibers.

rons, and motor (efferent) neurons. Sensory input comes from *mechanoreceptors* within the muscular layers and *chemoreceptors* within the mucosa. Mechanoreceptors monitor distention of the gut wall, whereas chemoreceptors in the mucosa monitor chemical conditions in the gut lumen (Fig. 26–4).

Intrinsic motor nerves supply muscles and glands within the gut wall. Motor innervation of gut smooth muscle is less intimate than that found in skeletal muscle; there is no direct synaptic-type junction between GI nerve endings and smooth muscle fibers. Rather, axons end in arborizations containing many vesicular structures called *varicosities* (see Fig. 26–4). The varicosities contain *neuroregulatory* substances that are secreted by the nerves in response to action potentials and affect the activities of nearby muscle or glandular cells. There are two general types of efferent neurons: *cholinergic* and *noncholinergic*. Generally, the cholinergic neurons are excitatory, increasing muscle contractions and gland secretions. As implied by their name, cholinergic nerves secrete *acetylcholine* as a neuroregulatory substance. The noncholinergic neurons are inhibitory, in general, and contain various neuroregulatory substances, all of which are peptide in nature. The most important of the neuroregulatory peptides is *vasoactive intestinal peptide* (VIP). As its name implies, VIP has an effect on the intestinal blood vessels, inducing a relaxation of vascular smooth muscle. More importantly, however, it also appears to have a relaxing effect on smooth muscle of the gut wall. VIP and other neuroregulatory peptides are discussed later under the more general topic of regulatory peptides.

The Gut Also Receives Extrinsic Innervation from the Autonomic Nervous System

The parasympathetic and sympathetic nervous systems form the link between the intrinsic nervous system of the gut and the CNS. Most of the GI tract receives parasympathetic innervation by way of the vagus nerve, except the terminal portions of the colon, which receive parasympathetic innervation from the sacral cord by way of the pelvic nerve (Fig. 26–5). By classic description, the parasympathetic nervous system is composed of pre- and postganglionic fibers. However, this division of parasympathetic fiber types is not clearly defined for the gut, because extrinsic, pregan-

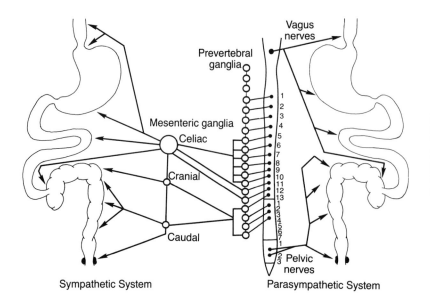

Figure 26–5. The distribution of autonomic nerve fibers to the gut. The spinal cord is represented in the center with the sympathetic system extended to the left and the parasympathetic system to the right.

glionic fibers of the parasympathetic system become integrated with fibers of the intrinsic nervous system. Parasympathetic, preganglionic fibers reach the gut and synapse on cell bodies of the intrinsic system, so in that way the intrinsic ganglia of the gut serve as peripheral autonomic ganglia of the parasympathetic system. However, the intrinsic nervous system must be perceived as being much more than postganglionic parasympathetic neurons. The intrinsic neurons receive input from sources other than preganglionic parasympathetic fibers, including afferent neurons and interneurons of the intrinsic system. Thus, the classic description of the organization of the parasympathetic nervous system does not strictly apply to the gut (Fig. 26–6). *Acetylcholine* is the neurotransmitter agent between the preganglionic parasympathetic fibers and the intrinsic neurons.

Extrinsic sympathetic fibers entering the gut are postganglionic, in contrast to the extrinsic parasympathetic fibers. Postganglionic sympathetic fibers arise from cells in the prevertebral ganglia and follow the splanchnic nerves and vascular arteries into the gut wall (see Fig. 26–5). Some sympathetic fibers synapse on neurons of the intrinsic system, whereas others exert a direct effect on GI muscles and glands. Those sympathetic fibers that exert a direct effect do so in a manner similar to the intrinsic fibers, i.e., by the release of neurosecretory substances in the vicinity of their target cells. The neurosecretory substance of the postganglionic sympathetic cells is *norepinephrine.*

The Gastrointestinal System Has an Intrinsic Endocrine System

The GI system has an extensive number and variety of endocrine cells. These cells are morphologically similar, but they produce a wide variety of hormones and hormone-like substances. Whereas endocrine cells are usually grouped together into glands, the GI endocrine cells are distributed diffusely throughout the gut epithelium. Typically, the GI endocrine cells are columnar with a broad base and a narrow apex. They are positioned individually among the other mucosal cells in both the glandular and absorptive areas of the mucosa. The narrow apex of the endocrine cells is exposed to the lumen of the gut, allowing them to "sample" or "taste" the luminal contents. The base of these cells contains *secretory granules,* storage forms of hormones. This anatomical arrangement provides a mechanism for the cells to sense changes in luminal contents and to respond by releasing hormones into the submucosal area, where they may be absorbed into the blood stream. The hormones are not secreted into the lumen of the gut (Fig. 26–7).

Hormones released into the submucosa may be picked up by the blood vascular system and transported out of the gut to distant sites, or they may simply diffuse through the extracellular fluid to have their effects on local target cells. By strict definition, a hormone is a substance that is transported through the blood from its site of production to its distant site of effect, so technically those products of the GI endocrine cells that reach nearby target

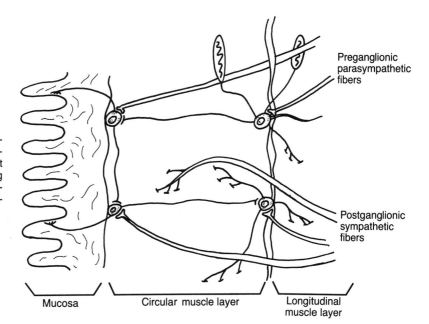

Figure 26–6. The interface between the autonomic and GI intrinsic nervous systems. Note that parasympathetic fibers reaching the intrinsic system are preganglionic, whereas sympathetic fibers are postganglionic.

Preganglionic
parasympathetic
fibers

Postganglionic
sympathetic
fibers

Mucosa   Circular muscle layer   Longitudinal
muscle layer

cells by diffusion through the extracellular fluid should not be called hormones. They are called *paracrines*, in contrast to *endocrines*; the latter is a synonym for hormone. There are many different active molecules produced by the various GI endocrine cells; some function as endocrines, some as paracrines, and several probably function in both manners. All of the GI endocrine cell products—endocrines and paracrines—are peptides and can be referred to collectively as *regulatory peptides*.

Each type of endocrine cell has a characteristic distribution within the GI tract. *Gastrin-producing cells*, for example, are found primar-

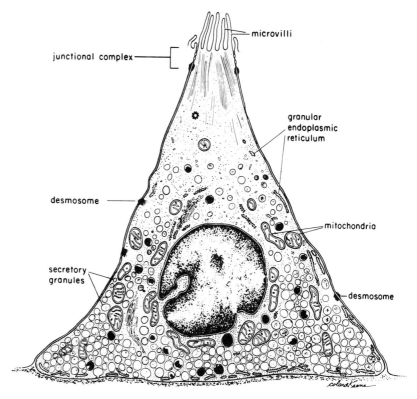

Figure 26–7. Schematic illustration of a GI endocrine cell. All of the GI endocrine cells have a similar structure, but each cell produces only one type of hormone. Note the narrow apex that is exposed to the intestinal luminal contents and the broad base for storage of secretory granules. (From Johnson LR, Christensen J, Jacobsen ED, et al (eds): Physiology of the Gastrointestinal Tract, Vol 1, 2nd ed. New York, Raven Press, 1987.)

microvilli

junctional complex

granular
endoplasmic
reticulum

desmosome

mitochondria

secretory
granules

desmosome

Table 26–1
DESCRIPTION OF MAJOR GASTROINTESTINAL HORMONES

Hormone	Site of Production	Action		Release Stimulus
Gastrin	Distal stomach	Primary:	Stimulates acid secretion from stomach glands	Protein in the stomach; high gastric pH; vagal stimulation
		Secondary:	Stimulates gastric motility, growth of the stomach epithelium	
Secretin	Duodenum	Primary:	Stimulates bicarbonate secretion from the pancreas	Acid in the duodenum
		Secondary:	Stimulates biliary bicarbonate secretion	
Cholecystokinin (CCK)	Duodenum to ileum, with highest concentration in the duodenum	Primary:	Stimulates enzyme secretion from the pancreas	Protein and fats in the small intestine
		Secondary:	Inhibits gastric emptying	
Gastric Inhibitory Polypeptide (GIP)	Duodenum and upper jejunum	Primary:	Inhibits gastric motility and secretory activity	Carbohydrate and fat in the small intestine
		Secondary:	Stimulates insulin secretion, provided sufficient glucose is present; may be the most important action in many species	
Motilin	Duodenum and jejunum	Primary:	Probably regulates the motility pattern of the gut in the period between meals	Acetylcholine
		Secondary:	May regulate the tone of the lower esophageal sphincter	

ily in the distal portion of the stomach, and few are found elsewhere in the gut. *Cholecystokinin-producing cells* are found in the small intestine, especially in the proximal region. Thus, whereas endocrine cells are distributed throughout the GI tract, production of individual hormones may be confined to specific areas. This is not always the case, however, as in the instance of *enteroglucagon-producing cells*, which are distributed along the entire length of the gut. The sites of production and actions of the major GI regulatory peptides are listed in Table 26–1.

The GI regulatory peptides influence various gut functions and in many instances form part of regulatory feedback loops. An example is the feedback loop involving gastrin and gastric acid. After a meal, gastrin-producing cells, which are located in the stomach, secrete gastrin that stimulates gastric acid production and lowers the stomach pH. The gastrin-producing cells monitor the pH of the distal stomach, and when the pH is reduced to a critical point,

gastrin secretion is inhibited, removing the stimulus for production of more gastric acid and stabilizing the stomach pH. Thus, the pH of the stomach is regulated closely by the actions of the gastrin-producing endocrine cells. Other specific examples of GI regulatory peptide effects are discussed in subsequent chapters in the context of the actions they regulate (Fig. 26–8).

Regulatory Peptides Exert a Tropic Effect on Gastrointestinal Epithelial Cells

In addition to regulating cell functions, several GI regulatory peptides exert *tropic*, or growth-regulating, effects on epithelial cells of the GI system. For example, gastrin promotes growth of the gastric mucosa, and enteroglucagon and cholecystokinin promote growth of the intestinal mucosa. This is one mechanism by which the gut can adapt to increased digestive requirements, i.e., as appetite and food intake increase, GI regulatory peptide produc-

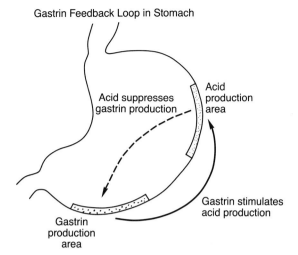

Gastrin Feedback Loop in Stomach

Acid suppresses gastrin production

Acid production area

Gastrin stimulates acid production

Gastrin production area

Figure 26–8. Example of a feedback loop. This is a negative feedback loop in that acid production, which is stimulated by gastrin, suppresses gastrin secretion.

tion is stimulated, and the gut mucosa hypertrophies to meet the increased functional demand.

Regulatory Peptides May Originate from Neurons, As Well As from Endocrine Cells

All products of GI endocrine cells are regulatory peptides, but not all regulatory peptides of the GI system come from endocrine cells. The neuroregulatory substances produced by the noncholinergic neurons of the intrinsic nervous system are also peptides and have mechanisms of action much like the endocrine

Table 26–2
KNOWN AND SUSPECTED REGULATORY PEPTIDES OF THE GUT

Established Endocrines

Gastrin
Cholecystokinin
Secretin
GIP*
Motilin

Probable Endocrine or Paracrine Substances

Vasoactive Intestinal Peptide
Somatostatin
Pancreatic Polypeptide
Enteroglucagon
Neurotensin
Peptide YY
Bombesin

*Originally named gastric inhibitory peptide; some physiologists now believe glucose-dependent insulinotropic peptide would be a more appropriate name.

and paracrine substances. These substances of neuronal origin are grouped also in the category of regulatory peptides, and are sometimes referred to specifically as *neurocrines*. There are some regulatory peptides that appear to be produced by both neurons and endocrine cells.

Table 26–2 is a list of known or suspected regulatory peptides of gut origin; the list is probably incomplete. Some peptides, such as substance P and bombesin, have strange, nondescriptive names that reflect historical incidents in their discovery. Others, like vasoactive intestinal peptide (VIP) and gastric inhibitory peptide (GIP), have names that describe their first-discovered action, but do not describe what is now known to be their primary action. GI regulatory peptide function is an area of active research and rapidly expanding knowledge. The *clinical* use of GI hormones and their analogs is just beginning to occur in human and veterinary medicine. As GI regulatory peptide physiology becomes better understood, these substances will probably become an important part of the treatment of GI disease.

Bibliography

Berne RM, Levy MN: Physiology. St. Louis, CV Mosby, 1983, pp 743–753.
Go VLW, Michener S, Roddy D, Koch M: Clinical relevance of regulatory gastrointestinal peptides. Clin Biochem 17:82–88, 1984.
Johnson LR (ed): Gastrointestinal Physiology. St. Louis, CV Mosby, 1985, pp 1–22.
Johnson LR, Christensen J, Jacobsen ED, et al (eds): Physiology of the Gastrointestinal Tract, Vol 1, 2nd ed. New York, Raven Press, 1987, pp 1–334.
Stevens CE: Comparative Physiology of the Vertebrate Digestive System. Cambridge, Cambridge University Press, 1988, pp 125–158, 220–237.
Tache Y: Nature and biological actions of gastrointestinal peptides: Current status. Clin Biochem 17:77–81, 1984.

PRACTICE QUESTIONS FOR CHAPTER 26

1. Which statement is the most accurate anatomical description of the intrinsic nervous system of the gut?

   a. Intrinsic neuronal fibers and their cell bodies are diffusely spread throughout the length and thickness of the stomach and intestine.

b. Intrinsic neuronal fibers traverse the length of the stomach and intestine in discrete nerve bundles.
c. Intrinsic neuronal cell bodies are aggregated in a discrete "gut brain" that is positioned near the pylorus.
d. Intrinsic neuronal cell bodies lie in discrete planes within the thickness of the gut wall and are diffusely distributed throughout its length.
e. Intrinsic neuronal fibers exist only in the longitudinal muscle layer of the stomach and intestine.

2. Which statement is true regarding the parasympathetic fibers that innervate the cells of the intrinsic nervous system?

a. The fibers exit the CNS from lumbar segments of the spinal cord.
b. The fibers have VIP as a neurotransmitter.
c. The fibers are inhibitory.
d. The fibers are preganglionic.
e. There are no parasympathetic fibers that innervate cells of the intrinsic nervous system.

3. Which statement is true regarding the GI endocrine cells?

a. Secretory activity is influenced by the luminal contents of the gut.

b. Hormones are secreted directly into the gut lumen and affect the activity of glands "downstream" from the point of secretion.
c. Endocrine cells are aggregated into discrete bundles known as intestinal glands.
d. Secretory activity is influenced by nervous activity of the intrinsic nervous system.
e. Both a and d are true.

4. Assume that substance A is secreted by one gland, and it stimulates a second gland or cell type to secrete substance B. If substance B, in turn, stimulates the further production of substance A, how would this feedback loop be described?

a. Negative
b. Positive

5. It is important for clinicians to understand GI endocrinology because

a. GI hormones are involved in abnormal, as well as normal, gut activity.
b. some tumors can produce copious and unrestricted amounts of GI hormones.
c. GI hormones and their analogs will probably become important agents of therapy in GI disease.
d. All of the above

27

Movements of the Gastrointestinal Tract

1. Slow waves of electrical depolarization are a unique feature of gut smooth muscle
2. When spreading slow waves reach primed smooth muscle cells, action potentials and contraction result
3. Coordinated motility of the lips, tongue, mouth, and pharynx prehend food and propel it down the gastrointestinal tract
4. Motility of the esophagus propels food from the pharynx to the stomach
5. The function of the stomach is to process food into a fluid consistency and release it into the intestine at a controlled rate
6. The proximal stomach stores food awaiting further gastric processing in the distal stomach
7. The distal stomach grinds and sifts food entering the small intestine
8. Control of gastric motility differs in the proximal and distal stomach
9. The rate of gastric emptying must match the small intestine's rate of digestion and absorption
10. Between meals the stomach is cleared of undigestible material
11. Vomiting is a complex reflex coordinated from the brainstem
12. Motility of the small intestine has a digestive and interdigestive phase
13. The ileocecal sphincter prevents movement of colon contents back into the ileum
14. Motility of the colon causes mixing, retropulsion, and propulsion of ingesta
15. In the carnivore colon, absorption and storage occur
16. Despite anatomical differences in herbivore colons, similar motility patterns are found
17. The anal sphincter has two layers with separate innervation
18. The rectosphincteric reflex is important in defecation

The walls of the gastrointestinal (GI) tract, at all levels, are muscular and capable of movement. Movements of the GI muscles have direct actions on ingesta in the gut lumen. There are several functions of GI movements: (1) to propel ingesta from one location to the next; (2) to retain ingesta at a given site for digestion, absorption, or storage; (3) to physically break up food material and mix it with digestive secretions; and (4) to circulate ingesta so that all portions come into contact with absorptive surfaces. The dynamics of fluid movement in the gut are not as well understood as in other organ systems, particularly the cardiovascular system. The heart and great vessels behave similarly to most mechanical pumping systems; there is a central pump that pushes fluid through a conduit of relatively fixed diameter. Because of this configuration, the cardiovascular system more or less conforms to physical laws that are well established and studied reasonably easily; sophisticated quantitative analyses of cardiovascular function can be made clinically. In contrast to the heart, in the gut the fluid pump and conduit are the same organ. This makes study of the fluid dynamics of the gut extremely complex. At this time, the mathematically defined physical laws of fluid dynamics, as applied to the gut, are of little clinical usefulness. Therefore, the physiology of GI motility is usually applied clinically on a qualitative, rather than quantitative, basis.

Movement of the gut wall is referred to as *motility,* and motility may be of a propulsive, retentive, or mixing nature. The time it takes material to travel from one portion of the gut to another is referred to as the *transit time.* An increase in propulsive motility decreases transit time, whereas an increase in retentive motility increases transit time. Selectively increasing retentive motility and reducing propulsive motility is an important aspect of diarrhea therapy.

Slow Waves of Electrical Depolarization Are a Unique Feature of Gut Smooth Muscle

In both the longitudinal and circular layers, GI smooth muscle cells are arranged in a network of interconnected, indistinct bundles, so that each muscle layer is a continuous, interlocking sheet of muscle cells. The individual muscle cells are connected to each other by *gap junctions* or *nexuses.* These junctions create an electrical connection between the cells and allow changes in membrane potential to be transferred from cell to cell. The arrangement permits the gut musculature to function as a *syncytium* (i.e., a multinucleate mass of protoplasm produced by the merging of cells) that allows waves of electrical activity to spread over the muscle layers, much like the transmission of electrical activity in heart muscle.

The first level of control of GI motility lies in the intrinsic electrical properties of the

smooth muscle mass. Smooth muscle cells of the gut, like other excitable cells, maintain an electrical potential difference across their cell membranes, the inner surface being electrically negative compared to the outer surface. The events responsible for cellular membrane potentials are similar in most cells and involve selective transport of ions into or out of the cell. These mechanisms are described in Chapter 3.

The membrane potentials of GI smooth muscle cells, in contrast to many other types of excitable cells, fluctuate spontaneously. In the resting state, the baseline membrane potential is usually -70 to -60 mV (Fig. 27–1). But the membrane potential may spontaneously depolarize or hyperpolarize from this baseline level by as much as 20–30 mV (see Fig. 27–1). Thus, under resting conditions, the depolarization is only partial, and the membrane potential never reaches 0 mV. Because the cells are connected electrically, the variation in membrane potential is spread, or propagated, over large areas of muscle. In the intestine, the spontaneous, rhythmic changes in membrane potential occur most rapidly in the duodenum. Because of this, the duodenum acts as a pacemaker, initiating changes in membrane potential that are propagated

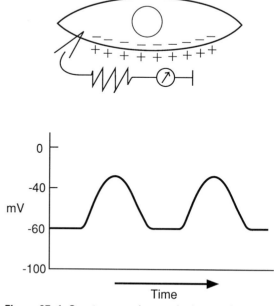

Figure 27–1. Spontaneous changes in the membrane polarity of GI smooth muscle cells. The upper figure represents a single cell with a voltmeter measuring the transmembrane electrical potential. The graph illustrates spontaneous changes in electrical potential (mV) that would be measured across the cell membrane.

aborally (away from the mouth) along the length of the small intestine (Fig. 27–2). These aborally moving waves of partial depolarization are called *slow waves*, or alternatively *basic electrical rhythm*, and they are similar to an excitatory postsynaptic potential (EPSP) in nerve cell membranes (see Chapter 3). In the small intestine of the dog, slow waves occur with a frequency of about 20 times per minute. In the stomach and colon they are considerably less frequent, occurring about five times per minute. However, the slow waves are present throughout the smooth muscle portions of the GI tract. The frequency of slow waves varies among the domestic species, but their presence does not.

The slow waves are an intrinsic property of the GI smooth muscle. Whereas their amplitude and, to a lesser extent, their frequency can be modulated by the nervous or endocrine systems, the presence of the slow waves, in most areas of the gut, is not dependent on influences from outside the smooth muscle. The link between slow waves and muscle contractions is under control, however, of nervous and endocrine factors.

When Spreading Slow Waves Reach Primed Smooth Muscle Cells, Action Potentials and Contraction Result

Slow waves have an important relationship with muscle contractions, but they are not the direct stimulus for contractions. Slow waves are constantly passing over GI smooth muscle,

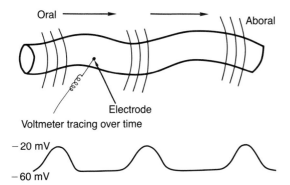

Figure 27–2. The partial membrane depolarizations of GI smooth muscle cells occur in a coordinated manner, creating waves of depolarization that sweep over large segments of muscle. Electrodes placed on or near the surface of the muscle record changes in potential as waves of depolarization pass toward or away from them. Coordinated changes in membrane potential among cells are necessary for these waves to be measured, because random changes among cells would cancel each other out, and no changes would be recorded by electrodes placed extracellularly.

whether or not it is actively contracting. GI smooth muscle cells, like other muscle cells, contract in association with action, or spike, potentials. These potentials are characterized by complete depolarization of the membrane for a short period of time. (A more complete discussion of action potentials can be found in Chapter 3.) Action potentials in the GI smooth muscle occur only at the crest of slow waves. Thus, muscle contractions can occur no more frequently than the frequency of the slow waves. This can be seen in the activity of muscle in the stomach of the dog. Slow waves in the canine stomach occur with a frequency of about five times per minute. The crest of each slow wave may or may not be accompanied by action potentials. Therefore, during a given minute, the muscle in a localized area may contract between zero and five times. If the passing slow waves generate no action potentials, the muscle does not contract at all. If there are action potentials associated with one slow wave, the muscle contracts once. Action potentials on two slow waves result in two contractions and so on up to a maximum of five contractions per minute, but no more than five, because there are no more slow waves.

The function of the slow waves appears to be to synchronize the contractions of the GI muscle mass. In order for the muscle to function efficiently, all, or many, of the muscle cells in one layer of a segment of gut must contract simultaneously. This can best be visualized by considering the circular muscle layer. The contents of the circle cannot be "squeezed" effectively unless all the muscles of the circumference contract simultaneously; it would have little effect on luminal pressure if one portion of the circle contracted while another portion relaxed. The nervous system cannot direct an individual circle of GI smooth muscle fibers to contract simultaneously, because there is no direct connection between the nervous system and the musculature, such as exists in the neuromuscular end-plates of skeletal muscle. Control of smooth muscle contraction is achieved by the combined effects of the intrinsic nervous system and the slow waves. The intrinsic nervous system releases neuroregulatory substances from nerve endings near muscle cells. The neuroregulatory substances sensitize the cells to make them more likely to generate an action potential and contract in the presence of a slow wave. When a slow wave passes over a sensitized group of cells, the entire group contracts. Thus, the nervous system "primes" the smooth muscle for contraction, while the slow waves signal the simultaneous contraction of a group of primed muscle fibers (Fig. 27–3).

Whether or not action potentials, and an associated muscle contraction, will occur as a given slow wave passes over an area of gut muscle is dependent on the height of the slow-wave crest. If the crest reaches a threshold value, a characteristic action potential, with short-term membrane depolarization and muscle contraction, occurs. The intrinsic nervous system regulates the likelihood of action potential occurrence by altering the baseline membrane potential and amplitude of the slow waves (see Fig. 27–3). Motor nerves that are stimulatory to the gut muscle raise the baseline and amplitude of the slow waves, whereas inhibitory nerves lower them, i.e., create more negative values. Parasympathetic stimulation (through cholinergic nerves of the intrinsic nervous system) tends to raise the slow-wave baseline and stimulate muscular activity in the gut, whereas sympathetic stimulation has the opposite effect.

The overall motility pattern of the gut is achieved by local variations in the activity of the intrinsic nervous system, in concert with the endocrine and autonomic nervous systems. Some areas of muscle may be "primed" for contraction, whereas others are not. Slow waves passing over primed areas incite action potentials and hence contractions; in un-primed areas the slow waves pass by, without stimulating muscle activity (see Fig. 27–3).

This discussion of control of GI muscle activity applies most directly to the small intestine. The general principles apply to both the stomach and colon also, but the system appears to be more intricate in those areas than in the small intestine.

Coordinated Motility of the Lips, Tongue, Mouth, and Pharynx Prehend Food and Propel It Down the Gastrointestinal Tract

Before digestion can begin, food must be directed into the GI tract. To ingest food, quadruped animals must first grasp it with their lips, teeth, or tongue. This involves highly coordinated activity of small, voluntary skeletal muscles. The muscles of the face, lips, and tongue appear to be among the most delicately controlled voluntary muscles of most domestic animals. The exact method of food prehension varies greatly among different species. For example, horses use their lips extensively, whereas cattle often use their tongues for grasping food. In all domestic animals, however, prehension is a highly coordinated process involving direct control by the central nervous system (CNS). Problems of prehension may develop because of abnormalities in the teeth, jaws, muscles of the tongue and face, cranial nerves, or CNS. The

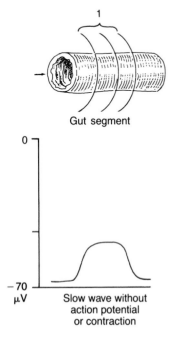

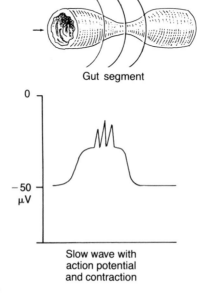

Figure 27–3. No muscle contraction occurs in the absence of action potentials *(1)*. Muscle contracts when the crest of the slow waves reaches a critical point of depolarization, allowing action potentials to occur *(2)*. The probability of action potentials' occurring during the passage of a slow wave over a segment of gut muscle is influenced by the degree of baseline depolarization. Norepinephrine lowers the baseline (increases its absolute value) whereas acetylcholine raises the baseline (decreases its absolute value).

facial, glossopharyngeal, and motor branch of the trigeminal cranial nerves controls the muscles of prehension.

Mastication, or chewing, involves the actions of the jaws, tongue, and cheeks and is the first act of digestion. It serves not only to break food particles down to a size that will pass into the esophagus, but it also moistens and lubricates food by thoroughly mixing it with saliva. Abnormalities of the teeth are a common cause of digestive disturbances in animals.

Swallowing involves voluntary and involuntary stages and occurs after food has been well masticated. In the voluntary phase of swallowing, food is molded into a bolus by the tongue and then pushed back into the pharynx. When food enters the pharynx, sensory nerve endings detect its presence and initiate the involuntary portion of the swallow reflex.

The involuntary actions of the swallow reflex occur primarily within the pharynx and esophagus. The pharynx is the common opening of both the respiratory and digestive tracts. The major physiological function of the pharynx is to assure that air, and only air, enters the respiratory tract and that food and water, and only food and water, enter the digestive tract. The involuntary portion of the swallow reflex is the action that directs food into the digestive system and away from the upper airway. This reflex involves the following series of highly coordinated actions (Fig. 27–4). Breathing stops momentarily. The soft palate is elevated, closing the pharyngeal opening of the nasopharynx and preventing food from entering the internal openings of the nostrils. The tongue is pressed against the hard palate, closing off the oral opening of the pharynx. The hyoid bone and larynx are pulled forward; this action serves to pull the glottis under the epiglottis, blocking the laryngeal opening. Concurrently, the arytenoid cartilages constrict, further closing the opening of the larynx and preventing the movement of food into the respiratory system. When all openings to the pharynx are closed, a wave of muscular constriction passes over the walls of the organ, pushing the bolus of food toward the opening of the esophagus. As the food reaches the esophagus, the upper esophageal sphincter relaxes to accept the material.

The complex reactions of swallowing are controlled by lower motor neurons located in various centers of the brainstem. Efferent nerve fibers from these centers travel in the

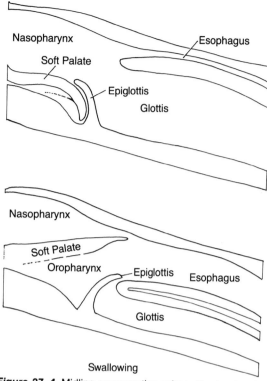

Figure 27–4. Midline cross-section schematic showing the position of the structures of the larynx and pharynx during breathing and swallowing.

facial, vagus, hypoglossal, and glossopharyngeal cranial nerves as well as the motor branch of the trigeminal nerve. Clinically, problems with prehension, mastication, and deglutition (swallowing) frequently are related to neurological lesions, either peripherally in the cranial nerves or centrally in the brainstem.

Motility of the Esophagus Propels Food from the Pharynx to the Stomach

The esophagus, like other tubular portions of the gut, contains an outer longitudinal and inner circular layer of muscle. The esophagus is unique with respect to other areas of the gut, however, in that much of its muscular wall is composed of striated, skeletal muscle fibers. In most domestic animals, the entire length of esophageal musculature is striated. In the horse, primate, and cat, however, a portion of the distal esophagus is smooth muscle. The striated-muscle portions of esophagus are under control of somatic (not parasympathetic) motor neurons in the vagus nerve, whereas the smooth muscle portions are under direct control of the intrinsic ner-

vous system and indirect control of the autonomic nervous system. A myenteric plexus
exists throughout the entire length of the
esophagus. In the area of striated muscle the
myenteric plexus probably serves a sensory
function and acts to coordinate the movements
of the striated-muscle portion with the esophageal smooth muscle segments and stomach.

In terms of motor activity, the esophagus
may be divided into an upper sphincter, body,
and lower sphincter. The upper esophageal
sphincter is called the *cricopharyngeal muscle*.
This muscle and the upper end of the esophagus are attached to the cricoid cartilage of the
larynx. When swallowing is not taking place
the muscle compresses the end of the esophagus against the cartilage of the larynx, tightly
closing the upper esophageal opening. During
swallowing, the cricopharyngeal muscle relaxes, and the larynx is pulled forward. Because the upper end of the esophagus is attached to the larynx, the forward motion of
the larynx tends to passively pull open the
upper esophageal orifice (see Fig. 27–4).

The body of the esophagus serves as a
relatively simple conduit, rapidly transferring
food from the pharynx to the stomach. Food
is propelled through the esophagus by propulsive movements known as *peristalsis*. Peristalsis consists of a moving ring of constriction
in the wall of a tubular organ. In the esophagus, these rings start at the cranial end and
progress toward the stomach. The rings reduce or obliterate the esophageal lumen, thus
pushing the bolus of food ahead of them in
much the same manner as you would push
material out of a soft rubber tube by stripping
it with your fingers. In addition to the constriction of the circular muscles, there may be
some contraction of longitudinal muscles just
ahead, or aboral, to the ring of circular muscle
contraction. This longitudinal muscle activity
would increase the size of the esophageal
lumen to accommodate the advancing food
bolus (Fig. 27–5). Peristalsis is a universal type
of GI propulsive motility that exists at all levels
of the gut.

During swallowing, the upper esophageal
sphincter relaxes as the pharynx constricts;
food is pushed into the upper portion of the
esophageal body, and a wave of peristalsis
propels the material toward the stomach. As
the food bolus reaches the distal end of the
esophagus, the lower sphincter relaxes, and
the ingested matter enters the stomach. If the
esophagus is not cleared of food material by
the primary wave of peristalsis, secondary

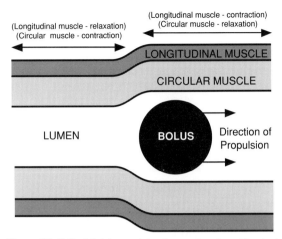

Figure 27–5. Peristalsis consists of a moving ring of luminal constriction preceded by an area of luminal distention. The area of constriction is created by contractions of the circular muscle, whereas the dilation is created by contractions of the longitudinal muscle. The net action is to propel a bolus of ingesta.

peristaltic waves are generated. One or more
secondary waves are almost always adequate
to push material into the stomach and clear
the esophagus. If food or foreign bodies become lodged in the esophagus, secondary
waves of peristalsis may lead eventually to
muscle spasms that constrict tightly around
the lodged material. These spasms frequently
interfere with attempts to remove the obstructing object.

When swallowing is not taking place, the
body of the esophagus is relaxed, but the
upper and lower sphincters remain constantly
constricted. The constriction of these sphincters is important because of the differences in
external pressure applied to the esophagus at
different points along its length. During the
inspiratory phase of breathing, the portion of
the esophagus within the thorax is subjected
to less-than-atmospheric pressure. If the two
esophageal sphincters were not tightly closed,
inspiration would cause aspiration of air from
the pharynx and reflux of ingesta from the
stomach into the body of the esophagus, in
the same manner as inspiration draws air into
the lung. Stomach contents would be drawn
into the esophagus, because inspiratory pressures in the thorax are less than intra-abdominal pressure. It is particularly important that
the lower esophageal sphincter remains closed
during inspiration, because the mucosa of the
esophagus is not equipped to resist the caustic
actions of gastric contents; thus, movement of
stomach contents into the esophagus would
cause damage to the esophageal mucosa.

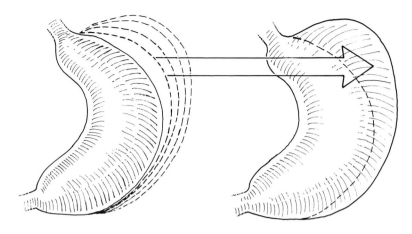

Figure 27–6. Adaptive relaxation refers to the stretching of the stomach wall that occurs as the organ fills during eating. This stretching occurs as a result of muscle relaxation and is accompanied by little or no change in intraluminal pressure.

In many species, the action of the lower esophageal sphincter is aided by the anatomical nature of the attachment of the esophagus and stomach. The esophagus enters the stomach obliquely, allowing distention of the stomach to block the esophageal opening in a valve-like fashion. During swallowing, the longitudinal muscle of the esophagus contracts, shortening the esophagus and opening the valve at the junction with the stomach. This anatomical arrangement, along with the lower esophageal sphincter, is particularly well developed in the horse, making reflux of stomach material into the esophagus extremely rare in this species. In many instances in which the intragastric pressure of the horse is pathologically raised, the stomach ruptures before vomiting or esophageal reflux takes place.

The Function of the Stomach Is to Process Food into a Fluid Consistency and Release It into the Intestine at a Controlled Rate

Among the animal kingdom there is tremendous diversity in the anatomy and motility patterns of the stomach. The following discussion applies best to the animals with the most simple stomachs, such as the dog and cat, but is probably also a reasonable description of the activity of the somewhat more complex stomachs of the pig, horse, and rat. The complex motility patterns of the ruminant stomach are discussed in Chapter 30.

The function of the stomach is to serve food to the small intestine. There are two important aspects of this function: rate of delivery and consistency of material. The stomach serves as both a storage vat to control the rate of delivery of food to the small intestine, and as a grinder and sieve that reduces the size of

food particles and releases them only when they are broken down to a consistency compatible with small intestinal digestion.

The stomach is divided into two physiological regions, each having a different impact on gastric function. The proximal region, at the esophageal end of the stomach, serves a storage function, retaining food as it awaits eventual entry into the small intestine. The distal region serves a grinding and sieving function, breaking solid pieces of food down into particles small enough for small intestinal digestion.

The Proximal Stomach Stores Food Awaiting Further Gastric Processing in the Distal Stomach

In the proximal stomach, there is little slow-wave activity. The major muscular activity in this region is of a weak, continuous-contraction nature. These *tonic* contractions tend to shape the gastric wall to its contents and provide gentle propulsion of material into the distal stomach. The major muscular reflex of the proximal stomach is *adaptive relaxation* (Fig. 27–6). This reflex is characterized by relaxation of the muscles as food enters the stomach. Because of this relaxation, the stomach can dilate to accept large quantities of food without an increase in intraluminal pressure. Thus, the proximal stomach serves as a food storage area. A consequence of the rather passive muscular activity of the proximal stomach is that little mixing occurs there. In fact, food boluses tend to become layered in the stomach in the order in which they are swallowed. As the stomach empties, tension on the wall of the proximal stomach increases slightly, pushing food into the gastric antrum, in which it can be processed for transport into the duodenum.

The Distal Stomach Grinds and Sifts Food Entering the Small Intestine

The muscular activity of the distal stomach and pylorus contrasts sharply with that of the proximal stomach. In the distal stomach, known as the *antrum*, there is intense slow-wave activity, and muscular contractions are frequently present. Strong waves of peristalsis begin at about the middle of the stomach and migrate, with the slow waves, toward the pylorus. As the waves of peristalsis near the pylorus, the pylorus constricts, blocking the gastric exit of all but the smallest particles (Fig. 27–7). Particles leaving the stomach during the digestive phase of activity are less than 2 mm in diameter. Those particles too large to pass the pylorus are crushed and ejected back into the antrum by the passing wave of peristalsis. Thus, the peristaltic actions of the distal stomach walls serve not only to propel food, but also, and perhaps more importantly, to grind and mix it.

Control of Gastric Motility Differs in the Proximal and Distal Stomach

The motility of the stomach, like other smooth muscle portions of the gut, is under both nervous and endocrine control. Fibers of the vagus nerve synapse on nerve cell bodies of the extensive gastric myenteric plexus and exert a high degree of control over gastric motility. The effects of vagal stimulation on the proximal and distal regions of the stomach are opposite; in the proximal stomach vagal activity suppresses muscular contractions and leads to adaptive relaxation, whereas in the distal stomach vagal stimulation causes intense peristaltic activity. Vagal stimulation of distal antral motility is mediated by acetylcholine, but vagal inhibition of proximal stomach motility is not. The identity of the inhibitory mediator is not well established, but it may be vascular inhibitory peptide (VIP).

Vagal action on the stomach is stimulated by events occurring within the CNS, as well as within the stomach and intestine. The anticipation of food consumption causes vagal stimulation of the stomach and thus primes the stomach to receive a meal. Reactions of the GI tract that originate in the CNS in response to anticipated food intake are often referred to as the *cephalic phase* of digestion. Vagal activity increases when food enters the stomach, as sensory receptors in the stomach create a positive feedback loop.

The exact role of hormones in regulation of gastric motility is not completely established. Gastrin, which is secreted from cells in the gastric antrum, appears to enhance gastric motility. Cholecystokinin (CCK), secretin, and gastric inhibitory peptide (GIP) appear to suppress gastric motility, at least in the dog. The roles of the various GI hormones are difficult to determine from available information, be-

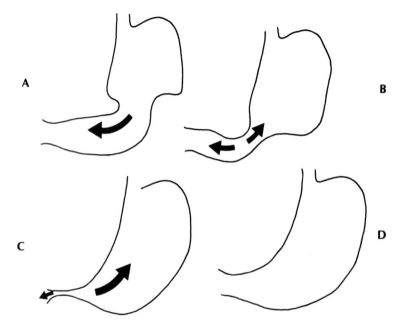

Figure 27–7. The grinding and churning activity of the distal stomach. (*A*) A wave of peristalsis begins at the junction of the proximal and distal areas of the stomach and moves toward the pylorus. (*B*) As the peristaltic wave approaches the pylorus, the pylorus constricts, causing some of the ingesta to be crushed within the peristaltic ring and propelled back toward the proximal stomach. (*C*) As the peristaltic wave reaches the pylorus, some finely ground and liquified material passes through into the duodenum, while the majority of material has been propelled back into the stomach. (*D*) Between contractions no gross movement of gastric contents occurs. (From Johnson LR (ed): Gastrointestinal Physiology. St. Louis, CV Mosby, 1985.)

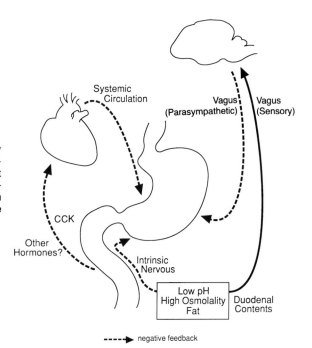

Figure 27–8. Inhibitory arcs of the enterogastric reflex. Low pH, high osmolality, and the presence of fat in the duodenum stimulate vagal, intrinsic, and hormonal reflexes that inhibit stomach emptying. After the duodenal pH and osmolality have moderated and some of the fat has been absorbed, the inhibitory influences on the stomach are removed.

cause many of the experimental results reported have been in response to administration of GI hormones at amounts far greater than those normally occurring.

The Rate of Gastric Emptying Must Match the Small Intestine's Rate of Digestion and Absorption

The rate at which food leaves the stomach must match the rate at which it can be digested and absorbed by the small intestine. Because some types of foods can be digested and absorbed more rapidly than others, the rate at which the stomach empties has to be regulated by the contents of the small intestine. Thus, there are reflexes that regulate gastric emptying and allow the stomach to serve as a storage site. These reflexes have their afferent receptors in the duodenum and are activated by low pH, high osmolality, and the presence of fat. It appears there are separate sensory receptors for each of these stimuli, but they have not been identified anatomically.

There are many reflexes that occur within the GI system. They are usually named by listing first the site of origin of the afferent stimulus followed by the site of the efferent response. Thus, reflex control of gastric emptying by the duodenum is referred to as the *enterogastric reflex*. "Entero-" is a prefix referring to the intestine.

The arc of the enterogastric reflex probably involves both the extrinsic and intrinsic nervous systems, as well as the endocrine system (Fig. 27–8). The extrinsic reflex pathway appears to involve afferent fibers of the vagus, which receive stimuli in the duodenum. These stimuli are integrated in the brainstem, and the response is mediated by vagal efferent fibers to the stomach. The intrinsic reflex arc involves receptors in the duodenum and nerve fiber connections in the intrinsic nervous system that directly affect gastric emptying.

A contribution of the GI endocrine system to the enterogastric reflex has long been suspected, but the exact hormones responsible for the reflex are not known. It is suspected that CCK and secretin may be important. Both hormones are secreted by cells in the duodenum; CCK is secreted in response to fat and secretin to low pH; both appear to have suppression of gastric emptying as secondary effects. GIP is a hormone produced in the duodenum in response to the presence of carbohydrate. In the dog, GIP may function as an inhibitor of gastric emptying, although stimulation of insulin secretion is probably its major action.

Enterogastric reflexes control gastric emptying by regulating stomach motility. The manner in which motility affects gastric emptying of solids is different from that for liquids. The rate at which solids are expelled from the stomach is regulated by the rate at which they are broken down into particles small enough to pass through the pylorus. This, in turn, is controlled by the motility of the antrum, or distal stomach; the greater the motility of the antrum, the faster material is broken down. Thus, antrum motility regulates the rate of release of solid material from the stomach. Liquid material leaves the stomach more quickly than solid matter, and the release of liquid may be less dependent on antral motility than it is on the motility of the proximal stomach.

There is little mixing activity in the proximal stomach. Because of this, liquids and solids tend to separate, the liquids to the outside and the solids to the center of the mass of food in the body of the stomach. Increased tension in the wall of the stomach body forces liquid into the antrum. Liquid may leave the antrum quickly, dependent on the activity of the pylorus. On the other hand, increased tension in the stomach body has little effect on the transport of solid material, because such material cannot leave the gastric body until sufficient space has been made available in the antrum. Thus, motility of the stomach body appears primarily responsible for the liquid-emptying rate, whereas motility of the antrum is most responsible for the solid-emptying rate. The effect of the pylorus itself on gastric emptying is not as great as might be expected; removal of the pylorus results in a slight increase in liquid-emptying rate and little increase in the rate of emptying of solid material. It appears that the distal portion of the antrum can account for much of the sieving action usually attributed to the pylorus. The rate of emptying of an isotonic liquid from the stomach is exponential and dependent on the initial volume of the liquid meal. Under usual circumstances, a liquid meal in the canine stomach has a half-life of about 18 minutes and is essentially gone by 1 hour. Solid material is emptied more slowly, and its rate is dependent on its fat content. Low-fat meat meals are usually gone from the stomach in 3–4 hours.

Between Meals the Stomach Is Cleared of Undigestible Material

It is obvious that often material ingested cannot be reduced to particles less than 2 mm in diameter. During the digestive phase of gastric motility, such material will not leave the stomach. To clear the stomach of undiges-

tible debris, a particular type of motility occurs between meals. This motility pattern is called the *interdigestive motility complex.* In association with this complex, the pylorus relaxes as strong waves of peristalsis sweep over the antrum, forcing less digestible material into the duodenum. This type of motility appears to have a "housekeeping" function in clearing the stomach of undigestible material.

The peristaltic waves of the interdigestive motility complex occur at approximately 1-hour intervals during the periods when the stomach is relatively empty of digestible material. Eating disrupts the complex and causes the resumption of the digestive motility pattern. Herbivores, which eat nearly constantly, have a slightly different pattern; the interdigestive motility complex occurs at approximately hourly intervals, even with digestible food present in the stomach.

Vomiting Is a Complex Reflex Coordinated from the Brainstem

Vomiting is a complex reflex activity with its integration, or coordination, centered in the brainstem. The act of vomiting involves many striated muscle groups and structures outside of the GI tract. Vomiting is associated with the following actions:

1. relaxation of the muscles of the stomach and lower esophageal sphincter and closing of the pylorus;
2. contraction of the abdominal musculature, creating an increase in intra-abdominal pressure;
3. expansion of the chest cavity while the glottis remains closed—this action lowers intrathoracic pressure;
4. opening of the upper esophageal sphincter.

The efferent limb of this reflex arc involves motor fibers in many different peripheral nerves.

Afferent stimulation of the vomiting reflex comes from a large number of receptors. Of particular importance are mechanoreceptors in the pharynx, and tension and chemoreceptors in the gastric and duodenal mucosa. Stimulation of these receptors sends signals to the *vomit center* in the brainstem. Thus, noxious tactile or chemical stimulation of the GI mucosa can result in vomiting that clears, or attempts to clear, the offending stimulus from the GI tract. Direct irritation of GI structures is not, however, the only stimulus for vomiting. The vomit center receives afferent input from a variety of organs; thus, vomiting is not always an indication of a primary GI problem.

An important structure outside of the GI tract that supplies afferent input in the vomit center is the *chemoreceptor trigger zone (CTZ)*. This is an area of the brainstem that lies in contact with the third ventricle. The CTZ is sensitive to the presence of some drugs and toxins in the blood. When stimulated, the CTZ sends signals to the vomit center and induces vomiting. Some of the products of inflammation stimulate the CTZ. Thus, inflammatory disease, even outside of the GI tract, can sometimes lead to vomiting. The semicircular canals of the inner ear are other important structures that supply afferent input to the vomit center. Constant stimulation of the semicircular canals may induce vomiting, as occurs in motion sickness. Other sites in the body may stimulate the vomit center also; thus, vomiting is a rather nondescript sign of disease.

Motility of the Small Intestine Has a Digestive and Interdigestive Phase

Motility of the small intestine occurs in two distinct phases: one during the digestive period following food intake, and another during the interdigestive period when little food is present in the gut. In the digestive phase there are two primary motility patterns: propulsive and nonpropulsive. The nonpropulsive pattern is referred to as *segmentation*. Segmentation results from localized contractions of circular muscle. Portions of small intestine, usually 3–4 cm long, contract tightly, dividing the gut into segments of constricted and dilated lumen. Within a few seconds, the constricted portions relax, and new areas constrict (Fig. 27–9). This action tends to "milk" gut

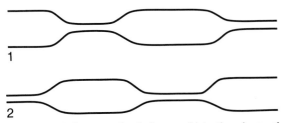

Figure 27–9. Segmentation in the small intestine. Areas of circular muscle constriction close the lumen and divide the gut into dilated segments containing ingesta. At periodic intervals the areas of constriction and dilation alternate, exerting a mixing and circulating action on the ingesta.

contents back and forth within the small intestine, mixing them with digestive juices and circulating them over the absorptive mucosal surfaces. This type of motility does not contribute much to the net aboral propulsion of ingesta. In fact, segmentation tends to slow down the aboral movement of material due to closure of the intestinal lumen in the constricted segments. Propulsive activity during the digestive phase consists of peristaltic contractions that migrate down the gut in phase with the slow waves. Digestive-phase peristaltic contractions, in contrast to interdigestive-phase peristalsis, pass over short segments of intestine and then die out. Thus, ingesta is pushed down the gut for a short distance and then subjected to additional segmentation contractions and mixing activity.

The interdigestive phase of small intestinal motility is characterized by waves of powerful peristaltic contractions that sweep over a large length of small intestine, sometimes traversing the entire organ. These waves are referred to as the *migrating motility complex (MMC)* or, alternatively, the *migrating myoelectric complex*. The MMC begins in the duodenum as groups of slow waves that stimulate intense action potential and muscle contraction activity. The complex migrates down the intestine at the rate of the slow waves. Some of the MMCs die out before reaching the ileum, but some travel the entire length of the small intestine.

The MMC probably has a housekeeping function and serves to push undigested material out of the small intestine. MMC may be important also in controlling the bacterial population in the upper gut. Normally the duodenum harbors a relatively small population of bacteria, and the population increases distally into the ileum, which has a moderately large number of bacterial organisms. The colon is heavily colonized by numerous species of bacteria. It is important for digestive function that this relative distribution of bacteria be maintained within the gut. The MMC may help to impede the migration of bacteria from the ileum to the duodenum.

The Ileocecal Sphincter Prevents Movement of Colon Contents Back into the Ileum

The *ileocecal sphincter* is at the junction of the small and large bowel and serves to prevent the movement of colon contents retrograde into the ileum. It consists of a well-developed

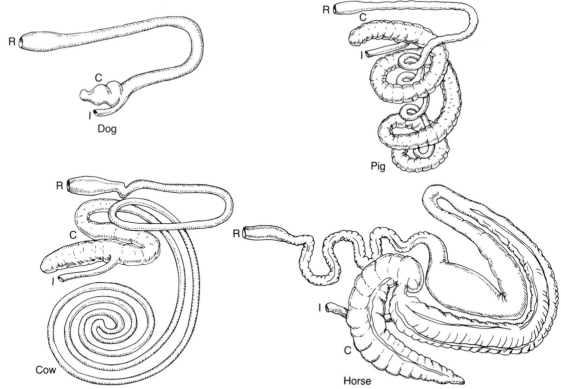

Figure 27–10. Variations of colon anatomy of four mammals. *I*, ileum; *C*, cecum; *R*, rectum. Animals with simple colons, like the dog, are not dependent on colonic fermentation to supply energy needs. Horses, with tremendous colonic development, rely on colonic fermentation for a large portion of their energy needs. Animals such as pigs and cattle are intermediate between the horse and dog in terms of the importance of colonic fermentation to digestive needs, and this intermediate position is noted in their colon development.

ring of circular muscle that remains constricted at most times. In addition to the muscular sphincter, in many species there is a flap of mucosa that acts as a one-way valve, further blocking movement of colon contents into the ileum. During periods of peristaltic activity in the ileum, the sphincter relaxes, allowing movement of material into the colon. When colonic pressure increases, the ileocecal sphincter constricts more tightly.

Motility of the Colon Causes Mixing, Retropulsion, and Propulsion of Ingesta

The colon acts in (1) absorption of water and electrolytes, (2) storage of feces, and (3) fermentation of organic matter that escapes digestion and absorption in the small intestine. The relative importance of these functions varies with the species, and tremendous differences in colon size and shape exist among animals. The major determinant of colon size is the importance of colonic fermentation to the energy needs of the animal. Those species,

such as the horse and rabbit, that make extensive use of fermentation products for nutritional needs, have large and complex colons. (The ruminant's fermentation chamber is in the stomach.) Other species, such as the dog and cat, do not rely on fermentation products and have relatively simple colons. Differences in colonic anatomy among four species with different needs for fermentative digestion are illustrated in Figure 27–10.

Considerable similarity appears to exist in colon motility patterns among animals, in spite of the anatomical diversity. Mixing activity is prominent in the colons of all species, because mixing and circulating is important to both absorptive and fermentative functions. Mixing is achieved by segmentation contractions, along with other types of motility. In many species, such as the horse and pig, colonic segmentation is pronounced and in some areas results in the formation of sacculations known as *haustra,* which are visible even after death.

A particular characteristic of colonic motility is retropulsion, or *antiperistalsis.* This is a type of peristaltic contraction that migrates orally, the opposite of normal peristaltic movement. This type of motility appears to result from colonic slow-wave activity that is somewhat more complex than that of the small intestine. The site of slow-wave origin in the colon, in contrast to the small intestine, is under control of the intrinsic nervous system. Under resting conditions in the colon, slow waves originate from "pacemakers" in one or more central sites. The pacemakers are not anatomical structures, but rather areas defined by activities of the intrinsic nervous system; thus, the pacemakers are not stationary, but can relocate in response to the need for different motility patterns. Antiperistaltic contractions occur in those segments in which slow waves migrate in an oral direction. Antiperistaltic contractions are retropulsive and impede the movement of ingesta, causing intense mixing activity and forcing material to accumulate in the proximal portions of the colon. Retropulsion appears to be particularly strong near the pacemakers and, therefore, the pacemakers represent sites of high resistance to the flow of colonic ingesta.

Because of continued inflow of material from the ileum into the colon, some ingesta escapes the retropulsive, antiperistaltic motility and moves into areas of propulsive, peristaltic activity and proceeds along the colon. In addition, there are periods of intense propulsive activity that involve the entire colon. These are called *mass movements* and frequently involve the distal translocation of the entire colonic content.

In the Carnivore Colon, Absorption and Storage Occur

The colon of the dog and cat is a relatively simple organ consisting of a short cecum, ascending part, transverse part, and descending part. During the resting phase, there is a colonic pacemaker at about the junction of the transverse and descending colons (Fig. 27–11). This gives rise to antiperistaltic activity in the proximal colon, with resultant accumulation of ingesta in the cecum and ascending colon areas. Moderate peristaltic activity usually occurs in the descending colon, whereas the distal colon and rectum are usually constricted and empty.

Material entering the carnivore colon is of a fluid consistency. It is thoroughly mixed in the ascending and transverse colons, and

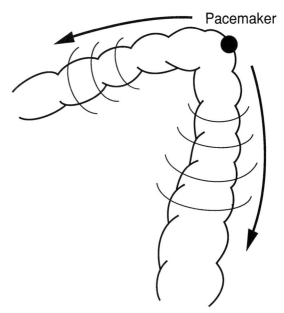

Figure 27–11. A pacemaker is present at the junction of the transverse and descending parts of the colon of the cat and probably in other mammals with similar colonic anatomy. Slow waves and peristaltic activity emanate in both directions from the pacemaker. Retrograde, or reverse, peristalsis in the proximal portions of the colon causes ingesta to be retained there, promoting the storage and absorptive functions of the colon.

much of the water and electrolytes are absorbed. By the time it reaches the descending colon, it is semisolid and becoming feces-like.

Despite Anatomical Differences in Herbivore Colons, Similar Motility Patterns Are Found

The functions of the herbivore colon are discussed more extensively in Chapter 30. Here it is important to point out the between-species comparisons in colon motility. In spite of the extreme between-species differences in colon anatomy, there are numerous similarities in colon motility.

The equine hindgut is complex and highly developed. The cecum is large and haustrated, and it is unique among most species because there is a distinct, sphincter-like orifice joining it to the colon. The colon is divided into a large and small portion, and the large colon is folded on itself so that there are three distinct flexures. The longitudinal muscles of the equine cecum and most areas of the colon are not evenly dispersed around the circumference of the gut. Instead, they form discrete bands, or *tenia*, that course along the longitudinal axis of the gut. The tenia divide the haustra longitudinally, giving the equine cecum and large colon a sacculated appearance.

Motility in the cecum consists of active segmentation and mixing, along with occasional mass movements that appear to transfer large amounts of ingesta to the colon. Motility in the colon consists of segmentation, antiperistalsis, and peristalsis. A colonic pacemaker appears to exist at the pelvic flexure and creates an area of high-flow resistance that retains material in the ventral portions of the large colon. Little is known about regulation of motility in the equine small colon. The characteristic ball-shaped form of equine feces probably represents intense segmentation-type motility in the small colon, where the feces are formed. The motility and function of the equine colon is discussed in more detail in Chapter 30.

In ruminants and swine the hindgut consists of a cecum of intermediate complexity, a spiral colon, and a straight colon. Less is known about the hindgut motility of the spiral-coloned animals than of other species. It seems that there is an area of high-flow resistance at the flexure, or central point, of the spiral colon. This may represent a pacemaker and result in generation of antiperistaltic motility in the centripetal portion of the colon.

The Anal Sphincter Has Two Layers with Separate Innervation

The anal opening is constricted by two sphincters: an internal sphincter of smooth muscle, which is a direct extension of the circular muscle layer of the rectum; and an external sphincter of striated muscle. The internal anal sphincter remains tonically contracted most of the time and is primarily responsible for anal continence. The internal sphincter receives parasympathetic innervation from the sacral spinal segments through the pelvic nerve, and sympathetic innervation from the lumbar spinal segments through the hypogastric nerve. In most species, sympathetic stimulation results in constriction of the sphincter, and parasympathetic stimulation results in relaxation.

The external sphincter maintains some degree of tonic contraction, but the consistent tone of the anus is primarily due to the internal sphincter. The external sphincter is innervated by general somatic efferent fibers having cell bodies in the cranial sacral spinal segments and coursing in the pudendal nerve.

The Rectosphincteric Reflex Is Important in Defecation

The entry of feces into the rectum is accompanied by the reflex relaxation of the internal anal sphincter, followed by peristaltic contractions of the rectum. This is known as the *rectosphincteric* reflex, and is an important part of the act of defecation (Fig. 27–12). The reflex normally results in defecation, but in trained animals its effects can be blocked by voluntary constriction of the external anal sphincter. When defecation is voluntarily prevented, the rectum soon relaxes to accommodate the fecal bolus, and the internal anal sphincter regains its tone. In humans, and presumably in dogs and cats, relaxation of the rectum and constriction of the internal sphincter is associated with fading of the urge to defecate, until another bolus of feces enters the rectum.

Uninhibited animals respond to the presence of feces in the rectum with a number of voluntary actions associated with defecation. In carnivores, the diaphragm and abdominal muscles contract to increase intra-abdominal pressure, and striated muscles of the anal canal relax as the animal assumes the defecation posture. These acts are important for complete evacuation of the rectum.

CLINICAL CORRELATION

EQUINE RABIES

HISTORY ☐ Owners report that their horse has not "been itself" for the past few days. Today, the animal is extremely depressed and stands with forelegs wide apart and head held low. The nostrils are soiled, and the owners report that water and feed come out of the nostrils when the animal attempts to eat or drink.

CLINICAL EXAMINATION ☐ From the history and presenting signs you recognize that the horse may have paralysis of muscles of the pharynx and larynx. Because these lesions are commonly associated with rabies in horses, you don a pair of plastic gloves and sleeves and proceed with your examination. To assess the function of the swallow reflex, you attempt to

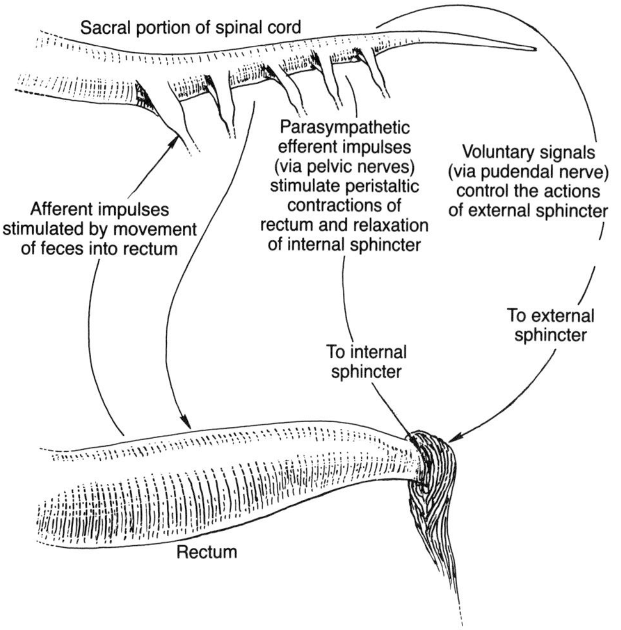

Figure 27–12. Arcs of the rectosphincteric reflex. The reflex is initiated by the movement of feces into the rectum and results in peristaltic movements of the rectal wall and relaxation of the internal anal sphincter. Fecal passage is the normal effect of the reflex, but voluntary constriction of the external anal sphincter can prevent the passage of feces and eventually override the reflex, apparently allowing trained animals to suppress the urge to defecate.

pass a stomach tube. You observe that the swallow reflex appears to be diminished, but that with some persistence the tube can be passed. This indicates that there is no physical obstruction in the pharynx or esophagus, and that the problem is of a functional nature. These findings support, but do not confirm, a diagnosis of rabies.

COMMENT □ Rabies in herbivorous animals may take a number of forms. One of the most common signs in cattle and horses is paralysis of the pharynx and larynx due to viral lesions in the brainstem nuclei supplying the appropriate cranial nerves. If rabies is suspected, no one should come into direct contact with the excretions of the animal, especially saliva.

TREATMENT □ In this case, treatment should consist of oral fluid and electrolyte therapy administered through an indwelling stomach tube. If there is no response to this conservative therapy, and if the animal's condition appears to deteriorate, euthanasia is necessary, and the head should be submitted for evaluation for a positive diagnosis of rabies.

Bibliography

Argenzio RA: Comparative physiology of the gastrointestinal system. *In* Anderson NV (ed): Veterinary Gastroenterology. Philadelphia, Lea & Febiger, 1980, pp 172–198.

Berne RM, Levy MN: Physiology. St. Louis, CV Mosby, 1983, pp 743–769.

Johnson LR (ed): Gastrointestinal Physiology. St. Louis, CV Mosby, 1985, pp 23–52.

Johnson LR (ed): Physiology of the Gastrointestinal Tract, 2nd ed. New York, Raven Press, 1987, pp 335–744.

Kerlin P, Zinsmeister A, Phillips S: Relationship of motility to flow of contents in the human small intestine. Gastroenterology 82:701–706, 1982.

Stevens CE: Comparative Physiology of the Vertebrate Digestive System. Cambridge, Cambridge University Press, 1988, pp 86–124.

Weems WA: Intestinal wall motion, propulsion, and fluid movement: Trends toward a unified theory. Am J Physiol 243:G177–G188, 1982.

PRACTICE QUESTIONS FOR CHAPTER 27

1. A unique feature of GI smooth muscle cells is that

   a. their resting transcellular electrical potential has the positive pole on the outside surface of the cell membrane.

   b. action potentials, or spikes of membrane depolarization, are not associated with muscle contractions.

   c. muscle contractions are stimulated by partial depolarization of the membrane.

d. there are spontaneous, rhythmic undulations in the electrical potential across the cell membrane.
e. contraction of the muscles is never influenced by nervous activity.

2. The term *slow waves* as applied to the gut refers to

a. slowly moving fronts of electrical activity that are propagated down the intrinsic nervous system.
b. slowly moving fronts of electrical activity that result from coordinated changes in cell membrane potential occurring throughout the smooth muscle of the intestinal wall.
c. slowly moving fronts of ingesta that proceed down the intestine in response to peristaltic movement.
d. slowly moving fronts of action potentials that are constantly passing over the gut smooth muscle.
e. slowly moving fronts of peristaltic contractions that pass uniformly over the entire small intestine during the digestive period.

3. An animal is presented to you with aspiration pneumonia (the result of food material entering the lower respiratory tract). Which of the following lesions would be a likely cause?

a. Loss of myenteric plexus function in the pharynx and upper esophagus
b. Loss of slow-wave activity in the pharynx and upper esophagus
c. A lesion in the brainstem
d. A lesion in the trachea
e. None of the above

4. The term *cephalic phase* is used in reference to a number of activities occurring in the GI tract. In general, the term means

a. the early phases of digestion, when food is nearest the head.
b. any actions stimulated directly by the presence of food in the stomach.
c. any actions stimulated directly by the presence of food in the mouth.
d. digestive events stimulated by the presence of food in the GI tract, but requiring reflexes integrated in the CNS.
e. digestive events that occur prior to the ingestion of food and in response to CNS stimulation that is brought on by the anticipation of eating.

5. Conditions in the duodenum, such as low pH or high-fat concentration, can reflexly inhibit gastric emptying. Which reflex arc is involved in this inhibition?

a. Parasympathetic nervous system
b. GI intrinsic nervous system
c. GI endocrine system
d. All of the above

28

Secretions of the Digestive Tract

THE SALIVARY GLANDS

1. Saliva moistens, lubricates, and partially digests food
2. Salivary secretions originate in the gland acini and are modified in the collecting ducts
3. Salivary glands are regulated by the parasympathetic nervous system
4. Ruminant saliva is a bicarbonate-phosphate buffer secreted in large quantities

GASTRIC SECRETION

1. Depending on the species, there may be two general types of gastric mucosa: *glandular* and *nonglandular*
2. The gastric mucosa contains many different cell types
3. The gastric glands secrete hydrochloric acid
4. Pepsin is secreted by gastric chief cells in an inactive form and subsequently activated in the gut lumen
5. The gastric glands are stimulated to secrete by the action of acetylcholine, gastrin, and histamine

THE PANCREAS

1. Pancreatic exocrine secretions are indispensable for the digestion of the complex nutrients, proteins, starches, and triglycerides
2. Acinar cells secrete enzymes, whereas centro-acinar cells and duct cells secrete a sodium bicarbonate solution
3. Pancreatic cells have cell-surface receptors stimulated by acetylcholine, cholecystokinin, and secretin

BILE SECRETION

1. The liver is an acinar gland with small acinar lumina known as canaliculi
2. Bile contains phospholipids and cholesterol maintained in aqueous solution by the detergent action of bile acids
3. The gallbladder stores and concentrates bile during the periods between feeding
4. Bile secretion is initiated by the presence of food in the duodenum and stimulated by the return of bile acids to the liver

Digestion and absorption can take place only in the aqueous milieu of digestive secretions. Synthesis and secretion of these fluids is a well-controlled process, regulated by endocrine as well as intrinsic and extrinsic neural events.

THE SALIVARY GLANDS

Saliva Moistens, Lubricates, and Partially Digests Food

As food is chewed, it is mixed with salivary secretions that allow it to be molded into a well-lubricated bolus that facilitates swallowing. In addition, saliva may have antibacterial, digestive, and evaporative cooling functions, depending on the species.

The antibacterial activity of saliva comes from antibodies and lysozyme. *Lysozyme* is an enzyme that has antibacterial properties. It may appear that the antibacterial properties of saliva are inefficient, because the mouth normally contains a large, thriving population of bacteria. However, saliva aids in keeping this population in check, and animals without salivary function are prone to infectious diseases of the oral cavity.

In omnivorous animals, such as rats and pigs, saliva contains a starch-digesting enzyme known as *salivary amylase*. This enzyme is absent usually from the saliva of carnivorous animals, such as dogs and cats. The saliva of some species also contains a fat-digesting enzyme known as *lingual lipase*. This enzyme is frequently present in young animals, such as calves, while they are on a milk diet; the enzyme disappears as they mature.

Salivary enzymes probably have their major digestive effect in the proximal stomach, because food is not retained in the mouth long enough to permit extensive digestion. The lack of mixing activity in the proximal stomach may be essential to the starch-digesting function of saliva. This is because the amylase enzyme is functional at neutral to slightly basic pH, as exists in saliva. The low pH of the distal stomach probably inactivates the enzyme; therefore, it may be important that food entering the stomach not be mixed with gastric secretions.

The evaporative cooling function of saliva is covered in Chapter 51.

Salivary Secretions Originate in the Gland Acini and Are Modified in the Collecting Ducts

Saliva is initially secreted into the lumen of the *acini* or end-pieces of the salivary glands. Water, electrolytes, enzymes, and mucus are secreted by the glandular cells lining the acini. As the secretion progresses through the collecting ducts, its composition is modified. The duct epithelium reabsorbs electrolytes, especially sodium and chloride, in a manner similar to the proximal tubules of the kidneys (Fig. 28–1). The final product, saliva, is hypotonic and has a sodium concentration several-fold less than extracellular fluid.

Most mammals have at least three pairs of salivary glands: the *parotid* glands, which lie just under the ear and behind the vertical ramus of the mandible; the *mandibular* glands, which are in the intramandibular space; and the *lingual* glands, which lie in the base of the tongue. Each of these glands drains into a main duct that has a single opening into the mouth. In addition to these major glands, there are minor glands in the tongue and buccal mucosa. These are small, indistinct glands that often have numerous secretory ducts emptying into the mouth. The concentration of mucus is different in the secretions of the various salivary glands. The parotid gland secretes a watery, or *serous* saliva, whereas many of the minor glands secrete a highly mucous saliva. Other glands secrete a

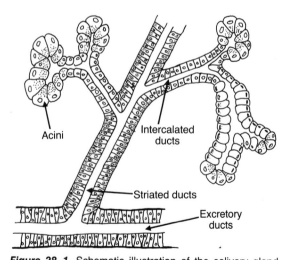

Figure 28–1. Schematic illustration of the salivary gland. Saliva initially is secreted by the acinar cells and then is modified as it passes through the intercalated, or collecting, ducts. Modification of acinar secretions by duct epithelia is a common physiological phenomenon among several types of glands, including the pancreas.

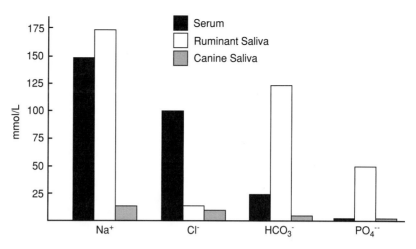

Figure 28–2. Electrolyte composition of blood serum and of canine and ruminant saliva. Note that the electrolyte concentration of canine saliva is much lower than that of serum, in contrast to the concentration in ruminant saliva. Also note the high concentrations of bicarbonate (HCO_3^-) and phosphate (PO_4^{--}) in ruminant saliva; these ions give ruminant saliva its alkalizing quality.

mixed type of saliva containing both mucous and serous material.

Salivary Glands Are Regulated by the Parasympathetic Nervous System

Autonomic, parasympathetic nerve fibers of the facial and glossopharyngeal nerves end on the secretory cells of the salivary gland acini and stimulate the cells by way of cholinergic receptors. All phases of salivary activity are stimulated by this mechanism, including electrolyte, water, and enzyme secretion. The anticipation of eating can initiate a parasympathetic response resulting in salivary secretion. In Pavlov's famous experiment, parasympathetic stimulation of the salivary gland was evoked in dogs by the sound of a ringing bell. The dogs had been trained to anticipate eating after hearing the bell. This well-known experiment was one of the first demonstrations that the central nervous system (CNS) could regulate digestive functions.

Salivary secretory cells also contain β-adrenergic receptors that are activated by sympathetic nerve stimulation or circulating catecholamines. This form of stimulation probably has little to do with normal digestive activity, but is related to the salivation and drooling that is seen in carnivores preparing to attack. Among digestive glands, the salivary glands are unique, because there is no endocrine regulatory component.

Ruminant Saliva Is a Bicarbonate-Phosphate Buffer Secreted in Large Quantities

The normal composition of ruminant parotid saliva is quite different from that of monogas-

trics. Bovine and canine saliva is compared in Figure 28–2. Ruminant saliva is isotonic and, compared to blood serum, has a relatively high concentration of bicarbonate and phosphate, and a relatively high pH. This well-buffered solution is necessary to neutralize acids formed by fermentation in the rumen, and ruminants secrete it in enormous quantities. An adult cow may secrete 100–200 L of saliva per day. This volume is approximately equivalent to the extracellular fluid volume of most adult cattle. It is obvious that much of the water and electrolyte secreted in saliva must be reabsorbed rapidly and recirculated through the total body water, or the cow would die of dehydration. In abnormal circumstances, such as blockage of the esophagus, in which the flow of saliva is diverted from the GI tract, cattle quickly become dehydrated and acidotic.

In general, the salivary glands of domestic animals are seldom involved in disease processes and infrequently require veterinary attention.

GASTRIC SECRETION

Depending on the Species, There May Be Two General Types of Gastric Mucosa: *Glandular* and *Nonglandular*

Most domestic animals have only a glandular mucosa, but horses and rats have an area in the proximal portion of their stomachs that is covered by nonglandular, stratified squamous epithelium. This area is visibly different from the glandular area, to which it adjoins with a sharp line of demarcation. The function of the nonglandular area of gastric mucosa is not known with certainty. It could be that the nonglandular area serves as a place where a small amount of fermentative (rumen-like) digestion could occur. Remember that there is little mixing activity in the proximal stomach, so food in the nonglandular area would be protected from the secretions of the gastric glands. These acid secretions kill bacteria and, thus, would prevent fermentation.

The glandular area of the stomach is divided into three regions: *cardiac mucosa, parietal mucosa,* and *pyloric mucosa.* These areas contain glands of similar structure but with different types of secretions, as described later. In most species, the cardiac mucosa forms a narrow band around the gastric opening of the esophagus. In the pig, however, the cardiac mucosa covers a substantial portion of the proximal stomach.

The Gastric Mucosa Contains Many Different Cell Types

The glandular mucosa of the stomach has frequent invaginations, or pores, known as *gastric pits.* The size of the pits is such that the pores leading into them can be seen with a hand-held magnifying glass. At the base of each pit is a narrowing, or isthmus, that continues into the opening of one or more gastric glands (Fig. 28–3).

The major surface areas of the stomach, as well as the lining of the pits, are covered with *surface mucous cells.* These cells elaborate a thick, tenacious mucus that is a special characteristic of the stomach lining. The mucous cells and their associated secretion are important for protecting the stomach epithelium from the acid conditions and grinding activity present in the lumen. When the mucous cells are injured, stomach ulcers result.

Each region of the mucosa contains glands with characteristic cell types. Within the parietal area, the glands contain *parietal* cells. These cells are clustered in the neck, or proximal area, of the gland. It is their function to secrete hydrochloric acid (HCl). Distributed among the parietal cells in the neck of the gland is another type of cell, the *mucous neck cells.* These mucous cells secrete a thin mucus, less viscous than that of the surface mucous cells. The mucous neck cells, in addition to their secretory function, appear to be the progenitor cells for the gastric mucosa. They are the only cells of the stomach lining that are capable of division. As they divide, they mi-

grate either down into the glands or up into the pits and onto the surface epithelium. As they migrate, they differentiate into any of the several types of mature cells of the gastric surface and glands. In the base of the gastric glands is yet a third type of cell, the *chief* cells. These secrete *pepsinogen,* precursor to the digestive enzyme *pepsin.*

The glands of the cardiac and pyloric mucosal regions resemble those of the parietal area in structure, but contain different cell types. The cardiac glands secrete only mucus. Their mucus is alkaline and probably serves to protect the adjacent esophageal mucosa from the acid secretions of the stomach. The pyloric glands have no parietal cells but contain the gastrin-producing G cells. According to most reports, pyloric glands do secrete pepsinogen.

The Gastric Glands Secrete Hydrochloric Acid

When the gastric glands are stimulated maximally, the HCl solution secreted into the lumen is isotonic and has a pH of less than 1. The hydrogen and chloride ions are both secreted by the parietal cells, but apparently by different cellular mechanisms. Hydrogen ion is secreted through a H^+, K^+ ATPase (adenosinetriphosphatase) pump located on the luminal surface of the cell. This enzyme exchanges hydrogen ions for potassium ions, pumping one potassium into the cell for each hydrogen secreted into the lumen. In the exchange process, one molecule of adenosine triphosphate (ATP) is hydrolyzed to adenosine diphosphate (ADP), representing an expenditure of energy. The potassium cations that accumulate within the cells are released back into the lumen in combination with chloride anions. This allows for the recycling of potassium ions as they are pumped back into the cells in exchange for hydrogen, resulting in the net secretion of hydrogen and chloride, with little net movement of potassium.

Hydrogen ions for secretion come from the dissociation of intracellular carbonic acid (H_2CO_3), leaving a bicarbonate ion (HCO_3^-) ion in the cell for each hydrogen ion secreted into the lumen (Fig. 28–4). Carbonic acid originates from water and carbon dioxide through the action of the enzyme *carbonic anhydrase,* an enzyme found in high concentration in the gastric mucosa.

As hydrogen cations are secreted, bicarbon-

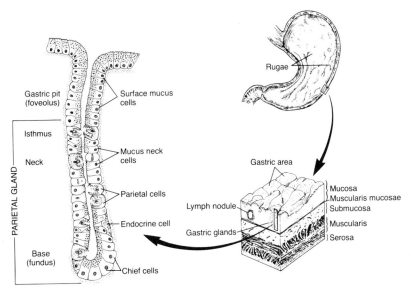

Figure 28–3. Anatomic illustration of glands of the stomach body. Other portions of the glandular stomach mucosa have similar structure, but may differ somewhat in the cell types present in the glands. The gland openings are large enough to be seen with a hand-held magnifying glass.

Gastric pit (foveolus)
Surface mucus cells
Isthmus
Mucus neck cells
Neck
Gastric area
Parietal cells
Lymph nodule
Endocrine cell
Gastric glands
Base (fundus)
Chief cells
Rugae
Mucosa
Muscularis mucosae
Submucosa
Muscularis
Serosa
PARIETAL GLAND

ate anions accumulate in the cell. To counterbalance this accumulation, bicarbonate anions are exchanged for chloride anions at the cell's nonluminal surface. In this manner, additional chloride is made available to the cell for secretion into the glandular lumen, and bicarbonate is secreted into the blood. During periods of intense secretion by the gastric glands, large amounts of bicarbonate are released into the blood. This alkalization of the blood is known as the "alkaline tide" and is associated with digestion. Normally, the alkaline tide is reversed when bicarbonate in the blood is consumed indirectly during the neutralization of gastric secretions as they enter the intestine (see the section on pancreatic secretions). Thus, on a total-body basis, gastric acid production results in only small and transient changes in blood pH; however, in disease states, where the secretions of the stomach are prevented from entering the intestine or are

lost from the body because of vomiting, the pH of the blood can rise to dangerously high values.

Pepsin Is Secreted by Gastric Chief Cells in an Inactive Form and Subsequently Activated in the Gut Lumen

Pepsin is usually referred to as a single compound, but actually it is a family of protein-digesting enzymes that are secreted from the gastric glands. They are formed in the chief cells as inactive proenzymes called *pepsinogens*. Pepsinogens are stored in the chief cells as granules until secreted into the lumen of the gastric glands. After secretion, pepsinogens are exposed to the acid contents of the stomach; this results in cleavage of a small portion of the protein molecule, which results in activation of the enzymes.

Digestive enzymes that are synthesized and stored as inactive proenzymes and activated in the lumen of the gut are known by the general name of *zymogens*. The general pattern of zymogen formation and activation is necessary, because the active enzymes could digest and destroy the cells that synthesize them.

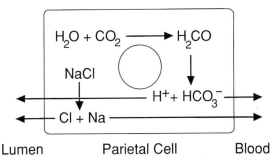

$$H_2O + CO_2 \longrightarrow H_2CO$$
NaCl
$$H^+ + HCO_3^-$$
Cl + Na

Lumen   Parietal Cell   Blood

Figure 28–4. The electrolyte movements during gastric acid secretion. The production of hydrogen and bicarbonate ions from water and carbon dioxide is stimulated by the action of the enzyme carbonic anhydrase, the activity of which is high in the gastric mucosa.

The Gastric Glands Are Stimulated to Secrete by the Action of Acetylcholine, Gastrin, and Histamine

Secretion of the gastric glands is stimulated by the anticipation of eating and the presence of undigested food in the stomach. When an animal anticipates eating, parasympathetic vagal impulses stimulate cells of the gastrointestinal (GI) intrinsic nervous system, which in turn release acetylcholine into the vicinity of G cells and parietal cells. These secretory cells have acetylcholine receptors on their surfaces and respond by secreting gastrin and HCl, respectively. Gastrin circulates in the blood stream and eventually finds its way to the parietal cells, which have gastrin receptors, in addition to acetylcholine receptors, on their surfaces. The combined actions of gastrin and acetylcholine on the parietal cells result in high rates of HCl flow. The response of the stomach to anticipatory stimuli originating in the brain is referred to as the "cephalic phase" of gastric secretion.

Food entering the stomach initiates the second, or "gastric phase," of gastric secretion. Distention of the stomach by food stimulates stretch receptors of the GI intrinsic nervous system; the system responds by direct nervous (acetylcholine) stimulation of the G and parietal cells. In addition, food acts as a buffer, raising the stomach pH. This removes the inhibiting effect of acid on G-cell secretion, further stimulating the production of gastrin, which leads to even greater enhancement of acid production by the parietal cells.

The role that histamine plays in gastric acid secretion is important but incompletely understood. There are histamine receptors on parietal cells, and it appears that maximal secretion by those cells is stimulated in the presence of all three mediators: acetylcholine, gastrin, and histamine. Histamine is produced in the gastric mucosa. It may be that gastrin and acetylcholine stimulate histamine production, and that histamine then enhances the effect of these mediators on parietal cells.

As gastric secretion and digestion proceed, the pH of the stomach decreases. When the stomach pH falls to about 2, gastrin secretion is depressed, and at a pH of 1, gastrin secretion is completely abolished; thus, the gastrin stimulus to the parietal cells is removed, and acid secretion is reduced (see Fig. 26–8).

In addition to the gastrin-mediated negative feedback on acid secretion in the stomach, there is also an intestinal negative feedback mechanism. As acid contents from the stomach flow into the duodenum and the duodenal pH is reduced, gastric acid production is suppressed. The exact mechanism by which duodenal acidification exerts a negative feedback on the parietal cells is not known with certainty. The hormone *secretin*, produced in the duodenum, may be involved, as well as neuronal reflexes acting through the GI intrinsic nervous system. Secretion of pepsinogen appears to be under the same regulatory influences as the secretion of HCl. However, regulation of pepsin secretion has received much less research than has the regulation of HCl secretion.

THE PANCREAS

Pancreatic Exocrine Secretions Are Indispensable for the Digestion of the Complex Nutrients, Proteins, Starches, and Triglycerides

The pancreas is composed of two functionally separate types of glandular tissue. A small, but important, portion of the pancreatic tissue is arranged into discrete islets within the parenchyma of the gland. These cells are collectively called the *endocrine pancreas*, because they secrete hormones into the blood stream. The endocrine pancreas is discussed in Chapter 33. The large majority of the pancreatic tissue is involved with the elaboration of digestive secretions. This portion is known as the *exocrine pancreas*, because its secretions are delivered into the intestinal lumen. It is the exocrine pancreas that we are concerned with here.

Acinar Cells Secrete Enzymes, Whereas Centro-Acinar Cells and Duct Cells Secrete a Sodium Bicarbonate Solution

The exocrine pancreas is a typical acinar gland in which the end-pieces, or acini, are connected by an arborizing system of ducts, so that the gland conceptually resembles a bunch of grapes. In general structure it resembles the salivary gland, as illustrated in Figure 28–1. The cells of the acini contain a generous portion of rough endoplasmic reticulum, upon which large amounts of secretory proteins, the digestive enzymes, are synthesized. Each pancreatic acinar cell can produce all of the more than 10 different enzymes secreted by the pancreas. A list of the major digestive enzymes of the pancreas is in Table 29–1. The functions of these enzymes are further discussed in Chapter 29. Protein-digesting enzymes, which are potentially harmful to the pancreatic cells, are synthesized as zymogens in a manner completely analogous to pepsinogen synthesis in the gastric glands. After synthesis, the enzymes and proenzymes are stored in vesicles, or *zymogen granules,* near the cellular apex. When the cells are stimulated, the zymogen granules fuse with the plasma membrane and release their contents into the lumen of the gland and eventually into the duodenal lumen, where they are converted to the activated form of the enzyme.

Specialized cells near the junction of the acini and ducts are called centro-acinar cells. These cells, and the lining cells of the ducts, produce a watery secretion rich in sodium bicarbonate. Within the cells, carbonic acid for the generation of bicarbonate ion is produced by the action of carbonic anhydrase on H_2O and CO_2. Carbonic acid (H_2CO_3) dissociates to form H^+ and HCO_3^-. Hydrogen ion is pumped from the cell in exchange for Na^+, allowing the accumulation of HCO_3^- within the cell. As HCO_3^- accumulates in the cell, it flows down its concentration gradient into the lumen of the pancreatic duct. In general, the ion transport activities of the pancreatic duct cells are opposite in direction to those of the parietal cells, as illustrated in Figure 28–4.

The ducts of the pancreatic lobules coalesce in an arborizing pattern to form either one or two main pancreatic ducts, depending on the species. The pancreatic duct(s) may empty directly into the duodenum or, as in the case of sheep, into the common bile duct. In the latter case, the pancreatic secretions enter the intestinal lumen along with bile.

Pancreatic Cells Have Cell-Surface Receptors Stimulated by Acetylcholine, Cholecystokinin, and Secretin

When binding sites on the surfaces of pancreatic acinar or duct cells are occupied, the cells are stimulated to secrete. Each type of cell, acinar and duct cells, appears to have receptors for the neurotransmitter substance acetylcholine as well as the GI hormones cholecystokinin (CCK) and secretin. Acetylcholine, released from nerve endings near the cells, stimulates secretion, as do CCK and secretin arriving in the blood. CCK is the primary hormonal stimulus for acinar cells, whereas secretin is the primary hormonal stimulus for duct cells. It appears, however, that maximal stimulation of the cells occurs when all receptors are occupied. Thus, acinar cells secrete most actively in the presence of all three ligands: acetylcholine, CCK, and secretin. In this manner, secretin is said to po-

tentiate, or increase, the action of CCK on acinar cells, and CCK potentiates the action of secretin on duct cells.

Nerve fibers ending in the vicinity of pancreatic acinar glands originate from cell bodies in the intrinsic nervous system. These neurons are stimulated to release acetylcholine by impulses arriving from other neurons of the intrinsic system, or by parasympathetic fibers arriving by way of the vagus nerve. Vagal stimulation of pancreatic secretion may arise as the result of several stimuli. The sight and smell of food induce centrally integrated vagal responses leading to pancreatic secretion; this is referred to as the *cephalic phase* of pancreatic secretion. Distention of the stomach causes a vagovagal reflex stimulating pancreatic secretion, and this is called the *gastric phase* of pancreatic secretion. The effects of the cephalic and gastric phases of pancreatic secretion are to "ready" the intestine for the imminent arrival of food by prior stimulation of pancreatic secretions.

The third, or *intestinal phase,* of pancreatic secretion is the most intense and involves endocrine as well as neuronal stimuli. This phase commences as food material from the stomach enters the duodenum. This leads to distention of the duodenum, which appears to produce intrinsic nerve impulses resulting in acetylcholine stimulation of pancreatic secretory cells. This stimulation reinforces and enhances the vagally mediated neuronal stimulation of the cephalic and gastric phases. The endocrine portion of the intestinal phase of pancreatic secretion occurs in response to the chemical stimulation resulting from the presence of gastric contents in the duodenum. Peptides in the duodenal lumen, arising from the digestion of food protein, stimulate CCK production from endocrine cells in the duodenum. Fats in gastric ingesta also stimulate CCK secretion, whereas the low pH of material entering the duodenum from the stomach stimulates the secretion of secretin.

This stimulatory pattern is logical and results in a coordinated pattern of digestion. Proteins (peptides) and fats stimulate, through CCK, the secretion of protein and fat-digesting enzymes. These enzymes function best in an alkaline environment, so the acid secretions of the stomach must be neutralized. Acid conditions in the duodenum stimulate pancreatic bicarbonate secretion through secretin, leading to alkalization of the ingesta. As food is digested and absorbed, and acid is neutralized, the stimuli for pancreatic secretion are re-

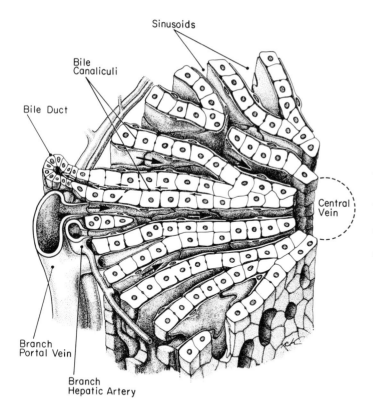

Sinusoids

Bile
Canaliculi

Bile Duct

Central
Vein

Branch
Portal Vein

Branch
Hepatic Artery

Figure 28–5. Hepatic microanatomy is complex and can be visualized in several ways. Note the relationship of the bile canaliculi to the bile ducts; the biliary system may be imagined as an acinar gland with the bile canaliculi forming a long, narrow acinus. (Modified from Ham AW: Textbook of Histology, 5th ed. Philadelphia, JB Lippincott, 1965.)

moved, and the rate of secretion diminishes to low, basal rates.

BILE SECRETION

One of the several functions of the liver is that of a secretory gland of the digestive system. Its secretion, bile, has an important role in fat digestion.

The Liver Is an Acinar Gland with Small Acinar Lumina Known As Canaliculi

The liver is composed of "plates" or one cell–thick layers of hepatocytes that are bathed on either side by blood from the hepatic sinusoids. Between each row of cells is a small space created by cavitations in the plasma membranes of two apposing cells. Within the plates of cells, these spaces join to form channels, or *canaliculi*, that connect to the bile ductules. Bile is secreted from the hepatocytes into the canaliculi from which it flows into the bile duct system. From a functional standpoint, the canaliculi may be perceived of as acini lined by hepatocytes and emptying into the biliary duct system, as schematically illus-

trated in Figure 28–5. The bile duct epithelium is metabolically active and capable of altering the composition of canalicular bile by adding additional water and electrolytes, especially bicarbonate.

Bile Contains Phospholipids and Cholesterol Maintained in Aqueous Solution by the Detergent Action of Bile Acids

Hepatocytes form bile acids from cholesterol. The chemical changes necessary to convert cholesterol to cholic acid, a representative bile acid, are shown in Figure 28–6. Cholesterol is almost totally insoluble in water, but the chemical changes involved in the conversion of cholesterol to bile acids result in a molecule with a water-soluble (*hydrophilic—* "water-loving") side and a lipid-soluble (*hydrophobic*—"water-hating") side. This combination hydrophobic-hydrophilic attribute is the characteristic property of a detergent. Because of this dual solubility, detergents can render lipids soluble in water. It is the function of the bile acids to emulsify dietary lipids and to solubilize the products of fat digestion.

Bile acids are produced in the smooth en-

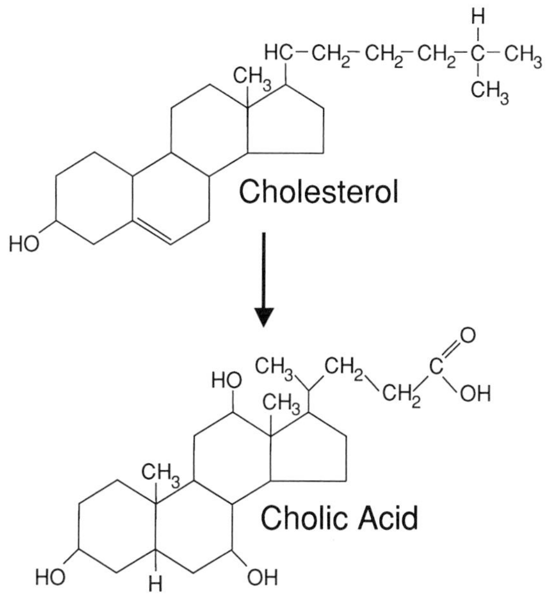

Figure 28–6. The conversion of cholesterol to cholic acid, a representative bile acid. Note the presence of two additional hydroxyl groups on the ring structure of cholic acid, compared to cholesterol. These hydroxyl groups enhance the water solubility and detergent action of the bile acid molecule. Other bile acids differ from cholic acid in the number and position of hydroxyl groups.

doplasmic reticulum of the hepatocytes. As they are secreted from the cells into the lumen of the canaliculi, bile acids "dissolve away" some of the cell membrane components: phospholipids and cholesterol. These constituents—phospholipids, cholesterol, and bile acids—are the major functional components of bile and are important for the digestion and absorption of fats. The mechanism by which bile aids in fat digestion is discussed in Chapter 30.

Bile acids are secreted into the canaliculi as their sodium salts. The presence of bile acid salts and sodium in the canaliculi draws water by osmosis into bile from the cells. The electrolyte composition of canalicular bile usually resembles plasma, but may be somewhat lower in chloride. As bile flows through the bile ducts, water and electrolytes are added. Bicarbonate may be secreted by the duct cells, so that the bicarbonate concentration of bile is often higher than in blood serum.

In addition to bile acids, phospholipids, and cholesterol, bile contains other lipid-soluble organic substances. Of these, the *bile pigments* are present in the highest concentration. Bile pigments are breakdown products of heme porphyrin, a portion of the hemoglobin molecule. The principal bile pigment is *bilirubin*,

which is produced during the normal process of red blood cell turnover. Bilirubin gives bile its characteristic green color. In the lumen of the gut, bilirubin is converted by bacterial action to other compounds. These secondary compounds are responsible for the characteristic brown color of the feces of nonherbivorous animals. Bile pigments serve no useful digestive function: the body simply uses bile, and ultimately feces, as an excretory route for the excretion of these waste products.

The liver serves as an excretory organ for many lipid-soluble substances in addition to bilirubin. The detergent action of the bile acids makes the liver an ideal excretory organ for these types of compounds, compared to the kidney. Substances metabolized and secreted by the liver include many important drugs and toxins. This is important clinically, because the actions of these agents can be potentiated by impaired liver function.

The Gallbladder Stores and Concentrates Bile During the Periods Between Feeding

When there is little or no food in the intestinal lumen, the *sphincter of Oddi*, at the union of the common bile duct and duodenum, is closed, and bile cannot enter the intestine and is diverted into the gallbladder. The gallbladder epithelium absorbs sodium, chloride, and bicarbonate from bile; water is absorbed passively. Thus, in the gallbladder the organic constituents of bile are concentrated while the volume of bile is reduced. In those species, such as horses and rats, that have no gallbladder, the sphincter of Oddi is apparently nonfunctional, and bile is secreted into the intestine during all phases of the digestive cycle.

Bile Secretion Is Initiated by the Presence of Food in the Duodenum and Stimulated by the Return of Bile Acids to the Liver

When food, especially fat-containing food, reaches the duodenum, the GI endocrine cells are stimulated to secrete CCK. CCK causes relaxation of the sphincter of Oddi and contraction of the gallbladder, forcing stored bile into the intestine. Bile acids aid in the digestion and absorption of fats in the jejunum (see Chapter 30), but are not absorbed themselves until they reach the ileum. After absorption in the ileum, the bile acids travel in the portal

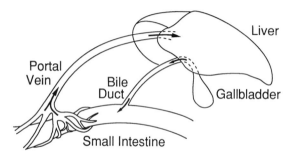

Figure 28-7. Bile acids and other molecules circulate in an enterohepatic cycle. Phases of the cycle include the portal vein, biliary system, and intestinal lumen.

blood to the liver. In the liver, bile acids are almost completely absorbed from the portal blood. As a result, almost no bile acids reach the vena cava, and consequently they are found only in low concentrations in the systemic circulation. The flow of bile acids from liver to intestine, to portal blood to liver, and back to intestine is known as *enterohepatic circulation* (Fig. 28-7).

Bile acids arriving at the liver, by way of the portal circulation, stimulate bile synthesis. Thus, a positive feedback system is initiated when the gallbladder contracts, i.e., the absorption of gallbladder bile from the intestine stimulates additional bile synthesis by the hepatocytes. Rapid bile synthesis continues as long as the sphincter of Oddi is open, and the gallbladder is contracted. When fats are digested, CCK secretion ceases, the sphincter of Oddi closes, and bile is diverted to the gallbladder. Because bile acids are no longer reaching the intestine, they are no longer being absorbed, and thus the stimulus for bile secretion is reduced, and bile flow slows down.

In addition to the effect of CCK on bile secretion, secretin influences secretion from the bile duct epithelium. Secretin stimulates water and bicarbonate secretion from the bile ducts in a manner similar to its effects on the duct cells of the pancreas. Thus, bile may participate in the neutralization of stomach acids.

Bibliography

Argenzio RA: Comparative physiology of the gastrointestinal system. *In* Anderson NV (ed): Veterinary Gastroenterology. Philadelphia, Lea & Febiger, 1980, pp 172–198.

Berne RM, Levy MN: Physiology. St. Louis, CV Mosby, 1983, pp 770–794.

Johnson LR (ed): Gastrointestinal Physiology. St. Louis, CV Mosby, 1985, pp 53–104.

Johnson LR (ed): Physiology of the Gastrointestinal Tract, 2nd ed. New York, Raven Press, 1987, pp 745–1208.

PRACTICE QUESTIONS FOR CHAPTER 28

1. In monogastrics, saliva produced during periods of rapid secretion has a higher electrolyte concentration than saliva produced during periods of slow salivary secretion. From your understanding of salivary gland physiology, which appears to be the most likely explanation?

   a. During periods of slow salivary secretion, the acinar cells are inactive, and low-electrolyte saliva is secreted by the duct cells.
   b. Parasympathetic stimulation of the acinar cells results in the elaboration of a more electrolyte-rich saliva.
   c. Gastrin stimulation increases the electrolyte concentration of saliva.
   d. During rapid secretion, fluid produced by the acinar cells is exposed to the actions of the duct cells for a shorter period of time than during slow rates of secretion.
   e. Different cell types within the acinus are responsible for salivary production, depending on the type of stimulus.

2. Some nutritionists are experimenting with a drug that increases salivary secretion in cattle. What effect do you think this would have on rumen pH?

   a. Increase rumen pH
   b. Decrease rumen pH
   c. No effect on rumen pH

3. Inhibition of the enzyme carbonic anhydrase is likely to have what effect on gastric pH?

   a. Decrease gastric pH
   b. Increase gastric pH
   c. No effect on gastric pH

4. Which of the following is NOT a potential stimulus for gastric acid secretion?

  a. Norepinephrine secretion resulting from stimulation of sympathetic nerves
  b. Vagal nerve activity resulting from the sight of food
  c. The presence of undigested protein in the pyloric antrum
  d. Acetylcholine release stimulated by gastric stretch receptors acting on nerves of the intrinsic system
  e. Histamine release from cells in the gastric mucosa

5. Which of the following is NOT a natural ligand for receptors in the pancreas?

  a. Cholecystokinin (CCK)
  b. Acetylcholine
  c. Gastrin
  d. Secretin

29

Digestion and Absorption: The Nonfermentative Processes

1. Digestion and absorption are separate, but related, processes
2. The small intestinal mucosa has a large surface area and epithelial cells with "leaky" junctions between them
3. At the intestinal surface, there is a microenvironment made up of glycocalyx, mucus, and an unstirred water layer.

DIGESTION

1. Breaking down food particle size by physical action is an important part of the digestive process
2. Chemical digestion results in the reduction of complex nutrients into simpler molecules
3. Luminal-phase carbohydrate digestion results in the production of short-chain polysaccharides
4. Luminal-phase digestion of carbohydrates applies only to starches, because sugars are all digested in the membranous phase
5. Proteins are digested by a variety of luminal-phase enzymes
6. Membranous-phase digestive enzymes are a structural part of the intestinal surface membrane
7. Membranous-phase digestion occurs within the microenvironment of the unstirred water layer, intestinal mucus, and glycocalyx
8. A specific membranous-phase enzyme exists for the digestion of each type of polysaccharide
9. Complete digestion of peptides to free amino acids takes place both on the enterocyte surface and within the cells

INTESTINAL ABSORPTION

1. Glucose is absorbed in combination with sodium
2. The movement of glucose across the basolateral membrane is by diffusion

3. The NA^+, K^+ ATPase system indirectly provides energy for the absorption of glucose

4. Free amino acids are absorbed by sodium co-transport

ABSORPTION OF WATER AND ELECTROLYTES

1. There are at least three distinct mechanisms of sodium absorption
2. Three major mechanisms exist for the absorption of chloride
3. Bicarbonate ion is secreted by several digestive glands and must be recovered from the gut if body acid-base balance is to be maintained
4. Potassium is absorbed, primarily, by passive diffusion through the paracellular route
5. The major mechanisms of electrolyte absorption are selectively distributed along the gut
6. All intestinal water absorption is passive, occurring because of the absorption of osmotically active solutes

INTESTINAL SECRETION OF WATER AND ELECTROLYTES

1. Passive increases in luminal osmotic pressure occur during hydrolytic digestion and result in water secretion
2. Active secretion of electrolytes from the crypt epithelium leads to intestinal water secretion

GASTROINTESTINAL BLOOD FLOW

1. Water and solute movement between the lateral spaces and villous capillaries is subject to the same forces that govern water and solute movement between the extracellular and vascular fluids in other tissues
2. Absorbed nutrients enter the capillaries by diffusion from the lateral spaces
3. A counter-current, osmotic-multiplier system may increase the osmolality of blood at the tips of the villi, further promoting absorption of water into the blood
4. Disturbances in the venous drainage from the intestine can markedly affect the mechanisms of capillary absorption in the villi

DIGESTION AND ABSORPTION OF FATS

1. Detergent action, as well as enzymatic action, is necessary for the digestion and absorption of lipids
2. Lipids are absorbed through the apical membrane by simple diffusion
3. Bile acids are reabsorbed from the ileum by a sodium co-transport system
4. Absorbed lipids are packaged into *chylomicrons* before leaving the enterocytes

GROWTH AND DEVELOPMENT OF THE INTESTINAL EPITHELIUM

1. The length of intestinal villi is determined by the relative rates of cell loss at the tips and cell replenishment at the base

DIGESTION IN THE NEONATE

1. During the first few hours of life, proteins are not digested, but absorbed intact
2. The major intestinal disaccharidase switches from lactase to maltase with maturity

PATHOPHYSIOLOGY OF DIARRHEA

1. Diarrhea occurs when there is a mismatch between secretion and absorption

Digestion and Absorption Are Separate, but Related, Processes

Digestion is the process of breaking down complex nutrients into simple molecules. On the other hand, absorption is the process of transporting those simple molecules across the intestinal epithelium (Fig. 29–1). The two processes are the result of different biochemical events occurring within the gut. Both processes are necessary for the assimilation of nutrients into the body; absorption cannot occur if food is not digested, and the process of digestion is fruitless if the digested nutrients cannot be absorbed. Disturbances of nutrient assimilation are common in veterinary medicine and may be caused by a variety of diseases, some of which affect digestion, whereas others affect absorption. The overt signs of failure of nutrient assimilation are often similar, but the biochemical lesions and specific therapies associated with maldigestive disease can be quite different from those associated with malabsorptive disease. Therefore, diagnosing the cause of failure of nutrient assimilation is a frequent challenge faced by veterinary clinicians, a challenge that requires a thorough understanding of the physiology of nutrient digestion and absorption. In this

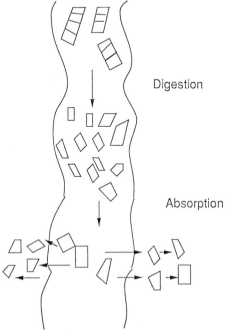

Digestion

Absorption

Figure 29–1. Digestion is the process of reducing macromolecules into their constituent monomers. Absorption is the transport of the resultant monomers across the intestinal epithelium into the blood stream.

chapter, the structural characteristics of the small intestinal epithelium that are of particular importance to the digestive and absorptive processes are reviewed first.

The Small Intestinal Mucosa Has a Large Surface Area and Epithelial Cells with "Leaky" Junctions Between Them

Contact between the small intestinal mucosa and the luminal contents is facilitated by an extensive intestinal surface area. Three levels of surface convolutions serve to expand the surface area of the small intestine (see Fig. 26–2). First, there are large folds of mucosa known as *plicae circulares* that add to the intestinal surface area of some animals, but are not present in all species. Second, the mucosal surface is covered with finger-like epithelial projections known as *villi*. These structures are present in all species and increase the intestinal surface area by some 10- to 14-fold, compared to a flat surface of equal size. Lastly, the villi themselves are covered with a brush-like surface membrane known as the *brush border*. The brush border is composed of submicroscopic *microvilli* that further increase the surface area (Fig. 29–2). At the base of the villi are gland-like structures known as *crypts of Lieberkühn* (Fig. 29–3). The villi and crypts are covered with a continuous layer of cellular epithelium.

The epithelial cells covering the villi and crypts are called *enterocytes*. Each enterocyte has two distinctly different types of cell membranes (Fig. 29–4). The cell surface facing the lumen is called the apex and is covered by the *apical membrane*. The apical membrane contains the microvilli. Under the light microscope, the microvilli give the cell surface a brush-like appearance, leading to the name brush border, which is synonymous with the apical membrane. Covering the apical membrane, and encasing the microvilli, is a jelly-like layer of glycoprotein known as the *glycocalyx*. Important digestive enzymes and other proteins are attached to the microvilli and project into the glycocalyx. Under the intense magnification of the electron microscope, these enzyme molecules, as well as other proteins, give the glycocalyx a fuzzy appearance (see Fig. 29–2). The apical membrane is a complex and unusual cellular membrane with a high protein content.

The remaining portion of the enterocyte plasma membrane, that part not facing the gut

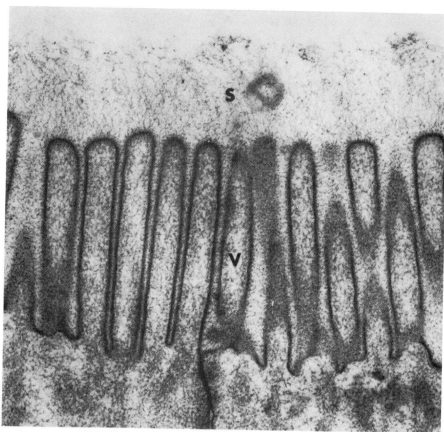

Figure 29–2. Electronmicrograph of the microvilli of the intestinal brush border. The brush border is composed of the apical membranes of enterocytes. Note the indistinct array of molecular material (S) that radiates away from the microvilli (V); membranous-phase digestion occurs within this array of molecular material, which includes the membrane-bound digestive enzymes. (From Johnson LR, Christensen J, Jacobsen ED, et al (eds): Physiology of the Gastrointestinal Tract, 2nd ed. New York, Raven Press, 1987, p 1215.)

lumen, is called the *basolateral membrane,* referring to the base and lateral sides of the cell. This membrane is not especially unusual and indeed has many similarities to cell membranes of other tissues. Although the basolateral membrane is not in direct contact with ingesta in the gut lumen, it serves an important role in intestinal absorption; nutrients that are absorbed into the enterocytes through the apical membrane must exit the cell through the basolateral membrane before gaining access to the blood stream.

The attachments between adjacent enterocytes are called *tight junctions.* These connections serve a special function in the process of digestion and absorption. The tight junctions form a narrow band of attachment between adjacent enterocytes. The band is near the apical end of the cells and divides the apical membrane from the basolateral membrane. The junctions may be called "tight," but from

a molecular standpoint, they are rather loose. This is especially true in the duodenum and jejunum, where the tight junctions are loose enough to allow the free passage of water and small electrolytes. However, organic molecules will not penetrate the tight junctions.

The narrow nature of the tight junctions leaves the majority of the basolateral membrane unattached to its neighboring membrane on the adjacent enterocyte. This arrangement creates a potential space between enterocytes. This area between the lateral surfaces of the enterocytes is called the *lateral space.* The lateral spaces are normally distended and filled with extracellular fluid. At the end of the lateral spaces nearest the apical membrane, the extracellular fluid is separated from the fluid of the intestinal lumen only by the tight junctions. At the opposite end of the lateral spaces, the fluid is separated from the blood by only the endothelium of the intestinal capillaries. Both

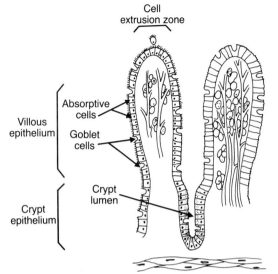

Figure 29–3. The intestinal epithelium is a one-cell-thick layer that is continuous over the villi and crypts of Lieber-kühn.

the tight junctions and the capillary endothelium are permeable barriers that allow the free passage of water and small molecules. Thus, there is relatively free flow of water and most electrolytes between the fluid in the lumen of the intestine, the extracellular fluid in the lateral spaces, and the blood.

At the Intestinal Surface, There Is a Microenvironment Made Up of Glycocalyx, Mucus, and an Unstirred Water Layer

Liberally interspersed among the entero-cytes are *goblet cells,* which secrete a rich layer of mucus that covers the mucosa. At the brush border surface, the mucus blends into the glycocalyx, the two layers forming a viscous coating that tends to trap molecules near the apical membrane. In addition to the mucus and glycocalyx layers, there is an area near the intestinal surface known as the *unstirred water layer.* With respect to the unstirred water layer, the intestine can be likened to a large stream or river, i.e., the water in the center flows relatively rapidly, whereas the water near the edge or bank is quiet and flows slowly. Because of the same fluid-friction phenomena that causes the water on the banks of rivers to be less turbulent and flow at a slower rate than water in center stream, the water very near the intestinal surface is quiet and flows at a much slower rate than water in the

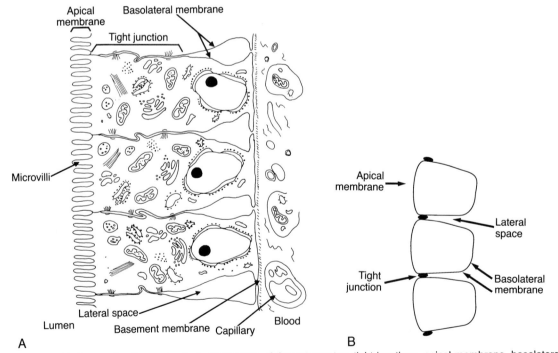

Figure 29–4. Understanding the anatomical relationships of the enterocytes, tight junctions, apical membrane, basolateral membrane, and lateral spaces is critical to understanding the physiology of intestinal absorption. (*A*) An anatomical illustration of the intestinal epithelium. (*B*) A stylized sketch of the epithelium. It is important to understand the relationship between part A and part B of this diagram.

central part of the lumen. The unstirred water layer, mucus, and glycocalyx form an important diffusion barrier through which nutrients must pass before entering the enterocytes.

DIGESTION

Breaking Down Food Particle Size by Physical Action Is an Important Part of the Digestive Process

The overall process of digestion is the physical and chemical breaking down of food particles and molecules into subunits suitable for absorption. Physical reduction of food particle size is important, not only because it allows food to flow through the relatively narrow digestive tube, but also because it increases the surface area of the food particles, thus increasing the area exposed to the actions of digestive enzymes. Physical reduction of food particle size begins with mastication (chewing) but is completed by the grinding action of the distal stomach. In the distal stomach, the physical action of grinding is aided by the chemical action of pepsin and hydrochloric acid. The chemical actions of these stomach secretions break down connective tissue and thus aid in breaking apart food particles, especially foods of animal origin. The reduction of food particle size by physical means is essentially complete when food leaves the stomach, as described in Chapter 27 under motility of the distal stomach.

Chemical Digestion Results in the Reduction of Complex Nutrients into Simpler Molecules

In the case of each major nutrient, chemical digestion is accomplished by the process of *hydrolysis.* Hydrolysis, as its name implies, is the splitting of a chemical bond by the insertion of a water molecule. Glycosidic linkages in carbohydrates, peptide bonds in proteins, ester bonds in fats, and phosphodiester bonds in nucleic acids are all cleaved by hydrolysis during digestion. Hydrolytic splitting of these various chemical bonds is illustrated in Figure 29–5.

Hydrolysis in the digestive tract is catalyzed by the action of enzymes. There are two general classes of digestive enzymes: those that act within the lumen of the gut, and those that act at the membrane surface of the epithelium. Enzymes acting within the lumen originate from the major gastrointestinal (GI) glands, including the salivary gland, gastric glands, and especially, the pancreas. The secretions of these glands become thoroughly mixed with ingesta and exert their actions throughout the lumen of their associated gut segments; thus, the actions they catalyze are referred to as the *luminal phase* of digestion. In general, luminal-phase digestion results in the incomplete hydrolysis of nutrients, resulting in the formation of short-chain polymers from the original macromolecules (Fig. 29–6).

The hydrolytic process is completed by enzymes that are chemically bound to the surface

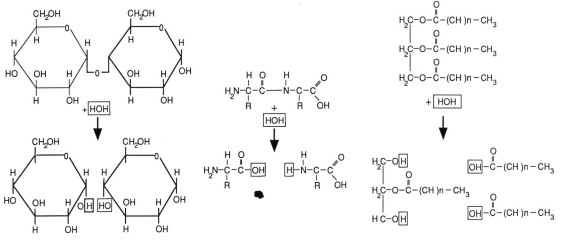

A Hydrolysis of glycosidic bond   **B** Hydrolysis of peptide bond   **C** Hydrolysis of two ester bonds in a triglyceride molecule

Figure 29–5. The major polymeric molecules forming food nutrients can be split into their constituent monomers by the insertion of a water molecule. This is referred to as *hydrolysis* and is the major action of the digestive enzymes.

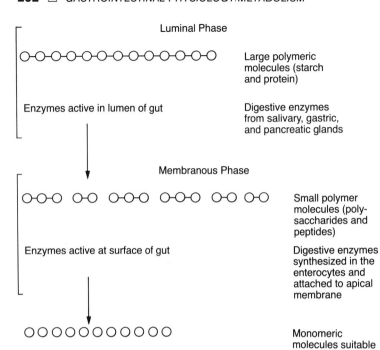

Figure 29–6. Luminal-phase and membranous-phase digestion.

epithelium of the small intestine. These enzymes break the short-chain polymers resulting from luminal-phase digestion into monomers that can be absorbed across the epithelium. This final phase, which occurs at the epithelial membrane surface, is referred to as the *membranous phase* of digestion. Membranous-phase digestion is followed closely by absorption.

Luminal-Phase Carbohydrate Digestion Results in the Production of Short-Chain Polysaccharides

Carbohydrates are nutrients containing carbon, hydrogen, and oxygen atoms arranged as long chains of repeating simple-sugar molecules. Dietary carbohydrates originate primarily from plants. There are three general types of plant carbohydrates: fibers, sugars, and starches. Fibers are the structural parts of plants and form an important energy source for herbivorous animals; however, plant fibers are not subject to hydrolytic digestion by mammalian enzymes and, therefore, cannot be digested directly by animals. Digestion of plant fibers is discussed under fermentative digestion in Chapter 30.

Sugars are energy-transport molecules in plants. Sugars, or *saccharides*, may be *simple* (made up of a single molecular unit, monosaccharides) or *complex* (made up of two or more repeating saccharide subunits, polysaccharides). *Glucose, galactose,* and *fructose* are the most important simple sugars in animal diets. These monosaccharides are present, preformed in small quantities, in normal diets; however, most monosaccharides absorbed from the gut arise from the enzymatic hydrolysis of more complex carbohydrates. Complex sugars are referred to as di-, tri-, and oligosaccharides, depending on the number of repeating simple-sugar subunits. Oligosaccharides contain several monomer units, usually between 3 and 10. Important complex sugars in animal diets are *lactose,* or milk sugar, and *sucrose,* or table sugar. Lactose is a disaccharide composed of glucose and galactose, whereas sucrose is a disaccharide composed of glucose and fructose. Other important complex sugars are *maltose, isomaltose,* and *maltotriose.* These latter three sugars are composed of two or three repeating glucose units (Fig. 29–7). They are seldomly present preformed in the diet, but rather are formed in the gut as intermediate products of starch digestion.

Starch is an energy-storage carbohydrate of plants and forms the major energy-yielding nutrient in the diets of many omnivorous animals, such as pigs, rats, and primates. There are two chemical forms of starch known as *amylose* and *amylopectin.* These are both long-chain glucose polymers, but amylose is a straight-chain molecule containing glucose

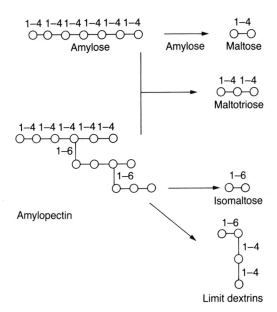

Figure 29–7. The two major forms of dietary starch are amylose and amylopectin. Amylose is composed of repeating glucose units joined by α [1–4] linkages. Amylopectin is a similar molecule except that there are branch points formed by α [1–6] linkages. Because of the different linkage points, various polysaccharides result from luminal-phase digestion, as illustrated.

monomers linked by α[1–4] glycosidic linkages. Amylopectin also contains glucose chains joined by α[1–4] glycosidic linkages, but the amylopectin chains are branched, having an α[1–6] linkage at each branch point (see Fig. 29–7). Although the chemical structure of starch is limited to these two molecular types, the physical structure and encapsulation of starches vary among plant sources. This variation results in the unique characteristics of starches from different sources, such as wheat, corn, or barley.

Luminal-Phase Digestion of Carbohydrates Applies Only to Starches, Because Sugars Are All Digested in the Membranous Phase

The enzyme involved in luminal starch digestion is α-amylase, which is actually a mixture of several similar molecules. Alpha-amylase arises from the pancreas in all species and, in addition, the salivary glands of some species (see Chapter 28). The α[1–4] linkages of either amylose or amylopectin are attacked by α-amylase. Characteristic of luminal-phase digestion, α-amylase does not break off, or cleave, single glucose units from the ends of the chain. Rather, the starch chains are broken

in their midsections, resulting in the production of polysaccharides of intermediate chain length, known as *dextrins*. These chains continue to be attacked until di- and trisaccharide units are formed: maltose and maltotriose, respectively. This digestive process proceeds for amylopectin in the same way as it does for amylose, except that the α[1–6] linkages at the chain branch points of amylopectin are not hydrolyzed. Because these branch points are not hydrolyzed, branch-chain oligosaccharides, known as *limit dextrins*, as well as an α[1–6]-linked disaccharide, known as *isomaltose*, are formed (see Fig. 29–7). The end result of luminal-phase carbohydrate digestion is the creation of many di-, tri-, and oligosaccharides from large starch molecules. These polysaccharide molecules are not hydrolyzed further in the luminal phase.

Proteins Are Digested by a Variety of Luminal-Phase Enzymes

Proteins are a source of amino acids, essential components of all animal diets. Dietary proteins come from both plant and animal sources. The general pattern of protein digestion is similar to carbohydrate digestion in that large molecular proteins are broken down into small peptide chains by luminal digestion. Subsequent digestion of the peptide chains to individual amino acids occurs to a large extent by membranous-phase digestion, although, in contrast to carbohydrate digestion, a portion of free monomers, i.e., amino acids, are released in the luminal phase. A major difference between protein and carbohydrate digestion is in the number of different enzyme types involved. The relatively large number of enzymes involved in protein digestion, compared to starch digestion, could be expected if one considers that starch molecules are made up of only one kind of monomer, glucose. Therefore, only one kind of carbohydrate bond has to be broken. On the other hand, proteins are made up of infinite combinations of up to 20 individual types of amino acids; the various proteolytic enzymes are necessary for digestion, because they differ in their efficiency in cleaving peptide bonds between specific kinds of amino acids. The major luminal-phase proteolytic enzymes are listed in Table 29–1. Most proteolytic enzymes are *endopeptidases*, meaning that they break proteins at internal points along the amino acid chains, resulting in the production of short-chain peptides from com-

Table 29–1
LUMINAL-PHASE ENZYMES OF PROTEIN DIGESTION

Enzyme	Action	Source	Precursor	Activator
Pepsin	Endopeptidase	Gastric glands	Pepsinogen	HCl, pepsin
Chymosin (Rennin)	Endopeptidase	Gastric glands	Chymosinogen	?
Trypsin	Endopeptidase	Pancreas	Trypsinogen	Enterokinase, trypsin
Chymotrypsin	Endopeptidase	Pancreas	Chymotrypsinogen	Trypsin
Elastase	Endopeptidase	Pancreas	Pro-elastase	Trypsin
Carboxypeptidase A	Exopeptidase	Pancreas	Pro-carboxypeptidase A	Trypsin
Carboxypeptidase B	Exopeptidase	Pancreas	Pro-carboxypeptidase B	Trypsin

plex proteins. Endopeptidases produce essentially no free amino acids. Two *exopeptidases,* which release individual amino acids from ends of peptide chains, are secreted also from the pancreas and are active in luminal-phase digestion.

The proteolytic enzymes are secreted from the stomach glands or pancreas in the form of inactive *zymogens* (see Chapter 28 for a discussion of zymogens), which are activated in the stomach or intestinal lumen, respectively. These enzymes must be secreted in an inactive form, because otherwise the active enzymes would digest the cells in which they are synthesized. Activation of the zymogens occurs in the gut lumen. The stomach enzymes, pepsinogen and chymosinogen, are activated by hydrochloric acid (HCl) in the stomach. Pepsinogen is activated also by pepsin in an autocatalytic feedback loop. Trypsinogen from the pancreas is activated by *enterokinase,* an enzyme elaborated by the duodenal mucosal cells. The active enzyme, trypsin, then serves

as an autocatalytic agent to activate additional trypsinogen, as well as the other pancreatic protein-digesting enzymes. The cascade of intraluminal zymogen activation is illustrated in Figure 29–8.

Luminal-phase protein digestion begins in the stomach. Gastric digestion of protein is facilitated not only by the stomach enzymes, but also by HCl, which has hydrolytic properties of its own. The acid environment of the stomach is suited to the action of pepsin, which has its optimal activity at pH 1–3. Gastric hydrolysis of protein is probably important to the physical, as well as chemical, digestion of protein, because most connective tissue of animal origin is protein in nature; digestion of connective tissue aids in breaking food down into particles small enough to pass the pylorus. Although stomach action is important in initiating protein digestion, it is not essential; animals without stomachs can digest proteins, provided they have a functional pancreas and are fed small, frequent meals of soft, moist

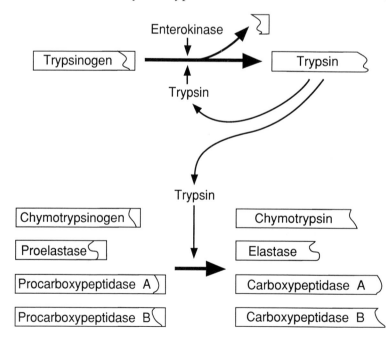

Figure 29–8. The activation of pancreatic zymogens. Note that trypsinogen is activated by trypsin, as well as by the duodenal enzyme enterokinase. The autocatalytic action of trypsin on trypsinogen forms a positive feedback loop that assures the rapid and complete activation of trypsinogen in the gut. Trypsin then activates the other zymogens.

food. Luminal-phase digestion of proteins is completed in the small intestine by the action of pancreatic enzymes.

Membranous-Phase Digestive Enzymes Are a Structural Part of the Intestinal Surface Membrane

Membranous-phase digestion, like its luminal counterpart, occurs because of the hydrolytic action of enzymes. The difference between the two phases is that membranous-phase enzymes are chemically bound to the surface membrane of the intestine, thus the enzyme substrates must be in contact with the epithelium before hydrolysis can occur. These membrane-bound digestive enzymes are synthesized within the enterocytes, and are subsequently transported to the luminal surface of the apical membrane. They remain attached to the surface by a short anchor segment while the large, catalytic portion of the enzyme molecule projects away from the surface, toward the gut lumen.

Membranous-Phase Digestion Occurs Within the Microenvironment of the Unstirred Water Layer, Intestinal Mucus, and Glycocalyx

The unstirred water layer, mucus, and glycocalyx form a diffuse zone separating the mucosal surface from the lumen of the intestine. The membranous-phase digestive enzymes project from the apical membrane into this surface layer. The quiet surface layer forms a microenvironment in which membranous-phase digestion occurs. Peptides and polysaccharides in the intestinal lumen must diffuse into the surface layer before membranous-phase digestion can take place. Furthermore, most of the products of membranous-phase digestion never diffuse away from the surface environment back into the lumen of the intestine: instead, they are absorbed, soon after formation, into the underlying epithelial cells. This arrangement is efficient, because it assures that the final products of carbohydrate and protein digestion are formed near their site of absorption, avoiding the need for long diffusion distances (Fig. 29–9).

A Specific Membranous-Phase Enzyme Exists for the Digestion of Each Type of Polysaccharide

The membranous-phase enzymes of carbohydrate digestion have as their substrates di-

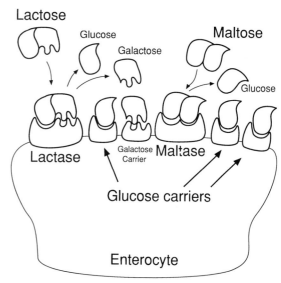

Figure 29–9. The relationship of membranous-phase digestion to absorption. The enzymes responsible for digestion and the carrier molecules responsible for absorption are both part of the apical membrane. The products of digestion are thus formed in the immediate vicinity of the carrier proteins, preventing the need for long diffusion distances. Specific enzymes and carrier molecules are present for the various substrates, as illustrated.

etary polysaccharides, such as sucrose and lactose, as well as the polysaccharide products of luminal-phase starch digestion, including maltose and isomaltose. The specific membranous-phase enzymes are named according to their substrates and include *maltase, isomaltose, sucrase,* and *lactase.* The sole product of maltose and isomaltose digestion is glucose, whereas in addition to glucose, fructose and galactose are produced from the digestion of sucrose and lactose, respectively. All polysaccharides are digested to monosaccharides prior to absorption (Fig. 29–10).

Complete Digestion of Peptides to Free Amino Acids Takes Place Both on the Enterocyte Surface and Within the Cells

Membranous-phase digestion of peptides is in some respects similar to that of carbohydrates; peptide-digesting enzymes, or *peptidases,* are present on the enterocyte-surface membrane and extend into the glycocalyx. These enzymes hydrolyze the peptide products of luminal-phase protein digestion, yielding free amino acids. Some of the longer chain peptides are incompletely digested, yielding dipeptides and tripeptides. A large portion of dietary amino acids are absorbed directly in

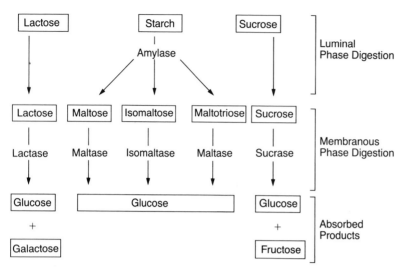

Figure 29–10. Luminal- and membranous-phase digestion of carbohydrate. Note that specific enzymes exist for each polysaccharide and that a limited number of monomers are formed eventually from a relatively large number of starches and polysaccharides.

the form of dipeptides and tripeptides. This mode of absorption is in contrast to carbohydrates, in which only monomeric, simple sugars may pass the apical membrane. Di- and tripeptides that are absorbed intact are subsequently hydrolyzed by the action of intracellular peptidases, which results in the formation of free amino acids that are then available for passage into the blood. Thus, the final digestion of peptides to free amino acids may occur at either of two sites: on the surface membrane of the enterocyte, or within the cell. In either case, the final product of protein digestion is free amino acid (Fig. 29–11).

INTESTINAL ABSORPTION

Absorption refers to the movement of the products of digestion across the intestinal mucosa and into the vascular system for distribution. Absorption can occur through one of two routes. First, nutrients may pass completely through the enterocytes, entering at the apical membrane and leaving through the basolateral membrane into the lateral spaces; this is called *transcellular absorption*. Alternatively, nutrients may move through the tight junctions directly into the lateral spaces; this is called *paracellular absorption*. Transcellular and paracellular absorption works in a complementary manner to produce an efficient absorptive process (Fig. 29–12).

Glucose Is Absorbed in Combination with Sodium

The absorption of glucose provides an important and well-studied example of a mech-

anism of nutrient absorption found in the intestine, as well as several other body tissues. As glucose is produced at the intestinal surface by the digestion of polysaccharides, it quickly attaches to special transport proteins (see Fig. 29–9). These transport proteins, like the membranous-phase digestive enzymes, are located

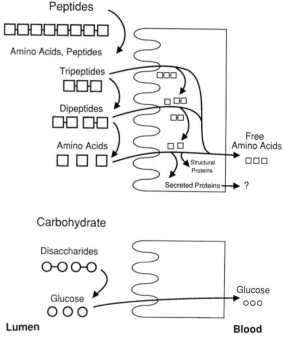

Figure 29–11. Membranous-phase digestion of peptides. Note that tripeptides and dipeptides may be hydrolyzed to their constituent amino acids either on the apical membrane or within the enterocyte. This is in contrast to carbohydrate digestion, in which all disaccharide hydrolysis occurs at the apical membrane. Regardless of at which site the final hydrolysis of peptides occurs, the product absorbed into the blood is free amino acid (see Fig. 29–16).

Lumen   Blood

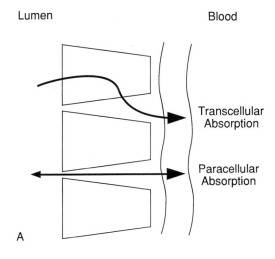

Transcellular
Absorption

Paracellular
Absorption

A

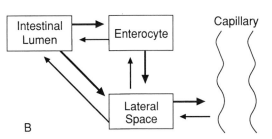

B

Figure 29–12. Transcellular and paracellular absorption.
(*A*) Substances move from the intestinal lumen to the
capillary by either transcellular (through the enterocyte) or
paracellular (through the tight junction) absorption. (*B*) The
intestinal lumen, enterocytes, and lateral spaces form three
separate pools that may contain nutrients in different concentrations. Note that nutrients move into the capillaries
from the lateral spaces and that reverse transport (from the
capillary to the intestinal lumen) is possible for some substances.

dition, the role of sodium co-transport extends
beyond its direct role in the absorption of its
specific substrates; it has a major indirect effect
on the absorption of water and electrolytes
other than sodium.

To better understand the physiologically eloquent and clinically important process of sodium co-transport, it may be necessary to
review several of the earlier chapters of this
book. Be sure you understand the process of
diffusion across membranes (Chapter 1), the
difference in composition of intracellular and
extracellular fluid (Chapters 2, 3), the electrical
polarity across cell membranes (Chapters 1,
3), the function of the Na^+, K^+ adenosinetriphosphatase (ATPase) pump, and the function
of selective ion channels (Chapters 1, 3). In
considering sodium co-transport, first remember that molecules diffuse across membrane
barriers in response to chemical and electrical
gradients. In some respects, the situation with
regard to sodium co-transport is no different
than in the case of simple diffusion; there is
movement of molecules from an area of higher
concentration to lower concentration and
movement of positively charged ions to areas
of negative electrical polarity. A concentration

on the apical membrane. The proteins have
specific binding sites for glucose and sodium
ions, and when each binding site is occupied,
the entire complex, i.e., transport protein,
glucose, and sodium ion, migrates across the
apical membrane from outer to inner surface
(Fig. 29–13). Once on the intracellular surface
of the apical membrane, the transport protein
releases its glucose and sodium load into the
intracellular fluid; the protein returns to the
outer surface of the membrane, ready to repeat
the transfer process.

Transport of glucose by this process will not
occur unless sodium is present, hence the
process is referred to as *sodium co-transport.*
Sodium co-transport is especially important,
because it provides the absorptive mechanism
for glucose; however, several other nutrients
are absorbed by this mechanism also. In ad-

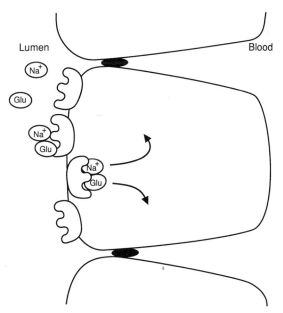

Figure 29–13. Sodium-glucose co-transport. Transport is
mediated by a protein in the apical membrane. The protein
has ligand sites for sodium ion and glucose; when both
sites are occupied, the protein alters its configuration so
that the sodium and glucose are released on the inner face
of the apical membrane. The protein, then free of its ligands,
reverses its orientation, ready to transport another sodium-
glucose pair.

gradient is created by the high sodium ion concentration in the gut lumen and the low sodium concentration in the enterocytes. The relatively high sodium concentration in the luminal fluid is maintained by sodium-rich digestive secretions, e.g., saliva, pancreatic juice, and so forth, whereas the low sodium concentration within enterocytes is maintained by the Na^+, K^+ ATPase pump located in the basolateral membrane. This is the same Na^+, K^+ ATPase pump found in the plasma membranes of most cells of the body and is responsible for the normally low intracellular sodium concentration.

In addition to maintaining a low sodium concentration within the enterocytes, the Na^+, K^+ ATPase pump also creates a transmembrane electrical potential difference, with the negative pole oriented to the inside of the cell. Because of the combined chemical concentration and electrical potential differences, there is a strong gradient favoring the movement of the positively charged sodium ion from the intestinal lumen into the enterocyte. This provides the stimulus for glucose-sodium co-transport. As sodium enters the cells, it is immediately expelled by the pump system, thus the chemical and electrical sodium gradients are maintained, and sodium absorption continues (Fig. 29–14).

At the beginning of the absorptive process, after consumption of a carbohydrate meal, the situation with respect to glucose is similar to that for sodium. That is, there is a high concentration of glucose on the luminal side of the apical membrane, due to the rapid diges-

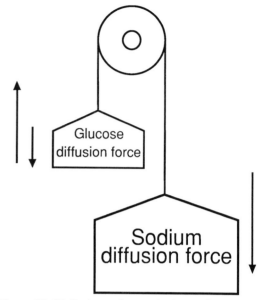

Figure 29–15. During co-transport, glucose is transported against an unfavorable concentration gradient. This diagram illustrates that the large sodium concentration difference across the apical membrane provides energy to transport glucose against its concentration gradient.

tion of polysaccharides, and a low intracellular glucose concentration, which is the normal, resting condition of cells. At this early phase there is a chemical gradient favoring movement of glucose across the apical membrane into the enterocytes; however, as absorption proceeds, the transfer of glucose into the cells increases the intracellular glucose concentration while reducing the luminal concentration, eventually eliminating the favorable absorption gradient. However, glucose absorption is coupled to sodium absorption, so as long as sodium is being absorbed, glucose will come along with it. In contrast to the glucose gradient, the sodium absorption gradient is maintained by the Na^+, K^+ ATPase pump, even in the face of rapid sodium absorption. The electrochemical gradient for sodium absorption is so great that it provides the energy to move glucose against its concentration gradient and into the cells. Energetically, you might conceive of this situation as the two unequal weights illustrated in Figure 29–15; as sodium flows "down" its electrochemical gradient, it pulls glucose "up" its chemical gradient. This mechanism is so efficient that near the end of the absorptive period glucose is moved against a strong concentration gradient, resulting in the nearly complete removal of glucose from

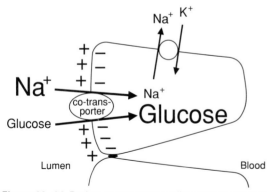

Figure 29–14. During co-transport, sodium moves down its electrochemical gradient. The favorable gradient for sodium movement is maintained by the continuous action of the Na^+, K^+ ATPase pump. During absorption, the glucose concentration difference appears to become unfavorable for transport, but absorption continues because of the sodium gradient (see Fig. 29–15).

the intestinal contents and the achievement of relatively high glucose concentrations in the enterocytes.

The Movement of Glucose Across the Basolateral Membrane Is by Diffusion

During absorption, the concentration of glucose in the enterocytes increases until at some point it exceeds the glucose concentration in the extracellular fluid of the lateral spaces. When this occurs, there is a favorable gradient for glucose diffusion out of the enterocyte into the lateral spaces, from which it can continue to diffuse into the blood of the intestinal capillaries. Back diffusion of glucose out of the lateral spaces, through the tight junctions, and into the gut lumen is prevented, because the tight junctions are impermeable to glucose. The net, or total effect, of glucose-sodium co-transport is that glucose is transported from the lumen of the gut into the blood, even at the end of the absorptive period when the intestinal glucose concentration is much lower than the blood glucose concentration.

The Na⁺, K⁺ ATPase System Indirectly Provides Energy for the Absorption of Glucose

While glucose is being absorbed during periods when the luminal concentration is less than the intracellular concentration of the enterocytes, it must be moved "up hill" against its concentration gradient. This represents chemical work and means that there must be an energy input. As pointed out earlier, the sodium electrochemical gradient provides the direct supply of energy to run the absorptive process. This energy is supplied in turn by the Na⁺, K⁺ ATPase pump. This enzyme pump uses the biological energy represented by adenosine triphosphate (ATP) to expel sodium from the cell and thus provides the transcellular sodium electrochemical gradient that directly promotes the absorption of glucose. In the process of removing sodium from the cells, ATP is converted to adenosine diphosphate (ADP), signifying the utilization of biological energy. The energy demand for intestinal absorption is high. In a rapidly growing animal on high feed intake, the total energy needed for intestinal absorption may amount to 50% of the animal's total energy needs at rest.

Sodium co-transport is an eloquent physiological system; only one mechanism for direct utilization of ATP is necessary to drive the absorptive process, not only for glucose, but as discussed later, for several other molecules that are also absorbed by sodium co-transport. Furthermore, the Na⁺, K⁺ ATPase pump is an enzyme system necessary for many aspects of cellular function, not only transport functions. Thus, the body uses one enzyme system to support a variety of cellular processes.

Free Amino Acids Are Absorbed by Sodium Co-Transport

The products of membranous-phase protein digestion are free amino acids and di- or tripeptides. The amino acids are absorbed by sodium co-transport in a manner completely similar to glucose, except that specific amino acid transport proteins are involved (Fig. 29–16). There are several distinct transport proteins that participate in the sodium co-transport of amino acids. These include specific transport proteins for acidic, basic, and neutral amino acids.

The absorption of di- and tripeptides is less well understood than that of amino acids. There is no question that absorption of these short peptides accounts for a significant portion of the total amount of amino acids that pass the apical membrane, but the mechanism of absorption is still under study. Some investigators believe that sodium co-transport may be involved in the transport of peptides, as well as free amino acids.

In addition to glucose and amino acids, other molecules are absorbed also by sodium co-transport. Examples include galactose, bile acids, and some vitamins, such as thiamine. In each case, there is a specific sodium co-transport protein for each type of molecule absorbed.

ABSORPTION OF WATER AND ELECTROLYTES

Conservation of the body's supply of water and electrolytes, primarily sodium, potassium, chloride, and bicarbonate, is a high priority in sustaining life. The gut plays a major role in this conservation, not only because it is the portal of entry for replenishment of the nutrients, but also because water and electrolytes in GI secretions must be efficiently reclaimed to maintain body composition. The most immediate clinical ramifications of GI disease

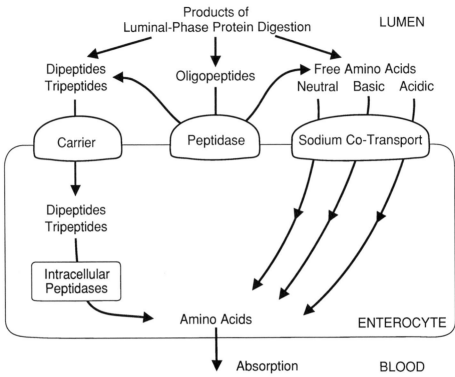

Figure 29–16. At least three different sodium co-transport proteins exist for the transport of amino acids: those for neutral, basic, and acidic amino acids. A sodium co-transport process might be involved in the absorption of di- and tripeptides, but this is not well established.

usually involve the loss of water and electrolytes. Here, the absorption of the major ions and electrolytes is discussed sequentially.

There Are at Least Three Distinct Mechanisms of Sodium Absorption

The first of these mechanisms is the sodium co-transport system, as discussed earlier in reference to glucose and amino acid absorption (Fig. 29–17). This mechanism accounts for the absorption of a major portion of sodium during the absorptive phase of digestion.

The second sodium absorption mechanism is *chloride-coupled* sodium absorption (Fig. 29–17B). Some researchers feel that this is a type of sodium co-transport in which chloride, in a manner analogous to glucose, is a coupling molecule for a transport protein. Presently, however, most investigators appear to believe that the sodium absorption occurring in direct association with chloride absorption is mechanistically different than co-transport. Therefore, this type of absorption is referred to here as chloride-coupled sodium transport.

Chloride-coupled sodium absorption appears to result from two separate ion transporters working in concert to facilitate the movement of sodium and chloride across the apical membrane. To initiate this process, carbonic acid is formed within the enterocyte from water and carbon dioxide. This reaction is catalyzed by carbonic anhydrase, as occurs in other tissues. The carbonic acid dissociates to hydrogen and bicarbonate ions. An ion exchange channel in the apical membrane then trades intracellular hydrogen ion for intraluminal sodium ion. Simultaneously, another ion exchange channel trades intracellular bicarbonate for intraluminal chloride, because both hydrogen ion and bicarbonate ion are removed from the cell in equal proportions; the pH of the cell is maintained. Once in the intestinal lumen, the hydrogen and bicarbonate ions can reassociate to form water; thus, there is no net generation of ions.

The chloride-coupled sodium absorption mechanism is usually most active in the ileum and colon, where the sodium concentration in the gut is usually relatively low compared to the duodenum and jejunum. After entering the cell, sodium is transported to the lateral spaces through the Na$^+$, K$^+$ ATPase pump; chloride, on the other hand, remains in the

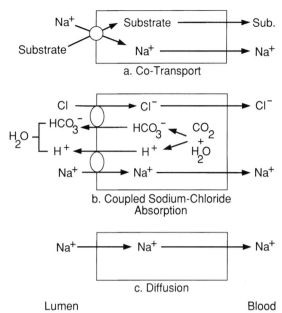

Lumen   Blood

Figure 29–17. Three mechanisms of sodium absorption. (a.) Sodium co-transport with organic molecules is a major means of sodium uptake during active digestion and absorption. (b.) Chloride-coupled sodium absorption is also an important means of sodium absorption and requires the action of carbonic anhydrase and the existence on the apical membrane of bicarbonate-chloride and sodium-hydrogen exchange mechanisms. (c.) Simple diffusion of sodium across the apical membrane may occur because of the large favorable concentration gradient, but it is a relatively minor means of sodium absorption.

enterocyte until its concentration is high enough to promote the diffusion of chloride through special channels in the basolateral membranes. The rate of absorption of sodium and chloride by this mechanism appears to depend on the permeability of the chloride channels; when the permeability is high, chloride passes rapidly out of the enterocyte, allowing continued chloride absorption. Conversely, when chloride channels are relatively closed, the intracellular chloride concentration increases, diminishing chloride absorption by the creation of an unfavorable concentration gradient.

The third mechanism of sodium absorption is simple diffusion (Fig. 29–17C). The large electrochemical gradient that can exist for sodium from lumen to enterocyte appears to allow for some direct, uncoupled movement of sodium across the apical membrane. Whereas some sodium absorption probably occurs by this mechanism, its overall importance in body sodium homeostasis is probably not large.

Three Major Mechanisms Exist for the Absorption of Chloride

One mechanism of chloride absorption is chloride-coupled sodium absorption, as discussed earlier (Fig. 29–18A). Another mechanism is paracellular chloride absorption that occurs in association with sodium co-transport of glucose and amino acids (Fig. 29–18B). Paracellular chloride transport occurs because of an electrical gradient. Sodium co-transport leads to the net movement of positive electrical charges (sodium ions) across the apical membrane, because neither glucose nor most amino acids are charged molecules. As the sodium cations are transferred to the lateral spaces, the spaces develop a positive polarity with respect to the gut lumen. Chloride from the gut lumen passes directly into the lateral spaces through the tight junctions, because the tight junctions are readily permeable to small anions. This provides a major mechanism for the absorption of chloride ion while maintaining electrical neutrality, although a small electrical potential is maintained across the gut surface with the lumen positive with respect to the lateral spaces.

The last mechanism of chloride absorption is by direct exchange for bicarbonate (Fig. 29–18C) without coupled sodium absorption. With this mechanism, there is a net movement of bicarbonate into the gut lumen, resulting in an increase in gut pH.

Bicarbonate Ion Is Secreted by Several Digestive Glands and Must Be Recovered from the Gut if Body Acid-Base Balance Is to Be Maintained

Much bicarbonate is absorbed effectively by the neutralization of HCl from the stomach. (See Chapter 28 for an explanation of the counter-balancing effects of gastric acid secretion and pancreatic bicarbonate secretion.) However, considerable bicarbonate remains in the intestine after the neutralization of stomach acid. This remaining bicarbonate is reabsorbed, primarily in the ileum and colon by the ion exchange mechanism.

Bicarbonate anions in the gut are electrically balanced, primarily, with sodium cations and reabsorbed essentially as sodium bicarbonate. In the absorptive process, hydrogen and bicarbonate ions are first generated within the enterocytes from water and carbon dioxide. Hydrogen ion is then exchanged for sodium

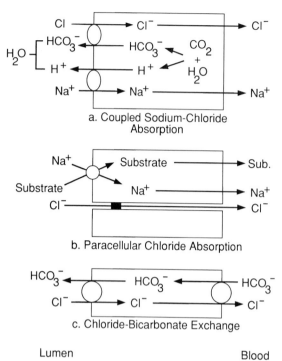

a. Coupled Sodium-Chloride Absorption

b. Paracellular Chloride Absorption

c. Chloride-Bicarbonate Exchange

Lumen   Blood

Figure 29–18. Three mechanisms of chloride absorption. (*a.*) Chloride-coupled sodium absorption is directly related to sodium uptake. (*b.*) Paracellular chloride absorption is indirectly related to sodium absorption that occurs during co-transport. (*c.*) Chloride-bicarbonate exchange occurs especially in areas where bicarbonate secretion into the intestinal lumen is important.

ion across the apical membrane. Within the cell, sodium ion is electrically balanced by the remaining bicarbonate ion, whereas the bicarbonate ion remaining in the gut lumen is neutralized by the secreted hydrogen ion (Fig. 29–19). The result is that sodium is transferred through the membrane. However, luminal bicarbonate is converted to water and carbon dioxide in the gut lumen, whereas bicarbonate anion is being regenerated intracellularly. The net effect is the absorption of sodium bicarbonate. This mechanism is essentially one half of chloride-coupled sodium absorption, except the bicarbonate ion remains within the enterocyte rather than being exchanged for chloride.

Potassium Is Absorbed, Primarily, by Passive Diffusion Through the Paracellular Route

Potassium, although a highly important ion in the body, is present in abundance in most animal diets. This is in contrast to sodium, which is present in nutritionally inadequate amounts in most natural animal feeds. Therefore, frequently the concentration of potassium in the material entering the intestinal lumen is relatively high, compared to sodium. In addition, dietary potassium is concentrated in the gut lumen because of the absorption of other nutrients, electrolytes, and water, unaccompanied by active potassium absorption. Thus, the potassium concentration within the gut lumen increases as digestion and absorption of other osmotically active molecules proceeds. As potassium reaches relatively high concentrations in the intestinal lumen, a concentration gradient favorable for the diffusion of potassium across the intestinal epithelium is created. Furthermore, the concentration gradient is enhanced by the normally low concentration of potassium in the lateral spaces. The primary mechanism of potassium absorption is paracellular passive diffusion, which occurs in response to this concentration gradient (Fig. 29–20). A clinical ramification of this absorptive mechanism is that potassium absorption is directly coupled to water absorption. In diarrhea conditions, where net absorption of water is impaired, potassium absorption is impaired also, because potassium in the gut lumen is diluted so that a concentration gradient favorable for passive diffusion of potassium never develops.

The Major Mechanisms of Electrolyte Absorption Are Selectively Distributed Along the Gut

The activity of the assorted electrolyte absorption mechanisms discussed earlier varies along the length of the gut. The distribution of activity is listed in Table 29–2.

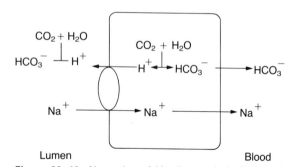

Lumen   Blood

Figure 29–19. Absorption of bicarbonate is facilitated by sodium-hydrogen exchange at the apical membrane. The bicarbonate ion is regenerated by the action of carbonic anhydrase.

All Intestinal Water Absorption Is Passive, Occurring Because of the Absorption of Osmotically Active Solutes

Water moves through the intestinal mucosa by either the paracellular or transcellular routes, but always by osmosis. A general discussion of osmosis is in Chapter 1 and should be reviewed by those who do not have a clear understanding of the process. The intestinal mucosa is freely permeable to water, allowing it to move in whatever direction is dictated by changes in osmotic pressure. As electrolytes and other soluble nutrients are actively absorbed, water is drawn along passively from lumen to intestinal capillaries. As discussed later, water may move also into the intestinal lumen at times, when the intraluminal osmotic pressure is high.

INTESTINAL SECRETION OF WATER AND ELECTROLYTES

In addition to the water and electrolytes that are secreted into the intestine by the pancreas, liver, and other glandular organs, a considerable portion of GI water and electrolyte secretion occurs directly from the intestinal surface. All water secretion is osmotic, but the osmotic gradient driving water secretion may occur in response to either passive or active processes.

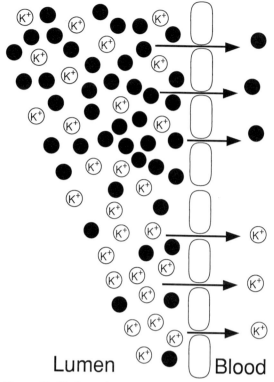

Figure 29–20. Potassium is absorbed by simple diffusion through the paracellular route. Water absorption in the upper intestine results in an increase in potassium concentration in the lower intestine, creating a favorable diffusion gradient for potassium. Note that the removal of water (solid black circles) in the upper part results in a relative increase in the number of potassium ions in the lower part.

Passive Increases in Luminal Osmotic Pressure Occur During Hydrolytic Digestion and Result in Water Secretion

Food entering the intestine may be hyperosmotic because of its composition, e.g., salty foods or those with high sugar contents. On the other hand, food may become hyperosmotic following digestion. Digestion of foods creates many osmotically active molecules from one giant precursor molecule; thus, the osmotic activity of ingesta is increased initially by digestion. When starchy meals, for example, first enter the duodenum, intraluminal digestion creates thousands of osmotically active di- and trisaccharide molecules from single starch molecules. These osmotically active saccharide molecules draw water from the lateral spaces into the intestinal lumen. Water in the lateral spaces is quickly replaced by water from the intestinal capillaries, so that water is essentially drawn into the intestine from the blood vascular system. As digestion proceeds, the saccharide molecules are absorbed, thus reducing the number of particles and lowering the osmotic pressure of the intestinal lumen. As solute molecules are absorbed, water follows them osmotically back through the epithelium and, hence, into the blood vascular system. *The cardinal rule of water movement in the intestine is that water moves in whatever direction necessary to keep ingesta iso-osmotic*, entering the gut when ingesta is hyperosmotic and leaving the gut when ingesta is hypo-osmotic. This has important clinical implications in the pathophysiology of diarrhea, as discussed later.

Active Secretion of Electrolytes from the Crypt Epithelium Leads to Intestinal Water Secretion

In contrast to the absorptive function of the villous cells, the crypt cells have a secretory function. This secretory function appears to

Table 29–2
DISTRIBUTION OF ELECTROLYTE ABSORPTIVE MECHANISMS THROUGHOUT THE GUT

Mechanism	Duodenum	Jejunum	Ileum	Colon
Sodium co-transport	+ + + +	+ + + +	+	–
Chloride-coupled sodium absorption	+	+	+ +	+ + +
Chloride-bicarbonate exchange	–	–	+ +	+ + +
Bicarbonate absorption	–	–	– / +	+ + +
Potassium absorption	–	–	+	+ + +

be due to a chloride transport mechanism. This mechanism appears similar to chloride-coupled sodium transport, as occurs in the villous enterocytes, except that the direction of transport is reversed. In the crypt cells, the chloride-coupled sodium transport mechanism is on the basolateral membrane, in contrast to its position on the apical membrane of the villous cells. The effect of this is to pump sodium and chloride into the crypt enterocytes from the lateral spaces. As these ions are transported into the enterocytes, sodium is quickly pumped out by the Na^+, K^+ ATPase pump. In contrast, chloride is trapped within the cells, reaching relatively high intracellular concentrations. Under appropriate stimuli, chloride channels in the apical membranes of the crypt cells are opened, and the pent-up chloride from within the cells flows down its concentration gradient into the lumen of the crypt. (Ion channels and their regulation in cellular membranes are discussed in Chapter 1). Movement of the chloride anion into the crypts creates an electrical attraction for sodium cations, which move into the crypts from the lateral spaces through the paracellular route. Water follows sodium and chloride osmotically; thus, chloride, sodium, and water are secreted from the crypt epithelium (Fig. 29–21).

The triggering mechanism that activates water secretion from the crypts is the opening of the chloride gates in the crypt-enterocyte apical membrane. Much study has been devoted to determining the factors controlling chloride gate opening in crypt cells. It appears that one important factor in regulating chloride gates is the activity of the adenylate cyclase enzyme and the intracellular concentration of adenosine $3':5'$-cyclic phosphate (cyclic AMP, or cAMP). (The role of adenylate cyclase and cAMP in cellular regulation is discussed in Chapter 1). As cAMP concentrations increase, chloride gates open, and water and electrolyte secretion is stimulated. The physiological, or normal, activator(s) of adenylate cyclase on crypt cells is not known for sure, but one such

activator may be the intestinal regulatory peptide VIP (vasoactive intestinal peptide). Of perhaps greater medical significance is the existence of pathological, or abnormal, activators of crypt-cell adenylate cyclase. These are discussed later under the pathophysiology of diarrhea.

The physiological function of water and electrolyte secretion by the crypts is not completely understood. It can be speculated that such secretion may have a function in maintaining the concentration of sodium and water near the villous surface during sodium co-transport–stimulated absorption. It may be that at certain times during digestion the amount of sodium near the absorptive surface of the villi becomes insufficient to promote the maximal absorption of glucose and amino

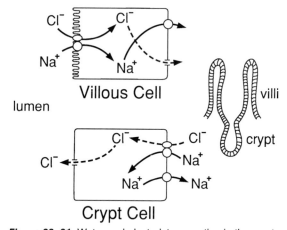

Figure 29–21. Water and electrolyte secretion in the crypts are effected by the secretion of chloride from the apical membrane of crypt enterocytes. Sodium moves into the lumen by the paracellular route and electrically balances chloride secretion. Water follows osmotically, with the net effect being that of secretion of a sodium-chloride solution into the crypt lumen. In the crypts, the coupled sodium-chloride absorption mechanism appears to exist on the basolateral membrane with chloride gates present on the apical membrane. The opening of the chloride gates on the crypt-cell apical membranes initiates crypt secretion. The membrane position of the coupled sodium-chloride transport process reverses itself, moving from the basolateral membrane to the apical membrane as the cells mature and move up the villi.

acids by sodium co-transport. If this is the case, crypt secretion could provide a mechanism to supply additional sodium for villous absorption. Under this hypothesis, water, sodium, and chloride would circulate from the crypt to the villi and back during the process of glucose and amino acid absorption by sodium co-transport.

GASTROINTESTINAL BLOOD FLOW

Water and Solute Movement Between the Lateral Spaces and Villous Capillaries Is Subject to the Same Forces That Govern Water and Solute Movement Between the Extracellular and Vascular Fluids in Other Tissues

Water and all other nutrients, whether they are absorbed through the trans- or paracellular routes, enter the extracellular fluid of the lateral spaces before entering the vascular system. Therefore, the movement of extracellular fluid components into capillaries is of particular importance to intestinal absorption. The physical laws determining the distribution of water between the intra- and extravascular fluid are the same in the villi as in other tissues. These Starling laws (which can be reviewed in Chapters 1 and 22) simply state that the movement of water is determined by the algebraic sum of osmotic and hydrostatic* forces. For example, consider the forces moving water and nutrients from the lateral spaces into the capillaries.

Absorbed Nutrients Enter the Capillaries by Diffusion from the Lateral Spaces

The collective action of the various intestinal absorptive mechanisms concentrate solutes (nutrients) in the lateral spaces. When the concentrations of individual solutes in the spaces exceed their concentrations in blood, a gradient favoring the diffusion of nutrients from lateral spaces into the capillaries is established. The movement of solutes by diffusion into the capillaries creates an osmotic force that draws water into the capillaries (water follows solute). In addition, the oncotic force (the osmotic force exerted by plasma proteins, see Chapters 1, 22) also tends to draw water

*Hydrostatic = the force created by water pressure.

into the capillary lumen. Moreover, hydrostatic pressure in the lateral spaces may force water directly into the capillaries. Lateral-space hydrostatic pressure can be created by the osmotic effect of absorbed solutes. As these solutes attract water from the intestinal lumen, the lateral spaces become distended, developing a small amount of hydrostatic pressure. There are two exits for the relief of this pressure: the tight junctions and the capillary endothelium, with the endothelium presenting the route of least resistance to water flow. Thus, water under slight pressure within the lateral spaces tends to flow into the capillaries, rather than into the intestinal lumen (Fig. 29–22).

A Counter-Current, Osmotic-Multiplier System May Increase the Osmolality of Blood at the Tips of the Villi, Further Promoting Absorption of Water into the Blood

The villous vascular system consists of an arteriole rising up the central portion of the villi and dividing at the tip into many capillar-

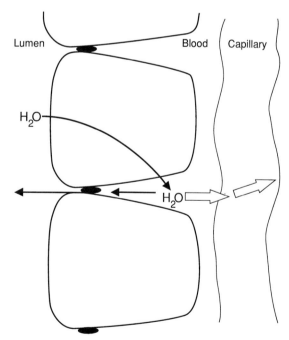

Figure 29–22. Water enters the lateral spaces because of osmotic effects created by absorbed solutes. This creates a hydrostatic pressure head in the lateral spaces. Under pressure, the lateral-space solution can exit through the tight junctions or through the basement membrane of the capillaries. Under normal conditions, the route of least resistance is into the capillaries, resulting in little movement of water from the lateral space into the intestinal lumen.

ies, which course down the outer portion of the villous stroma, between the mucosa and artery. This arrangement provides for direct counter-current flow of blood, i.e., blood coming down the venules passes close to blood flowing in the opposite direction up the arteriole. Because blood in the venules contains absorbed nutrients, its osmolarity could be expected to be slightly higher than that of blood entering the villi in the arteriole. This slight difference in osmolarity can be multiplied and perpetuated by the counter-current flow characteristics of the arterial and venous blood supplies. These conditions create a potential for the creation of an osmotic gradient along the villi; some authors calculate osmolalities near the tips of the villi to be as high as 600 mosm, approximately twice that of blood entering the base of the villi. (The characteristics of a counter-current osmotic multiplier are further explained in Chapters 40 in reference to the renal loop of Henle.) The existence of the villous counter-current osmotic multiplier is still somewhat controversial, and its presence may depend on the species in question. The effect of this osmotic multiplier system would be to accentuate all of the osmotic forces that result in the movement of water from lumen to lateral spaces and from lateral spaces to capillaries.

Disturbances in the Venous Drainage from the Intestine Can Markedly Affect the Mechanisms of Capillary Absorption in the Villi

With the exception of blood from the terminal colon and rectum, all venous blood from the GI tract is collected into the hepatic portal vein and passes through the liver before entering the vena cava and returning to the heart (Fig. 29–23). This system exists so that the nutrient-rich blood leaving the intestine may be modified by the liver so that the nutrient concentration of blood reaching general body tissues can remain relatively constant. This particular vascular arrangement of the GI system results in blood passing through two capillary beds, one in the gut wall and one in the liver, before returning to the heart. In most tissues, arterial hydrostatic pressure forces blood through the capillary beds. In the liver, however, this is not the case, because most of the arterial hydrostatic pressure has been dissipated during flow of blood through the intestinal capillaries. Two circumstances

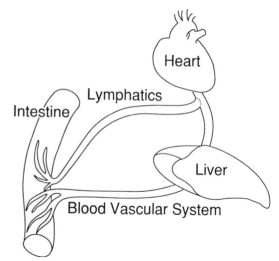

Figure 29–23. All blood exiting the gut flows through the liver before returning to the heart. Lymphatic drainage from the gut bypasses the liver, entering the blood stream through the thoracic duct.

tend to overcome this problem and allow hepatic blood flow to occur:

1. the capillaries (referred to as sinusoids) of the liver are comparatively large and, thus, offer little resistance to flow; therefore, they can function in a low pressure system.

2. the venous outflow of the liver goes directly into the thoracic vena cava.

The bellows-like action of the thorax transmits a negative pressure to the thoracic vena cava, which tends to aspirate blood from the hepatic veins and abdominal vena cava. Under normal circumstances these conditions allow blood to flow readily from the intestine through the liver. However, small changes in circulatory function can have a large impact on GI blood flow. If the pumping capacity of the heart becomes reduced, such as in early heart failure, it cannot remove returning blood quickly, and this results in an accumulation of blood and an increase in pressure in the thoracic vena cava. This increase in pressure interferes with the flow of blood out of the liver, which in turn reduces blood flow out of the intestine, making the GI system particularly susceptible to right-sided heart failure. Diffuse liver disease can reduce intestinal blood flow also. In this condition the resistance to blood flow in the liver is increased due to pressure on the sinusoids. Small increases in hepatic flow resistance can have large effects on intestinal blood flow, because the pressure gradient across the hepatic portal vein is normally small. When the flow of blood out of the intestine is impaired, hydrostatic pressure in the capillaries of the villi is increased; this tends to offset the osmotic and hydrostatic forces promoting water absorption and, thus, water absorption is impaired.

DIGESTION AND ABSORPTION OF FATS

Detergent Action, As Well As Enzymatic Action, Is Necessary for the Digestion and Absorption of Lipids

Lipids, or fats, present a special digestive problem to the animal, because they do not dissolve in water, the major medium in which most body processes, including digestion, occur. Detergent action is necessary to emulsify or dissolve lipids, so that they may be subjected to the actions of water-soluble, hydrolytic enzymes in the gut. The problem of solubility makes the mechanics of digestion and absorption of lipids somewhat different than that of proteins and carbohydrates. For that reason, lipid assimilation is covered here as a separate section.

Lipids make up a large portion of the diets of carnivores, whereas they usually form a minor portion of the natural diets of adult herbivores. Nonetheless, it appears that herbivorous species have the capacity to digest and absorb lipids in quantities considerably higher than found in their natural diets, and frequently supplemental lipids are added to the diets of performance horses and high-producing dairy cows. The neonates of all mammalian species have a high capacity for lipid digestion and absorption, because milk has a high fat content.

The primary dietary lipid is *triglyceride*, which may originate from either plant or animal sources. Other important dietary lipids include *cholesterol* and *cholesterol ester* from animal sources, waxes from plant sources, and *phospholipids* from both plant and animal sources. The structures of these dietary lipids are illustrated in Figure 29–24. In addition, the lipid-soluble vitamins A, D, E, and K are absorbed along with the other dietary lipids.

Lipid assimilation can be divided into four phases: *emulsification, hydrolysis, micelle formation,* and *absorption.* Emulsification is the process of reducing lipid droplets to a size that forms stable suspensions in water or water-based solutions. In the gut, the emulsification phase begins in the stomach as the lipids are warmed to body temperature and subjected to the intense mixing, agitating, and sieving actions of the distal stomach. This distal-stomach activity tends to break lipid globules up into droplets that pass into the small intestine. In the small intestine, emulsification is completed by the detergent action of bile acids and phospholipids. (See Chapter 28 for a discussion of bile formation and secretion.) These bile products reduce the surface tension of the lipids and allow the droplets to become even further divided and reduced in size (Fig. 29–25).

While in the bile-coated, or emulsified droplet stage, the lipids are subject to the actions of hydrolytic enzymes. Hydrolysis of triglyceride, the major dietary lipid component, occurs because of the combined action of the pancreatic enzymes *lipase* and *co-lipase.* Lipase is an enzyme secreted, in its active form, from the pancreas. However, lipase cannot attack directly the emulsified lipid droplets in the gut, because it cannot penetrate the coat of bile products surrounding the droplets. The function of co-lipase, a relatively short peptide, is to "clear a path" through the bile products, giving lipase access to the underlying triglycerides. Lipase cleaves the fatty acids off each end of the triglyceride molecule, but does not attack the central fatty acid, resulting in the formation of two *free,* or *nonesterified, fatty acids* and a *monoglyceride* from each molecule of triglyceride hydrolyzed (Fig. 29–26).

Other lipid-digesting pancreatic enzymes include *cholesterol esterase* and *phospholipase.* The products of these enzymes are nonesterified fatty acids, cholesterol, and lysophospholipids.

The products of hydrolytic lipid digestion (fatty acids, monoglycerides, and so forth) combine with bile acids and phospholipids to form *micelles,* small water-soluble aggregations of bile acids and lipids. Micelles are considerably smaller than the emulsified fat droplets from which they are derived (see Fig. 29–25). The soluble micelles allow the lipids to diffuse through the gut lumen into the unstirred water layer and into close contact with the absorptive surface of the apical membrane (Figs. 29–26, 29–27).

Lipids Are Absorbed Through the Apical Membrane by Simple Diffusion

The process of lipid absorption into the enterocytes is incompletely understood. It is

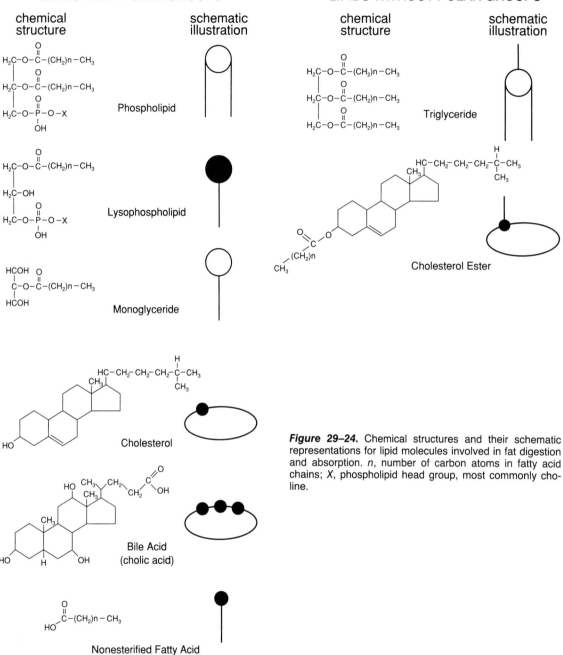

Figure 29–24. Chemical structures and their schematic representations for lipid molecules involved in fat digestion and absorption. *n*, number of carbon atoms in fatty acid chains; *X*, phospholipid head group, most commonly choline.

probable that it occurs by simple diffusion. As the micelles come close to the surface of the enterocytes, the various lipid components diffuse the short distance through the glycocalyx to the apical membrane. Whereas an elaborate mechanism is necessary for the transport of saccharides and amino acids through the apical membrane, no such transport systems are necessary for lipid absorption. The apical membrane, as other cellular membranes, is composed primarily of phospholipids (see Chapter 1 for a description of cellular membranes). The products of lipid digestion are soluble in the phospholipid matrix of the membrane and, thus, may diffuse freely through the apical membrane and into the cell. Lipid absorption from micelles is illustrated in Figure 29–27.

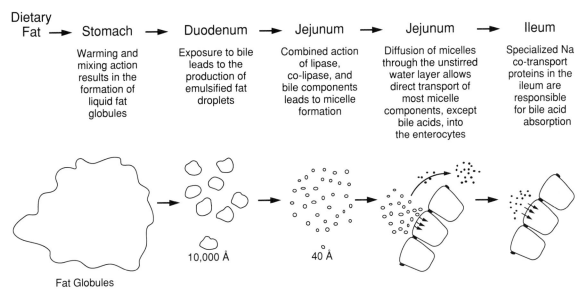

Dietary Fat →	Stomach →	Duodenum →	Jejunum →	Jejunum →	Ileum
	Warming and mixing action results in the formation of liquid fat globules	Exposure to bile leads to the production of emulsified fat droplets	Combined action of lipase, co-lipase, and bile components leads to micelle formation	Diffusion of micelles through the unstirred water layer allows direct transport of most micelle components, except bile acids, into the enterocytes	Specialized Na co-transport proteins in the ileum are responsible for bile acid absorption

10,000 Å   40 Å

Fat Globules

Figure 29–25. The sites and reactions involved in fat digestion and absorption.

Figure 29–26. A portion of the surface of a bile-coated, emulsified fat droplet. Bile components reach the surface of the droplet through micelles (*A*) coming from the gallbladder. Co-lipase clears bile constituents from an area of the surface of the droplet, allowing the attachment of lipase. Lipase catalyzes the formation of fatty acids and monoglycerides from triglycerides. The surface components and products of lipase action combine to form micelles (*B*) containing fatty acids and monoglycerides, as well as bile constituents.

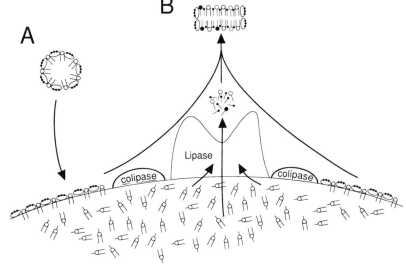

A

B

Lipase

colipase   colipase

Bile-coated, emulsified droplet

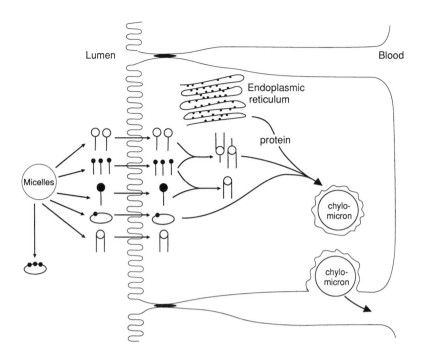

Figure 29–27. Lipid absorption from micelles with subsequent formation of chylomicrons. As micelles come into close proximity with the apical membrane, lipid constituents, except bile acids, diffuse through the membrane into the cell. Once in the enterocyte, triglycerides are re-formed from fatty acids and monoglycerides. Triglycerides are then packaged into the core of chylomicrons for transport out of the cell. The chylomicron surface is coated with phospholipids, cholesterol, and proteins.

Bile Acids Are Reabsorbed from the Ileum by a Sodium Co-transport System

All components of the micelle diffuse into the enterocytes except the bile acids. Bile acids remain in the lumen of the gut, being separated from the other micellar elements as absorption proceeds. By the time bile acids reach the ileum, they are in a relatively free state, devoid of other lipids. Localized in the ileum is a specific bile-acid transport system. This system operates by sodium co-transport and results in the nearly complete reabsorption of bile acids. After absorption, bile acids are transported directly back to the liver by the portal vasculature. The liver efficiently extracts bile acids from the portal blood, so normally the concentration of bile acids in the nonportal blood (systemic circulation) is small. The bile acids extracted by the liver are recycled into the bile. This recycling process occurs repeatedly, so the entire mass of bile acids within the body is circulated through the intestine several times per day.

Absorbed Lipids Are Packaged into *Chylomicrons* Before Leaving the Enterocytes

After passing the apical membrane, the absorbed lipids are quickly picked up by carrier molecules and transported intracellularly to the endoplasmic reticulum. Once on the en-doplasmic reticulum, the major lipids are re-esterified to form triglyceride and phospholipids. The re-esterified lipids are then packaged with cholesterol and minor dietary lipids into structures known as *chylomicrons*. Chylomicrons are spherical structures with a core of triglyceride and cholesterol ester and a surface of phospholipid and cholesterol. The phospholipid and cholesterol are arranged with their hydrophobic (water-repelling) ends facing the core lipids and their hydrophilic (water-attracting) ends facing the surface of the chylomicron particle (Fig. 29–28). This arrangement of surface lipid results in the chylomicron being water-soluble. A small number of special protein molecules are present also on the chylomicron surface. These proteins help to stabilize the surface and also to direct the metabolism of the particle.

After formation, chylomicrons are expelled from the basolateral membrane into the lateral spaces. Unlike most other nutrients entering the lateral spaces, chylomicrons are too large to pass through the basement membrane of the intestinal capillaries and, thus, cannot be absorbed through the intestinal blood system. Rather, chylomicrons travel through the intestinal lymphatics, which eventually form a major abdominal lymph duct that passes through the diaphragm and into the *thoracic duct*. The thoracic duct is the major lymph-collecting vessel of the body and empties into the vena cava. Through this means, chylomicrons even-

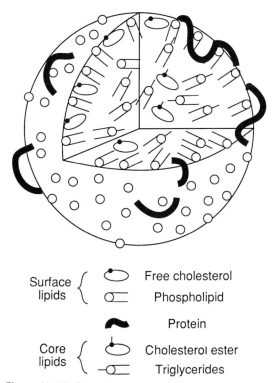

Surface lipids	⟨ ◯ Free cholesterol
	◯ Phospholipid
	~ Protein
Core lipids	⟨ ◯ Cholesterol ester
	◯ Triglycerides

Figure 29–28. Chylomicron structure. Special proteins and lipids with polar groups form the surface coat, whereas nonpolar lipids form the core of the particle.

tually reach the blood vascular system. During absorption of lipid, intestinal lymph turns from its normal water-clear character to a milky white color because of the presence of chylomicrons. After a fatty meal, this milky white color can even be seen in blood plasma. In normal animals this white color in blood plasma, known as *lipemia*, is transient, disappearing within 1–2 hours after digestion of the meal. The metabolic fate of the chylomicrons is discussed in Chapter 31.

GROWTH AND DEVELOPMENT OF THE INTESTINAL EPITHELIUM

The Length of Intestinal Villi Is Determined by the Relative Rates of Cell Loss at the Tips and Cell Replenishment at the Base

Replication of enterocytes occurs in the crypts. Crypt enterocytes are highly mitotic and regenerate rapidly. In fact, the intestinal crypt cells are one of the most rapidly regenerating cells of the body, representing the single greatest need for protein synthesis in

nongrowing animals. As crypt cells multiply, they migrate onto the base of the villi, pushing other villous cells ahead of them, so that there is a continuous progression of cells migrating up the villi. As the cells migrate they mature, changing from relatively undifferentiated cells in the crypts to highly specialized absorptive cells on the villi. As the cells reach the tops of the villi, they are lost because of age and exposure to gut contents. The rate at which cells are lost at the tips of the villi, compared to the rate at which they are replaced by cells from the crypts, determines the length of the villi.

The rate of cell replication in the crypts appears to be stimulated by several of the GI hormones. When appetite and feed intake increases, there is an overall increase in the secretion of GI hormones. This increase leads to an increase in crypt cell proliferation, which is accompanied by an increase in villi length. Appetite and feed intake may increase because of conditions of increased energy need, such as lactation, exercise, and cold environmental temperatures. Under these conditions of increased feed intake and GI hormone secretion, there is a corresponding increase in villi length. The increased villi length provides a greater digestive and absorptive capacity to match the need created by increased feed intake. Thus, the functional capacity of the intestine is adjusted to match the nutrient needs of the animal.

DIGESTION IN THE NEONATE

During the First Few Hours of Life, Proteins Are Not Digested, but Absorbed Intact

In general, a major function of digestion is to destroy proteins by hydrolysis. Under most circumstances this is a benefit to the animal, not only from a nutritional and digestive standpoint, but also from a toxicological and allergic standpoint; potentially toxic or allergenic proteins are destroyed before they are absorbed into the body. In the special case of some neonates, however, there is a need to absorb proteins intact. In most livestock species, including horses, cattle, sheep, and swine, essentially no antibodies are passed from the mother to fetus through the placenta, in contrast to some other animals such as primates. Thus, young livestock are born without the immunological protection of their mother's antibodies. In these species, antibodies from the mother must be acquired through ingestion of colostrum, the special mammary secretion present at the time of birth. At birth in these animals, the digestive tract is altered from the adult state in order to absorb the antibody proteins intact, rather than after digestion.

There are three primary alterations: (1) acid secretion from the stomach is delayed for several days after birth; (2) there is a similar delay in the development of pancreatic function, thus, acid and trypsin digestion of proteins is avoided; and (3) there is a specialized intestinal epithelium capable of engulfing soluble proteins in the intestinal lumen and discharging them into the lateral spaces. This epithelium has the same villous structure as the mature epithelium, but the villi are covered with special enterocytes capable of protein absorption. Immediately after birth this special epithelium starts to disappear, and it is essentially gone after 24 hours. The loss of the protein-absorptive function in the neonate is referred to as *gut closure.*

The Major Intestinal Disaccharidase Switches from Lactase to Maltase with Maturity

Lactose from milk is the major carbohydrate in the diets of neonatal and young mammals; thus, all mammals are born with high intestinal lactase activity. In contrast, maltase activity, necessary for digesting the products of luminal starch digestion, is weak or absent for several weeks after birth. As the animals progress toward weaning, lactase activity wanes and maltase activity increases, allowing the animals to shift from lactose to starch as a carbohydrate source. In many species of adult animals, lactase activity is practically nonexistent.

PATHOPHYSIOLOGY OF DIARRHEA

Diarrhea refers to an increase in the frequency of defecation or the volume of feces. Here we are mainly concerned with the volume of feces. Fecal volume increases in diarrhea, primarily because of an increase in water content. The amount of water passed in feces is the algebraic sum of GI water input and

water absorption. As discussed earlier, water in the gut results from ingested water, water secreted by gastric glands, and water secreted or lost directly through the mucosal epithelium. Under most circumstances, the amount of water secreted into the gut greatly exceeds the amount ingested. Normally, the amount absorbed is just slightly less than the sum of the amounts secreted and ingested, leaving a small remainder for passage in the feces (Fig. 29–29A).

Diarrhea Occurs When There Is a Mismatch Between Secretion and Absorption

The amount of water in the feces is the result of the balance betweeen secretion and absorption. *Malabsorptive diarrhea* occurs when absorption is inadequate to recover a sufficient portion of water that is secreted, as illustrated in Figure 29–29C. Malabsorptive diarrhea usually occurs because of the loss of GI epithelium. In most instances, such losses occur

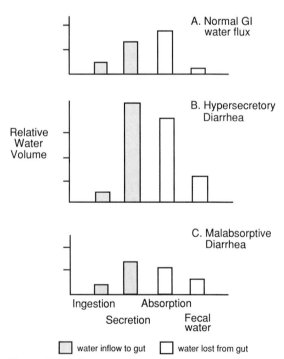

Figure 29–29. Pathophysiology of diarrhea. The bars represent the relative amounts of water entering or leaving the gut. Fecal volume is the sum of the water ingested and secreted minus the water absorbed. Therefore, fecal volume is dependent not on the amount of water entering the gut, but rather on the balance between water influx and efflux.

because of viral, bacterial, or protozoal infections; viral infections often cause particularly severe destruction of villous epithelium. These infections result in the loss of enterocytes from the villi. As pointed out previously, villous length is determined by the relative rates of cell loss and cell replacement (Fig. 29–30). Intestinal infections result in decreased villous length, because the rate of cell loss is increased relative to the rate of cell replacement. Short villi cause impaired absorption for two reasons: (1) there is an absolute loss of absorptive intestinal surface area, and (2) the cells that are lost are the mature cells from the upper regions of the villi. It is these mature cells that possess the enzymes of membranous-phase digestion and the transport proteins for sodium co-transport; loss of these cells results in impaired digestion and absorption of nutrients. Because nutrient absorption is necessary for the osmotic absorption of water, water absorption is diminished by impaired nutrient absorption.

Secretory diarrhea occurs when the rate of intestinal secretion increases and overwhelms the absorptive capacity. Most cases of hypersecretory diarrhea result from inappropriate secretion from the small intestinal crypts. This occurs when the normal secretory mechanism of the crypt epithelium (as discussed earlier) is abnormally stimulated. Toxins, known as *enterotoxins,* are produced by some types of pathogenic bacteria. These toxins bind to enterocytes and stimulate adenylate cyclase activity and the production of cAMP within the cells, resulting in opening of the chloride gates and the secretion of water and electrolytes from crypt epithelium. If the stimulation is mild, the gut may respond with increased absorption, and diarrhea will not result. However, when the secretion exceeds the capacity of the gut to increase absorption, as illustrated in Figure 29–29B, diarrhea results. Hyperse-

cretory diarrhea has devastating effects on the water electrolyte and acid-base status of animals, especially neonates. Hypersecretory diarrhea due to enterotoxin producing *Escherichia coli* is an extremely common disease of neonatal calves and pigs, causing large economic losses to the cattle and swine industries.

CLINICAL CORRELATIONS

CALF DIARRHEA WITH DEHYDRATION AND ACIDOSIS

HISTORY □ You are asked to examine a 2-day-old calf. The owner reports that she appeared normal the night before, but this morning she is recumbent and will not rise. In addition, she shows no interest in suckling a bottle.

CLINICAL AND LABORATORY EXAMINATION □ The calf's body temperature is subnormal. The mouth is dry, and the eyes are sunken into the orbits. The ears, tail, and distal legs are cool to the touch. The tail and perineum of the calf are wet. As you remove your thermometer the calf passes a stream of liquid feces. The feces are nearly clear and slightly yellow; they have the consistency of water. Simple laboratory tests indicate that the packed cell volume is 50% (normal 30–35%), and the serum total-solids concentration is 7.5% (normal 5.5–6.5%).

COMMENT □ The calf has diarrhea, and the physical examination and laboratory findings indicate a state of advanced dehydration. Loss of body fluid volume is so severe that the calf appears to be in or near a state of hypovolemic shock. Although you cannot be absolutely sure from the information you collect while examining

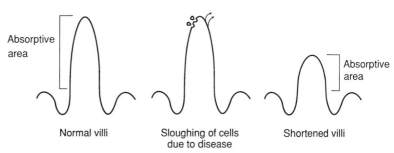

Figure 29–30. Shortening of villi because of increased cell loss. Many infectious diseases result in an increased rate of cell sloughing from the villi. As cells are lost, the villus shrinks to fill in the gap in the epithelial coat. If villous height is to be maintained in the presence of rapid loss of enterocytes, the rate of recruitment of new cells, generated in the crypts, must be increased. Therefore, when the rate of cell loss exceeds the capacity for cell replacement, shortened villi with reduced absorptive surfaces and relatively immature enterocytes occur.

Absorptive area

Absorptive area

Normal villi

Sloughing of cells due to disease

Shortened villi

the calf at the farm, the severity of dehydration, the rapidity of onset, and the age of the calf all suggest a hypersecretory diarrhea due to enterotoxigenic *Escherichia coli* bacteria. Animals with such clinical signs are usually severely acidotic, although blood pH is seldom measured in field cases. Diarrhea, acidosis, and dehydration occur because toxins produced by the bacteria stimulate opening of chloride gates in the apical membranes of crypt cells, stimulating copious secretion of water and electrolytes, including bicarbonate. The sodium co-transport system on the villi is unaffected by the bacterial toxin, but the simultaneous presence of glucose and sodium in the lumen is necessary to promote co-transport, which can offset some of the fluid and electrolyte losses caused by hypersecretion from the intestinal crypts.

TREATMENT □ Vascular volume expansion and correction of acidosis are primary concerns in such cases. A calf such as this should receive 2 L of alkalizing fluids by rapid intravenous (IV) administration. An additional 2 L or more should be given IV over the next 24 hours. Frequently, the response of calves to such treatment is remarkable, and calves that appear almost dead can be saved often by vigorous fluid therapy. After the initial replacement of lost fluids by IV therapy, further dehydration due to ongoing fluid losses can be prevented by oral administration of glucose and sodium-containing fluids.

JUVENILE PANCREATIC ATROPHY

HISTORY □ You are presented with a thin, 3-year-old German shepherd. The owners report that the dog appeared normal up until 6 months ago. At that time they noticed that he started losing weight and began to develop the disgusting habit of eating his own feces. Recently, the weight loss has become more severe, even though he has had a good appetite and seems normal otherwise. Lately they have noted that he seems to pass a large amount of feces, and the fecal material is soft, gray, and has a clay-like consistency.

CLINICAL AND LABORATORY EXAMINATION □ Physical examination reveals an extremely thin dog with a dull, uneven hair coat. Other physical findings are unremarkable, and the dog seems bright and friendly. You hospitalize the animal for further testing, and note

that he readily eats two cans of commercial dog food per day. Laboratory analysis of feces collected over a 24-hour period reveals that the dog is passing 25 g of fat in the feces per day (normal is less than 5 g, assuming a normal type of diet).

COMMENT □ This degree of fat malabsorption is characteristic of pancreatic exocrine insufficiency. Because there is insufficient pancreatic lipase, fats cannot be hydrolyzed to fatty acids for absorption; thus, they pass unabsorbed through the gut. Several other laboratory tests are available for assessing pancreatic exocrine function. Other tests have as their basis such things as the examination of blood for the presence of orally administered markers that require pancreatic enzymes for digestion and absorption, or the direct examination of feces for the presence of pancreatic enzymes or undigested nutrients.

TREATMENT □ Feeding highly digestible diets mixed with commercially prepared pancreatic enzymes is frequently successful in promoting adequate nutrient absorption in animals with juvenile pancreatic atrophy. Digestion may not be completely normal, but is sufficient for the dogs to attain a normal body weight. Treatment must be continued for life. You may wonder how orally administered pancreatic enzymes can make it through the proteolytic environment of the stomach without being destroyed. Undoubtedly, some of them are destroyed but enough appear to make it through the stomach to be effective.

Bibliography

Argenzio RA, Whipp SC: Pathophysiology of diarrhea. *In* Anderson NV (ed): Veterinary Gastroenterology. Philadelphia, Lea & Febiger, 1980, pp 220–232.

Berne RM, Levy MN: Physiology. St. Louis, CV Mosby, 1983, pp 795–820.

Johnson LR (ed): Gastrointestinal Physiology. St. Louis, CV Mosby, 1985, pp 105–150.

Johnson LR, Christensen J, Jacobson ED, et al (eds): Physiology of the Gastrointestinal Tract, 2nd ed. New York, Raven Press, 1987, pp 1209–1698.

Stevens CE: Comparative Physiology of the Vertebrate Digestive System. Cambridge, Cambridge University Press, 1988, pp 125–158, 191–219.

Strombeck DR: Small Animal Gastroenterology. Davis, CA, Stonegate Publishing, 1979, pp 136–178, 201–222.

PRACTICE QUESTIONS FOR CHAPTER 29

1. Finding triglycerides and starch in the feces of a thin dog with a normal feed intake would suggest

   a. malabsorption.
   b. maldigestion.

2. Which statement about the tight junctions is false?

   a. Tight junctions encircle the enterocyte near its apical end.
   b. Tight junctions form the dividing line between the apical membrane and the basolateral membrane.
   c. Tight junctions are impermeable to water.
   d. Tight junctions separate the lateral space from the intestinal lumen.
   e. Tight junctions are the only points that attach enterocytes together.

3. Which of the following molecules is consumed during the process of hydrolytic digestion?

   a. Glucose
   b. Alanine
   c. Dipeptides
   d. Fatty acids
   e. Water

4. A drug that blocks the activity of the Na^+, K^+ ATPase pump could be expected to have what effect on sodium-glucose co-transport?

   a. Increases sodium-glucose co-transport
   b. Decreases sodium-glucose co-transport
   c. No effect on sodium-glucose co-transport

5. During sodium absorption by glucose co-transport,

   a. chloride is absorbed by the paracellular route.
   b. chloride absorption is not affected.
   c. chloride is absorbed in exchange for bicarbonate.
   d. chloride absorption is coupled with potassium absorption.
   e. chloride is absorbed in exchange for hydrogen ion.

6. Before entering the intestinal capillaries, all nutrients pass through the

   a. apical membrane.
   b. tight junction.
   c. lateral space.
   d. basolateral membrane.
   e. enterocyte cytoplasm.

30

Digestion: The Fermentative Processes

1. Fermentation is the metabolic action of bacteria
2. The sites of fermentative digestion must be conducive to microbial growth

THE MICROBIAL ECOSYSTEM OF FERMENTATIVE DIGESTION

1. The microbes responsible for fermentative digestion include bacteria, fungi, and protozoa
2. Cooperation and interplay between the many species of microbes give rise to a complex ecosystem in the forestomach and hindgut

SUBSTRATES AND PRODUCTS OF FERMENTATIVE DIGESTION

1. Plant cell walls are important substrates for fermentative digestion and important nutrient sources for many species
2. Nutrients other than cell walls are also subject to fermentative digestion
3. Anaerobic conditions in the rumen result in metabolic activities leading to the production of *volatile fatty acids*
4. Volatile fatty acids are important energy substrates for the host animal
5. Fermentative digestion of protein results in the deamination of a large portion of amino acids
6. When protein and energy availability in the forestomach are well matched, there is rapid microbial growth and efficient protein utilization
7. Microbial protein can be synthesized in the rumen from nonprotein nitrogen sources

RETICULORUMEN MOTILITY AND THE MAINTENANCE OF THE RUMEN ENVIRONMENT

1. The physiological functions of the rumen serve to maintain an environment favorable to fermentation patterns that are beneficial to the host
2. Rumen fermentation is maintained by selectively retaining actively fermenting material while allowing unfermentable residue to pass on to the abomasum
3. Gravity and reticulorumen motility combine to create the selective flow of particulate matter out of the rumen
4. *Functional specific gravity* determines the rate at which particulate matter (solids) moves through the zones of the reticulorumen
5. Digestibility and physical characteristics of feed have important influences on both the rate of particle passage from the rumen and the rate of feed intake

6. Rumination, or cud chewing, has an important effect on particle size reduction and the movement of solid material through the rumen
7. Water moves through the rumen at a much faster rate than particulate matter
8. Rumen dilution rate has important influences on fermentation and microbial cell yield

CONTROL OF RETICULORUMEN MOTILITY

1. Reticulorumen motility is controlled by the central nervous system and affected by intraluminal conditions

OMASAL FUNCTION

1. Passage of material from the reticulum to the omasum occurs during reticular contraction

VOLATILE FATTY ACID ABSORPTION

1. Volatile fatty acids, representing 60–80% of the energy needs of the animal, are absorbed directly from the forestomach epithelium

RUMEN DEVELOPMENT AND ESOPHAGEAL GROOVE FUNCTION

1. Tremendous changes in forestomach size and function occur with dietary changes in early life
2. The esophageal groove functions to divert the flow of ingested milk past the forestomach and into the abomasum

EQUINE LARGE HINDGUT FUNCTION

1. The equine hindgut has a tremendous capacity for fermentation
2. Type of substrate and fermentation patterns are essentially identical for forestomach and hindgut fermentation
3. The motility functions of the cecum and colon serve to retain material for fermentation and to separate particles based on size
4. The rate of fermentation and volatile fatty acid production in the equine colon is similar to that of the rumen
5. There are tremendous variations in hindgut anatomy and function among the many species of veterinary interest

Fermentation Is the Metabolic Action of Bacteria

In fermentative digestion molecular substrates are broken down by the action of bacteria and other microorganisms. Enzymatic hydrolysis of large molecules is an essential part of fermentative digestion, just as it is for glandular digestion. The major difference between the two processes is that the enzymes of fermentative digestion are microbial in origin, rather than coming from the host animal. Other major differences between fermentative and glandular digestion are rates of reactions and the extent of alteration of the substrate molecules. In general, the rate of fermentative digestion is much slower than that of glandular digestion, and the substrates are altered to a much greater degree.

The Sites of Fermentative Digestion Must Be Conducive to Microbial Growth

Fermentative digestion occurs in specialized compartments that are positioned either before or after the stomach and small intestine. Fermentative compartments positioned prior to the stomach are called *forestomachs* and are most highly developed in the ruminants and cameloids. There are tremendous species variations in the size and development of the forestomach fermentation compartments; many species have distinct, but less developed, forestomachs than ruminants. In some species, including the horse, pig, and rat, there is no anatomically distinct forestomach; however, there is a nonglandular portion of the proximal stomach in which some fermentative digestion may occur.

Fermentation compartments positioned distal to the small intestine are the cecum and colon, often collectively called the *hindgut*. As with the forestomachs, there are tremendous anatomical differences in the hindguts of various species. This variation can be so great as to make it appear that the cecum and colon are functionally different organs in different species; however, when evaluated critically, it can be seen that there are important similarities in hindgut function among species.

The forestomach and hindgut can support fermentative digestion, because their pH, moisture, ionic strength, and oxidation-reduction conditions are maintained in a range compatible for the growth of suitable microbes. In addition, the flow of ingesta through these areas is comparatively slow, allowing microbes time to maintain their population size. The importance of these factors can be seen by comparing the forestomach and colon to the stomach and small intestine. In the stomach, bacterial numbers are kept low by the acid pH, whereas in the small intestine bacterial numbers are kept in check by the constant flushing action of ingesta and secretions.

In general, the fermentative patterns of the hindgut appear to be similar to those in the forestomach, although forestomach fermentation, especially that of the rumen, appears to be the better studied of the two. The following discussion concerns rumen digestion specifically, but comments concerning hindgut digestion are included. A specific discussion of digestion in the equine cecum and colon follows at the end of the chapter.

THE MICROBIAL ECOSYSTEM OF FERMENTATIVE DIGESTION

The Microbes Responsible for Fermentative Digestion Include Bacteria, Fungi, and Protozoa

The bacterial population associated with fermentative digestion is vast, with at least 28 different functionally important species occurring in the rumen. Some of the major species found in the rumen are listed, with their preferred substrates, in Table 30–1. Total bacterial numbers in the forestomach or hindgut normally range from 10^{10} to 10^{11} cells per gram of ingesta. Most of these bacteria are strict anaerobes that cannot survive in the presence of oxygen, although facultative organisms are present also. In the rumen, fungi are present,

Table 30–1
GROUPING OF RUMEN BACTERIAL SPECIES ACCORDING TO THE TYPE OF SUBSTRATES THAT ARE FERMENTED

Major Cellulolytic Species
Bacteroides succinogenes
Ruminococcus flavefaciens
Ruminococcus albus
Butyrivibrio fibrisolvens

Major Hemicellulolytic Species
Butyrivibrio fibrisolvens
Bacteroides ruminicola
Ruminococcus sp.

Major Pectinolytic Species
Butyrivibrio fibrisolvens
Bacteroides ruminicola
Lachnospira multiparus
Succinivibrio dextrinosolvens
Treponema bryantii
Streptococcus bovis

Major Amylolytic Species
Bacteroides amylophilus
Streptococcus bovis
Succinimonas amylolytica
Bacteroides ruminicola

Major Ureolytic Species
Succinivibrio dextrinosolvens
Selenomonas sp.
Bacteroides ruminicola
Ruminococcus bromii
Butyrivibrio sp.
Treponema sp.

Major Methane-Producing Species
Methanobrevibacter ruminantium
Methanobacterium formicicum
Methanomicrobium mobile

Major Sugar-Utilizing Species
Treponema bryantii
Lactobacillus vitulinus
Lactobacillus ruminus

Major Acid-Utilizing Species
Megasphaera elsdenii
Selenomonas ruminantium

Major Proteolytic Species
Bacteroides amylophilus
Bacteroides ruminicola
Butyrivibrio fibrisolvens
Streptococcus bovis

Major Ammonia-Producing Species
Bacteroides ruminicola
Megasphaera elsdenii
Selenomonas ruminantium

Major Lipid-Utilizing Species
Anaerovibrio lipolytica
Butyrivibrio fibrisolvens
Treponema bryantii
Eubacterium sp.
Fusocillus sp.
Micrococcus sp.

Church DC (ed): The Ruminant Animal. Digestive Physiology and Nutrition. Englewood Cliffs, NJ, Prentice Hall, 1988, p 126.

and more recent research has suggested that they may play an important role in the digestion of plant cell walls.

There is also a large population of protozoa in the rumen, as well as in the cecum and colon. Protozoal numbers average about 10^5 to 10^6 cells per gram of rumen contents. Although this number is considerably smaller than the number of bacteria, the relatively larger size of the individual protozoans, compared with bacteria, results in a total rumen bacterial cell mass approximately equal to the protozoal cell mass, under most dietary conditions. Most of the rumen protozoa are ciliated and belong to the genus *Isotricha* or *Entodinium*, although flagellate species are present also, especially in young ruminants. Like the other organisms of the rumen, the protozoa are anaerobic. The digestive abilities, or capacities, of protozoa and bacteria are similar; thus, either type of organism can perform most of the fermentative functions of the rumen. Protozoa ingest large numbers of bacteria and hold rumen bacterial numbers in check. However, none of the actions of protozoa appear essential to rumen function, because ruminants can survive well without protozoa. Thus, the role of protozoa in the total ecological picture of the rumen is uncertain. One potentially important function of protozoa may involve their ability to slow down the digestion of rapidly fermentable substrates, such as starch and some proteins. Protozoa are capable of ingesting particles of starch and protein and storing them in their bodies, protected from bacterial action. The starch and protein remain engulfed until digested by the protozoa, or until the protozoa die or are swept from the rumen into the lower digestive tract. Thus, protozoa may have the effect of delaying, or prolonging, the digestion of these substrates. Especially in the case of starch, this protozoal effect may be beneficial to the host by modulating or delaying the digestion of rapidly fermentable substrate.

Cooperation and Interplay Between the Many Species of Microbes Give Rise to a Complex Ecosystem in the Forestomach and Hindgut

The digestive process in the rumen or colon involves the interplay between the many species of bacteria and other microbes. The ecosystem of fermentative digestion is extremely complex, with the waste products of one microbial species serving as substrate for another. For example, *Ruminococcus albus* and *Bacteroides ruminicola* appear to exist synergistically. *R. albus* digests cellulose (is *cellulolytic*) but cannot ferment protein. *B. ruminicola*, on the other hand, can digest protein but cannot digest cellulose. When grown together, cellulose digestion by *R. albus* provides hexoses for the energy needs of *B. ruminicola*, whereas protein digestion by *B. ruminicola* provides ammonia and branched chain fatty acids for the growth needs of *R. albus*. In addition to substrate needs, growth factor needs are also supplied synergistically within the rumen ecosystem. As an example, B vitamins are necessary for the growth of several rumen microbes, and yet these nutrients are generally not necessary in ruminant diets. This is because of tremendous cross-feeding between species of microbes, which produce various B vitamins and those microbes that require them.

In spite of tremendous ecological complexity, however, the entire pattern of fermentation may be viewed as a holistic process, without consideration of the roles and interactions of individual microbial species. Fermentative digestion is examined here in that light, with the actions of the entire rumen biomass considered as an overall digestive process, irrespective of the specific needs and actions of individual microbial species.

SUBSTRATES AND PRODUCTS OF FERMENTATIVE DIGESTION

Plant Cell Walls Are Important Substrates for Fermentative Digestion and Important Nutrient Sources for Many Species

Forages, or the foliage of plants, are the major feedstuff of large herbivores and an important substrate for fermentative digestion. Some appreciation of the physical and chemical nature of plants is important to understand the fermentative digestion of forages. This understanding may be aided by a brief comparison of plant and animal tissue structure. At the cellular level, a major difference between plants and animals is the existence of a *cell wall*. The cell wall is a complex of various carbohydrate molecules. The structural parts of plants, the leaves and stems, contain a large portion of cell-wall material. This material gives the plants their rigid framework and protects them from weather and other elements during growth. The cell-wall structure of plants can be roughly compared to the connective tissue structure of animals. Long fiber-like molecules of *cellulose* serve a strength-giving role similar to collagen, whereas *hemicellulose, pectin,* and *lignin* serve to cement the cellulose together, much as hylouronic acid and chondrotin sulfate do in animal connective tissue. With the exception of lignin, all of these cell-wall molecules are carbohydrate in nature.

Cellulose is composed of nonbranching chains of glucose monomers joined by $\beta[1{-}4]$ glycosidic linkages. This is in contrast to the $\alpha[1{-}4]$ linkages in starch. Pectin and hemicellulose are chemically more heterogenous than cellulose, and are composed of various proportions of several sugars and sugar acids. None of the cell-wall materials are subject to hydrolytic digestion by mammalian glandular digestive enzymes. However, cellulose, hemicellulose, and pectin are subject to the hydrolytic action of a complex of microbial enzymes known as *cellulase.* This enzyme system releases monosaccharides and polysaccharides from the complex carbohydrates of cell walls, but the saccharides released are not directly available for absorption by the animal. Rather, they are further metabolized by the microbes, as discussed later. Lignin, a heterogeneous group of phenolic chemicals, is resistant to the action of either mammalian or microbial enzymes, and only a small portion of lignin is digested by either process. Lignin is important, not only because it is indigestible itself, but also because it tends to encase the cell-wall carbohydrates, reducing the digestibility of the carbohydrates by protecting them from the action of bacterial cellulase. The lignin concentration of plants increases with age and ambient temperature; thus, young, cool-season plants are more digestible than mature plants grown in hot weather.

Nutrients Other Than Cell Walls Are Also Subject to Fermentative Digestion

The fermentative digestion of plant cell-wall material and its importance to herbivore digestion is well known. It must not be forgotten, however, that essentially all protein and carbohydrate nutrients that can provide substrate for energy and growth in mammals can also support the similar needs of microbes. There-fore, nearly all dietary protein and carbohydrate is potentially subject to fermentative digestion. This is especially important in the case of ruminants in which food is exposed to fermentative digestion in the forestomach, prior to its arrival at sites of glandular digestion. This temporal arrangement leads to the fermentative digestion of many nutrients that would have otherwise been available to the animal through glandular digestion. Thus, forestomach fermentative digestion, which provides for the efficient use of plant cell walls, can potentially lead to the inefficient use of other nutrients because of microbial alteration.

Anaerobic Conditions in the Rumen Result in Metabolic Activities Leading to the Production of *Volatile Fatty Acids*

When carbohydrate material enters the rumen or colon, it is attacked by hydrolytic, microbial enzymes. In the case of insoluble carbohydrates, attack requires the physical attachment of bacteria to the surface of the plant particle, the enzymes themselves being part of the surface coating of the bacteria. Enzymatic action liberates glucose, other monosaccharides, and short-chain polysaccharides into the fluid phase, outside of the microbial cell bodies. Although free in solution, these products of microbial enzyme action do not become immediately available to the host animal; rather, they are quickly subjected to further metabolism by the microbial mass. Glucose and other sugars are absorbed into the cell bodies of the microbes. Once into the microbial cells, glucose enters the glycolytic, or Embden-Meyerhof, pathway. This is the same glycolytic pathway that exists in mammalian cells, and as in mammalian tissues, catabolism of glucose through this pathway yields two molecules of pyruvate for each molecule of glucose. In the process, two molecules of oxidized nicotinamide-adenine denucleatide (NAD^+) are reduced to NAD hydrogen (NADH), and two molecules of adenosine triphosphate (ATP) are formed from adenosine diphosphate (ADP). The potential energy represented by the ATP formed in this reaction is not directly available to the host animal, but is the major source of energy for maintenance and growth of microbes.

If fermentative digestion were to occur under aerobic conditions, which it does not, the pyruvate produced by the glycolytic process would enter the citric acid (Krebs) cycle and

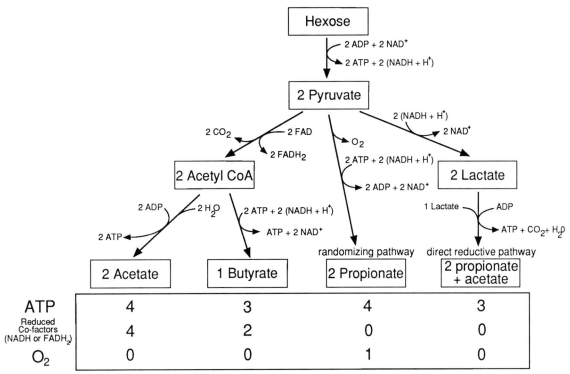

Figure 30–1. Pathways of volatile fatty acid production by the rumen or colonic biomass. The production of methane is necessary for the production of oxidixed cofactors in the pathways leading to acetate and butyrate production, but not in the pathways leading to propionate production. The production of oxygen by the randomizing pathway results in the net production of oxidized cofactors.

be metabolized to carbon dioxide and water, as occurs under the aerobic conditions of mammalian cells. Furthermore, in an aerobic system the NADH produced would be oxidized in the cytochrome oxidase system with additional production of ATP and the regeneration of NAD. But fermentative digestion is not an aerobic system; on the contrary, it is a reductive, highly anaerobic environment. Therefore, a different mechanism must be provided for the oxidation of NADH and other reduced cofactors such as flavin adenine dinucleotide hydrogen ($FADH_2$). If such a mechanism were not available, all of the oxidized

cofactors present would soon be reduced, and metabolism would come to a halt. Because no atmospheric oxygen is available, some other compound must serve as an electron sink for the oxidation of enzyme cofactors.

In fermentative digestion, pyruvate can act as an electron sink, being further reduced to provide for regeneration of NAD and the general removal of excess electrons, with an additional yield of ATP. In addition, carbon dioxide can be reduced to methane, accepting electrons for the regeneration of NAD and flavin adenine dinucleotide (FAD). The metabolic pathways of these reactions are illus-

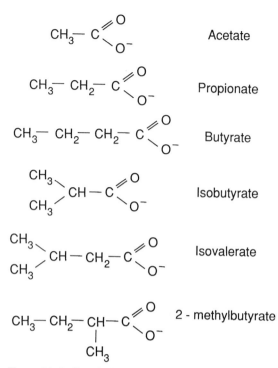

Figure 30–2. Chemical structures of the major volatile fatty acids produced by fermentative digestion.

trated in Figure 30–1. These pathways lead to the major end products of the fermentative digestion of carbohydrate, the *volatile fatty acids* (VFAs). The primary VFAs are *acetic acid, propionic acid,* and *butyric acid.* Frequently, the VFAs are referred to as their dissociated ions: acetate, propionate, and butyrate. Some quantitatively minor, but metabolically important, additional VFAs are valeric, isovaleric, isobutyric, and 2 methyl butyric acids. The chemical structure of the VFAs is shown in Figure 30–2.

From Figure 30–1 it can be seen that production of propionic acid from pyruvate results in the efficient regeneration of NAD with no net production of NADH. In fact, production of available oxygen by the *randomizing branch* of the propionic-acid pathway leads to oxidation of excess NADH originating from the acetic or butyric acid pathways, as illustrated (see Fig. 30–1). The production of acetic acid leads to the efficient generation of ATP, but, in contrast to propionic acid, does not result in the regeneration of NAD from NADH. In the case of the acetic acid pathway, excess NADH is produced. In this case, NAD is regenerated by the formation of free hydrogen, which is subsequently used to reduce carbon dioxide to methane and water (see

lower portion of Fig. 30–1). Thus, there is a direct relationship between acetic acid production and methane production; as the amount of pyruvate entering the acetic acid pathway increases, there must be a concomitant increase in methane production. Likewise, there is a reciprocal relationship between methane production and propionic acid production; as pyruvate is diverted to propionic acid production, there is less need for methane syntheses. These relationships are illustrated in the stoichiometric equations of Table 30–2. It should be appreciated that these reactions do not fully describe the flow of hydrogen, or reducing substances, in rumen or colonic metabolism. The chemical reactions of fermentation are extremely complex and interdependent, and NADH can donate its electrons to reactions other than those described in Table 30–2, such as the synthesis of microbial protein or the saturation of unsaturated fatty acids.

In the rumen, methane production is facilitated by methanogenic bacteria, such as *Methanobacterium ruminantium.* This is a fragile bacterium that is sensitive to changing conditions in the rumen. When conditions are unfavorable for the survival of *M. ruminantium*, methane production is reduced, shifting the metabolic pathways toward propionic acid production. Some conditions that suppress methanogenic species include high levels of

Table 30–2
THEORETICAL STOICHIOMETRIC CARBON-HYDROGEN BALANCE EQUATIONS DESCRIBING CONVERSION OF GLUCOSE IN THE RUMEN

Case 1

glucose → 2 acetate + 2 CO_2 + 8 H
glucose → butyrate + 2 CO_2 + 4 H
glucose + 4 H → 2 propionate + 2 H_2O
CO_2 + 8 H → CH_4 + H_2O

Net*

3 glucose → 2 acetate + butyrate + 2 propionate +
  3 CO_2 + CH_4 + 2 H_2O

Case 2

3 glucose → 6 butyrate + 2 CO_2 + 24 H
glucose → butyrate + 2 CO_2 + 4 H
glucose + 4 H → 2 propionate + 2 H_2O
3 CO_2 + 24 H → 3 CH_4 + 6 H_2O

Net

5 glucose → 6 acetate + butyrate + 2 propionate +
  5 CO_2 + 3 CH_4 + 6 H_2O

Van Soest PJ: Nutritional Ecology of the Ruminant. Ithaca, NY, Cornell University Press, 1982
*Note that in Case 1, acetate to propionate ratio is 1:1 and methane to glucose is 1:3, whereas in Case 2 acetate to propionate is 3:1 and methane to glucose is 3:5.

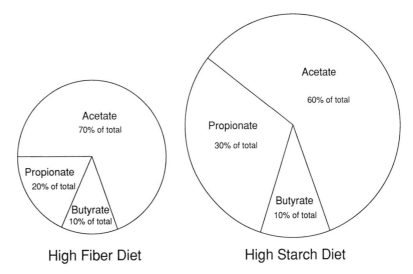

Figure 30–3. VFA production on high forage and high starch diets. Although the percentage of acetate is lower on the high starch diet than on the high forage diet, the total amount of acetate produced is greater on the high starch diet than on the high forage diet. In contrast, propionate increases in both amount and proportion on the high starch diet.

feed intake, finely ground or pelleted feeds, and high grain or starch diets. Under these circumstances, the rate of methane production is reduced, resulting in a reduced rate of acetic acid production with a concomitant increase in the propionic acid production rate.

The proportional rates at which acetic, propionic, and butyric acids are produced are reflected in their relative concentrations in the rumen fluid. The relative concentrations of the VFAs have important nutritional and metabolic consequences and, although seldom measured medically, VFA concentrations are frequently reported in research literature. Typically, the ruminal concentration ratios of acetic:propionic:butyric acids range, respectively, from 70:20:10 for high-forage diets to 60:30:10 for high-grain diets. It must be appreciated that these values represent relative proportions and not absolute amounts. The total amount of VFA produced on a high-starch diet is usually much higher than that produced on a high-fiber diet, such that total acetic acid production may be higher on a high-starch diet than on a high-fiber diet, even though the acetic acid production relative to the other VFA may be reduced. This principle is illustrated in Figure 30–3.

Volatile Fatty Acids Are Important Energy Substrates for the Host Animal

The elegance and beauty of the symbiotic relationship represented by fermentative digestion can be appreciated by considering the metabolism of VFAs. These molecules are the end products, indeed the waste products, of anaerobic microbial metabolism, just as car-

bon dioxide is the waste product of aerobic metabolism. If the VFAs were allowed to accumulate, they would suppress or alter the fermentative process by lowering the pH of the gut or forestomach. However, the host animal maintains conditions for fermentation both by buffering pH changes and also by removing VFAs from the gut by absorption. The benefit derived by the host is from the chemical energy that is contained in the VFAs. These bacterial "waste products" represent spent compounds within the framework of the anaerobic fermentation system, but they still contain considerable energy that can be derived from aerobic metabolism. In ruminants and other large herbivores, the VFAs are the major energy fuels, serving to a large extent the role played by glucose in omnivorous monogastrics. The metabolic fates of the VFAs are discussed further in Chapter 31.

Fermentative Digestion of Protein Results in the Deamination of a Large Portion of Amino Acids

To this point, the discussion of fermentative digestion has centered primarily on carbohydrate, but as previously mentioned, other energy-yielding substrates are subject to microbial attack also. Proteins are particularly vulnerable, because they are composed of carbon compounds that can be further reduced to provide energy for anaerobic microbes. As proteins enter fermentative areas of the gut, they are attacked by extracellular microbial proteases. The majority of these enzymes are "trypsin-like" endopeptidases that form short-chain peptides as end products. These peptides are formed extracellularly and absorbed into the microbial cell bodies, in a manner similar to the formation and absorption of glucose from carbohydrate. Within the microbial cells, the peptides can be utilized either for the formation of microbial protein or further degraded for the production of energy through the VFA pathways (Fig. 30–4). To enter the VFA pathways, the individual amino acids are first deaminated to yield ammonia and a carbon skeleton. The carbon structures of many of the amino acids can fit directly in to various steps of the VFA pathways, leading to the production of the three major VFAs. The three branch-chain amino acids (BCAA) are exceptions, however, and lead to the production of branch-chain VFAs by the following reactions:

$$valine + 2\ H_2O \rightarrow isobutyrate + NH_3 + CO_2$$

$$leucine + 2\ H_2O \rightarrow isovalerate + NH_3 + CO_2$$

$$isoleucine + 2\ H_2O \rightarrow 2\text{-methylbutyrate} + NH_3 + CO_2$$

These branch-chain VFAs are important growth factors for several species of bacteria, as described later.

Although many species of rumen microbes appear capable of using preformed amino acids, which they derive from absorbed peptides, for the synthesis of protein, there are several species that cannot. These species must synthesize amino acids from ammonia and the various carbon metabolites of the VFA pathways. For synthesis of the BCAA, however, the branched-chain VFAs are required. Among the ammonia-requiring, branch-chain fatty acid–requiring species are some of the important cellulose-digesting bacteria.

When Protein and Energy Availability in the Forestomach Are Well Matched, There Is Rapid Microbial Growth and Efficient Protein Utilization

Because a large part of preformed dietary protein is fermented in the rumen, ruminant animals are dependent, to a large degree, on microbial protein to meet their own protein needs. Microbial protein reaches the abomasum and small intestine when microbes are washed out of the rumen and into the lower tract. Digestive efficiency is optimized in ruminants by conditions that result in the maximul delivery of microbial protein to the host animal. These conditions are best met by rapidly growing populations of microbes. The microbial growth rate is dependent on the supply of nutrients and the rate at which microbes are washed from the rumen. Here, the nutrient supply is considered; factors affecting the rate of microbial removal are discussed later in this chapter.

The overall reaction in the rumen may be

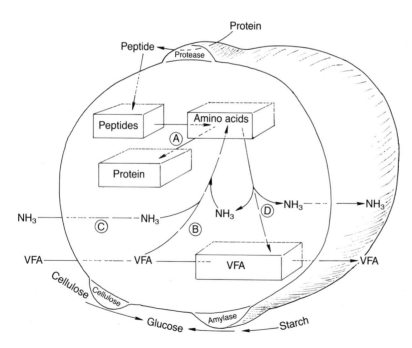

Figure 30–4. Protein metabolism by rumen microbes. Protease enzymes on the microbe surfaces generate peptides that are then taken up by many types of organisms. Absorbed peptides contribute to an intracellular pool of amino acids from which microbial proteins are synthesized (*A*). Another source of amino acids is from intracellular synthesis (*B*), using ammonia and VFA. Many microbes appear capable of deriving their amino acids from either extracellular peptides or intracellular synthesis; however, several types of bacteria appear incapable of using peptides for an amino acid source and are thus dependent on an extracellular source of ammonia (*C*) for amino acid synthesis. Amino acids not used for protein synthesis can be metabolized to VFA and ammonia (*D*).

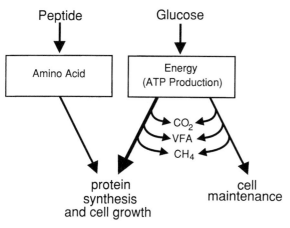

a. Peptide and glucose availability well matched

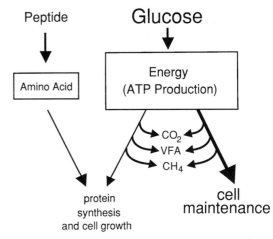

b. Excess glucose, relative to peptide

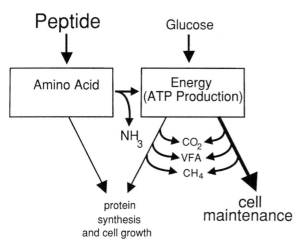

c. Excess peptide, relative to glucose

Figure 30–5. The efficiency with which dietary energy is used for protein synthesis in the rumen depends on the balance between energy and nitrogen sources. The proportion of energy used for protein synthesis and cell maintenance (as indicated by the size of the arrows) changes in relation to the balance of peptide (nitrogen) and glucose supplies.

greatly simplified, for the purposes of this discussion, to equation I:

(I) glucose + peptide = microbes + VFA + NH_3 + CH_4 + CO_2

where glucose and peptide represent ruminally available carbohydrate and protein, respectively. In this context, "available" means available to the microbes for fermentation; carbohydrate or protein that is not susceptible, or accessible, to microbial attack is not included. Glucose was chosen to represent carbohydrate, and peptide to represent protein, because all carbohydrates must be broken down to simple sugars and proteins to peptides prior to becoming available to bacteria.

The term "peptide" in this equation could be replaced by other forms of nitrogen, but for now the discussion is confined to peptide as a nitrogen source. Peptide is the only nitrogen-containing substrate on the left in the equation, but there are two nitrogen-containing products on the right: microbes (as protein) and NH_3. Both substrates, glucose and peptide, contain carbon, oxygen, and hydrogen, and thus can contribute to the formation of microbial carbon, VFA, CH_4, and CO_2.

Equation I will always balance, but the distribution of products varies based on the relative concentrations of substrates, as illustrated in Figure 30–5A–C. For microbial cells to be produced, both energy and nitrogen are required; energy can come from either glucose or peptide, but nitrogen must come from peptide. When glucose and peptide availability are appropriately matched (see Fig. 30–5A), energy for cellular growth comes primarily from glucose, with peptides directed toward microbial protein synthesis. Under these conditions, the products of equation I favor microbial cells with little ammonia production. Glucose fermentation with accompanying VFA production is high in order to meet the large energy demands necessary to support the rapid growth of the microbial mass. Ammonia production is low, because most peptide nitrogen is being incorporated into microbial protein.

When the availability of glucose is high, relative to peptide (see Fig. 30–5B), there is ample energy but insufficient nitrogen to support adequate protein synthesis, and thus microbial replication is not maximal. In this case, microbial energy utilization becomes inefficient as energy is utilized for the maintenance of nondividing cells, rather than for the energy-requiring synthetic processes of growing cells. The maintenance energy needs of the microbes still drive some fermentation of glucose with moderate VFA production, but production of both microbial cells and ammonia is limited because of lack of nitrogen.

The last possible case is that in which peptide availability exceeds glucose availability (see Fig. 30–5C). In this case there is ample nitrogen to support growth, but growth is limited owing to insufficient energy supplies. These conditions force the microbes to utilize peptides to meet energy needs instead of to synthesize proteins. Microbial growth rate is low, and VFA production is moderate, because fermentation is driven only by the maintenance energy needs of the microbes. Much of the VFA production comes from the carbon portions of the peptides, whereas the amine groups are shunted to ammonia production; thus, the products of equation I favor ammonia.

The relationship between available glucose (carbohydrate) and peptide (or nitrogen) has a tremendous impact on the production of microbial cells and, thus, a profound impact on the nutrition of the host. This relationship, as illustrated in Figure 30–5A–C, is quantified by expressing microbial growth in terms of grams of microbial dry matter produced per mole of energy-producing substrate utilized. This value is referred to as *microbial yield* and is usually designated by a capital "Y" subscripted with the energy substrate to which it

is referenced. A convenient, but somewhat theoretical, substrate with which to reference microbial cell yield is ATP. Microbial yield is then written as $Y_{ATP} = x$, where x is the grams of microbial dry matter produced per mole of ATP utilized. The value of Y_{ATP} varies between about 10 and 20 grams of microbes per mole of ATP. Nitrogen availability, either from peptide or nonprotein sources, has an important affect on the Y_{ATP} value. When microbial growth is limited by *low* nitrogen availability, a large portion of available ATP is used for maintenance, rather than cell growth; thus, the number of cells produced per ATP is small, and the Y_{ATP} value is low.

Microbial Protein Can Be Synthesized in the Rumen from Nonprotein Nitrogen Sources

If there is sufficient available carbohydrate, most rumen microbes, even those capable of utilizing preformed peptides, can synthesize protein from ammonia (see Fig. 30–4). Thus, protein can be produced in the rumen from such nonprotein sources as ammonia, nitrates, and urea. From a nutritional and economical point of view, this has been exploited by including inexpensive nonprotein nitrogen sources in place of expensive protein in ruminant diets, allowing the microbes to synthesize protein for the amino acid needs of the host. This process can be exploited physiologically also by the recycling of endogenous urea.

Urea is the nitrogenous waste product of protein catabolism and is formed in the liver. In ruminant animals, hepatic urea production is from two sources: (1) nitrogen arising from the deamination of endogenous amino acids, and (2) nitrogen absorbed as ammonia from the rumen (Fig. 30–6). Ammonia absorption from the rumen is proportional to the ruminal ammonia production rate, which is subject to the influences of ruminal carbohydrate and protein availability, as discussed earlier. Ammonia, which is toxic to most cells, is absorbed from the rumen and delivered to the liver through the hepatic-portal blood vascular system. The liver extracts ammonia from the portal blood efficiently; thus, little of the potentially toxic ammonia reaches the systemic circulation.

In monogastrics, urea is excreted from the

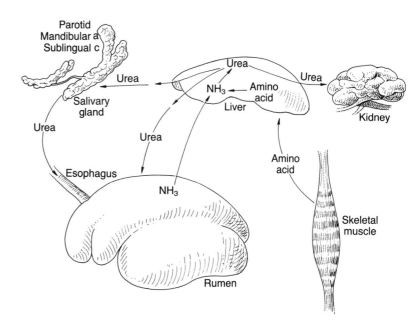

Figure 30–6. Interorgan nitrogen cycling in ruminants. The diagram shows the effects of rumen ammonia concentration on the formation and utilization of urea. When rumen ammonia concentrations are high, the net movement of nonprotein nitrogen is toward the liver, resulting in high urea production rates and poor nitrogen conservation. When rumen ammonia concentrations are low, the net movement of nonprotein nitrogen is from liver to rumen, resulting in protein production from endogenous urea.

body nearly exclusively by the kidneys. In ruminants, however, urea may be excreted also into the rumen (see Fig. 30–6). Such excretion can occur by direct absorption into the rumen from the blood or by urea excretion into saliva. In either case, the urea reaches the rumen, where it is quickly transformed to ammonia, and enters the general pool of rumen nitrogen from which microbial proteins are synthesized.

The direction of nonprotein nitrogen flow, either into the rumen as urea or out of the rumen as ammonia, depends on rumen ammonia concentrations. During times of high ruminal nitrogen availability, relative to carbohydrate, this system results in high blood urea concentrations and the extensive loss of precious nitrogen through urinary excretion, making ruminants nutritionally inefficient under these dietary conditions. However, during times of high carbohydrate availability, relative to nitrogen, the major flow of urea nitrogen is from the blood into the rumen. Under these circumstances, in which ruminal ammonia concentrations are low, most of the blood urea is from endogenous protein catabolism. A portion of this urea, which in monogastrics would be unavailable for protein synthesis, is excreted into the rumen, where it can be resynthesized into protein that will contribute eventually to the amino acid needs of the host. Thus, under conditions of low dietary protein, ruminants are efficient conservers of nitrogen.

RETICULORUMEN MOTILITY AND THE MAINTENANCE OF THE RUMEN ENVIRONMENT

The Physiological Functions of the Reticulorumen Serve to Maintain an Environment Favorable to Fermentation Patterns That Are Beneficial to the Host

The host animal has no direct control over the metabolism of the microbes in its gut. Yet, there are important physiological factors that influence the gastrointestinal (GI) fermentation process. In order for the host to assure that the proper type of fermentation patterns occur, it must maintain within the rumen (or colon) conditions that promote the growth and favorable metabolic patterns of the most beneficial bacteria and other microbes. There are several requirements that must be met by the host for proper fermentation to occur:

1. substrate for fermentation must be supplied;
2. temperature must be maintained at or near 37°C;
3. ionic strength (osmolality) of the rumen fluid must be kept within an optimal range (near 300 mosm);
4. a negative oxidation/reduction potential must be maintained (-250 to -450 mV);
5. undigestible waste (solid material) must be removed;
6. the rate of removal of microbes must be

compatible with the regeneration times of the most favorable microbes;

7. acid products of anaerobic fermentation (VFA) must be buffered or removed.

The first of these requisites, delivery of substrate, requires only eating; others—temperature and ionic strength—are met by the same homeostatic mechanisms that maintain these physiological conditions within the host body in general. Maintenance of oxidation/reduction potential requires only that oxygen be kept away from the fermentation site. The remaining requisites for fermentation, however, have required the development of special physiological functions associated with the forestomachs (or hindgut). These specialized functions include the motility patterns characteristic of the reticulorumen, the direct absorption of VFA, and the production of tremendous amounts of saliva.

Rumen Fermentation Is Maintained by Selectively Retaining Actively Fermenting Material While Allowing Unfermentable Residue to Pass on to the Abomasum

The walls of the reticulorumen are muscular, possess an extensive intrinsic nervous system, and are capable of highly complex and coordinated motility patterns. The selective ruminal retention of fermenting material, and release of unfermentable residue, is accomplished by these motility patterns. An understanding of reticulorumen anatomy is necessary to comprehend the effects of reticulorumen motility patterns. In Figure 30–7 note the division of the reticulorumen into compartments, or *sacs*. These divisions are created by muscular pillars that project into

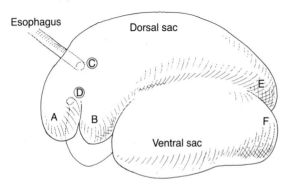

Figure 30–7. Rumen anatomy. *A*, reticulum; *B*, cranial sac; *C*, cardia; *D*, reticulo-omasal orifice; *E*, caudal-dorsal blind sac; *F*, caudal-ventral blind sac.

the lumen of the organ. It should be appreciated that the reticular fold and rumen pillars, in addition to the walls themselves, are motile. During reticulorumen contractions, the pillars elevate and relax alternately, either accentuating or reducing the divisions within the lumen of the reticulorumen. It may be difficult for students who are accustomed to visualizing the reticulorumens of embalmed specimens to appreciate, but at times during contractions the excursions of the walls and pillars are so great that the total shape of the reticulorumen is distorted; sacs and compartments become nearly obliterated, and pillars elevate to the extent that compartmental divisions become nearly complete. When the magnitude of these contractions is recognized, it is not difficult to appreciate the tremendous effect that reticulorumen motility has on the flow of rumen ingesta.

Two patterns of reticulorumen motility are generally described: *primary* or *mixing contractions*, and *secondary* or *eructation contractions*. Primary contractions start with a double, or biphasic, contraction of the reticulum. In the first phase of this reticular contraction, the organ is reduced to about one half its relaxed size, whereas the second contraction is strong, nearly obliterating the lumen of the reticulum. The next action of the primary contraction pattern is a caudal-moving peristaltic contraction of the dorsal sac. Upon completion of the dorsal sac contraction, there is a similar caudal-moving contraction of the ventral sac, followed by a cranial-moving contraction of the dorsal sac. The primary contraction pattern is completed by a cranial-moving contraction of the ventral sac (Fig. 30–8). The primary contraction pattern serves to mix ingesta and to aid in the separation of large and small particles. Secondary contractions, when they occur, follow immediately after the primary contractions. The secondary contractions consist of a cranial-moving wave that starts in the caudal-dorsal blind sac and continues over the dorsal sac (see Fig. 30–8). The function of the secondary contraction is to force gas toward the cranial portion of the rumen. As the secondary contraction moves gas toward the cardia, the cranial sac relaxes, and the cranial pillar elevates, allowing liquid ingesta to move away from the cardia so that gas can enter the esophagus and be eructated. Secondary contractions are important, because large amounts of gas, primarily CO_2 and CH_4, are formed during fermentation, and these must be removed rapidly to prevent rumen distention.

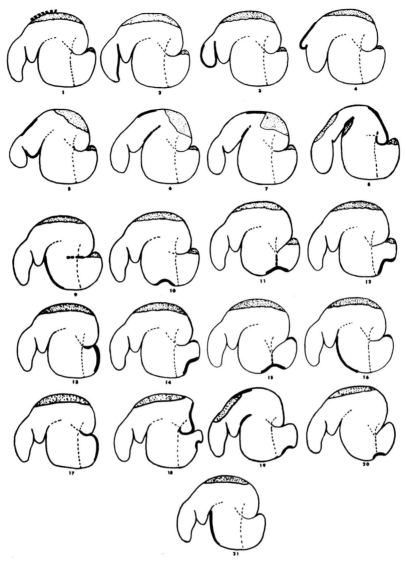

Figure 30–8. Conraction sequence in reticulorumen. These drawings were derived by taking tracings directly from radiographs. The stippled regions represent gas and the heavy lines indicate regions actively contracting. Drawings 1–16 represent the sequence of events in a primary contraction in a normally fed sheep. Drawings 17–21 represent the sequence of events in a secondary or eructation contraction. The individual drawings represent the following events: (1) resting stage: double-dotted line represents points of attachment of rumen to dorsal abdominal wall; (2) initiation of sequence with elevation of reticulorumenal fold; (3) end of first phase of reticular contraction; (4) end of second phase of reticular contraction—note dilation of cranial sac; (5–7) contraction of cranial sac followed by contraction of cranial pillar and dorsal sac; (8) contraction of caudal-dorsal blind sac and caudal pillar, causing displacement of gas cap cranially toward reticulum, under cranial pillar, and into caudal-ventral blind sac; (9) contraction of longitudinal pillar and cranial ventral rumen—in the fasted sheep the sequence frequently ceases at this point, and the occurrence of the remaining steps in the sequence is variable depending on the degree of filling of the reticulorumen; (10–12) wave of contraction migrating caudally onto the caudal-ventral blind sac, associated with a ventral displacement of the caudal pillar; (13) contraction of the pole of the caudal-ventral blind sac displacing gas cap around the caudal pillar; (14–16) cranial migration of contraction if no secondary contraction sequence occurs; (17) when a secondary contraction follows a primary, the terminal contraction of the caudal-ventral blind sac may be maintained over a prolonged period or may be repeated simultaneously with a second contraction of the caudal pillar; (18) contraction of caudal pillar and dorsal blind sac start to push gas cap cranially—contraction starts to move cranially across caudal-ventral blind sac; (19) contraction has moved rapidly across dorsal rumen and cranial pillar has moved for the second time—eructation occurs at this point if it is going to; (20–21) contraction migrates cranially onto ventral rumen, causing contraction of ventral coronary pillars and second ventral displacement of the caudal pillar—cycle terminates with a contraction of the cranial ventral rumen. (From Ruckebusch Y, Thivend P: Digestive Physiology and Metabolism in Ruminants. Westport, CT, AVI Publishing, 1980, p 40.)

In general, reticulorumen contractions occur with a frequency of one to three per minute: contractions occur most frequently during eating and disappear entirely during deep sleep. The rate and strength of contractions are dependent on the character of the diet; coarse, fibrous feeds stimulate the most frequent and strongest contractions. Secondary contractions usually occur in association with half of the primary contractions, although this relationship is variable and may be more or less frequent depending on the rate of gas formation. Reticulorumen contractions have an important influence on the flow of fluid and particulate matter through the rumen.

Gravity and Reticulorumen Motility Combine to Create the Selective Flow of Particulate Matter Out of the Rumen

Rumen ingesta are stratified and segregated by the effects of gravity and reticulorumen motility. In cattle receiving forage diets, there are distinct zones or phases of rumen ingesta. In the dorsal rumen there is a gas cap, or zone, created by the fermentation gases. Below this there is a *solid zone* composed of intertwined particles of fermenting forage. The solid zone is sometimes referred to as the *rumen mat* because of the braided or woven nature of its particles. The solid zone is kept afloat by buoyancy created by air trapped in the feed particles and also by small bubbles of fermentation gases that form around bacteria that adhere to the plant material as fermentation takes place. At the bottom of the rumen there is a *liquid zone* with a water-like consistency. The area between the solid and liquid zones is the *slurry zone*. The slurry zone has indistinct boundaries and forms a continuum of consistency from the liquid to the solid zones. These four major zones are created primarily by the effect of gravity; two additional functional zones are created by the motility patterns. These are the *ejection zone* and the *zone of potential escape*, which comprise the dorsal and ventral areas, respectively, of the reticulum and cranial sac (Fig. 30–9).

Functional Specific Gravity Determines the Rate at Which Particulate Matter (Solids) Moves Through the Zones of the Reticulorumen

As forage is consumed by ruminants, the particles are only partially comminuted by the

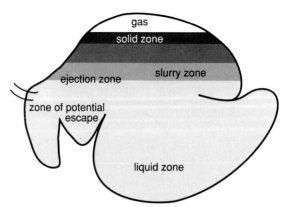

Figure 30–9. The rumen is stratified into indistinct zones, varying in consistency of ingesta. The dorsal solid zone contains relatively undigested forage material and continues imperceptibly into the slurry and liquid zones. The ejection zone is near the cardia and is the area that receives newly swallowed feed; contractions of the reticulum eject feed material from this area into the solid zone. As material becomes digested, it sinks into the liquid zone, eventually returning from the liquid zone to the cranial sac and reticulum. Once in the reticulum and cranial sac, material is in a zone of potential escape from which it may enter the reticulo-omasal orifice.

initial mastication and thus arrive at the reticulum as a tangled, masticated bolus of fairly long forage pieces. The bolus has a functional specific gravity of less than one because of air that is trapped both within and between the feed particles. (The term *functional* is applied to specific gravity in this context to indicate that the effects of trapped air are taken into consideration.) Because of the low specific gravity, the bolus floats in the ejection zone until a reticulum contraction occurs, at which time the pressure exerted by the reticular contraction washes, or ejects, the bolus from the reticulum into the solid zone of the dorsal sac. In the dorsal sac, bacteria become adhered to the forage particles, and fermentation starts to occur with the formation of small bubbles of fermentation gases that help to keep the functional specific gravity of the particles low. Motility in the dorsal sac serves to mix ingesta and the solid zone in a counterclockwise circle (when viewed from the left, Fig. 30–10). As the ingesta are mixed, the particles begin to break up because of fermentative destruction of structural carbohydrates in the plants. As fermentation proceeds, particle size is reduced; entrapped air escapes; there is a reduced rate of fermentation gas formation; and functional specific gravity of the feed particles increases.

As functional specific gravity increases, particles tend to sink and separate into the slurry zone in the ventral sac of the rumen, where further fermentation and size reduction occurs. In the ventral sac, the motility pattern creates a clockwise movement of ingesta (see Fig. 30–10). As the flowing ingesta move against the cranial pillar of the rumen, material that still has a relatively low functional specific gravity tends to remain in suspension in the slurry zone, and is retained in the circulating mass within the ventral sac. Material that has become relatively dense tends to fall over the cranial pillar and into the cranial sac, thus into the zone of potential escape. During contractions of the cranial sac, dense material can move into the reticulum from which it can exit the rumen through the reticulo-omasal orifice.

The effectiveness of the particle separation system in the rumen can be appreciated by considering particle sizes at different points in the digestive process. Long forage material is reduced in size by initial mastication to particles of 1–2 cm or less in length. Most of the material in the dorsal rumen is of similar particle size. Particle size diminishes in the more ventral portions of the rumen. Most particles that move through the reticulo-omasal orifice are 2–3 mm long. The selection of small particles for passage into the omasum occurs even though the reticulo-omasal orifice, when dilated for food passage, is probably in the order of 2 cm in diameter, indicating that size discrimination is not based on sieving action at the orifice.

Digestibility and Physical Characteristics of Feed Have Important Influences on Both the Rate of Particle Passage from the Rumen and the Rate of Feed Intake

From the earlier discussion it can be appreciated that feed does not leave the rumen until it is broken down into small particles. Microbial action and remastication (as discussed later) are primarily responsible for particle size reduction in the rumen, and the rate of breakdown of fiber is primarily a function of its digestibility. Poorly digestible fiber takes longer to be broken down sufficiently to enter the zone of potential escape, compared to fiber of greater digestibility. This means that poorly digestible fiber remains in the rumen longer than fiber of higher digestibility. Because there are fixed limits to the volume of the rumen, rate of feed intake cannot exceed the rate of ingesta outflow; therefore, intake of poorly

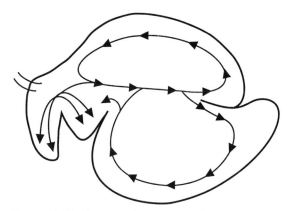

Figure 30–10. Patterns of movement of rumen ingesta. Rumen motility results in more or less circular patterns of ingesta movement.

digestible feeds is always less than intake of highly digestible feeds. Feed preparation can influence this relationship. Chopping, or grinding, of poorly digestible forages increases their rate of passage from the rumen, because there is less particle size reduction necessary before pieces can pass into the omasum. This usually increases the amount of the material that an animal can eat, because rumen throughput is increased; however, digestibility is decreased often, because the time of exposure to microbial action is reduced. Thus, physical form (length) and digestibility each have an effect on rate of passage from the rumen and also on feed intake. In general, forage material of relatively high digestibility has a rumen half-life of approximately 30 hours, whereas poorly digestible material has a half-life of up to 50 hours.

Rumination, or Cud Chewing, Has an Important Effect on Particle Size Reduction and the Movement of Solid Material Through the Rumen

Rumination is the act of remasticating rumen ingesta. The initial act of rumination is regurgitation, which occurs just prior to the initiation of a primary rumen contraction. When regurgitation occurs, there is an extra contraction of the reticulum, which takes place just before the regular biphasic reticular contraction that initiates the primary cycle. Simultaneous with the extra reticular contraction, the cardia relaxes, and there is an inspiratory excursion of the ribs with the glottis closed. The latter action creates a negative pressure within the thorax, favoring the movement of food into the esophagus. When food enters the esophagus, there is a reverse peristaltic wave that propels the material cranially into the mouth. As soon as the food bolus reaches the mouth, excess water is expressed by action of the tongue; the water is swallowed, and remastication of the material begins. The duration of remastication depends on the character of the diet, with course material appearing to require more time for remastication than finely ground or highly digestible feeds.

Regurgitated material for remastication comes from the dorsal portion of the reticulum, which has particle size and functional specific gravity characteristic of the slurry zone. Thus, the ingesta selected for rumination is not the coarsest material in the rumen, but rather material that has already been through the digestive actions of the solid zone. This appears to be an efficient system in which some of the structural material of the plant is softened by soaking, and removed or weakened by microbial action in the solid zone. The partially fermented material then reaches the slurry zone and is subject to remastication, causing further comminution and exposing additional fermentable substrate that may not have been directly exposed to previous microbial action.

Rumination may serve also to aid the particle separation process: as the regurgitated bolus reaches the mouth, it is squeezed by the tongue and cheeks before mastication begins. Water and small particles are expressed from the bolus by this squeezing action and swallowed, prior to mastication of the remaining bolus. Thus, this squeezing or expressing action tends to separate small particles from large particles. The small particles, when reswallowed, tend to sink into the zone of potential escape, whereas the larger particles, swallowed after remastication, are ejected back into the slurry zone.

Rumination occurs during times when the animal is not actively eating, usually during times of rest, but not during times of deep sleep. The time spent ruminating is dependent on the type of diet and appears to range from almost none on high grain diets to a maximum of about 10 hours/day on high forage diets. Feed intake level also influences the amount of rumination time, with high intakes stimulating increased rumination.

Water Moves Through the Rumen at a Much Faster Rate Than Particulate Matter

The flow of water has important effects on rumen dynamics. In order for small particles

and soluble material to exit the rumen, liquid from the liquid zone of the ventral sac, cranial-ventral blind sac, and reticulum must constantly be moving through the reticulo-omasal orifice. This means that water must be constantly flowing through the mass of solid material. In effect, the reticulorumen functions like a giant strainer holding the fermenting mass of particulate matter while water flows through it, washing small particles and soluble material away. Therefore, the transit rate of water must be considerably greater than the transit rate of particulate matter through the rumen. The relative differences in the rates of movement of solid and liquid phase material through the rumen can be appreciated from their respective rumen half-lives: 30–50 hours for particulate matter and about 15–20 hours for liquid.

The rate of liquid flow through the rumen is measured often as the dilution rate, which is expressed as a percent of total liquid that leaves the rumen in an hour. The term *dilution rate* comes from the way liquid turnover is measured; some soluble marker substance is mixed into the rumen and its concentration measured as soon as it is thoroughly dispersed into the liquid phase. Then, samples are taken over time, and the rate at which the marker substance becomes diluted is measured. The rate of dilution is dependent on the rate at which water containing marker leaves the rumen and is replaced with new, unmarked water; thus, the dilution rate is an indirect measure of the rate of water flow through the rumen. Normal dilution rate values vary with diet and feed intake and are usually in the range of 5–30%/hour. One other point should be appreciated from the concept of dilution rate; water only leaves the rumen as it is replaced from some other source.

Nearly all water that enters the rumen does so through the esophagus, either from salivary flow, drinking, or succulent feeds. Thus, the dilution rate is dependent on rates of salivation and drinking. Salivation rate is influenced by chewing time and feed type; feeds such as long-stemmed dry roughages that require relatively high rates of mastication stimulate large salivary flow rates and high dilution rates. Salivation occurs during rumination as well as during initial mastication; therefore, those feeds, such as forages, that stimulate high rates of rumination also stimulate high dilution rates. Conversely, feeds, like concentrates, that do not stimulate extensive rumination result in relatively low dilution rates. The rate of drinking is influenced by the rate of feed intake and the salt, or electrolyte, content of the diet. Thus, high rates of intake or diets with high electrolyte contents stimulate high dilution rates.

Little water enters the rumen by way of the mucosa. The mucosa of the forestomachs is stratified squamous and is aglandular; thus, there is no direct fluid secretion. Some water can enter the rumen through osmosis, but under normal conditions this appears to be little. Normal rumen osmolality is about 280 mosm/L, compared to a normal of approximately 300 mosm/L in blood and extracellular fluid. Thus, the usual osmotic flow of water is out of the rumen. After consumption of relatively digestible feeds, rumen osmolality increases briefly due to VFA production; however, it appears that osmolalities in excess of 340 are necessary for water to flow osmotically into the rumen. Under normal conditions, osmolalities this high are not sustained for long and, thus, there is usually little osmotic flow of water into the rumen.

Rumen Dilution Rate Has Important Influences on Fermentation and Microbial Cell Yield

Small particles, including microbes, leave the rumen with the liquid phase. Therefore, high dilution rates result in rapid microbial removal and reductions in microbial cell concentrations. Because high microbe concentrations suppress microbial cell division, growth of microbes is stimulated by high dilution rates. High growth rates are nutritionally desirable, because a higher portion of the energy available to the microbes is used for growth instead of for maintenance, as occurs in older, relatively stable microbial populations. Thus, high dilution rates usually increase Y_{ATP} values, provided that adequate protein is available to support cell growth.

In addition to its effect on Y_{ATP}, dilution rate may affect the microbial makeup of the rumen biomass, and also have some influence on the fermentation pattern. The rate of microbial wash-out increases with the dilution rate. At high dilution rates, those species with slow growth rates diminish in population size, because their replication rate is not great enough to match the rate at which they are removed. Thus, selection pressure favors species with faster growth rates during times of high rumen dilution rates. Exceptions to this pattern occur, because some microbes are able to attach themselves to the particulate matter in the solid and slurry zones. Such microbes then exit the rumen dependent on the kinetics of particle size reduction, rather than on dilution rate. In general, the changes occurring in the rumen microbial population with high dilution rates appear to favor acetic acid production and to increase the acetic acid to propionic acid ratio.

CONTROL OF RETICULORUMEN MOTILITY

Reticulorumen Motility Is Controlled by the Central Nervous System and Affected by Intraluminal Conditions

In the dorsal vagal nucleus of the brainstem, there is a motility control center for the regulation of reticuloruminal motility. This center issues afferent fibers to the forestomach through the vagus nerve. There is an extensive intrinsic nervous system within the reticulorumen, but vagal innervation is necessary for coordination of normal motility patterns. When the vagal nerves are destroyed, motility of the rumen musculature ceases initially, but returns within several days; however, the motility that develops after vagotomy is erratic, uncoordinated, and incapable of supporting the normal flow of ingesta through the reticulorumen. Vagotomized ruminants do not survive.

The dorsal vagal nucleus receives afferent stimuli that affect the control of forestomach motility. Important afferent signals come from the lumen of the reticulorumen and serve to monitor distention, ingesta consistency, pH, VFA concentration, and ionic strength. Rumen volume, or distention, appears to be monitored by stretch receptors in the walls and, especially, in the pillars. Moderate distention increases rumen motility and rumination. Increased motility and rumination have the effect of increasing the rate at which particles are broken down, which leads to an increased passage rate. Thus, rumen throughput is enhanced when increased intake expands rumen volume. Severe distention, as occurs pathologically in bloat, causes cessation of rumen motility.

Consistency of ingesta also has an important influence on rumen motility. Consistency is determined largely by diet type. When the diet consists of succulent plants, grain, or finely chopped forage, there is little material in the solid zone, or rumen mat, and the slurry zone is fluid. This type of fluid ingesta offers little resistance to the movement of the rumen pillars; thus, the rumen musculature has to apply relatively little force to mix and circulate the rumen contents. Tension receptors in the reticuloruminal muscle appear to monitor the force necessary to move the pillars through the ingesta. Highly fluid rumen ingesta are associated with low muscle tension and have a negative influence on reticulorumen motility. At the other dietary extreme, when animals are eating dry, long-stem hay, the rumen contents are solid and create a large and highly interwoven rumen mat. Resistance to movement of the pillars through the solid mass of ingesta is high and results in the stimulation of tension receptors, resulting in a positive feedback on motility. Because motility rate is directly related to the rate of particle breakdown, this appears to be a self-regulatory mechanism that increases the rate of particle comminution when diets with large particle size are fed.

Chemoreceptors appear to exist in the walls of the rumen and reticulum. These receptors monitor pH, VFA concentration, and ionic strength (or osmolality). The pH of the reticulorumen is normally slightly acid, reflecting the acidity of the VFA, but extreme acid conditions are undesirable. Increasing VFA concentrations or decreasing pH results in a suppression of rumen motility. Normal rumen pH is in the range of 5.5–6.8, depending on the type of diet. When the rumen pH falls much below 5.0, motility is severely depressed. This response appears to be protective in nature, because fermentation tends to be enhanced by motility-induced mixing; thus, suppression of motility slows down fermentation, allowing VFA absorption to catch up with VFA production.

Osmolality may influence rumen motility also, although motility appears less sensitive to osmotic changes than to pH changes. Normal osmolality in the rumen is about 280 mosm, but increases during active fermentation. Osmotically active solutes in the rumen include organic acids as well as salivary and dietary electrolytes. As organic acid formation increases during fermentation, osmolality increases also, which tends to reduce motility. The rumen epithelium creates a relatively impermeable barrier to water, so that wide swings in rumen osmolality can occur without large shifts in water between the rumen and vascular compartment. At abnormally high osmolalities, however, water can be drawn into the rumen.

OMASAL FUNCTION

Passage of Material from the Reticulum to the Omasum Occurs During Reticular Contraction

The omasum is composed of a body and a canal. The body is filled with multiple muscular folds, or *leaves*, that project from the greater curvature into the lumen. The canal, which is located on the lesser curvature, connects the reticulum to the abomasum. Ingesta moves into the omasum during reticular contractions. The omasal orifice usually remains open, but dilates especially during the second phase of the reticular contraction, during which ingesta flow rapidly into the omasal canal. After the reticular contraction, the omasal orifice closes briefly as the canal contracts, forcing newly arrived ingesta up into the leaves. Intermittently, the body and leaves of the omasum contract, forcing the material from the body of the organ into the canal and on into the abomasum. Proper functioning of the omasum and reticulum appears to be particularly important to the passage of ingesta out of the rumen. Occasionally, traumatic injury due to ingested foreign bodies causes severe adhesions of the reticulum and omasum to the body wall. In addition, damage to vagal fibers entering the organs may occur. In such cases, motility of the rumen proper may continue normally, but the ability to move food out of the forestomachs and into the abomasum is severely impaired. The rumen becomes greatly distended with finely comminuted feed, and the entire rumen becomes a slurry zone. In spite of the distended rumen, there is little movement of ingesta into the abomasum, and the animals eventually suffer severe inanition. This condition is variably known as *omasal transport failure* or vagal indigestion; there is usually little that can be done to correct it.

The structure of the omasum, with its many leaves and large mucosal surface area, suggests that it has an absorptive function, but the exact nature of this function is still incompletely understood. One important possibility is that it exists to remove residual VFAs and bicarbonate from ingesta before material is transported to the abomasum. VFAs appear

to cause unfavorable reactions in the abomasum, so it is important that the major portion of them are removed prior to abomasal entry. Also, it appears desirable to absorb, prior to abomasal entry, any bicarbonate remaining in the ingesta. Bicarbonate remaining in ingesta entering the abomasum would serve only to neutralize abomasal hydrochloric acid (HCl), causing the abomasal glands to work harder to maintain appropriate abomasal pH.

VOLATILE FATTY ACID ABSORPTION

Volatile Fatty Acids, Representing 60–80% of the Energy Needs of the Animal, Are Absorbed Directly from the Forestomach Epithelium

VFAs are bacterial waste products and, if allowed to accumulate, will suppress fermentation. Furthermore, the VFAs are tremendously important energy substrates for the host, supplying 60–80% of the dietary energy to ruminants on most types of diets. Therefore, it is important from both the standpoint of digestion and host metabolism that an efficient and high-capacity mechanism for VFA absorption be present. The forestomach epithelium supplies such a system, absorbing nearly all of the VFA, with only small amounts escaping to the lower digestive tract. In addition, the absorptive process aids in maintaining rumen pH by removing acid from the forestomach ingesta and contributing bicarbonate in the process.

The epithelium responsible for this tremendous absorption is structurally much different from other absorptive epithelia of the GI system. However, there is an interesting nature to this epithelium that may impart to it functional characteristics similar to the absorptive epithelium of the small intestine and colon. The forestomach surface is of the stratified squamous type and, similar to the stratified squamous epithelium of the skin and other surfaces, consists of several layers of cells of varying maturity. The deepest layer is the *stratum basale* from which cells divide and migrate into the *stratum spinosum*. Cells of the stratum spinosum begin the process of keratinization and continue into the *stratum granulosum*, which is covered by the outermost and most keratinized layer, the *stratum corneum*. Although seemingly completely different from

the columnar epithelium of the small intestine, an interesting similarity between forestomach and intestinal epithelia is noted when the cellular attachments and intercellular spaces of the forestomach are examined (Fig. 30–11).

The cells of the stratum granulosum are tightly joined by junctions that may functionally resemble the tight junctions of the enterocytes (see Chapter 29 for a description of enterocyte tight junctions). Deeper in the epithelium, the cells of the stratum spinosum and stratum basale are separated by intercellular spaces that increase in size as the basement membrane is approached. These intercellular spaces are reminiscent of the lateral spaces of columnar absorptive epithelia. Add to these observations the intercellular bridges that characterize the forestomach epithelium, and an interesting analogy to columnar absorptive epithelia can be constructed. It appears that VFAs, electrolytes, and water are

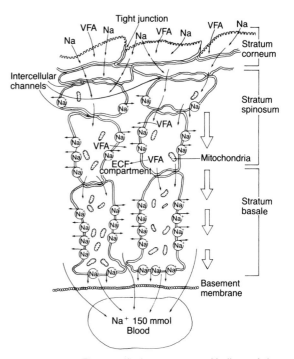

Figure 30–11. The stratified squamous epithelium of the rumen, although anatomically much different, shares functional similarities with the columnar epithelium of the intestine. Note the tight junctions of the cells of the stratum corneum and the lateral space-like compartment between adjacent cells of the stratum spinosum and stratum basale. Although the cells of the stratum spinosum are metabolically inactive, the intercellular channels allow the metabolic actions of the stratum basale to be reflected in the more superficial layers.

initially absorbed through the stratum corneum and passed cell to cell by way of intercellular bridges to the cells of the stratum spinosum and stratum basale, from which the absorbed substances are passed into the intercellular spaces before entering the capillaries. This arrangement appears to impart to the forestomach epithelium the same three-compartment characteristics of the columnar absorptive epithelia, with solutes passing from lumen to cell to lateral spaces. Although the keratinized cells of the stratum corneum do not appear to retain adequate metabolic machinery (mitochondria, and so forth) to maintain appropriate gradients for diffusion, the cells of the stratum spinosum and basale do appear to be metabolically active. Because of the intercellular bridges, absorbed solute can be transferred directly from the outer keratinized cells to the deeper, more metabolically active cells. Thus, the metabolic activity deep in the epithelium appears to maintain conditions for absorption at the epithelial surface.

The molecular mechanism of VFA absorption is incompletely understood, but appears to involve local alterations in pH near the absorptive surface. Differences in pH can have an important influence on VFA absorption because of shifts in the dissociation state of the VFA molecules. The pKa of the VFA is approximately 4.8, well below the normal pH of the rumen; thus, most of the VFAs exist in the rumen in the dissociated, or ionic, form. However, sodium-hydrogen ion exchange by the epithelial cells may decrease the local pH at the absorptive surface. Such a drop in pH would lead to a shift in the VFA from the ionic to the free-acid state. Cell membranes are permeable to VFA free acids, and absorption proceeds because of the concentration gradient between the lumen and cells. The high CO_2 tension in the rumen, due to the production of fermentation gases, may also enhance the conversion of VFA to the free acid state. Note from Figure 30–12 that in the process of absorbing one VFA molecule, one molecule of bicarbonate is generated in the lumen; thus, VFA absorption helps to buffer rumen pH both by generating base as well as by removing acid.

All of the VFAs appear to be absorbed by the same mechanism, but they are handled differently within the epithelial cells. Some acetate appears to be completely oxidized within the cells, with the remainder absorbed unchanged. Most propionate is absorbed, but a small portion is converted to lactate by the

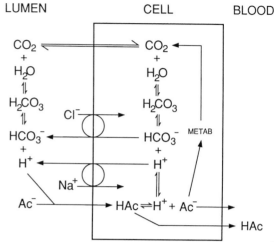

Figure 30–12. Volatile fatty acid absorption is promoted by the conversion of VFA anions to free acids in the microenvironment near the epithelial surface. This diagram illustrates two proposed means, one intracellular and one extracellular, by which hydrogen ions could be locally generated to effect the formation of VFA free acids; both mechanisms could exist simultaneously.

epithelial cells. Butyrate is modified extensively and essentially all changed to β-*hydroxybutyrate* before absorption. Beta-hydroxybutyrate is an important metabolite that is known as a *ketone body*. Ketone bodies are metabolites that frequently have special medical significance, and are discussed in greater detail in Chapter 31. It is important to point out here that in ruminants the rumen itself is an important source of ketone bodies. This is in contrast to monogastrics in which ketone bodies arise exclusively from the partial oxidation of long-chain fatty acids.

The rumen epithelium is arranged in *papillae*, which are finger-like projections that serve to increase the absorptive surface area. Whereas these papillae serve the same area-expansion function as the villi of the small intestine, they are much larger and easily visible to the unaided eye. The size and shape of the papillae are quite dynamic and responsive to changes in diet. Papillary growth is stimulated by VFAs, especially butyrate and propionate. Diets with high digestibility result in high rumen VFA concentrations, which stimulate the growth of long papilla. In contrast, animals receiving little feed or diets of low digestibility have short rumen papilla. It is important to adapt animals gradually when changing them from diets of low digestibility to those of high digestibility. Part of the reason for this may be to allow time for sufficient adjustment of papillary size, so that VFA absorption will match VFA production.

RUMEN DEVELOPMENT AND ESOPHAGEAL GROOVE FUNCTION

Tremendous Changes in Forestomach Size and Function Occur with Dietary Changes in Early Life

At birth the forestomach is about equal in size to the abomasum in both lambs and calves. This is in stark contrast to the normal adult proportions, in which the forestomach accounts for more than 90% of the total stomach volume. Enlargement of the forestomach occurs rapidly after birth, but the rate is dependent on diet type. When young ruminants are given access to solid feeds soon after birth, forestomach development rate is maximal. In cattle, the period of forestomach development is arbitrarily divided into the nonruminant period, from 0–3 weeks, and the transitional period from 3–8 weeks. Approximate adult distribution of stomach proportions is achieved usually by 8 weeks, assuming the calves have access to solid feeds. Calves can be seen eating grain and forage at less than 2 weeks old, and are frequently seen to ruminate by 3 weeks of age, indicating considerable forestomach development by this time. Withholding solid feed dramatically reduces the rate of rumen development. In calves that are given diets of only milk or milk replacer, forestomach development remains rudimentary for 14–15 weeks or more.

Forestomach epithelial development parallels the general development of the organ. At birth the epithelium is low with small or nonexistent papillae. Exposure of the epithelium to VFAs appears to stimulate papillary development and general organ development as well. Highly digestible feeds, such as concentrates, result in the greatest VFA production and fastest epithelial development. Some dietary forage may aid in muscular development of the forestomachs, but calves and lambs should receive most of their solid feed as grain, because their energy needs are high compared to their ability to ferment forages.

At birth the forestomach is sterile, but is quickly colonized by environmental bacteria, mostly facultative organisms. As bacterial fermentation proceeds in the anaerobic confines of the forestomach, the electromotive force becomes low, as the typical reductive environment of the rumen is created by bacterial action. This environment creates conditions necessary for the growth and establishment of the strict anaerobes. The development of forestomach bacterial flora occurs independently of any special inoculation process, and indeed, it is impossible to prevent it from occurring except by raising calves under gnotobiotic conditions. Protozoal inoculation, in contrast to bacterial inoculation, appears to require some exposure to cattle: calves raised in complete isolation will not develop protozoal fauna. It appears that aerosol spread of protozoa can occur, because no direct physical contact among cattle is necessary to establish a protozoal fauna.

The Esophageal Groove Functions to Divert the Flow of Ingested Milk Past the Forestomach and into the Abomasum

For proper rumen development in the suckling animal, it is important for milk to be diverted away from the developing rumen. This is accomplished by the actions of the *reticular groove* (also called the *esophageal groove*). This structure is a gutter-like invagination traversing the wall of the reticulum from the cardia to the reticulo-omasal orifice. When stimulated, muscles of the groove contract, causing it to shorten and twist. The twisting action causes the lips of the groove to close together, forming a nearly complete tube from the cardia to the omasal canal. Milk entering the cardia when the groove is contracted is directed into the omasum, with 10% or less entering the rumen. Milk quickly traverses the omasum and enters the abomasum. Reticular groove closure is a reflex action with efferent impulses arriving from the brainstem through the vagus nerve. Afferent stimuli arise centrally and from the pharynx. Anticipation of suckling invokes central stimulation of reticular groove closure, which may be considered a cephalic phase. Fluid, especially sodium-containing fluid in the pharynx, stimulates afferent fibers that reinforce the cephalic phase of groove closure. The posture of the calf or lamb when suckling does not appear to have a large influence on reticular groove function, but rapid drinking from an open pail, in contrast to suckling from a nipple, frequently results in inefficient groove function and spillage of milk into the rumen.

Milk in the rumen results in the formation of improper fermentation patterns.

The reticular groove has its primary function in suckling animals, and the activity of the groove reflex appears to diminish after weaning and with advancing age. However, the groove reflex is stimulated by ADH (antidiuretic hormone, see Chapter 41), indicating that it may have some physiological function in adult life. ADH is secreted by the posterior pituitary in response to dehydration or increases in plasma osmolality. ADH is associated with thirst, and its stimulation of the reticular groove means that when water-deprived animals drink, a large portion of the water may bypass the rumen. This may be a functional mechanism to assure that water arrives quickly at the site of most rapid absorption, the small intestine.

EQUINE LARGE HINDGUT FUNCTION

The Equine Hindgut Has a Tremendous Capacity for Fermentation

A general function of the cecum and colon, as mentioned in Chapter 29, is to recover fluid and electrolytes from ingesta leaving the ileum. In many herbivorous species, this function has been expanded to include fermentative digestion. As is seen, absorptive and fermentation functions complement each other in the colons of nonruminant herbivores. This leads to an elegantly interactive system of fermentation and absorption; however, it also leads to an interdependence between the two processes, meaning that disturbances in fermentation can result in important abnormalities in absorption, and vice versa.

Type of Substrate and Fermentation Patterns Are Essentially Identical for Forestomach and Hindgut Fermentation

Structural and nonstructural carbohydrates, as well as proteins, form the major substrates for hindgut fermentation. However, the passage of material through the stomach and small intestine prior to its arrival at the cecum and colon may have some important effects on fermentative digestion. First, hindgut fermentation may be aided by prior gastric action. The effects of soaking and acid exposure on plant particles in the stomach may increase

their susceptibility to microbial attack and, thus, increase their rate of digestion in the hindgut. Second, some of the readily available carbohydrate, particularly sugars and starches, may be digested and absorbed prior to arrival in the cecum. Most evidence indicates, however, that glandular digestion of carbohydrate in the horse is not extremely efficient, and that substantial amounts of starch and sugars reach the cecum. It further appears that cell-wall carbohydrate interferes with the digestion or absorption of nonstructural carbohydrate, so that diets high in cell-wall content result in relatively little starch digestion and absorption in the equine small intestine. Even on a high grain diet, up to 29% of dietary starch may reach the cecum and colon.

Protein, as well as carbohydrate, is absorbed in the small intestine, potentially leading to a deficiency of nitrogen for colonic microbes. However, there is extensive urea recycling into the colon and cecum, in a manner similar to that occurring in the rumen (see Fig. 30–6). Thus, urea plus protein escaping small intestinal digestion supplies the nitrogen needs of the microbes. In contrast to the ruminant, there is no efficient means of recovering the microbial protein synthesized in the hindgut, and most of it passes out in the feces. Some experiments have shown a small amount of amino acid absorption from the equine cecum or colon, but the amount does not compare to microbial protein availability in the ruminant.

The Motility Functions of the Cecum and Colon Serve to Retain Material for Fermentation and to Separate Particles Based on Size

The functions of the hindgut in maintaining fermentation are similar to those of the rumen: favorable conditions must be maintained to support optimal fermentation. As in the rumen, these include substrate supply, pH and osmolality control, anaerobiosis, retention of fermenting material, and the continual removal of waste products and the residue of spent fermentation substrate. Separation of fermenting material from residue appears to be accomplished by selective retention of particles based on size, just as it was in the rumen; however, the means by which size separation and discriminate passage are accomplished are quite different for the cecum and colon compared to the forestomach. Anatomical characteristics and motility patterns in the cecum and colon are responsible for selective retention of long particles, allowing sufficient exposure for microbial digestion to occur. In general, the fermentative digestive process in the horse is not as efficient as that of the ruminant, and digestible energy values for forages are usually lower for horses than for cattle.

Before discussing the motility of the equine cecum and colon, a brief review of the anatomy of equine hindgut is important. A diagram of the equine digestive system, separated from its mesenteric attachments and laid out in a linear fashion, is in Figure 30–13. The hindgut commences with the cecum, which is separated from the large colon by a well-defined orifice. The large colon is folded on itself three times, forming four major anatomical divisions, the *right* and *left ventral*, and *left* and *right dorsal colon* segments. Ingesta enter the right ventral colon and course to the left ventral colon, from which the material enters the left dorsal portion through the *pelvic flexure*. From the left dorsal colon, material moves to the right dorsal colon before entering the small colon. A description of the arrangement of the large colon in the abdomen can be found in textbooks of anatomy. For the purposes of physiological study, note in Figure 30–13 the tremendous size and volume of the cecum and colon, compared to the small intestine. Note also the differences in diameter that occur throughout the colon, particularly the reductions in diameter that occur at the pelvic flexure and at the junction of the large and small colons. The sac-like evaginations that occur in the wall of the cecum and most segments of the colon are called *haustra*. Functionally, the equine hindgut can be divided into four sections: cecum, ventral colon, dorsal colon, and small colon.

Ingesta reach the cecum after a relatively short time in the stomach and small intestine. A large portion of soluble ingesta usually reaches the cecum by 2 hours after ingestion, whereas solids take somewhat longer, depending on particle size and consistency. The material in the cecum and throughout the large colon has a high water content and a slurry-like consistency.

The majority of cecal motility is of a mixing nature, with frequent low amplitude contractions that transport ingesta from haustrum to haustrum and back in a mixing pattern. The mixing action of the cecum maintains the cecal contents in a homogeneous state. About once every 3–4 minutes there is a strong contraction

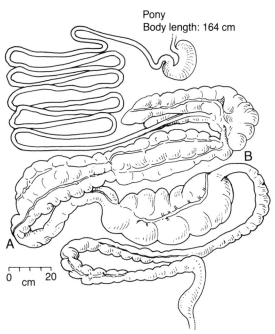

Pony
Body length: 164 cm

0   20
  cm

Figure 30–13. The equine gut. Note the tremendous development of the colon, compared to the small intestine. Note also the relative areas of constriction at the junctions of the ventral and dorsal colons (*A*) and the large and small colons (*B*).

of cecal muscles in a mass-movement type of action (see Chapter 29 for a description of "mass movement") in which the *body* and *apex* of the organ shorten and constrict, lifting ingesta into the *base*. Constriction of the base forces material through the *ceco-colic* orifice and into the right ventral colon. The motility pattern serves to functionally separate the cecum from the ventral colon with no apparent mixing of contents between the two hindgut segments. Thus, there is no retrograde flow of material from the colon to the cecum, so the composition of ingesta in these two organs is usually somewhat different.

Three types of motility patterns exist in the right and left ventral colon: haustral segmentation, propulsive peristalsis, and retropulsive peristalsis. Segmentation serves a mixing function that aids in promoting fermentation and bringing VFAs in contact with the mucosa for absorption. Mixing occurs throughout the ventral colon, and the right and left segments may be considered as one functional unit with homogeneous ingesta. Propulsive activity, or aboral peristalsis, in the ventral colon originates near the cecum and appears to occur as a continuation of the cecal mass movements. Peristaltic activity in the proximal ventral colon propels ingesta distally into the left ventral colon. In the left ventral colon, retropulsive or antiperistaltic movements are encountered, which resist the flow of ingesta and result in the retention of material in the ventral colon, allowing time for microbial digestion and preventing the washout of microbial species. In addition, the retropulsive actions of the left ventral colon aid in creating differential flow rates of liquid and particulate matter through the colon. The antiperistaltic motility appears to originate from a pacemaker in the *pelvic flexure,* the area of restricted diameter where the left ventral and dorsal colons meet.

The motility of the ventral colon can be roughly compared to the stomach, with the pelvic flexure and distal left ventral colon acting as the pylorus and antrum, respectively. The pumping action of cecal mass movements combined with the propulsive action of the proximal ventral colon continually moves ingesta toward the pelvic flexure. In the distal ventral colon, however, antiperistaltic activity and the narrow diameter of the pelvic flexure retard the movement of material, causing it to be retained in the ventral colon. The squeezing action of the pelvic flexure mimics the action of the pylorus in selectively retaining relatively large particulate matter, while allowing liquid and small particles to pass. As particle size is reduced by fermentative action and the mixing activity of the colon, particles eventually become small enough to flow with the fluid phase and leave the colon. The action of the pelvic flexure is not as efficient as that of the pylorus, and some large particles do escape the ventral colon. In addition, there are periods during which propulsive movements occur in the left ventral colon and pelvic flexure. These factors allow the movement of particulate matter into the left dorsal colon.

The actions of the dorsal colon appear to mimic those of the ventral colon. Impedance to ingesta flow is created by the size restriction at the junction of the right dorsal colon and small colon. In addition, there may be retropulsive motility originating in the area of the distal right dorsal colon, near the junction with the small colon. These actions tend to impede the movement of ingesta through the dorsal colon, subjecting the material to another round of fermentative digestion, as occurred in the ventral colon. The delay in the flow of ingesta created by the combined actions of the ventral and dorsal colons results in significant retention of material, with most particulate matter taking from 24–96 hours to pass the large

colon. The efficiency of the large colon in retaining and separating ingesta of different particle sizes can be seen in Figure 30–14.

Understanding the motility of the equine colon is important, because problems of colon impaction in horses are common. Impactions usually occur near or within the pelvic flexure. This probably happens because the pelvic flexure is a site of flow restriction and differential flow of solid and liquid material. It is easy to imagine how the normal motility pattern could allow solid material to accumulate in this area and cause obstructions to occur.

The general understanding of small colon motility is limited, but it appears to exist primarily of segmentation and propulsion. The characteristic fecal balls of horses are formed by segmentation within the small colon.

The Rate of Fermentation and Volatile Fatty Acid Production in the Equine Colon Is Similar to That of the Rumen

In the equine colon, efficient means of buffering and VFA absorption must be present. Salivary buffering, as occurs in ruminants, cannot aid in buffering the colon, because of the changes in ingesta pH that occur over the course of gastric and small intestinal transit. In the horse, large quantities of fluid, rich in bicarbonate and phosphate buffers, are secreted by the ileum and transferred to the cecum, thus mimicking the actions of the salivary glands in ruminants. In addition, because of the glandular nature of the colonic mucosa, there is more direct addition of bicarbonate and other electrolytes to the lumen fluid in the cecum and colon than in the rumen.

Large fluxes of water traverse the cecal and colonic mucosa during the course of digestion. When horses are meal-fed, feed starts to enter the cecum about 2 hours after eating, and VFA production rapidly commences. As feed is transported from the cecum, VFA production continues in the large colon. During the period of active VFA production, large quantities of water enter the hindgut from the blood through the mucosa. Although this water flux may be in response to increased osmolality created by the generation of osmotically active VFA molecules, it is more likely because of direct fluid secretion from the crypts of the colonic epithelium (see Chapter 28 for a description of colonic epithelium). Secretion of sodium-, bicarbonate-, and chloride-contain-

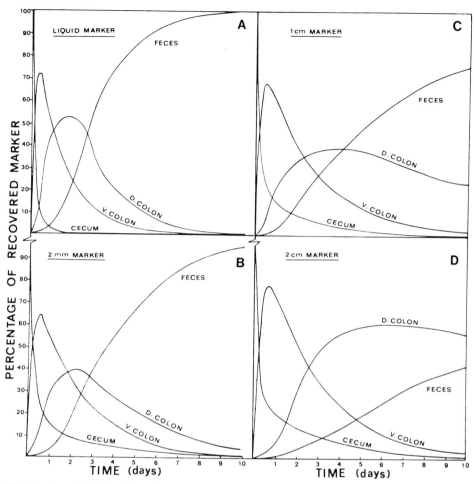

Figure 30–14. Retention of liquid and particles of various sizes in the compartments of the equine large intestine. Marker liquid and marked particles of various sizes, as indicated, were placed in the cecum of ponies and the distribution of marked materials among colon segments was measured at 2-hour intervals. The lines of the graph were mathematically fitted to the data. Each line indicates the percentage of marker in a given segment at any time. Note in graph *A* that at 7 days postinfusion nearly all of the liquid marker had been recovered in the feces, with little or none remaining in the intestinal segments. Increasing particle size has a relatively small effect on movement of particles out of the cecum. In contrast, as particle size increases there is significant retention of material in the colon and slow passage to the feces. (From Argenzio RA, Lowe JE, Pickard DW, Stevens CE: Digesta passage and water exchange in the equine large intestine. Am J Physiol 226:1035–1042, 1974.)

ing fluid from the colonic mucosa appears to occur in response to high concentrations of VFA in the lumen. This secretory response, in combination with the ileal secretions, is responsible for buffering of the lumen contents. Figure 30–15 illustrates the magnitude of water fluxes that occur during hindgut digestion in the pony. Note that there is considerable in-

ward and outward movement of water across the mucosa in each of the major fermentation compartments, ventral and dorsal colons, and cecum. Inward (into the lumen) water movement results from mucosal secretion, whereas outward water movement occurs in association with absorption of VFA.

The molecular mechanisms of VFA absorption in the equine colon appear to be identical to those in the rumen (see Fig. 30–12). Note from the figure that sodium absorption accompanies VFA absorption, and that bicarbonate is generated in the lumen. The absorption of VFA and sodium leads to osmotic absorption of water, probably through the transcellular pathway. The dynamics of water and electrolyte absorption in the gut may be reviewed in Chapter 29.

The function of the small colon is to recover water, electrolytes, and VFAs that were not absorbed in the large colon. There appears to be little VFA production in the small colon, but considerable absorption of water, sodium, and phosphate occurs there.

The large water and electrolyte fluxes that occur in the colon make horses vulnerable to colonic diseases. Colonic disease in the horse has consequences in terms of fluid and electrolyte loss that are more characteristic of small intestinal disease in many other animals.

There Are Tremendous Variations in Hindgut Anatomy and Function Among the Many Species of Veterinary Interest

All of these variations cannot be discussed here, but it should be remembered that, in addition to *Equidae*, rabbits, rats, guinea pigs, and swine depend on hindgut fermentation for a significant portion of their energy needs. It must also be appreciated that ruminants have a reasonably extensive hindgut, and that fermentative digestion occurs there, even after material has been through the rumen.

The basic scientific understanding of colonic function in general is not as advanced as that of small intestinal function. This dichotomy probably exists because problems of the small intestine occur as more important and life-threatening diseases of humans than do problems of the colon. However, interest in colonic physiology and pathophysiology among basic scientists and physicians has increased. Veterinary physiologists have long been interested in colonic function and have become leaders in the exploration of this area.

CLINICAL CORRELATIONS

GRAIN ENGORGEMENT TOXEMIA

HISTORY □ In mid-January a cattle feeder has asked you to examine a lot of 400-kg steers.

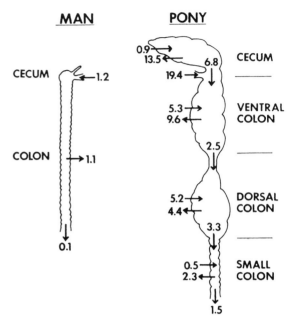

Figure 30–15. Net movement of water through the large intestine of a 70-kg man and a 160-kg pony. Values are in liters per day. Note the relatively large amount of fluid delivered to the pony's colon from the ileum (19.4 L/day), compared to humans. Also note the inward and outward movement of fluid in the various compartments of the pony's large intestine. (From Argenzio RA, Lowe JE, Pickard DW, Stevens CE: Digesta passage and water exchange in the equine large intestine. Am J Physiol 226:1035–1042, 1974.)

The steers have been on free-choice grain from a self-feeder for several weeks. Three days ago a blizzard prevented the caretaker from delivering feed to the feeders, and they were empty for 36 hours. Yesterday, they were filled, and all the steers ate ravenously. Today two of the 40 steers are dead, and many appear depressed and uncoordinated, and have diarrhea.

CLINICAL AND LABORATORY EXAMINATION □ Two steers are isolated for physical examination. They are depressed and have to be coaxed to move. Their heart rates are all above 100 (normal <80), and their body temperatures are less than 101.0°F (normal 101.5–103.0). Their rumens appear distended, and there is no evidence of rumen motility. The eyes are sunken in the orbits, and the oral mucosa is dry and sticky, indicating clinical dehydration. Necropsy examination of a dead steer reveals a greatly distended rumen, filled with grain and fluid. A pH-paper test indicates that the rumen fluid pH of the dead animal is below 4.5, but above 3 (normal 5.5–7.0).

COMMENT □ Ruminants may be fed large

amounts of grain if they are accustomed to it and receive it on a regular and frequent basis. In this case, even though the steers had been accustomed to a high grain diet, the lack of grain for more than a day followed by a large grain intake set up conditions for grain engorgement toxemia.

In grain engorgement, there is an abundant supply of starch, leading to the rapid growth and proliferation of rumen streptococci. These bacteria produce VFA rapidly, causing the rumen pH to diminish. As the rumen pH becomes lower, conditions become unfavorable for the growth and survival of cellulose-fermenting organisms and favorable for the growth of lactic acid–producing bacteria. This leads to the accumulation of lactic acid, a stronger acid than the VFA. Thus, rumen pH becomes even lower, killing many of the normal microflora. Some of the lactic acid becomes absorbed, which leads to a reduced blood pH and a life-threatening situation. Moreover, the large ruminal concentration of lactic acid and VFA results in a high osmotic pressure, drawing water out of the vascular fluid compartment and into the rumen. This leads to systemic hypovolemia, which may proceed to hypovolemic shock.

TREATMENT □ This is a grave situation, and it is likely that the farmer will lose additional steers. Treatment is aimed at expanding the intravascular fluid volume, correcting the systemic acidosis, and re-establishing a normal rumen environment. Severely affected steers should be evaluated to determine if their prognosis is good enough to warrant the expense of therapy: if not, euthanasia should be employed. Initial treatment should consist of rapid intravenous administration of large quantities of alkalizing fluid. Following the correction of fluid and acid base disturbances, ideally the rumen should be emptied, either by entubation with a large-bore stomach tube or by rumenotomy. In some cases, oral administration of antifermentation agents, such as oil of turpentine, mineral oil, or antibiotics, along with an alkalizing agent is an acceptable alternative to emptying the rumen. After the rumen environment is brought back to normal, it may be helpful to reinoculate the rumen with material taken from the rumen of a normal animal.

IMPACTION COLIC

HISTORY □ You are presented with a 20-year-old gelding that has been showing signs of abdominal discomfort (colic) for 16 hours. When left alone in his stall, the horse lies down, frequently preferring to lie on his back. There is little fresh manure in the stall. When taken out of the stall, he leads normally, but then lies down and rolls whenever he is released from the lead rope.

CLINICAL AND LABORATORY EXAMINATION □ The heart rate is slightly elevated at 60; respiratory rate and temperature are normal. The hydration state, as well as the color and perfusion of the mucus membranes, are normal. Simple laboratory evaluation reveals the packed cell volume to be 41% (normal 35–45%) and the plasma total solids to be 7.8 g/dL (normal 6.5–8.0 g/dL). Borborygmi (intestinal sounds) are softer and less frequent than normal, especially on the left side. Examination by rectal palpation reveals the pelvic flexure to be firm with a dough-like consistency; normally, the contents of the pelvic flexure have a fluid consistency. When you examine the teeth, you find that the molar surfaces are irregular, and one of the molars has a crack extending from the table surface to below the gum line.

COMMENT □ The pelvic flexure is a site of flow restriction and particle size separation. As water moves through the pelvic flexure, large forage particles accumulate and are retained for further fermentation and mixing in the ventral colon. A horse with poor teeth may not chew its forage adequately, resulting in many large particles. These particles tend to accumulate in the pelvic flexure and may cause an impaction and obstruction, as occurred in this case. Treatment involves the oral administration of softening agents, such as mineral oil. Drugs such as dioctyl sodium sulfosuccinate, which stimulate water secretion from the intestinal mucosa, are also beneficial. Prevention in this case involves correction of the dental problems, so that forage is more thoroughly chewed. Feeding pelleted feeds may be beneficial also.

Bibliography

Argenzio RA: Functions of the equine large intestine and their interrelationship in disease. Cornell Vet 65:303–330, 1975.

Church DC: The Ruminant Animal: Digestive Physiology and Nutrition. Englewood Cliffs, NJ, Prentice Hall, 1988, pp 14–298.

Hungate RE: The Rumen and its Microbes. New York, Academic Press, 1966.

McDonald W, Warner ACI (eds): Digestion and Metabolism in the Ruminant. Armidale, Australia, University of New England Publishing, 1975.

Phillipson AT (ed): Physiology of Digestion and Metabolism in the Ruminant. Newcastle upon Tyne, Oriel Press, 1970.

Ryckebusch Y, Thivend P: Digestive Physiology and Metabolism in Ruminants. Westport, CT, AVI Publishing, 1980.

Stevens CE: Comparative Physiology of the Vertebrate Digestive System. Cambridge, Cambridge University Press, 1988, pp 159–190.

Van Soest PJ: Nutritional Ecology of the Ruminant. Portland, OR, Durham and Downey, 1982, pp 152–275.

PRACTICE QUESTIONS FOR CHAPTER 30

1. In which of the following respects is fermentative digestion different from glandular digestion?

    a. Enzymes are not involved in fermentative digestion.
    b. Chemical bonds are not split by hydrolysis in fermentative digestion.
    c. Only carbohydrates are digested by fermentative digestion.
    d. Substrates are more extensively altered in fermentative digestion than in glandular digestion.
    e. Proteins are digested to amino acids by fermentative digestion and dipeptides by glandular digestion.

2. When comparing hindgut and forestomach fermentation, which of the following statements is true?

    a. The microbial populations are considerably different, but the products of digestion are the same.
    b. The microbial populations are the same, but the products of digestion are considerably different.
    c. Both the microbial populations and digestion products are similar.
    d. Structural carbohydrates of plants are not digested by hindgut fermentation.
    e. A nitrogen source is not required by the microbes of the hindgut.

3. The three VFAs—acetate, propionate, and butyrate—are

    a. net reaction products of the fermentative action of entire rumen biomass.
    b. the individual products of cellulose, starch, and hemicellulose digestion, respectively.
    c. the individual products of bacterial, protozoal, and fungal digestion, respectively.
    d. volatile products that leave the rumen with the gas phase during eructation.
    e. intermediate metabolites that are passed between microbial species.

4. Matching protein and energy availability in the rumen is an important nutritional goal in feeding ruminants. Which of the following is not a reason that protein and energy availability should be matched in ruminant diets? Well-matched diets result in

    a. most efficient use of energy for microbial growth.
    b. maximal delivery of protein to the host.
    c. maximal conservation of dietary amino acids, so that the dietary amino acid profile closely resembles that presented to the host for absorption.
    d. a minimal amount of dietary protein being lost because of formation of excess ammonia.
    e. the lowest possible rumen ammonia concentrations.

5. Which of the following is true of both methane and propionate?

    a. They are waste products of anaerobic fermentation but contain potential energy that is recoverable by the host.
    b. They are highly oxidized molecules.
    c. They are eructated from the rumen.
    d. Their formation results in the generation of NAD from NADH.
    e. They are toxic to monogastrics.

31

Postabsorptive Nutrient Utilization

1. Homeostatic mechanisms exist to balance the supply and demand of nearly all nutrients

THE FURNACE

1. The tricarboxylic acid (or Krebs) cycle is the major energy-yielding pathway of fuel utilization in the body

THE FUELS

1. The major metabolic fuels consist of glucose, amino acids, and fatty acids; various storage and transport forms exist for these compounds
2. Glucose is the central fuel in the energy metabolism of most animals
3. Amino acids are important fuels, in addition to being the building blocks of protein
4. Fatty acids are the major form of energy storage in the animal body

NUTRIENT UTILIZATION DURING THE ABSORPTIVE PHASE

1. During the absorptive phase, the liver takes up glucose and converts it into glycogen and triglyceride
2. The conversion of glucose to fatty acids is an irreversible process
3. Transport of fatty acids out of the liver is through chylomicron-like particles known as very low-density lipoproteins
4. Amino acids can be classified into groups based on metabolic characteristics
5. Amino acids are extensively modified during absorption
6. Many amino acids are removed by the liver on "first pass," never reaching the systemic circulation
7. Some amino acids taken up by the liver are used for protein synthesis
8. Most amino acids taken up by the liver are converted to carbohydrates
9. Not all amino acids are subject to hepatic destruction
10. Metabolism at the tissue level is coordinated with hepatic metabolism and results in the deposition of fuel into storage tissues during the absorptive period
11. Insulin promotes the synthesis of protein and the deposition of glycogen in muscle
12. Insulin-stimulated uptake of amino acids by muscle results in a net increase in muscle protein synthesis

13. During the absorptive phase, triglyceride accumulation in adipose tissue occurs by two mechanisms: uptake from very low-density lipoproteins, and direct lipid synthesis from glucose

NUTRIENT UTILIZATION DURING THE POSTABSORPTIVE PHASE

1. Hepatic metabolism switches from glucose utilization to glucose production during the postabsorptive phase
2. Fuel mobilization in peripheral tissues occurs when blood insulin concentration declines
3. Muscle reacts to a metabolic demand for glucose by mobilizing amino acids to support hepatic gluconeogenesis
4. Muscle release of amino acids is related to reduced glucose and amino acid uptake
5. The complex pattern of muscle amino acid catabolism and release is necessary to accommodate the liver's limited capacity for branch-chain amino acid uptake and to facilitate the removal of amino nitrogen from the muscle
6. The reaction of adipose tissue during the postabsorptive period is to mobilize fatty acids

NUTRIENT UTILIZATION DURING PROLONGED PERIODS OF ENERGY MALNUTRITION OR COMPLETE FOOD DEPRIVATION

1. During prolonged periods of fasting or undernutrition, glucose and amino acids are conserved by extensive utilization of fats and ketone bodies for energy production
2. A large portion of the fatty acids released from adipose are taken up directly by the liver
3. Hepatic ketone body formation is promoted by low glucose availability, a high glucagon to insulin ratio, and a ready supply of fatty acids
4. Glucagon plays an important role in the excessive production of ketone bodies during diabetes mellitus
5. Fatty acids cannot be used for glucose synthesis
6. Ketone bodies are formed in the mitochondria from acetyl CoA
7. Hepatic very low-density lipoproteins may be synthesized from adipose-derived fatty acid, as well as from newly synthesized fatty acid
8. Hormonal conditions direct the distribution of very low-density lipoprotein fatty acids in the body
9. Changes in growth hormone concentrations may aid in shifting peripheral fuel utilization from glucose and amino acids to ketone bodies and fatty acids

THE SPECIAL FUEL CONSIDERATIONS OF RUMINANTS

1. Ruminants exist in a perpetual state of gluconeogenesis because of their unique digestive process

The rate of absorption of nutrients from the gut is not constant; instead, it fluctuates greatly with food intake. Meals are digested at a rate dependent upon their chemical composition, irrespective of the nutrient needs of the animal. The nature of digestion dictates that nutrient absorption from the gut will be rapid during digestion, and then cease during interdigestive periods. In other words, the gut is not a storehouse for nutrients, and digestion is not modulated by the nutritional demands of the animal. The nutrient needs of the animal are not well matched to the wide fluctuations that occur in nutrient absorption from the gut. To the contrary, there is a vital need for a constant, steady supply of fuel-providing nutrients to maintain the basal metabolic functions of the body. In addition, there are times when the metabolic needs of the animal are greatly elevated, and these periods often do not coincide with the times of rapid absorption of nutrients from the gut. Therefore, there must be a sophisticated system for maintaining the supply of nutrients, particularly energy-supplying nutrients, and buffering both the short- and long-term "feast or famine" effects associated with the absorptive and postabsorptive periods of digestion.

Homeostatic Mechanisms Exist to Balance the Supply and Demand of Nearly All Nutrients

This chapter focuses on supply regulation of the major energy-supplying nutrients; however, other nutrients, including vitamins and minerals, also are subject to homeostatic regulatory mechanisms. Although many of these mechanisms directly involve the digestive system, space does not permit them all to be discussed in this book. Descriptions of the homeostatic mechanisms regulating the supply of minerals and vitamins can be found in some of the references listed at the end of this chapter.

Energy-supplying nutrients are referred to as metabolic fuels, and physiological mechanisms for maintaining the supply of fuels and matching it to demand is known as *fuel homeostasis*. Fuel homeostasis is maintained by several mechanisms: the insulin-glucagon axis, the hypothalamic-pituitary axis, and the central nervous system (CNS). This chapter includes a discussion on some of the ways in which fuel is stored during the absorptive period of digestion and subsequently mobilized when needed to supply energy needs. Chapter 1 on cell regulation should be reviewed, as well as the section on insulin and glucagon in Chapter 32, before reading this chapter.

THE FURNACE

The Tricarboxylic Acid (or Krebs) Cycle Is the Major Energy-Yielding Pathway of Fuel Utilization in the Body

The Krebs cycle and the major pathways leading into it are briefly outlined in Figure 31–1. It is assumed that most veterinary students have previously studied the *Krebs cycle, glycolysis,* and β-*oxidation of fats* in a basic course of biochemistry. Often in such courses, however, students become so intent on memorizing enzyme names and chemical changes in metabolites that the physiological signifi-

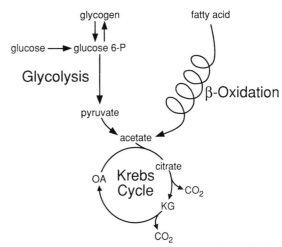

Figure 31–1. The relationship of the three major oxidative, catabolic pathways. *OA*, oxaloacetic acid; *KG*, α-ketoglutarate.

cance of the pathways is lost. For the purposes of this discussion it is important only that you follow the flow of the major carbon-containing nutrients into and out of the various pathways. The only specific metabolic steps that are emphasized are those points at which the flow of fuels is directed or regulated. As you read through this chapter, note that the Krebs cycle and associated pathways of intermediary metabolism are not only sites of fuel utilization and energy production, but also sites of transformation from one fuel type to another. These transformations are important in the overall scheme of fuel homeostasis.

THE FUELS

The Major Metabolic Fuels Consist of Glucose, Amino Acids, and Fatty Acids; Various Storage and Transport Forms Exist for These Compounds

Glucose is the digestion product of carbohydrate and is the basic metabolic fuel during periods of adequate nutrition in omnivorous monogastrics, such as dogs and rats. Although there are other important fuels in the body, glucose has special significance, because under most conditions, it is the only fuel that is consumed by the CNS. Therefore, maintaining a steady supply of glucose for brain metabolism is of paramount importance to the body. It is not surprising that an elegant system of homeostasis exists to regulate the availability of glucose to the brain and other tissues. Discussion of this system of maintaining glucose availability is a major objective of this chapter.

Glucose Is the Central Fuel in the Energy Metabolism of Most Animals

Glucose can be stored in the body as *glycogen*, a highly branched starch found in liver and skeletal muscle. Glycogen is the only direct storage form of glucose in the body, although glucose can be synthesized from other compounds. Directing glucose to and from glycogen depots is a major function of fuel homeostasis. When glucose is released from glycogen, the process is referred to as *glycogenolysis*.

The major means by which glucose is used as fuel is through the Embden-Meyerhof pathway, also referred to as *glycolysis*. Glycolysis is the series of biochemical steps that initiate the oxidation of glucose. Glycolysis leads directly into the *Krebs cycle*, the site of complete fuel oxidation and the major energy-yielding metabolic pathway of the body. For the study of fuel homeostasis, it should be appreciated that the process of glycolysis is, on an overall basis, reversible, meaning that glucose can be produced from the compounds that constitute the end products of glycolysis. Because of the close link between glycolysis and the Krebs cycle, any of the Krebs cycle intermediates can potentially move "backwards" into the glycolytic pathway to produce glucose. The synthesis of glucose from intermediates of the Krebs cycle and glycolysis is a critically important part of fuel homeostasis, and is referred to as *gluconeogenesis*. Although Krebs cycle activity occurs in virtually all tissues except red blood cells, the process of gluconeogenesis occurs only in the liver, and to a limited extent in the kidney.

Another pathway for glucose oxidation, in addition to glycolysis, is the *pentose-phosphate pathway*. This is a quantitatively minor pathway that does not have great impact on fuel homeostasis. However, it is an important metabolic pathway in erythrocytes; thus, erythrocytes have an absolute need for glucose, although the overall need for energy by these cells is small, compared to the rest of the body.

Amino Acids Are Important Fuels, in Addition to Being the Building Blocks of Protein

Amino acids are important fuels. Whereas these monomers are the building blocks of proteins, they are carbon-containing compounds also that can provide energy to the body. In addition, they are important substrates for gluconeogenesis, indicating that they (most amino acids) can be converted to glucose when the available glucose supply is short. Although it is sometimes said that there is no storage site of amino acids in the body, the protein of skeletal muscle could well be considered to have an amino acid storage function, in addition to its locomotor functions.

Fatty Acids Are the Major Form of Energy Storage in the Animal Body

Fatty acids are stored in adipose tissue in the form of *triglycerides* (also called *triacylglycerols*), which consist of three fatty acid molecules linked to a glycerol molecule by ester bonds (see Fig. 29–27). Triglycerides are an ideal form of energy storage for animals. They are highly reduced molecules (there is little oxygen compared to the amount of carbon and hydrogen), which means they are a concentrated energy source, having more than twice the caloric value per gram than carbohydrates or amino acids. In addition, adipose tissue contains little water, compared to protein or glycogen, the storage forms of the other two potential fuels. Thus, adipose tissue is undiluted by bulky water, allowing it to be a concentrated form of energy storage that permits animals to carry with them a maximul amount of energy at a minimal amount of weight. Fats, however, have a metabolic disadvantage; they are not water-soluble. Therefore, special transport systems are necessary so that fats may be distributed among the tissues through the blood and lymph systems. In addition, fatty acids cannot be converted to glucose, so they cannot, under usual circumstances, contribute to the energy supply of the CNS. However, fatty acids can be converted to *ketone bodies*. Ketone bodies are fat-derived, water-soluble metabolites that serve as glucose substitutes. Ketone bodies can pass the blood-brain barrier, and during prolonged periods of dietary energy deprivation, they can provide a large portion of the energy supply to the CNS, at least in some species. It does appear, however, that they cannot totally replace glucose in this function, and that a small amount of glucose is always needed by the CNS.

In monogastric species, ketone bodies are

formed exclusively in the liver and are utilized by a wide variety of tissues. Some tissues, including cardiac muscle, use ketone bodies in preference to glucose. In ruminants, the ketone body β-hydroxybutyrate is formed from butyrate in the rumen epithelium; thus, ketone bodies arising from normal digestion are important energy metabolites in ruminant species. Elevated serum concentrations of ketone bodies are characteristic of several diseases associated with abnormalities of fuel homeostasis. This may lead students to conclude that ketone bodies are abnormal, or even toxic, metabolites. In fact, when present in physiological concentrations, ketone bodies are important fuels that occupy an integral part of the scheme of fuel homeostasis. The chemical structure of the three major ketone bodies is illustrated in Figure 31–2.

NUTRIENT UTILIZATION DURING THE ABSORPTIVE PHASE

As absorption takes place, metabolic events in the liver and peripheral organs are coordinated to direct nutrients into storage molecules and storage sites. The general scheme of metabolism during the absorptive phase is illustrated in Figure 31–3.

During the Absorptive Phase, the Liver Takes Up Glucose and Converts It into Glycogen and Triglyceride

When a meal is ingested, insulin secretion begins to occur even before maximal absorption of glucose. This secretion is stimulated by the action of gastric inhibitory peptide (GIP) (see Chapter 26) and perhaps other enteric hormones. Early insulin secretion assures that

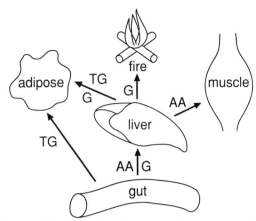

Figure 31–3. Metabolism during the absorptive period is characterized by the movement of potential fuels into depot sites and the utilization of glucose as a fuel. *AA*, amino acid; *G*, glucose; *TG*, triglyceride.

the liver and other tissues will be "primed" and ready for the arrival of glucose from the gut. A large portion of the glucose absorbed postprandially is taken up by the liver, because the liver receives a large portion of total blood flow and has a high capacity for glucose uptake. Under the influence of insulin, glucose in the liver is diverted into glycogen synthesis. The net effect is that glucose from the gut is diverted into glycogen and stored there during absorptive periods, thus keeping blood glucose concentrations from becoming excessively high. Insulin exerts its stimulatory effect on hepatic glycogen synthesis by stimulating intracellular metabolic pathways, which result in the formation of glycogen. These effects are discussed further in reference to the counterbalancing effects of glucagon.

The amount of glycogen that can be stored in the liver is limited, and under normal conditions probably never exceeds 10% of the total weight of the liver. In humans this represents about 100 grams of glycogen, and it is likely that a proportionally similar limit exists for the storage of glycogen in the livers of other species. This amount of glycogen does not account for all of the glucose taken up by the liver during the digestion and absorption of a large carbohydrate meal; therefore, there must be some additional mechanism for the disposal of excess glucose. If there were no such alternatives for glucose disposal, other than glycogen, blood glucose levels could rise out of control after glycogen concentrations had reached their maximum. Fatty acid synthesis offers an alternative mechanism for glucose removal.

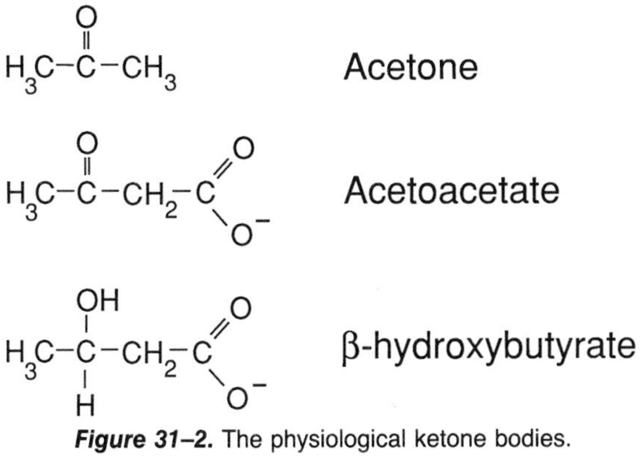

Figure 31–2. The physiological ketone bodies.

The Conversion of Glucose to Fatty Acids Is an Irreversible Process

The synthesis of fatty acids from glucose begins with glycolysis. This pathway leads to the production of two pyruvate molecules for each molecule of glucose consumed. Pyruvate can then enter the mitochondria and be activated to *acetyl coenzyme A* (acetyl CoA) for entry into the Krebs cycle. However, the Krebs cycle is for energy generation, and during the absorptive period there is more than enough acetyl CoA and Krebs cycle activity to provide for energy needs; therefore, there is excess acetyl CoA that must be shunted away from the Krebs cycle. The acetyl CoA combines with *oxaloacetate* to form *citrate* in what is essentially the first reaction of the Krebs cycle. However, instead of continuing through the Krebs cycle reactions, during the absorptive period much of the citrate is transported out of the mitochondria into the cytosol. Once in the cytosol, each citrate molecule contributes two carbons toward the synthesis of fatty acids. The remaining portion of the citrate molecule cycles

back into the mitochondria for further use. Thus, citrate serves as a carrier molecule to transport two carbon acetate units, originally from glucose, out of the mitochondria for the synthesis of fatty acids in the cytosol (Fig. 31–4).

Several important steps in this conversion of glucose carbon to fatty acids are promoted by insulin and are discussed in greater detail later. It is important to recognize that the conversion of glucose to fatty acids is irreversible; thus, carbohydrate can form fat, but fat cannot form carbohydrate. The discussion here concerns hepatic metabolism, and the liver is an important site of fatty acid synthesis in several species. Direct synthesis of fatty acids occurs also in adipose tissue. The relative importance of liver and adipose as sites of fatty acid synthesis varies with species, as is further discussed later.

Transport of Fatty Acids Out of the Liver Is Through Chylomicron-Like Particles Known as Very Low-Density Lipoproteins

Once formed in the liver, fatty acids must be transported either to adipose tissue for storage or to other tissues, such as muscle, for direct utilization for energy production. Because fatty acids are insoluble in blood, some special transport mechanism for their distribution is necessary. This mechanism is through the hepatic formation of triglyceride-rich serum lipoproteins, also known as *very low-density lipoprotein* or *VLDL*. The name VLDL is given because of the very low density of the triglyceride-rich lipoproteins compared to other lipoproteins that exist in blood serum. In the synthesis of VLDL, fatty acids are first esterified to form triglycerides, and the triglycerides are wrapped in a coat of phospholipid, cholesterol, and specific proteins (Fig. 31–5). It should be recognized that this is essentially the same mechanism by which fatty acids were transported out of the enterocytes after absorption from the gut. In the latter case, the lipoproteins were called chylomicrons. The VLDLs of the liver are smaller than chylomicrons, but have a similar structure and function. The mechanisms by which VLDL and chylomicrons deliver fatty acids to peripheral tissues are further discussed in relation to peripheral tissues.

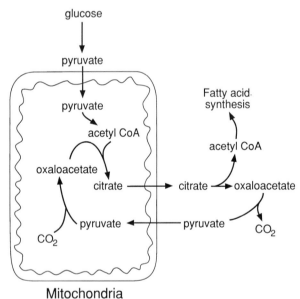

Figure 31–4. The hepatic synthesis of fatty acid from carbohydrate requires the passage of carbohydrate carbons through the mitochondria. Citrate forms a shuttle to transport the carbons of acetyl coenzyme A (acetyl CoA) out of the mitochondria, because acetyl CoA cannot pass directly through the mitochondrial membrane. The formation of citrate from oxaloacetate and acetyl CoA is the first reaction of the Krebs cycle; thus, fatty acid formation is an alternative to Krebs cycle oxidation when there is more than enough acetyl CoA to provide for cellular energy through Krebs cycle activity.

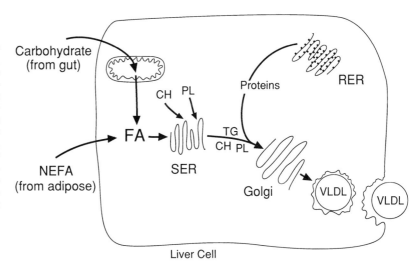

Figure 31–5. Very low-density lipoprotein (VLDL) formation. Fatty acids for triglyceride formation may come either from synthesis from carbohydrate or amino acids, or from adipose tissue fatty acids arriving at the liver in the form of NEFA. Note the similarity to chylomicron formation (see Fig. 29–27). *NEFA,* nonesterified fatty acids; *FA,* fatty acids; *CH,* cholesterol; *PL,* phospholipids; *TG,* triglycerides; *SER,* smooth endoplasmic reticulum; *RER,* rough endoplasmic reticulum; *VLDL,* very low-density lipoprotein.

Amino Acids Can Be Classified into Groups Based on Metabolic Characteristics

The discussion of amino acid absorption and metabolism is complicated by the fact that not all amino acids are subject to the same reactions. For this discussion, the amino acids are placed into two groups, each containing two subgroups (Table 31–1). The major groups are the nutritionally dispensable and indispensable amino acids. Within the dispensable amino acid group, glutamate, aspartate, and alanine are separated out as *transport amino acids;* within the indispensable amino acid group, leucine, isoleucine, and valine form a special group known as the *branch-chain amino acids* (BCAA). The transport amino acids are utilized in several reactions in which amino groups are transferred from molecule to molecule or organ to organ.

Amino Acids Are Extensively Modified During Absorption

The profile of amino acids in the portal vein is considerably different than that of the diet, indicating that amino acid destruction and transformation occurs during the absorptive process. Essentially all of the glutamate and much of the aspartate in the diet is removed by the intestinal epithelial cells during absorption, so that the portal blood is nearly devoid of glutamate and contains little aspartate. Much of the nitrogen from glutamate and aspartate are transferred to pyruvate to form the amino acid alanine, which is present in high concentrations in portal blood. The metabolism of the transport amino acids in the intestinal epithelium is a good example of the way in which amino groups can be gained and lost, and how the metabolism of amino acids is interfaced with the metabolism of carbohydrate. Glutamate and aspartate are

Table 31–1
METABOLIC CLASSIFICATION OF AMINO ACIDS

Indispensable Amino Acids		Dispensable Amino Acids	
Branch-chain Amino Acids	*Others*	*Transport Amino Acids*	*Others*
Leucine	Arginine*	Alanine	Cysteine
Isoleucine	Histidine	Glutamine	Glycine
Valine	Lysine	Glutamic acid	Proline
	Methionine	Asparagine	Glycine
	Phenylalanine	Aspartic acid	Tyrosine†
	Threonine		Serine
	Tryptophan		

*Indispensable for cats, not required in the diets of many other species.
†Dietary adequacy depends on a supply of phenylalanine.

similar to two Krebs cycle intermediates, α-ketoglutarate and oxaloacetate, differing only by the presence of an amino group or a keto-oxygen. Carbohydrates and amino acids having this relationship are said to be *analogs;* thus, α-ketoglutarate is the keto-analog of glutamate, and pyruvate is the keto-analog of alanine (Fig. 31–6). All amino acids can form keto-analogs, and all keto-analogs can be readily converted back to their parent amino acids.

Many Amino Acids Are Removed by the Liver on "First Pass," Never Reaching the Systemic Circulation

The hepatic-portal circulation is arranged in a way that all nutrients leaving the gut through the blood pass through the liver before entering the systemic circulation (see Fig. 29–23). This places the liver in a "sentinel" position from which it can modify the nutrient composition of portal blood before the blood is distributed to other tissues. The function of the liver in modifying portal blood composition is well illustrated in the case of amino acid absorption. A large portion of amino acids absorbed into portal blood is removed as the blood passes the liver, never reaching the general circulation. Figure 31–7 illustrates that in the dog only about 23% of the amino acids reaching the liver during the absorptive period pass into the general circulation, thus aiding in keeping blood amino acid concentrations stable during periods of amino acid absorption. Blood amino acid concentration, like blood glucose concentration, is usually kept relatively constant.

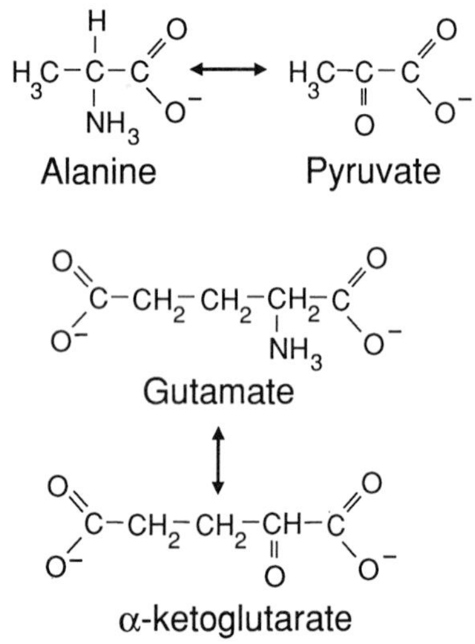

Some Amino Acids Taken Up by the Liver Are Used for Protein Synthesis

The liver is an important site of protein synthesis, making its priority position for amino acid uptake seem reasonable. Figure 31–7 shows that approximately 20% of the portal blood amino acid supply is used for protein synthesis in the liver, although this proportion varies with dietary protein intake. Nearly all of the serum proteins are synthesized in the liver, including such critical proteins as albumin and the blood-clotting factors. Although the liver-derived serum proteins serve many important functions, one function they do not serve is that of amino acid transport. The direct amino acid supply for protein synthesis in nonhepatic tissue comes from free amino acids in the blood, not from preformed serum proteins.

Most Amino Acids Taken Up by the Liver Are Converted to Carbohydrates

Most amino acids entering the liver undergo *deamination,* which means that the amino groups are removed and the molecules converted to their keto-analogs. The keto-analogs enter the pathways of carbohydrate metabolism, from which they may be completely metabolized for energy, converted to glucose or glycogen, or shunted to fatty acid synthesis. All of these reactions proceed in the same manner as previously described for carbohydrate metabolism. The sites at which the various amino acids enter the carbohydrate pathways are illustrated in Figure 31–8.

To many students, deamination of amino acids for the production of carbohydrate or energy may seem like a waste of expensive dietary protein; however, consider that there are some species in which the deamination of amino acids is important for homeostasis of glucose and other fuels. The natural diets of the true carnivores, such as cats and mink, for example, contain a large portion of protein and little carbohydrate. Yet, the glucose needs of these animals are no less than those of other animals, so it is highly important that they synthesize glucose from amino acids. Ruminants are a similar case, because most carbohydrates are digested by fermentative digestion and absorbed as volatile fatty acids

Figure 31–6. Example of amino acids and their keto-analogs. All amino acids can reversibly form keto-analogs.

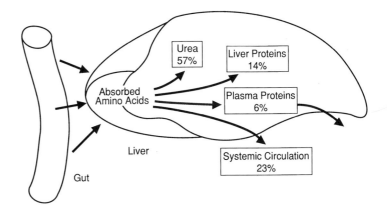

Figure 31–7. The fate of dietary amino acids reaching the canine liver.

(VFAs), rather than glucose. Ruminants, like carnivores, depend on amino acids for some of their glucose needs, although a large portion of ruminant glucose requirements may be met through conversion of propionate.

To allow for carbohydrate production and the deamination of excess amino acids, the endocrine reactions to high protein meals are somewhat different from those of meals containing substantial amounts of carbohydrate. During the digestion of high protein meals, insulin and glucagon secretion does not occur in its usual reciprocal pattern. Insulin secretion is stimulated by amino acids, as well as by glucose. Glucagon secretion, which is inhibited by glucose, is stimulated by amino acids, as long as glucose concentrations are moderately low. This relationship means that during the digestion of a high protein, low carbohydrate meal, there is simultaneous secretion of insulin and glucagon. One of the effects of insulin is the increased cellular uptake of amino acids, as well as glucose. Thus, the effect of insulin in this situation is to increase transport of amino acids into tissues. However, if insulin secretion were the only action stimulated by amino acid absorption, the animal would risk insulin-stimulated hypoglycemia when consuming high protein, low carbohydrate diets. An important action of glucagon is to stimulate gluconeogenesis through the deamination of amino acids in the liver. This assures that adequate glucose will be available to counterbalance the effects of amino acid–stimulated insulin secretion. The relationship of insulin and glucagon secretion during the absorption of diets with different carbohydrate and protein concentrations is illustrated in Figure 31–9.

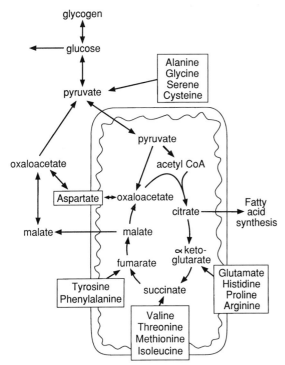

Figure 31–8. The sites of entry of various amino acids into the scheme of carbohydrate metabolism. This figure illustrates the means by which glucose can be synthesized from amino acids in the process of gluconeogenesis. In the case of the dispensable amino acids, the reactions are reversible, allowing for amino acid production from carbohydrate.

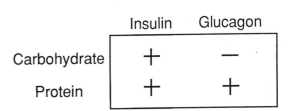

Figure 31–9. The influence of dietary carbohydrate and protein on insulin and glucagon secretion.

Not All Amino Acids Are Subject to Hepatic Destruction

During the absorptive period, amino acids for peripheral (nonhepatic) protein synthesis must come from that portion of amino acids escaping hepatic destruction. As seen from Figure 31–7, this only amounts to about 23% of the amino acids absorbed from the gut. Although this may seem like a meager portion of amino acids to be allocated for protein synthesis by all body tissues except liver, there are several considerations that make it seem more appropriate. First, amino acids are selectively taken up by the liver, so that the distribution of individual amino acids in blood leaving the liver is not the same as that in blood reaching the liver. The indispensable amino acids, especially the BCAA, are not avidly extracted by the liver, whereas some of the dispensable amino acids, alanine for example, are extensively taken up by hepatic tissue. The dispensable amino acids can be synthesized by protein-producing tissues; thus, the removal of dispensable amino acids by the liver is not rate limiting for tissue protein synthesis. Secondly, it must be pointed out that the proportion of amino acids taken up by the liver, and the fate of the amino acids that are taken up, is not constant, but can be adjusted according to the body's protein needs. Low protein diets lead to reduced hepatic amino acid uptake, reduced protein synthesis, and reduced amino acid destruction by the liver.

Metabolism at the Tissue Level Is Coordinated with Hepatic Metabolism and Results in the Deposition of Fuel into Storage Tissues During the Absorptive Period

The overall effects of hepatic metabolism during the absorption of a meal are for the removal of glucose and amino acids, and the synthesis of protein and fat. Complementary changes occur in peripheral tissues, so that additional glucose and amino acids are removed by skeletal muscle and adipose tissue. In addition, fatty acids secreted by the liver as VLDL triglyceride are deposited in adipose tissue, as are the triglycerides of chylomicrons.

Insulin Promotes the Synthesis of Protein and the Deposition of Glycogen in Muscle

The absorptive period is dominated by the effects of insulin. In skeletal muscle, the largest tissue mass of the body, insulin promotes the uptake of glucose and amino acids, thus tending to moderate the increase in blood concentration of these nutrients during absorption of a meal. The uptake of glucose by muscle is associated with glycogen synthesis, just as it is in the liver. Muscle glycogen, in contrast to liver glycogen, cannot be made directly available to augment blood glucose concentrations during periods of low glucose availability. Thus, muscle glycogen is primarily for metabolism in the muscle, although at certain times muscle glycogen can indirectly provide substrate for hepatic gluconeogenesis.

Insulin-Stimulated Uptake of Amino Acids by Muscle Results in a Net Increase in Muscle Protein Synthesis

The term *net increase* is used in reference to muscle protein synthesis, because muscle protein is in a state of dynamic equilibrium, i.e., a constant state of flux. Protein molecules are continuously being broken down and their amino acids added to an intracellular amino acid pool. Simultaneously, new proteins are constantly being made, deriving their amino acids from the same pool (Fig. 31–10). The size of the amino acid pool depends on the relative rates of entry and exit of amino acids. Amino acids enter the pool from the blood during the absorptive phase and at all times from the breakdown of protein. Exit of amino acids from the pool occurs because of protein synthesis and oxidative catabolism. In the absorptive phase of digestion, the amino acid pool is large, because amino acids are being taken up from the blood. In addition, few of the amino acids leaving the pool are directed toward oxidative catabolism, because there is plenty of available glucose for oxidation and energy generation. The result is that the amino acid pool is large, and a high portion of amino acids are directed to protein synthesis. When the rate of protein synthesis exceeds the rate of protein breakdown, there is a net increase in amount of muscle protein. Thus, during the absorptive phase, amino acids are stored in muscle protein, protein that has a functional

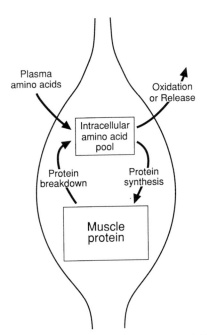

Figure 31–10. The intracellular amino acid pool. The size of the pool depends on the rate of amino acid uptake from plasma and muscle protein relative to the rates of amino acid loss owing to oxidation, export to plasma, and protein synthesis.

role not only for locomotion and posture, but also as amino acid storage.

During the Absorptive Phase, Triglyceride Accumulation in Adipose Tissue Occurs by Two Mechanisms: Uptake from Very Low-Density Lipoproteins, and Direct Lipid Synthesis from Glucose

Triglyceride fatty acids are transferred from chylomicrons and VLDL to adipose tissue by the action of *lipoprotein lipase (LPL)*. This enzyme resides on endothelial surfaces of capillaries and, when activated, binds to chylomicrons and VLDL, catalyzing the hydrolysis of fatty acids from their core triglycerides and allowing the transfer of those fatty acids to the surrounding tissues. The sensitivity of LPL to specific hormones varies in different tissues. Adipose tissue LPL is stimulated by insulin; thus, during the absorptive phase, fatty acids from the triglycerides of chylomicrons and VLDL are selectively transferred to adipose tissue. It should be apparent then that under the influence of insulin, during the absorptive phase, excess carbohydrate and amino acids are converted to fatty acids in the liver, and that those fatty acids are subsequently trans-

ported, through VLDL triglyceride, to the adipose tissue. Similarly, it should be seen that chylomicron triglyceride arising from intestinal fatty acid absorption is also selectively transported to adipose tissue, under the influence of insulin.

Adipose tissue fatty acids may arise also from direct synthesis, in addition to uptake from chylomicrons and VLDL. Adipose tissue cells are metabolically active and, under the influence of insulin, take up glucose. Within the adipocytes, glucose can be converted to fatty acids by the same metabolic mechanisms by which fatty acids were synthesized in the liver. In addition, acetate from fermentative digestion also can serve as substrate for fatty acid synthesis in adipose tissue (see later under "special fuel considerations of ruminants"). It should now be appreciated that there are two major sites of fatty acid synthesis in the body, the liver and adipose tissue. The relative importance of these sites varies with species.

NUTRIENT UTILIZATION DURING THE POSTABSORPTIVE PHASE

The postabsorptive phase refers to the relatively brief periods (usually a few hours) between meals in well-fed animals. It is characterized by short-term changes that mobilize nutrients from storage pools in order to maintain fuel availability for metabolically active tissue. The general scheme of postabsorptive metabolism is illustrated in Figure 31–11.

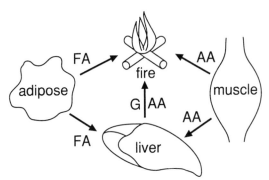

Figure 31–11. Postabsorptive metabolism is characterized by movement of fuels out of depot sites for immediate use. Glucose (*G*) arising either from glycogenolysis or gluconeogenesis is a major fuel, although some fatty acid (*FA*) is consumed also. Amino acid (*AA*) forms the substrate for gluconeogenesis.

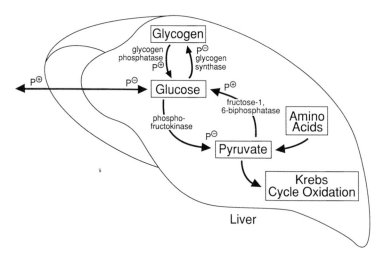

Figure 31–12. The effects of phosphorylation on four key enzymes of glucose production and utilization. All four enzymes are phosphorylated under the influence of cAMP. Note, however, that the enzymes that favor glucose formation are stimulated by phosphorylation (P$^+$), whereas those that favor glucose utilization and storage are inhibited by phosphorylation (P$^-$).

Hepatic Metabolism Switches from Glucose Utilization to Glucose Production During the Postabsorptive Phase

As the absorption of a meal is completed, the rate of glucose absorption from the gut wanes, and blood glucose concentration diminishes, removing the stimulus for insulin production and stimulating glucagon secretion. The primary target organ of glucagon is the liver, in which it creates marked metabolic changes. Through stimulation of specific cell surface receptors on hepatocytes, glucagon activates adenyl cyclase, leading to the phosphorylation of numerous cellular enzymes (see Chapter 1 for a more complete discussion of phosphorylation and dephosphorylation reactions). Some enzymes are activated by phosphorylation, whereas others are inactivated, and unless the overall scheme of substrate flow is considered, the whole phosphorylation-dephosphorylation system appears to be quite random and to make little sense. However, when the actions of the individual enzymes are considered in light of their effect on the flow of energy substrate through the liver, the system is revealed to be an elegant and incredibly well-orchestrated mechanism for the maintenance of fuel homeostasis.

Those enzymes that stimulate mobilization and utilization of fuels are activated by phosphorylation, whereas those stimulating storage of fuels are inactivated by phosphorylation. It must be understood that many enzymes of intermediary metabolism serve a passive role, catalyzing reactions that can go in either direction, depending on substrate concentrations. There are a relatively small number of regulatory enzymes that usually stand at the head of metabolic pathways and determine the substrate concentrations to which the other, unregulated enzymes are exposed. By its effect on several key regulatory enzymes, glucagon—a stimulator of phosphorylation—places the liver in a fuel-mobilization state, whereas insulin—an inhibitor of phosphorylation—promotes an hepatic metabolic pattern that favors fuel storage, as discussed in the previous section on absorptive-phase metabolism.

The opposing actions of insulin and glucagon on hepatic metabolism are evident from their actions on two key regulatory enzyme pairs: *glycogen synthase* and *glycogen phosphatase*, and *phosphofructokinase* and *fructose-1,6-biphosphatase*. The first of these pairs regulates glycogen synthesis and breakdown, whereas the second regulates glycolysis and gluconeogenesis, respectively. The actions of these enzymes and their regulatory effects are illustrated in Figure 31–12. Glycogen synthase and phosphofructokinase are inhibited by phosphorylation and, thus, stimulated by insulin. Glycogen phosphatase and fructose-1,6-biphosphatase are stimulated by phosphorylation and, thus, stimulated by glucagon. The actions of insulin and glucagon on these antagonistic enzyme pairs emphasize the importance of the insulin: glucagon ratio to which the liver is exposed. Neither hormone elicits an "all-or-none" reaction, but rather alters the balance of opposing reactions by influencing the relative activity of antagonistic enzymes. Thus, the fuel mobilizing/storing activity of the liver is dependent upon which hormone is most dominant. For this reason, the ratio of insulin to glucagon appears to be more important to liver metabolism than the absolute concentration of either hormone.

Under the influence of glucagon, glycogen phosphatase is activated by phosphorylation, promoting glycogenolysis and the elevation of intracellular glucose concentrations. As glucose accumulates, it is prevented from cycling back into glycogen, because the major enzyme catalyzing that reaction, glycogen synthase, is blocked by phosphorylation. In addition, the flow of glucose into glycolysis is also blocked by phosphorylation inhibition of phosphofructokinase (Fig. 31–12). Thus, the normal pathways for glucose utilization within the hepatocyte are all inhibited by glucagon, allowing glucose from glycogen breakdown to accumulate in the cells. Eventually, intracellular glucose escapes into the extracellular fluid and on into the blood. In this manner, hepatic glycogen is mobilized to elevate and maintain blood glucose concentrations when they begin to decline.

The liver stores of glycogen are relatively limited and cannot maintain blood glucose concentrations for long. Estimates in humans are that hepatic glycogen will serve blood glucose needs for 6–12 hours under conditions of low exertion and only about 20 minutes under conditions of heavy exertion. Values for animals are probably similar. Therefore, there must be some means, in addition to glycogen mobilization, to maintain the body's glucose supply during periods of exertion or when the period between meals is prolonged. Under these conditions of increased demand, glucose is provided by gluconeogenesis. Gluconeogenesis is promoted by the phosphorylation-stimulated enzyme fructose-1,6-biphosphatase. This enzyme essentially puts the glycolytic pathway into reverse, leading to glucose production from the same molecules that are intermediates in its oxidative destruction. Important substrates include pyruvate and all of the intermediates of the Krebs cycle.

At this point it is important to remember that most of the Krebs cycle intermediates or pyruvate can be supplied by the deamination of amino acids. The entry point of the various amino acids into the scheme of carbohydrate metabolism is illustrated in Figure 31–8. Pyruvate and all of the Krebs cycle intermediates can flow backwards* through the oxidative

pathway, resulting in the production of glucose. Thus, amino acids provide a large store of precursors for glucose formation through gluconeogenesis. The end result of glucagon stimulation is to promote the production of glucose through glycogenolysis and gluconeogenesis, turning the liver into a glucose-synthesizing organ.

Fuel Mobilization in Peripheral Tissues Occurs When Blood Insulin Concentration Declines

The pattern of metabolism in the peripheral tissues changes in the postabsorptive period to support the liver's capacity to maintain fuel supplies.

Muscle Reacts to a Metabolic Demand for Glucose by Mobilizing Amino Acids to Support Hepatic Gluconeogenesis

Mobilization of amino acid from muscle appears to be stimulated, to a large degree, by a relative lack of insulin; thus, mobilization occurs when blood glucose concentrations are low. Amino acids mobilized from skeletal muscle come from the intracellular amino acid pool referred to earlier (see Fig. 31–10). However, the mobilizing reactions are complex, and the distribution of amino acids leaving the muscle does not reflect the distribution of amino acids in the intracellular pool, as is explained later.

Muscle Release of Amino Acids Is Related to Reduced Glucose and Amino Acid Uptake

The postabsorptive decline in serum insulin has a twofold effect on muscle; the entry of amino acids from the serum into the intracellular amino acid pool is diminished, and in addition, the entry of glucose into muscle cells for energy production declines. Reduced amino acid entry results in conditions favoring net protein degradation to maintain the cellular amino acid pool size. Reduced glucose entry results in increased utilization of amino acids from the pool for energy production.

The pattern of utilization of amino acids for energy by muscle may, at first, seem unnecessarily complex, with selective use and extensive transformation of amino acids occurring. BCAAs serve as primary sources of energy in muscle cells during the postabsorptive state,

---

*Not all of the reactions of gluconeogenesis are the exact reverse of the corresponding reactions in glycolysis; however, the net result of gluconeogenesis is the reverse of glycolysis.

because these amino acids account for approximately one third of all muscle amino acid. Catabolism of BCAA begins with deamination and the formation of the α keto-acids of the BCAA. The α keto-acids then enter the Krebs cycle for energy production. Deamination of the BCAA requires that some acceptor be available to receive the amino group, and this acceptor is ultimately pyruvate, resulting in the formation of alanine. The source of pyruvate can be muscle glycogen, blood glucose, or the metabolic products of BCAA α keto-acids. When metabolism of BCAA α keto-acids serves as the supply of pyruvate for alanine synthesis, the net reaction is that of conversion of BCAA to alanine (Fig. 31–13). Thus, the overall metabolic activity in muscle during the postabsorptive state is that of destruction of BCAA and formation of alanine. The alanine formed is released from the muscle cells into the blood, from which it may be taken up by the liver for gluconeogenesis.

The Complex Pattern of Muscle Amino Acid Catabolism and Release Is Necessary to Accommodate the Liver's Limited Capacity for Branch-Chain Amino Acid Uptake and to Facilitate the Removal of Amino Nitrogen from the Muscle

To the student, it may appear that a simpler system of amino acid transfer to the liver would suffice. Why are amino acids not just released from muscle-cell amino acid pools into the blood and transported to the liver for glucose synthesis? The answer to this lies in the limited uptake capacity of the liver for BCAA and the need to transport amino nitrogen out of the muscle. Remember that BCAAs, the predominate amino acids of skeletal muscle, are not taken up readily by the liver; thus, if BCAAs were not transformed to alanine, there would be limited amino acid transfer to the liver.

In addition, alanine is a convenient means by which nitrogen from the deamination of muscle amino acid can be transported to the liver. This is important, because free amino groups liberated by the catabolism of amino acids in muscle could lead to the formation of toxic levels of ammonia, if not removed. Ammonia is detoxified in the body by formation of urea, but urea formation only occurs in the liver. Thus, alanine forms a gluconeogenic precursor that also transports nitrogen to the liver for urea synthesis. Figures 31–13 and 31–14 illustrate the role of alanine in the transport of amino acid nitrogen and carbon to the liver for urea and glucose synthesis, respectively.

The regulation of muscle-protein mobilization is influenced to a large extent by the lack of insulin. However, the adrenal-cortical hormone cortisol has an important effect of stimulating protein breakdown and amino acid

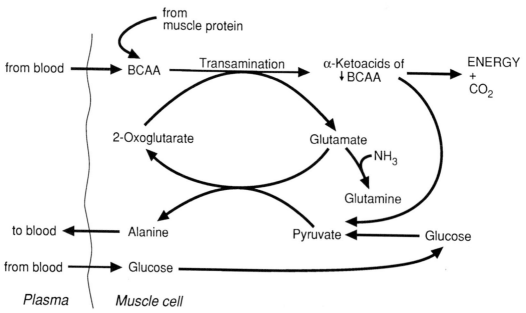

Figure 31–13. Catabolism of branch-chain amino acids (BCAA) by muscle cells. The pyruvate for export of amino groups may be derived from glucose or the amino acids themselves.

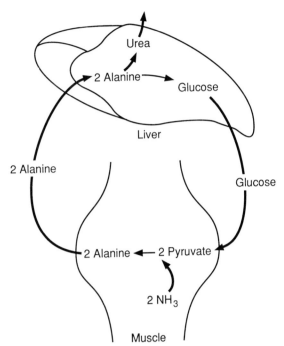

Figure 31–14. Alanine arising from BCAA catabolism in muscle is converted to glucose and urea in the liver. The glucose produced can potentially return to the muscle for alanine production. Thus, the cycle of alanine to glucose forms a shuttle to transport nitrogen from the muscle to the liver for urea synthesis.

mobilization. Through the mobilization of muscle protein and stimulation of hepatic gluconeogenesis, cortisol exerts one of its major effects, that of increasing blood glucose concentration. Under normal conditions, glucagon, the other major gluconeogenic hormone, exerts its effects on the liver and does not appear to have a direct effect on muscle.

The Reaction of Adipose Tissue During the Postabsorptive Period Is to Mobilize Fatty Acids

Fatty acids are released from adipose tissue because of the action of the phosphorylation-stimulated enzyme, *hormone-sensitive lipase* (*HSL*). This enzyme is stimulated by the relative lack of insulin in the postabsorptive period; insulin suppresses HSL action by promoting its dephosphorylation. Glucagon may have some adipose tissue activity in promoting triglyceride breakdown by stimulating the phosphorylation and activation of HSL. More likely, however, glucagon's effects are restricted to the liver, and the normal stimulation of HSL comes from epinephrine or norepinephrine; norepinephrine originates from

sympathetic nerves in the adipose tissue. The exact means by which sympathetic nerve activity in adipose is coordinated with body fuel availability are not well established, but it does appear that the catecholamine hormones and neuroregulators are the primary positive stimulus for breakdown of adipose triglyceride. However, the negative stimulus provided by the absence of insulin may be the most important regulator of adipose fat mobilization.

Stimulation of HSL in the postabsorptive state leads to the release of fatty acids from adipose tissue into the blood. Fatty acids in blood are reversibly bound to albumin, because they are not otherwise soluble in water. Albumin-bound fatty acids in blood are usually referred to as *nonesterified fatty acids* (*NEFA*) to distinguish them from triglyceride fatty acids in chylomicrons and lipoproteins. NEFA in blood may be used directly for energy by many tissues. However, a large portion of the fatty acids are taken up by the liver and used either for ketone body production or VLDL synthesis, as discussed in the next section.

NUTRIENT UTILIZATION DURING PROLONGED PERIODS OF ENERGY MALNUTRITION OR COMPLETE FOOD DEPRIVATION

During Prolonged Periods of Fasting or Undernutrition, Glucose and Amino Acids Are Conserved by Extensive Utilization of Fats and Ketone Bodies for Energy Production

From the previous discussion of postabsorptive metabolism, it can be appreciated that amino acids form an important depot for glucose precursors and energy-producing substrate. During prolonged fasting or undernutrition, however, it would not be advantageous for animals to rely heavily on their skeletal muscle for energy and glucose production, because soon this would lead to severe weakness as the skeletal muscle protein was consumed. Thus, protective mechanisms have developed by which skeletal muscle is preserved during periods of insufficient energy intake. Shifts away from glucose in body fuel utilization and toward the use of adipose fat stores are necessary for protein sparing. The general scheme of metabolism during prolonged catabolic periods is illustrated in Figure 31–15.

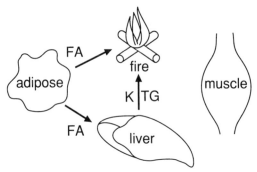

Figure 31–15. During prolonged periods of food deprivation or energy deficiency, the ketone bodies (*K*), fatty acids (*FA*), and triglycerides (*TG*) become the major fuels. Glucose oxidation becomes minor, thus sparing muscle protein that otherwise would be needed for gluconeogenesis.

A Large Portion of the Fatty Acids Released from Adipose Are Taken Up Directly by the Liver

During prolonged periods of undernutrition, low glucose availability leads to rapid mobilization of adipose fatty acids in the form of NEFA. Although NEFA are metabolized by many tissues, a large portion of them are extracted from the blood by the liver. This is due to the large portion of total blood flow reaching the liver as well as an efficient hepatic NEFA extraction mechanism. Once in the hepatocytes, there are three potential metabolic paths that fatty acids may follow. The first is complete oxidation for energy production; however, the hepatic requirements for energy are such that only a minor amount of the total fatty acid supply during adipose mobilization needs to be used for complete oxidation. The second pathway is esterification with triglyceride production, and the third is the production of ketone bodies. Triglyceride synthesis is discussed further later; here, ketone body production is the focus.

Hepatic Ketone Body Formation Is Promoted by Low Glucose Availability, a High Glucagon to Insulin Ratio, and a Ready Supply of Fatty Acids

Ketone body formation occurs within the hepatic mitochondria, and the rate of ketone body synthesis is controlled by the regulated transport of fatty acids across the mitochondrial membrane (Fig. 31–16). Fatty acids enter mitochondria in combination with a molecule known as *carnitine*, and transport is dependent on an enzyme known as *carnitine palmitoyltransferase I* (*CPT I*). The activity of this en-

zyme, along with the availability of fatty acid, is the primary determinant of the rate of ketone body formation. CPT I activity is regulated in an interesting fashion, being inhibited by an intermediate of the fatty acid synthesis pathway, *malonyl CoA*. Malonyl CoA concentrations are high when there is an excess of glucose, and when glucose is being used for fatty acid synthesis, i.e., when the liver is responding to insulin. When glucose supplies are low, or glucagon concentrations are high relative to insulin, little fatty acid is synthesized in the liver. Thus, malonyl CoA concentrations are low, and CPT I is fully active when the insulin:glucagon ratio is low.

Under conditions of active CPT I, most available fatty acid is transported into the mitochondria for ketone body synthesis. This well-orchestrated, but somewhat complex, regulatory system is important, because the liver can both produce and consume fatty acids. If there were not a way of "turning off" fatty acid destruction during periods of synthesis, a futile cycle of synthesis and destruction would occur. The inhibition of CPT I by

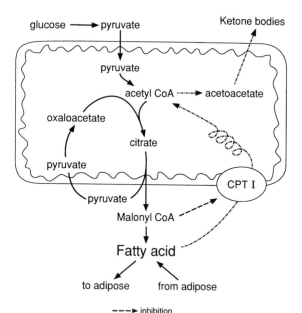

Figure 31–16. The liver is a site of both destruction and synthesis of fatty acids. To keep both processes from occurring simultaneously, fatty acid destruction is inhibited during periods of fatty acid synthesis. The pathway of fatty acid synthesis is indicated by the solid lines, whereas that of fatty acid destruction is indicated by the irregular broken line. Oxidative destruction is suppressed by the action of malonyl CoA, an intermediate in the synthesis of fatty acid. Malonyl CoA blocks the transport of fatty acids into the mitochondria at the translocation enzyme carnitine palmitoyltransferase I (*CPT I*).

malonyl CoA provides a system that blocks the metabolic destruction of newly synthesized fatty acid, while still providing a mechanism for the utilization of fatty acids derived from adipose tissue in times of insufficient energy supply. The overall pattern of metabolism results in a reciprocal relationship between glucose availability and ketone body production. Although ketone bodies are produced in the liver, they cannot be used there for energy production. Therefore, all ketone bodies are transported to peripheral tissues for utilization. When the concentration of ketone bodies in the blood becomes abnormally high, some are excreted in the urine.

Glucagon Plays an Important Role in the Excessive Production of Ketone Bodies During Diabetes Mellitus

If untreated, diabetes mellitus in animals, especially dogs, leads to high concentrations of ketone bodies in the blood. Diabetes mellitus occurs because of a lack of insulin, but the hepatic production of ketone bodies occurs because of the unrestrained action of glucagon. Even though serum concentrations of glucose are high in diabetes mellitus, the inability of the pancreas to secrete insulin leads to a low insulin:glucagon ratio; thus, the liver is functioning solely under the direction of glucagon. Glucagon inhibits fatty acid production from glucose; thus, malonyl CoA concentrations are low, and CPT I activity is high. Because of the lack of insulin to suppress adipose HSL, blood NEFA concentrations are high. The combination of high NEFA availability and unrestrained CPT I activity results in rapid transport of fatty acids into the mitochondria with extensive ketone body production, even though blood glucose concentrations are high.

Fatty Acids Cannot Be Used for Glucose Synthesis

It is important to understand that the metabolism of fat within the mitochondria cannot contribute directly to gluconeogenesis. Once across the mitochondrial membrane, fatty acids undergo β-*oxidation*, which results in the successive removal of two carbon acetyl CoA units from the carbon chains of the fatty acids. The resulting acetyl CoA can enter the Krebs cycle through condensation with oxaloacetate. Because any of the Krebs cycle intermediates

can lead to glucose production, it may appear at first that acetyl CoA from fatty acid β-oxidation can lead to the production of glucose. However, this is not the case; there is no *net* production of oxaloacetate associated with the consumption of acetyl CoA by the Krebs cycle (Fig. 31–17). Existing oxaloacetate combines with acetyl CoA to form citrate in the initial step of the cycle. At the end of the cycle, the original oxaloacetate is reformed, as the two carbons from the acetyl CoA are converted to carbon dioxide. No new oxaloacetate can be produced by this process.

Ketone Bodies Are Formed in the Mitochondria from Acetyl CoA

Not all mitochondrial acetyl CoA must enter the Krebs cycle. In fact, when fatty acids are rapidly entering the mitochondria, there is far more acetyl CoA available than necessary for Krebs cycle activity. It is this excess acetyl CoA, originating from fatty acids, from which the ketone bodies are synthesized (see Fig. 31–16). Ketone bodies are able to freely leave the mitochondria.

Ketone bodies affect fuel homeostasis at the peripheral tissue level, where in many tissues, they serve as a substitute for glucose. In this

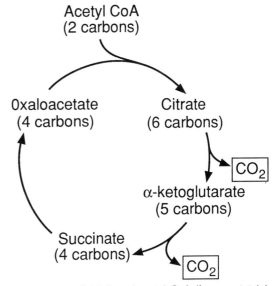

Figure 31–17. Oxidation of acetyl CoA (from acetate) by the Krebs cycle. The two carbons of acetyl CoA result in the formation of carbon dioxide; there is no net synthesis of oxaloacetate. Because it is oxaloacetate that forms the precursor for glucose synthesis, acetyl CoA (and thus acetate) cannot lead to glucose formation.

way, they conserve available glucose and reduce the need for gluconeogenesis.

Hepatic Very Low-Density Lipoproteins May Be Synthesized from Adipose-Derived Fatty Acid, As Well As from Newly Synthesized Fatty Acid

In the section on absorptive-phase metabolism, the hepatic production of VLDL is discussed. During the absorptive phase, triglyceride for VLDL synthesis comes from fatty acids synthesized from glucose. During catabolic periods, VLDLs may continue to be produced, but fatty acids derived from serum NEFA are used for VLDL synthesis (see Fig. 31–5). This may initially appear to be an unnecessary and inefficient metabolic step. Why should fatty acids from adipose tissue be transported to the liver for VLDL formation, when they can be directly metabolized for energy by the tissues? The need for VLDL synthesis occurs because of the need for a better transport system. The capacity of the serum to transport NEFA is limited, because NEFA must circulate bound to albumin, and the NEFA-binding capacity of albumin is finite and may become nearly saturated during periods of rapid adipose mobilization. VLDLs provide a transport system for fatty acids that is not dependent on albumin, and thus is not limited in the amount of fatty acid that can be accommodated by albumin.

Hormonal Conditions Direct the Distribution of Very Low-Density Lipoprotein Fatty Acids in the Body

During the absorptive phase, VLDLs are directed to adipose tissue by the action of lipoprotein lipase (LPL), an insulin-stimulated enzyme. LPL also exists in muscle tissue, but it is not dependent on insulin stimulation for activity. Thus, during periods of low glucose availability, adipose tissue LPL is inhibited because of a lack of insulin, but muscle tissue LPL is fully active. This leads to the selective direction of VLDL fatty acids to muscle tissue during times of adipose mobilization.

Changes in Growth Hormone Concentrations May Aid in Shifting Peripheral Fuel Utilization from Glucose and Amino Acids to Ketone Bodies and Fatty Acids

The fat mobilization-induced changes in hepatic metabolism are only effective in conserving protein because of changes that occur in glucose and amino acid utilization in peripheral tissues. As ketone bodies, NEFA and VLDL triglycerides become the major energy supplies; there is less tissue demand for glucose or amino acids as energy substrate. Endocrine alterations, in addition to low insulin concentrations, may aid in promoting this switch in peripheral fuel utilization. In several species, growth hormone concentrations increase during a prolonged period of energy deprivation. Growth hormone is antagonistic to insulin, thus promoting an increase in serum glucose concentration, even in the face of normal or near-normal serum insulin levels. In addition, growth hormone may have some direct effect on conserving protein and mobilizing lipid.

THE SPECIAL FUEL CONSIDERATIONS OF RUMINANTS

Ruminants Exist in a Perpetual State of Gluconeogenesis Because of Their Unique Digestive Process

The large majority of carbohydrate digestion in ruminants occurs in the forestomach through fermentative digestion. The result is that almost no digestible carbohydrate enters the intestine for glandular digestion and absorption as glucose. This means that ruminants exist in a constant state of potential glucose deficiency. In order to cope with this situation, ruminants have developed efficient systems of both production and conservation of glucose.

Essentially, all of the glucose available to ruminants on most types of diets originates from gluconeogenesis. Quantitatively, the most important glucose precursor is the volatile fatty acid propionate. Propionate contributes to glucose synthesis after entering the Krebs cycle at the level of succinate. The reactions involved in conversion of propionate to succinate are illustrated in Figure 31–18. Note that succinate is a four-carbon Krebs cycle intermediate that can lead to net formation of oxaloacetate, the entry metabolite for gluconeogenesis. The other VFAs, acetate and butyrate, also enter the Krebs cycle; however, like the long-chain fatty acids from adipose tissue, acetate and butyrate enter the cycle as acetyl CoA. As previously discussed, acetyl

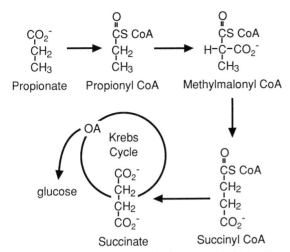

Figure 31–18. Gluconeogenesis from propionate involves its initial conversion to succinate. Succinate is a four-carbon Krebs cycle intermediate that can lead to net glucose synthesis.

CoA cannot lead to the net production of oxaloacetate or glucose. Therefore, of the major energy sources of the ruminant—acetate, propionate, and butyrate—only propionate can support glucose production.

Nearly all propionate absorbed from the rumen is extracted from the portal blood by the liver, never entering the systemic circulation. Hepatic extraction of propionate means that all propionate is used for gluconeogenesis. In addition to propionate, amino acids from intestinal absorption also provide substrate for gluconeogenesis. The use of dietary amino acid for gluconeogenesis is discussed earlier in relation to amino acid–stimulated glucagon release in the section on absorptive-phase metabolism.

In addition to constant gluconeogenesis, ruminants also support their glucose needs by efficiently conserving glucose. Fatty acids, which in some animals, such as primates, rats, and dogs, are synthesized in the liver, are only synthesized in the adipose of ruminants. Furthermore, glucose is essentially not used for fatty acid synthesis. Rather, fatty acids are synthesized from acetate, which is the most abundant energy source in ruminants. The only glucose used by adipose tissue is for the synthesis of the glycerol backbone for triglycerides. In lactating animals, fatty acids produced in the udder for milk fat are synthesized from either acetate or ketone bodies, never from glucose.

Some important metabolic diseases of ruminants occur during periods when their system

of glucose homeostasis is stressed. Dairy cows are especially vulnerable at peak lactation, because the synthesis of lactose, milk sugar, requires glucose. In high-producing cows, nearly all of the glucose they produce goes to lactose synthesis, whereas the remainder of their tissues function on alternative fuels. Sheep experience a similar stress on glucose synthesis in late gestation. The energy needs of the fetus and placenta can only be met by glucose (or glucose-derived lactate) and amino acids. Sheep, in comparison to many other animals, have a high fetal-mass to body-size ratio; thus, their fuel homeostatic mechanisms are particularly stressed by pregnancy. Failure of the glucose homeostatic mechanism frequently occurs under these circumstances, resulting in conditions known as lactational ketosis in dairy cows and pregnancy toxemia in ewes.

CLINICAL CORRELATION

HEPATIC LIPIDOSIS IN A CAT

HISTORY □ You are asked to examine a 3-year-old intact female cat. She had been apparently normal, and in fact quite fat and happy until 2 weeks ago, when she disappeared from her owner's apartment for 4 days. When she returned, she seemed depressed and would not eat. Over the next few days she became progressively more listless, almost somnolent.

CLINICAL AND LABORATORY EXAMINATION □ The cat has a normal pulse, temperature, and respiratory rate, but she is depressed and responds little to handling. The ocular sclera (whites of the eyes) appear icteric, or jaundiced. The latter physical signs lead you to suspect liver disease, so you submit blood samples for biochemical analysis. Analysis of blood taken from the jugular vein reveals a higher-than-normal concentration of bile acids and bilirubin, confirming a diagnosis of liver disease. A needle-aspiration biopsy of the liver reveals hepatocytes that are distended with large droplets of nonstaining material, probably fat.

COMMENT □ The presence of significant concentrations of bile acids in blood, other than that in the hepatic-portal circulation, is evidence of reduced liver function. Recall that bile acids are absorbed from the ileum into the portal vein, in which they return to the liver. The normal liver extracts bile acids from portal blood efficiently, allowing only small amounts to escape into the systemic circulation; thus, elevated concentrations of bile acids in jugular blood are indicative of liver disease.

Hepatic lipidosis, or fatty liver, is a common disease of cats. It is brought on by a period of stress combined with either an unwillingness to eat or the lack of food availability. In either situation, the cats begin to mobilize large quantities of fat to support their metabolic energy needs. Normally, it would be expected that much of the mobilized nonesterified fatty acid (NEFA) would be taken up by the liver and converted to VLDL for export to energy-using tissues. In cats that develop fatty liver, the hepatic influx of NEFA appears to overwhelm the liver's capacity to synthesize and secrete VLDL, so fat accumulates in the liver. When the fat accumulation becomes severe, hepatic function is compromised, and the cats become systemically ill. Their appetites become severely depressed, and thus a downward spiral of events is created in which the hepatic lipidosis becomes more and more severe.

TREATMENT ☐ Treatment consists of reversing the state of negative energy balance by force-feeding the cats. Various methods of force-feeding exist; the most practical consists of the placement of indwelling gastric tubes. These are often passed through the nostrils, but may be placed by a number of different techniques, including direct intubation through the wall of abdomen. The latter technique is facilitated by use of a fiberoptic gastroscope. Once the cats are in positive energy balance, adipose mobilization ceases, and the liver eventually clears of fat. Tube feeding may have to continue for several days before the cats begin to eat on their own. Tube feeding has markedly improved the prognosis for this disease, although it is still a life-threatening condition.

Bibliography

Bauman DE, Currie WB: Partitioning of nutrients during pregnancy and lactation: A review of mechanisms in-volving homeostasis and homeorrhesis. J Dairy Sci 63:1514–1529, 1980.

Bondy PK, Rosenberg LE: Metabolic Control and Disease. Philadelphia, WB Saunders, 1979, pp 161–494.

Cahill GF: Starvation in man. Clin Endocrinol Metab 5:397–415, 1976.

DeGroot LJ (ed): Endocrinology. Philadelphia, WB Saunders, 1989, pp 2282–2293, 2367–2403.

Herdt TH: Fuel homeostasis in the ruminant. Vet Clin North Am (Food Anim Pract) 4:213–231, 1988.

Thomas JH, Gillham B: Will's Biochemical Basis of Medicine, 2nd ed. London, Wright, 1989.

PRACTICE QUESTIONS FOR CHAPTER 31

1. All of the following are metabolites that can be oxidized for fuel in the animal body. Which one is NOT important in the transport of energy between organs and organ systems?

   a. Triglyceride
   b. Ketone bodies
   c. Oxaloacetic acid
   d. Nonesterified fatty acids
   e. Amino acids

2. Which of the following reactions is NOT characteristic of the absorptive phase of digestion?

   a. Hepatic synthesis of glycogen
   b. Hepatic uptake of glucose
   c. Destruction of dietary amino acid
   d. Utilization of muscle-derived amino acid for gluconeogenesis
   e. Hepatic synthesis of triglyceride from glucose

3. Which of the following reactions in the liver could be expected to occur during both the digestive phase and a prolonged fast?

   a. Glycogen synthesis
   b. Fatty acid synthesis
   c. Ketone body synthesis
   d. Ketone body oxidation
   e. Triglyceride synthesis from fatty acids

4. Which of the following is true of both ketone bodies and nonesterified fatty acids?

a. They are water soluble.
b. They provide energy for muscle metabolism.
c. They circulate in blood bound to albumin.
d. They can provide energy to the brain.
e. They are formed exclusively in the liver.

5. Which of the following amino acids is NOT extensively catabolized by the liver?

a. Valine
b. Alanine
c. Glutamine
d. Asparagine
e. Glycine

GEORGE H. STABENFELDT

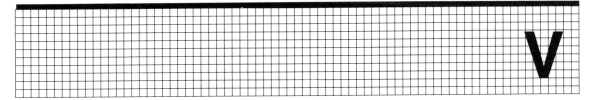

V

ENDOCRINOLOGY

32

The Endocrine System

GENERAL CONCEPTS

1. Hormones are chemicals produced by specific tissues that are transported by the blood vascular system to affect other tissues at low concentrations
2. The endocrine and nervous systems are integrated in their control of physiological processes

THE SYNTHESIS OF HORMONES

1. Protein hormones are initially synthesized as preprohormones, then cleaved in the rough endoplasmic reticulum to form prohormones and in the Golgi apparatus to form the active hormones, which are stored in granules before being released by exocytosis
2. Steroids are synthesized from cholesterol, which is synthesized by the liver—steroids are not stored, but are released as they are synthesized

THE TRANSPORT OF HORMONES IN THE BLOOD

1. Protein hormones are hydrophilic and carried in the plasma in dissolved form
2. Steroids and thyroid hormones are lipophilic and carried in plasma in association with both specific and nonspecific binding proteins, with the amount of unbound, active hormone being relatively small

HORMONE-CELL INTERACTION

1. Protein hormones have specific receptors on target tissue plasma membranes, whereas steroids have specific receptors within the cytoplasm or nucleus

POSTRECEPTOR CELL RESPONSES

1. Steroids interact directly with the cell nucleus through the formation of a complex with its cytosolic receptor, whereas protein hormones need a messenger, because they cannot enter the cell

METABOLISM OF HORMONES

1. Steroid hormones are metabolized by conjugation with sulfates and glucuronides, which makes them water-soluble

FEEDBACK CONTROL MECHANISMS

1. The most important feedback control for hormones is the negative feedback system in which increased hormone concentrations result in less production of the hormone, usually through an interaction with the hypothalamus or pituitary gland
2. Endocrine secretory patterns can be influenced by factors such as sleep or light, and can produce diurnal rhythms

THE HYPOTHALAMUS

1. The hypothalamus coordinates the activity of the pituitary gland through the secretion of peptides and amines

THE PITUITARY GLAND

1. The neurohypophysis has cell bodies that originate in the hypothalamus, with cell endings that secrete oxytocin and vasopressin
2. Oxytocin and vasopressin are synthesized in cell bodies within the hypothalamus and are carried by axon flow to the posterior lobe, where they are released
3. The main effects of oxytocin are on the contraction of smooth muscle (mammary gland and uterus); the effects of vasopressin are primarily on the conservation of water (antidiuresis) and secondarily on blood pressure
4. Plasma osmolality controls the secretion of vasopressin
5. The anterior pituitary produces the following hormones: growth hormone, prolactin, thyroid-stimulating hormone, follicle-stimulating hormone, luteinizing hormone, and adrenocorticotropic hormone
6. Adenohypophyseal activity is controlled by hypothalamic releasing hormones, which are released into the portal system that connects the median eminence of the hypothalamus and the anterior pituitary

GENERAL CONCEPTS

Hormones Are Chemicals Produced by Specific Tissues That Are Transported by the Blood Vascular System to Affect Other Tissues at Low Concentrations

The endocrine system has evolved to allow physiological processes to be coordinated and regulated. The system uses chemical messengers called *hormones*. The traditional definition of hormones has been as chemicals, produced by specific endocrine organs, that are transported by the blood vascular system and are able to affect distant target organs in low concentration. Whereas this definition is useful from a veterinary medical point of view, it should be recognized that there are substances, such as prostaglandins and somatomedins, that are produced by many tissues, yet are considered to be hormones.

Other types of control systems utilize chemical substances that are not transported in the blood vascular system to influence distant cell activity. These systems serve as means of local integration among, or between, cells. These systems are called (1) *paracrine effectors,* in which the messenger diffuses through the interstitial fluids, usually to influence adjacent cells—if the messenger acts on the cell of its origin, the substance is called an *autocrine effector* (Fig. 32–1); (2) *neurotransmitters,* which affect communication between neurons, or between neurons and target cells, with the substances being limited as to the distance traveled and the area of the cell influenced (Fig. 32–2); (3) *exocrine effectors,* in which chemicals are released from the body, e.g., hormones produced by the pancreas, which are released into the gastrointestinal (GI) tract.

The Endocrine and Nervous Systems Are Integrated in Their Control of Physiological Processes

The endocrine system interacts with the other main regulatory system, the *nervous system,* which coordinates activities that require rapid control. An example of the close interaction of the two systems is the reflex in which suckling causes the release of milk. Suckling

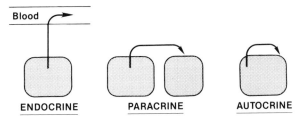

Figure 32–1. Types of cell communication via chemical mediators. (From Hedge GA, Colby HD, Goodman RL: Clinical Endocrine Physiology. Philadelphia, WB Saunders, 1987, p 29.)

initiates the transmission of nerve impulses from the mammary gland to the hypothalamus (by way of the spinal tract). Neurosecretory neurons within the supraoptic and paraventricular nuclei are stimulated to synthesize oxytocin. Oxytocin is transported along axons of these nerves and is released from nerve endings in the posterior pituitary into the blood vascular system. Oxytocin is carried to the mammary gland, where it causes contraction of myoepithelial cells. These cells surround the smallest unit of milk-secreting cells, called an *alveolus*. This results in the movement of milk into the large cisterns adjacent to the teat and, subsequently, into the teat.

The interaction between the nervous and endocrine systems can be even more direct, e.g., endocrine cells of the adrenal medulla are directly controlled by preganglionic neurons of the adrenal medulla; the medullary hormones are released immediately in response to stressful stimuli. The endocrine and nervous systems also share transmitters with substances such as epinephrine, dopamine, histamine, and somatostatin found in both endocrine and neural tissues.

The endocrine system is involved in control of physiological functions, including *metabolism, growth,* and *reproduction*. Metabolism can be divided into two parts: *energy* and *mineral*. The hormones that control *energy metabolism* include insulin, glucagon, cortisol, epinephrine, thyroid hormone, and growth hormone. The hormones that control *mineral metabolism* include parathyroid hormone, calcitonin, an-

giotensin, and renin. The hormones that control *growth* include growth hormone, thyroid hormone, insulin, estrogen and androgens (both reproductive hormones), and a large number of growth factors. The hormones that control *reproduction* include estrogen, androgen, progesterone, luteinizing hormone (LH), follicle-stimulating hormone (FSH), prolactin, and oxytocin.

One of the important characteristics of the endocrine system is the *amplification* of the signal. The action of one steroid molecule to activate a gene can result in the formation of many mRNA molecules, and each of these can induce the formation of many enzyme molecules. Also, one protein molecule can influence the formation of many adenosine 3':5'-cyclic phosphate (cAMP) molecules, and each of these can activate many enzymes. Amplification is the basis for the sensitivity of the endocrine system, which allows small amounts of hormones in plasma 10^{-11} to 10^{-12} mol) to produce significant biological effects. Another feature of hormone action is that *rates of existing enzyme reactions* are influenced, but not the initiation of new reactions. This implies that there are certain basal levels of enzyme activities even in the absence of hormones. Hormone action is relatively *slow and prolonged,* with the effects of hormones lasting minutes to days. This contrasts with the nervous system, in which the response is *rapid and short* (milliseconds to seconds).

THE SYNTHESIS OF HORMONES

Protein Hormones Are Initially Synthesized as Preprohormones, Then Cleaved in the Rough Endoplasmic Reticulum to Form Prohormones and in the Golgi Apparatus to Form the Active Hormones, Which Are Stored in Granules Before Being Released by Exocytosis

The major classes of hormones include *proteins* (e.g., growth hormone, insulin, adreno-

Figure 32–2. Comparison of functional arrangements of an ordinary neuron releasing its neurotransmitter (*NT*) into a synapse and a neurosecretory neuron relasing its neurohormone (*NH*) into a blood vessel. (From Hedge GA, Colby HD, Goodman RL: Clinical Endocrine Physiology. Philadelphia, WB Saunders, 1987, p 54.)

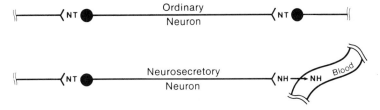

corticotropic hormone—ACTH); *peptides* (e.g., oxytocin and vasopressin); *amines* (e.g., dopamine, melatonin, epinephrine); and *steroids* (e.g., cortisol, progesterone, vitamin D). The protein and polypeptide hormones are initially synthesized on ribosomes as larger precursor proteins, which are referred to as *preprohormones* (Fig. 32–3). Synthesis of protein hormones begins in ribosomes, with the "pre" portion immediately attaching to the rough endoplasmic reticulum (RER), which pulls the ribosomes into close apposition with the RER. During synthesis, the preprohormone is secreted into the interior of the RER. The presence of a peptidase within the wall of the RER allows the "pre" portion of the molecule to be rapidly removed and the *prohormone* to leave the RER in vesicles that have been pinched off from the RER. These vesicles then move to the Golgi apparatus, where they coalesce with Golgi membranes to form secretory granules. The prohormone is cleaved during this process, so that most of the hormone is in its final form within the Golgi apparatus, although some prohormone can be found also.

Protein hormones are stored in granules within the gland until needed for release. Although some of the hormone is secreted on a continuous basis, most is secreted through the process of *exocytosis* of granules in response to a specific signal. The process of exocytosis requires adenosine triphosphate (ATP) and calcium. Increased cytoplasmic calcium results from intracellular release of calcium from mitochondria, or endoplasmic reticulum, or from the influx of extracellular calcium.

Steroids Are Synthesized from Cholesterol, Which Is Synthesized by the Liver—Steroids Are Not Stored, but Are Released as They Are Synthesized

Steroids represent a class of hormones that, unlike protein hormones, are lipophilic. In general, they fall under two categories: adrenocortical hormones (glucocorticoids, mineralocorticoids), and sex hormones (estrogen, progesterone, androgens). They have a common four ring, 17 carbon, skeleton that is derived from cholesterol (Fig. 32–4). Although the steroids can be synthesized *de novo* within the cell from the two carbon molecule acetate, the majority of steroids are formed from cholesterol, which is synthesized by the liver (Fig. 32–5). Low-density lipoproteins (LDL) enter steroid-producing cells through interaction with a membrane receptor. Cholesterol is released through the degradation of LDL by lysosomal enzymes. Cholesterol is either utilized immediately for steroid synthesis, or stored in granules in an ester form within the cell. The first step in the synthesis of all steroid hormones from cholesterol involves cleavage of the side chain of cholesterol to form pregnenolone, which occurs within the mitochondrion. Subsequent modifications of the steroid molecule may occur within the mitochondrion, or may involve movement to other compartments of the cell (Fig. 32–6). The control of movement of steroids among cell compartments during the synthesis process is not well understood.

The type of steroid hormone that is even-

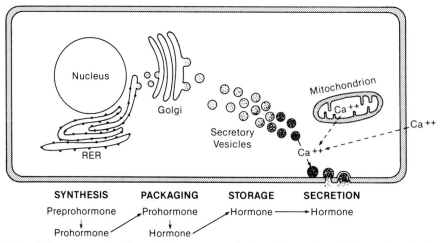

Figure 32–3. Subcellular components of peptide hormone synthesis and secretion. *RER*, rough endoplasmic reticulum. (From Hedge GA, Colby HD, Goodman RL: Clinical Endocrine Physiology. Philadelphia, WB Saunders, 1987, p 7.)

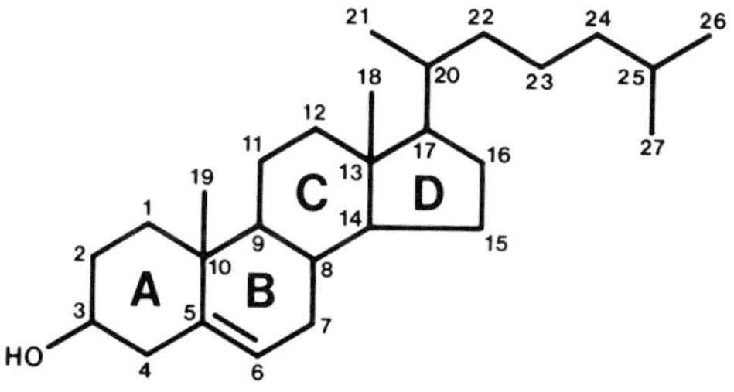

Figure 32–4. The ring structure and numbering system of the carbon atoms in steroid hormones, illustrated for the cholesterol molecule. (From Hedge GA, Colby HD, Goodman RL: Clinical Endocrine Physiology. Philadelphia, WB Saunders, 1987, p 9.)

THE TRANSPORT OF HORMONES IN THE BLOOD

Protein Hormones Are Hydrophilic and Carried in the Plasma in Dissolved Form

As previously defined, we are mainly concerned with hormones that are transported to target tissues in the blood vascular system. The means by which hormones are transported in the blood varies according to the solubility of the hormone. Protein and peptide hormones are *hydrophilic* and are carried in the plasma in dissolved form. The protein hormones may circulate in monomeric (single unit) or polymeric (multiple unit) form (e.g., insulin). Hormones that have subunits can appear in the circulation in subunit form, although this reduces the biological potency of the molecule.

Steroids and Thyroid Hormones Are Lipophilic and Carried in Plasma in Association with Both Specific and Nonspecific Binding Proteins, with the Amount of Unbound, Active Hormone Being Relatively Small

The transport of steroid and thyroid hormones is more complicated than that for protein hormones, because these hormones are *lipophilic* and, thus, have limited solubility in aqueous solutions. This group of hormones is transported in the blood through association with various types of proteins. Some of the proteins that bind steroids have a high affinity for a particular steroid, e.g., a globulin, *transcortin*, has a high affinity for cortisol and corticosterone, but also serves as an important transport vehicle for progesterone, even with a lower affinity for this hormone. The carrier proteins that have high affinities have low capacity. This contrasts with the general class of plasma proteins called *albumins*, which have low affinities for steroid hormones, but have a high capacity for steroid transport because of their high concentration in plasma.

A hormone must be in the free, or unbound, form before it can penetrate a target cell and elicit biological activity. This is accomplished by the establishment of an equilibrium between bound and free hormone in the plasma. The free form usually represents only about 1% of the total amount of hormone in

tually synthesized is dependent upon the presence of specific enzymes within the particular cell. For example, only cells of the adrenal cortex contain enzymes (hydroxylases) that result in hydroxylation of the eleventh and twenty-first carbon molecule, a process that is essential for the production of glucocorticoids and mineralocorticoids. The pattern for sex steroid biosynthesis is for pregnenolone to be modified in a sequence that involves progesterone, androgens, and finally, estrogens. Cells that synthesize androgens (e.g., Leydig's cells of the testis) have the enzymes required for the formation of pregnenolone and progesterone, as well as the modification of progesterone to androgen, but lack the enzymes required to modify androgens into estrogens. Whereas the sex steroid-forming cells do not have enzymes present that allow the formation of adrenal cortical hormones, the adrenal cortex contains the enzyme systems necessary for the formation of both adrenocortical hormones and sex hormones, although the former are emphasized. This results in the adrenal cortex's producing small amounts of sex steroids normally and larger amounts under certain pathophysiological conditions.

There is no provision for the storage of steroid hormones within the cell; they are secreted immediately after formation by simple diffusion across the cell membrane because of their lipophilic structure. Thus, synthesis and secretion of steroid hormones occur in a tightly coupled manner with the *rate of hormone secretion controlled by the rate of synthesis*. The only storage form of steroids within these cells involves that of the precursor molecule, cholesterol, as an ester.

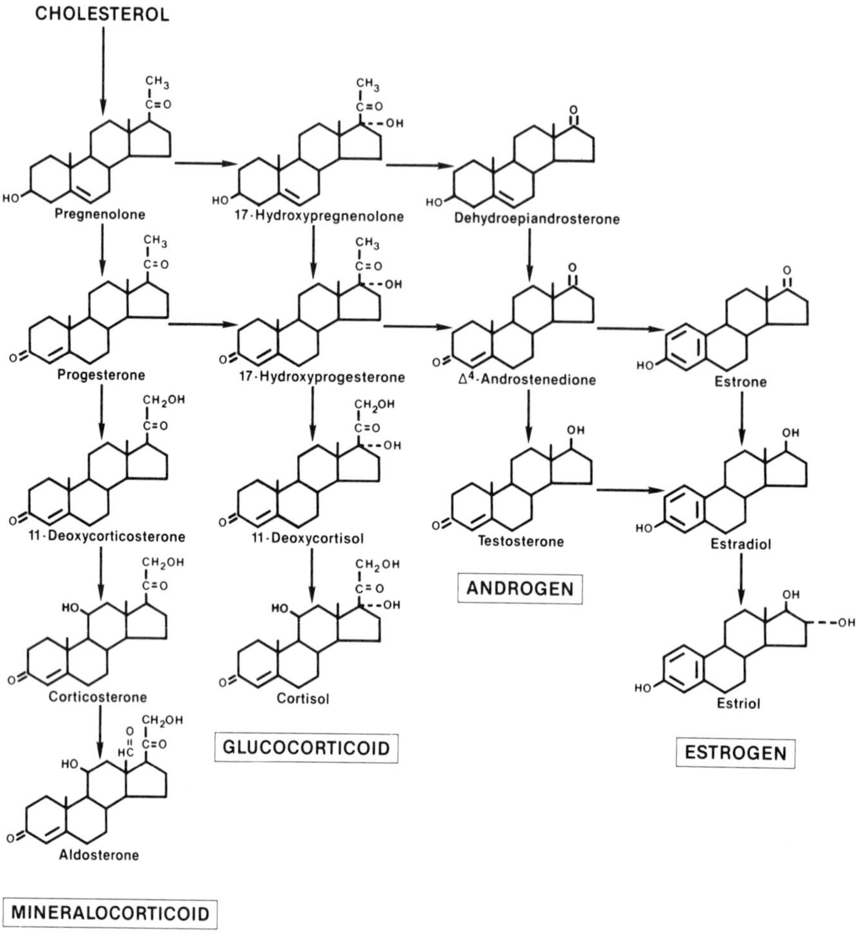

Figure 32–5. Pathways involved in the production of the major steroid hormones. (From Hedge GA, Colby HD, Goodman RL: Clinical Endocrine Physiology. Philadelphia, WB Saunders, 1987, p 12.)

the plasma (cortisol may be up to 10% in the free form). The system is responsive to utilization of the free form, with the free form replenished quickly by dissociation of bound hormone from the protein. The total amount of the hormone is usually reported, with the exception of thyroid hormone, in which attempts are usually made to estimate the amounts of bound and free. As indicated for steroid hormones, synthesis and release are tightly bound, and because metabolic clearance rates are usually constant, concentrations of steroids in plasma are usually a good reflection of the secretion rate. Under certain physiological conditions, such as pregnancy in humans, metabolism of estrogens can change because of the increased production of estrogen-binding proteins.

HORMONE-CELL INTERACTION

Protein Hormones Have Specific Receptors on Target Tissue Plasma Membranes, Whereas Steroids Have Specific Receptors Within the Cytoplasm or Nucleus

A central question in endocrinology is how do hormones and target cells of a particular tissue interact in a specific manner? The problem seems almost overwhelming for steroids, because they are lipid-soluble and able to permeate all cells of the body. The solution is that *target cells have receptors that are specific for a particular hormone.* For steroids, the receptors are located in the cytoplasm or nucleus of the target cells, whereas receptors for protein and peptide hormones are located on the plasma membrane of the cell. In addition to specificity,

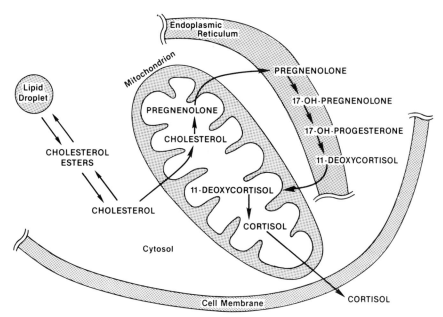

Figure 32–6. Subcellular compartmentalization of cortisol biosynthesis. (From Hedge GA, Colby HD, Goodman RL: Clinical Endocrine Physiology. Philadelphia, WB Saunders, 1987, p 13.)

receptors have a high affinity for their respective hormone. These characteristics of the receptor allows hormones to be in low concentration in the blood, yet effective in producing significant tissue response.

The greater the affinity of the receptor for the hormone, the longer the biological response. Termination of the action of a hormone usually requires dissociation of the hormone from the receptor. This occurs most often as a result of a decrease in plasma concentrations of the hormone; the binding of receptor and hormone is noncovalent, and declining hormone concentrations favor a chemical equilibrium of dissociation over association. Termination of hormone action can occur also as a result of internalization of the receptor-hormone complex through the process of endocytosis. The hormone is degraded by lysomal enzymes, whereas the receptor, protected because of its association with the vesicle membrane, can be recycled to the plasma membrane.

Receptors are present on cells in far greater numbers than is required for the elicitation of a biological response. Occupancy by a hormone of considerably less than 50% of the receptors usually elicits a maximal biological response. Even so, changes in receptor numbers can occur that affect the sensitivity of the cell, though not its maximal responsiveness. Changes in receptor number affect the probability that an interaction will occur between receptor and hormone. Stimulation of receptor

synthesis can occur by a hormone that is different from the hormone that interacts with the receptor. For example, predominant gonadotropin receptors on ovarian granulosa cells change from FSH to LH late in the ovarian follicle phase because of the influence of FSH. This allows the control of the ovarian follicle to pass from FSH to LH, which facilitates ovulation and the formation of a corpus luteum. Conversely, receptor numbers can decrease in conjunction with continued interaction of receptor and hormone. This often occurs in conjunction with administration of an agonist that has great affinity for the receptor, or in situations where amounts of hormone are pathologically elevated. The receptor numbers are *down-regulated* in this situation. The end result is that the animal becomes refractory to chronic therapy by the hormone in question.

POSTRECEPTOR CELL RESPONSES

Steroids Interact Directly with the Cell Nucleus Through the Formation of a Complex with its Cytosolic Receptor, Whereas Protein Hormones Need a Messenger, Because They Cannot Enter the Cell

The events that follow binding of the hormone and receptor depend upon whether a

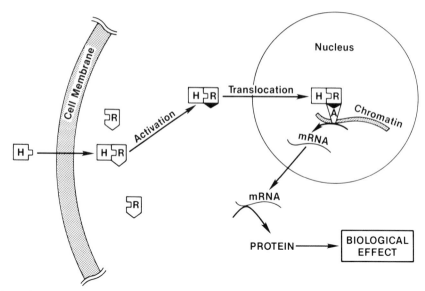

Figure 32–7. Subcellular mechanism of action of a lipophilic hormone (*H*) via an intracellar receptor (*R*). The H-R complex induces mRNA synthesis by binding to an acceptor site (*A*) on the chromatin. (From Hedge GA, Colby HD, Goodman RL: Clinical Endocrine Physiology. Philadelphia, WB Saunders, 1987, p 18.)

steroid or a protein peptide/hormone is involved. With steroids, the hormone is able to interact within the cell because of its ability to penetrate the lipoprotein plasma membrane (Fig. 32–7). The interaction of receptor and steroid hormone results in activation of the complex and subsequent translocation to the nucleus, where it interacts with specific sites on the chromatin. The result is the production of mRNA, which translocated to the ribosomes, directs synthesis of proteins that produce the desired biological result.

Protein/peptide hormones require an intermediary to act in their behalf, because they are not able to penetrate the plasma membrane of the cell; the intermediary substance is

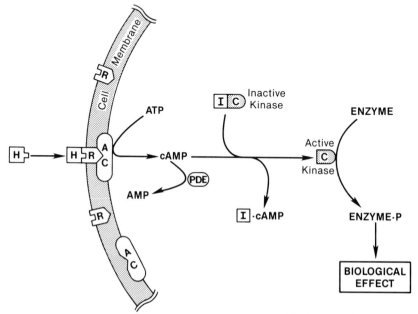

Figure 32–8. Subcellular mechanism of action of a hydrophilic hormone (*H*) via a membrane receptor (*R*), adenylate cyclase (*AC*), and cAMP. *I* and *C,* inhibitory and catalytic subunits of the kinase, respectively; *PDE,* phosphodiesterase. (From Hedge GA, Colby HD, Goodman RL: Clinical Endocrine Physiology. Philadelphia, WB Saunders, 1987, p 20.)

known as a *second* messenger (Fig. 32–8). The best documented second messenger is cyclic adenosine monophosphate (cAMP). cAMP is produced by the activation of an enzyme, adenylate cyclase, through interaction of the hormone and receptor in the plasma membrane. The activation of adenylate cyclase and the production of cAMP result in the phosphorylation of protein kinases, which are responsible for the biological response. Other second messengers include cytosolic calcium and its associated phosphodiesterase, calmodulin, as well as inositol triphosphate (IP_3) and diacylglycerol, products of phosphatidyl inositol metabolism. An important action of IP_3 is the stimulation of intracellular calcium release. One important response to diacylglycerol is the activation of phospholipase A and the formation of arachidonic acid, which leads to formation of members of the prostaglandin family of molecules. The biological response to a protein/peptide hormone-receptor interaction is more rapid than for steroids; pre-existing enzymes are activated, whereas the biological response to steroid requires the synthesis of enzyme protein.

METABOLISM OF HORMONES

Steroid Hormones Are Metabolized by Conjugation with Sulfates and Glucuronides, Which Makes Them Water-Soluble

Hormone activity is limited through the metabolism of hormones. The metabolism of steroids usually involves reduction of the molecule, followed by conjugation with sulfates and glucuronides, which increases the water solubility of the steroids, allowing them to be excreted in urine. The liver is the main organ responsible for this process. Thyroid hormones have iodine molecules removed during metabolism. Protein hormones are cleaved by peptidases, which is preceded by reduction of disulfide bonds if that is a characteristic of the molecule. Whereas a metabolite is usually less biologically potent than the original molecule, there is some evidence that conjugates of steroids can have significant biological activity. The question is raised regarding whether the conversion of hormones intracellularly, e.g., testosterone to dihydrotestosterone, represents metabolism, because dihydrotestosterone is more potent biologically than testoster-

one. Another example, the conversion of estradiol-17β to estrone by peripheral tissues, including adipose cells, is presented as a form of metabolism, yet estrone is a natural, and relatively potent, estrogen. Whereas one should be aware of situations in which the rate of clearance of a hormone can change, e.g., decrease as a result of increased hormone-binding plasma proteins during pregnancy or increase as the result of decreased hormone-binding plasma proteins in conjunction with liver disease, *metabolism of hormones is relatively constant,* and the concentration of a hormone usually reflects the other arm of the equation, i.e., the rate of synthesis of the hormone.

FEEDBACK CONTROL MECHANISMS

The Most Important Feedback Control for Hormones Is the Negative Feedback System in Which Increased Hormone Concentrations Result in Less Production of the Hormone, Usually Through An Interaction with the Hypothalamus or Pituitary Gland

The effects of hormones are proportional to their concentrations in blood, and it follows that control of these concentrations is an important aspect in assuring that normal physiological function is carried out. As indicated previously, the largest factor affecting hormone concentrations in blood is the secretion rate by a particular organ. *Feedback loop* control systems have evolved, in which concentrations of hormones are monitored at the controlling point in order to either increase, or decrease, secretion of a hormone by an endocrine organ. The most common feedback system is *negative feedback,* in which continuous monitoring allows the system to counteract changes in hormone secretion, or maintain a relatively constant environment.

An example of systems in which negative feedback control involves both the endocrine and nervous systems is shown in Figure 32–9. The hypothalamus, which controls secretion of tropic hormones in the anterior pituitary through the secretion of peptide-releasing hormones, has cells with a certain set-point by which they compare concentrations of hormone in the blood with the output of releasing hormones. If blood concentrations fall below

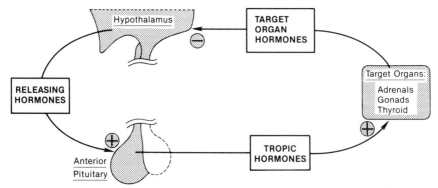

Figure 32–9. Negative feedback inhibition of tropic and releasing hormones by target organ hormones. (+) indicates stimulation and (−) indicates inhibition. In some cases, such inhibition occurs at the pituitary. (From Hedge GA, Colby HD, Goodman RL: Clinical Endocrine Physiology. Philadelphia, WB Saunders, 1987, p 25.)

the physiological set-point, an increase in releasing hormone output occurs that, in turn, increases production of tropic hormones by the anterior pituitary, and subsequently the secretion of the hormone by the target organ. Conversely, if the hormone concentration increases above acceptable physiological limits, a shutdown of releasing hormone production occurs within the hypothalamus, tropic hormone secretion by the anterior pituitary decreases, and production of the hormone by the target organ decreases. This type of control system is not an all-or-none affair, because changes and adjustments are being made continuously in order to maintain an optimal concentration of hormone.

In the negative feedback system, an increase in secretion of hormone results in a decrease in tropic hormone secretion. It is also possible to have a negative feedback system in which an increase in a physiological substance, e.g., glucose, causes an increase in a hormone, insulin, which plays an important role in glucose metabolism. This is considered to be a negative feedback system, because blood glucose concentrations are being dampened, or returned, toward normal levels through the action of insulin.

Positive feedback systems also exist, although they are much less common than negative feedback systems. One example is the preovulatory release of LH, in which the pulsatile rate of LH secretion greatly increases during the late stages of ovarian follicle development because of increased estrogen production by the follicle. In this situation, there is a definitive end point, i.e., ovulation results in a decline in the stimulus, estrogen, although the duration of the LH surge is likely determined within the hypothalamus, and therefore the LH response to estrogen is modulated.

Endocrine Secretory Patterns Can Be Influenced by Factors Such As Sleep or Light, and Can Produce Diurnal Rhythms

Endocrine secretion patterns can occur outside the control of negative feedback inhibition. Hormone patterns can change on an approximate 24-hour basis, a process referred to as a *diurnal* or *circadian* rhythm. Circadian is the preferred term, because diurnal refers to activity in the daytime; nocturnal should be used for those rhythms that are active at night. Most of the daily rhythms have some aspects of light, or lack of, as a major influence in the rhythm. Rhythmic changes in hormone patterns that occur at shorter intervals, often in the range of an hour, are called *ultradian* rhythms.

THE HYPOTHALAMUS

The Hypothalamus Coordinates the Activity of the Pituitary Gland Through the Secretion of Peptides and Amines

As indicated previously, the two major controlling systems are the nervous and endocrine systems. The interface between these systems occurs, for the most part, in the *hypothalamus*. The hypothalamus is an area of the diencephalon that forms the floor of the third ventricle and includes the optic chiasma, tuber cinereum, mammillary bodies, and the median eminence. Often not included in this classification are the infundibulum and the neurohypophysis (stalk of the posterior lobe and the posterior lobe, respectively), although both tissues represent extensions of the hypothalamus into the pituitary gland. The hypothalamus produces peptides and amines (discussed under control of the pituitary gland) that influence the pituitary gland to produce (1) *tropic hormones* (e.g., ACTH), which in turn influence the production of hormones by peripheral target endocrine tissues (e.g., cortisol), or (2) hormones that directly cause a biological effect in tissues (e.g., prolactin—PRL). The hypothalamus is also the center for the control of a large number of autonomic nervous system control pathways.

THE PITUITARY GLAND

The pituitary gland, or *hypophysis cerebri*, is composed of the *adenohypophysis* (pars distalis or anterior lobe), the *neurohypophysis* (pars nervosa or posterior lobe), the pars intermedia (intermediate lobe), and the pars tuberalis (Fig. 32–10). The adenohypophysis is formed from an area of the roof of the embryonic oral ectoderm called *Rathke's pouch*, which extends upward to meet the neurohypophysis, which extends downward as an outpouching of

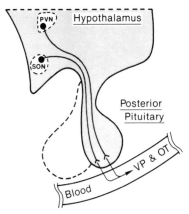

Figure 32–11. The hypothalamoneurohypophyseal system, which secretes vasopressin (*VP*) and oxytocin (*OT*). (From Hedge GA, Colby HD, Goodman RL: Clinical Endocrine Physiology. Philadelphia, WB Saunders, 1987, p 56.)

neural ectoderm from the floor of the third ventricle.

The Neurohypophysis Has Cell Bodies That Originate in the Hypothalamus, with Cell Endings That Secrete Oxytocin and Vasopressin

The neurohypophysis is composed of axons that have a neural origin largely within the *supraoptic* and *paraventricular nuclei* of the hypothalamus. The neurohypophysis is an extension of the hypothalmus into the pituitary, that is, the cell bodies are in the hypothalamus; the axons form the stalk of the posterior lobe, and the nerve endings are in the lobe proper (Fig. 32–11).

The *endocrine-secretory neurons* that constitute the neurohypophysis differ from neurons involved in the transmission of neural signals in several ways: (1) neurosecretory neurons do not innervate other neurons, even though they are innervated; (2) the secretory product of neurosecretory neurons is secreted into the blood; (3) the secretory product can act at distances greatly removed from the neuron. Also, as contrasted to anterior pituitary hormones, which influence other tissues to produce hormones, posterior lobe hormones can directly cause the desired tissue response.

The first indication of the physiological activity of the neurohypophyseal lobe was the finding of Oliver and Schafer in 1895 that the injection of whole pituitary extracts caused a rise in blood pressure. This effect was soon associated with the pars nervosa. This action represents the effects of one of the main neu-

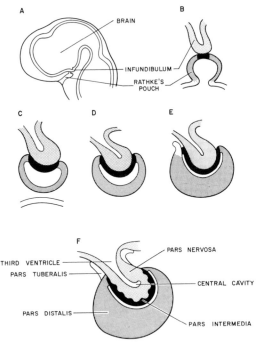

Figure 32–10. Diagrams showing progressive stages in the embryonic development of the pituitary gland. Rathke's pouch becomes detached from the oral epithelium at stage C. (Stage A is from Villee CA, Walker WF Jr, Smith FE: General Zoology, 2nd ed. Philadelphia, WB Saunders, 1963.) (From Turner CD, Bagnara JT: General Endocrinology, 6th ed. Philadelphia, WB Saunders, 1977, p 81.)

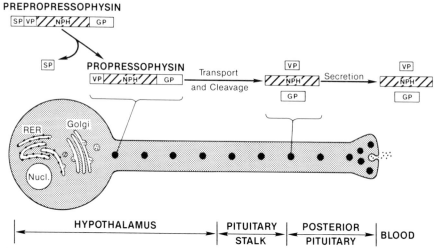

Figure 32–12. Diagram of a vasopressin-secreting neuron illustrating the subcellular components involved in synthesis and secretion. This process begins with the synthesis of prepropressophysin, which consists of (1) a signal peptide (*SP*); (2) vasopressin (*VP*); (3) neurophysin (*NPH*); and (4) a glycoprotein (*GP*). The production and release of oxytocin is identical except that no glycoprotein is involved. (From Hedge GA, Colby HD, Goodman RL: Clinical Endocrine Physiology. Philadelphia, WB Saunders, 1987, p 58.)

rohypophyseal hormones, *vasopressin*. The first indication of the existence of the other main neurohypophyseal hormone, *oxytocin*, was shown in 1915 by Gaines, wherein the injection of posterior pituitary gland extracts caused milk ejection. In 1941 Ely and Peterson showed that a denervated mammary gland could eject milk if perfused with blood that had been enriched with posterior pituitary extract. Both neurohypophyseal hormones were isolated and sequenced by du Vigneaud in 1954. These were some of the first proteins to have their amino acid sequences elucidated.

Oxytocin and Vasopressin Are Synthesized in Cell Bodies Within the Hypothalamus and Are Carried by Axon Flow to the Posterior Lobe, Where They Are Released

As indicated, the two important hormones produced by the neurohypophysis are vasopressin and oxytocin. Whereas it was previously thought that the two hormones were produced in separate nuclei, there is now evidence that both hormones are produced in both the supraoptic and paraventricular nuclei. The cell bodies that synthesize the hormones are large and, as such, are called *magnocellular nuclei*. The synthesis of vasopressin and oxytocin, as described previously for protein and peptide hormones, involves first the production of a preprohormone, *prepropressophysin* for vasopressin and *preprooxyphysin* for

oxytocin, at the level of the cell body within the hypothalamus (Fig. 32–12). The "pre" portion of the molecule is cleaved before the molecules are packaged into granules. During passage of the granules down the axon, the prohormone is cleaved to produce either oxytocin or vasopressin; the remaining peptide fragments are called *neurophysin I* or *neurophysin II*, respectively. Neurophysin I, which is released into the blood vascular system along with oxytocin has been quantified as an alternative means of following the release of oxytocin. At the moment, there is no known physiological function of the neurophysins.

The release of the posterior lobe peptide hormones is initiated in the hypothalamus as a result of depolarization of the cell body because of stimulation by neural afferents. The action potential generated extends down the axon to the nerve terminal, where the secretory granules containing the hormone are stored. The depolarization of the nerve cell membrane allows the influx of calcium ions, which initiates the release of hormone through the process of exocytosis.

The Main Effects of Oxytocin Are on the Contraction of Smooth Muscle (Mammary Gland and Uterus); the Effects of Vasopressin Are Primarily on the Conservation of Water (Antidiuresis) and Secondarily on Blood Pressure

The main effects of oxytocin involve the contraction of the myoepithelial cells, which surround the alveoli in the mammary gland and the myometrium of the uterus. These actions are covered in Chapters 37 and 38.

The main activity of vasopressin belies its name because its main effect is *antidiuretic,* or the enhancement of water retention by the kidney. As a consequence, the hormone is often called *antidiuretic hormone* (ADH). Vasopressin is the most important hormone for the control of water balance. Vasopressin also has a *pressor* effect, which involves the contraction of smooth muscle of the vascular system and therefore has an effect on blood pressure. The main form of vasopressin in most species is *arginine* vasopressin, whereas in pigs it is *lysine* vasopressin, and in birds *arginine vasotocin.*

Vasopressin activates the classic second messenger, cAMP, through binding with a cell membrane receptor (V_2) on the serosal surface of the kidney tubule cell (Fig. 32–13). Protein kinases are activated, which affect a cell membrane protein located in the mucosal surface of the kidney tubule cell. This allows water molecules to flow down a concentration gradient from an area of higher concentration in the renal filtrate to an area of lower concentra-

tion in the interstitium of the renal medulla. The pressor effect of vasopressin is initiated by interaction with receptors (V_1) in smooth muscle, which activates the inositol phosphate system.

Plasma Osmolality Controls the Secretion of Vasopressin

The control of vasopressin secretion as a result of changes in plasma osmolality is through *osmoreceptors* located in the hypothalamus as well as through receptors located in the esophagus and stomach that immediately sense water intake (Fig. 32–14). An increase in osmolality of body fluids increases the rate of action potential firing in the osmoreceptors, which in turn activate cells in the hypothalamus that synthesize vasopressin. This negative feedback system is sensitive to changes in osmolality, and the solute-to-water ratio is maintained within a few percent of the normal values. The regulation of the pressor effect of vasopressin, i.e., through blood volume, is by increasing the number of action potentials in

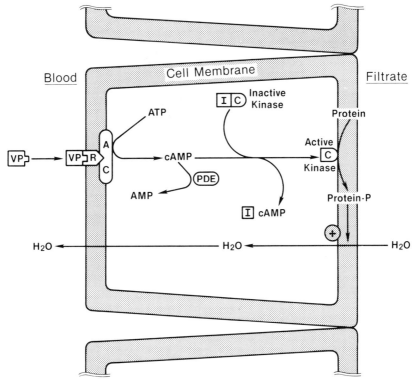

Figure 32–13. Antidiuretic mechanism of action of vasopressin (*VP*) on cells of the distal tubule and collecting ducts. *R,* receptor; *AC,* adenylate cyclase; *PDE,* phosphodiesterase. (From Hedge GA, Colby HD, Goodman RL: Clinical Endocrine Physiology. Philadelphia, WB Saunders, 1987, p 61.)

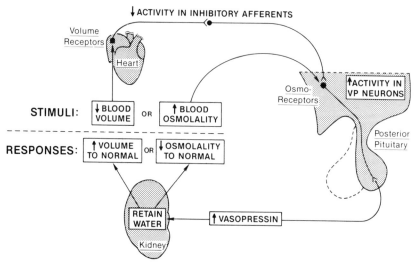

Figure 32–14. The major mechanisms regulating vasopressin (*VP*) secretion. A perturbation in either blood volume or osmolality will modify vasopressin secretion in order to restore these parameters to their normal values. However, this restoration requires appropriate adjustments in water intake by thirst as well as by the modulation of water retention depicted. Also, the two responses indicated may be affected by simultaneous changes in sodium balance. (From Hedge GA, Colby HD, Goodman RL: Clinical Endocrine Physiology. Philadelphia, WB Saunders, 1987, p 63.)

stretch receptors located in the atria. A decrease in blood volume activates the stretch receptors, which inhibit activity of neurons, vagal in origin, which inhibit the osmoreceptor cells. Blood volume changes that decrease blood pressure also affect vasopressin release through activation of *baroreceptors* in the carotid sinus and aortic arch.

The main clinical problem associated with vasopressin is hyposecretion. Vasopressin deficiency leads to the production of large amounts of dilute urine, a syndrome that is called *diabetes insipidus.* This condition is differentiated from that of *diabetes mellitus,* in which large amounts of glucose are present in urine, giving it a "sweet" taste (mellitus) or odor rather than the odorless, tasteless (insipid) urine of diabetes insipidus. *Hypothalamic diabetes insipidus* results from inadequate secretion of vasopressin, whereas *nephrogenic diabetes insipidus* results from abnormalities in the kidney that prevent it from responding to vasopressin. Deprivation of water or vasopressin administration in an animal can be used to differentiate the two types of diabetes insipidus. Animals with hypothalamic diabetes insipidus do not conserve water when deprived, but respond to vasopressin administration. Animals with *nephrogenic* diabetes insipidus respond to neither water deprivation or vasopressin administration, because the defect lies at the level of the kidney. One cause of hypothalamic diabetes insipidus is neoplasia.

Hypersecretion of vasopressin in the absence of osmotic or volumetric stimulation is called the syndrome of inappropriate ADH secretion (SIADH). Neoplastic processes are often involved in SIADH; ectopic tumors, often located in the lung, are the neoplasms most commonly involved in this syndrome.

The Anterior Pituitary Produces the Following Hormones: Growth Hormone, Prolactin, Thyroid-Stimulating Hormone, Follicle-Stimulating Hormone, Luteinizing Hormone, and Adrenocorticotropic Hormone

The adenohypophysis is comprised of the *pars distalis* and the *pars intermedia.* The major hormones produced by the anterior pituitary include *growth hormone* (GH—also called somatotropin); *prolactin* (PRL); *thyroid-stimulating hormone* (TSH); *follicle-stimulating hormone* (FSH); *luteinizing hormone* (LH); and *adrenocorticotropic hormone* (ACTH) (Table 32–1). GH and PRL are produced by acidophilic somatotropes and lactotropes, respectively, and are classified as *somatomammotropins.* GH and PRL are single-chain proteins that contain two and three disulfide bonds, respectively. There is overlap of activity between GH and PRL, which is based on the homology of amino acid sequence, i.e., about 50%. Of the two major

Table 32–1
SIX MAJOR HORMONES SECRETED BY THE ANTERIOR PITUITARY GLAND

Hormone	Abbreviation
Glycoproteins	
Follicle-stimulating hormone	FSH
Luteinizing hormone	LH
(interstitial cell-stimulating	(ICSH)
hormone)	
Thyroid-stimulating hormone	TSH
(thyrotropin)	
Somatŏmammotropins	
Growth hormone	GH
(somatotropin)	
Prolactin	PRL
Proopiomelanocortins	
Adrenocorticotropin	ACTH
(corticotropin)	

Modified from Hedge GA, Colby HD, Goodman RL: Clinical Endocrine Physiology. Philadelphia, WB Saunders, 1987, p 71.

somatomammotropins, GH is uniquely species-specific as to its activity.

TSH, produced by thyrotropes, and FSH and LH, produced by gonadotropes, are classified as *glycoproteins* because all three molecules have carbohydrate moieties. These hormones have α- *and* β-*subunits* that are linked by noncovalent binding. The β-subunit is identical (and interchangeable) among the three glycoproteins. The β-subunit, unique for each hormone, imparts the specific action of each hormone. Other members of this family of hormones that are not of anterior pituitary origin include *equine chorionic gonadotropin* (eCG—also called Pregnant Mares Serum Gonadotropin) and *primate chorionic gonadotropin* (hCG, mCG), which are produced by cells of the placental chorion.

ACTH and β-lipotropin belong to the *proopiomelanocortin* (POMC) family in that they originate from a common prohormone (Fig. 32–15). Cells in both the *pars distalis* and *pars intermedia* synthesize POMC molecules. The emphasis on the type of hormone produced is different, with ACTH produced by pars distalis corticotropes. In the pars intermedia, ACTH is cleaved by corticotropes to form *a-MSH*, the predominant hormone of this lobe, with the remaining peptide fragment known as *corticotropin-like intermediate lobe peptide* (CLIP); the physiological activity of CLIP is not known. In both the pars distalis and the pars intermedia, β-lipotropin is cleaved to form β-*endorphins* and γ-*lipotropin*. Endorphins have opioid activity and appear to modulate gonadotropin secretion.

Control of adenohypophyseal activity was not understood for a considerable length of time, first because the functional connection between the brain and the anterior pituitary was not understood. Popa and Fielding, Budapest medical student and university professor, respectively, in the 1930s described the blood vascular system that connects the hypothalamus with pituitary, but were unable to determine the direction in which blood flowed. In about 1950, Geoffrey Harris drew the important conclusion that the linkage involved blood passage from the hypothalamus to the anterior pituitary through the portal blood system previously described by Popa and Fielding (Fig. 32–16). The dorsal hypophyseal artery, which supplies nutrients and oxygen to the adenohypophysis (the ventral hypophyseal artery supplies the neurohypophysis), terminates in the *median eminence* as a capillary plexus. Blood from these plexuses are drained by two veins that empty into sinusoidal capillaries of the pars distalis, completing the *portal venous system* (one vein supplies the ventral, central part of the pars distalis, the other the dorsal, peripheral areas).

Adenohypophyseal Activity Is Controlled by Hypothalamic-Releasing Hormones, Which Are Released into the Portal System That Connects the Median Eminence of the Hypothalamus and the Anterior Pituitary

Whereas neurons that compose the neurohypophysis are influenced directly by neural input within the hypothalamus, the imposition of a blood vascular system between the hypothalamus and the adenohypophysis requires a different type of control system. The hypothalamus produces *regulatory* or *hypophysiotropic hormones*, which are transported to and released within the median eminence (comparable to posterior lobe hormones) (Fig. 32–17). These regulatory hormones then pass to the adenohypophysis via the portal venous system, where they stimulate the release of the various anterior pituitary hormones. The synthesis of adenohypophyseal regulatory hormones is controlled by both neural and hormonal inputs at the level of the hypothalamus. Some of the hypophyseal hormones have been found in other areas of the brain and extraneural sites, including the GI tract and the pancreas.

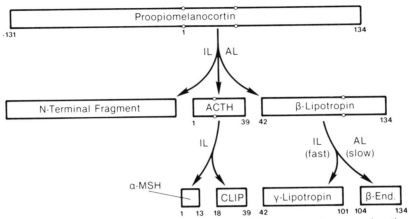

Figure 32–15. Cleavage of proopiomelanocortin to yield ACTH and related peptides. By convention, the numbering of the amino acids begins with the first one of ACTH and then increases positively toward the C-terminal and negatively toward the N-terminal. Cleavage occurs at pairs of basic amino acids indicated by the circles. *IL*, intermediate lobe; *AL*, anterior lobe; β-*End*, β-endorphin; *CLIP*, corticotropin-like intermediate lobe peptide. (From Hedge GA, Colby HD, Goodman RL: Clinical Endocrine Physiology. Philadelphia, WB Saunders, 1987, p 75.)

The initial isolation and identification of the hypothalamic hormones required large amounts of tissue as well as expertise in biochemistry. The first hypothalamic hormone identified, which controls ACTH release, was originally called *corticotropin-releasing factor* (now changed from *factor* to *hormone*). The initial work, done by Guillemin's group at the University of Houston in the early 1960s, required the collection, freezing, and transport of several hundred thousand sheep brains from abbatoirs located in the western United States, as well as the subsequent dissection of the hypothalami. The hypothalamic hormones that have been characterized, and the hormones they release, include (1) *corticotropin-releasing hormone (CRH)*, a 41 amino acid polypeptide that stimulates corticotropes to release all components of the proopiomelanocortin family of molecules; (2) *gonadotropin-releasing hormone (GnRH)*, a decapeptide that stimulates gonadotrope secretion of both FSH and LH; (3) *thyrotropin-releasing hormone (TRH)*, a tripeptide that stimulates thyrotrope secretion of TSH; (4) *dopamine*, a catecholamine precursor of norepinephrine that inhibits lactotrope secretion of PRL and thyrotrope secretion of TSH; (5) *somatostatin*, a tetradecapeptide that inhibits stomatotrope secretion of GH; and (6) *growth hormone-releasing hormone (GHRH)*, a 44

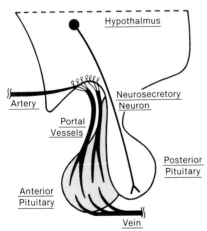

Figure 32–16. Diagram of the hypothalmopituitary unit contrasting the vascular connection between the brain and the anterior pituitary to the neuronal connection between the brain and the posterior pituitary. (From Hedge GA, Colby HD, Goodman RL: Clinical Endocrine Physiology. Philadelphia, WB Saunders, 1987, p 70.)

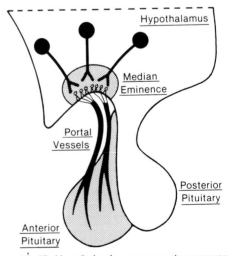

Figure 32–17. Hypothalamic neurosecretory neurons and hypothalamo-hypophyseal portal vessels. (From Hedge GA, Colby HD, Goodman RL: Clinical Endocrine Physiology. Philadelphia, WB Saunders, 1987, p 86.)

Table 32–2
MAJOR HYPOPHYSIOTROPIC HORMONES

Hormone	Abbreviation	Site of Origin
Thyrotropin-releasing hormone	TRH	PVN
Gonadotropin-releasing hormone	GnRH	POA
Growth hormone-inhibiting hormone (or somatostatin)	GHIH	AHA
Growth hormone-releasing hormone	GHRH	ARC
Corticotropin-releasing hormone	CRH	PVN
Prolactin-releasing factor	PRF	?
Prolactin-inhibiting hormone (or dopamine)	PIH	ARC

Modified from Hedge GA, Colby HD, Goodman RL: Clinical Endocrine Physiology. Philadelphia, WB Saunders, 1987, p 87.

amino acid polypeptide that stimulates somatotrope secretion of GH (Table 32–2). All of these hypophysiotropic hormones are peptides with the exception of the inhibitor of PRL secretion, dopamine.

As can be seen in Table 32–2, no hypothalamic hormone is listed for the stimulation of PRL secretion. There is some evidence that *vasoactive intestinal peptide* (VIP) may play an important physiological role in PRL secretion. The name of the peptide, VIP, indicates its initial site of discovery and again emphasizes that regulatory peptides ascribed to the hypothalamus are likely secreted and used for regulatory purposes on a local basis by many tissues.

Previously, only four of the anterior pituitary hormones (FSH, LH, TSH, and ACTH) were considered to be tropic, i.e., their main effect was stimulation of hormone secretion by specific endocrine organs located peripheral to the pituitary. More recently, GH has been

added to this list because GH stimulates the liver to produce somatomedins, which have a negative feedback effect on GH secretion. PRL remains as the only pars distalis hormone for which negative feedback inhibition has not been demonstrated through hormones produced by PRL-target tissues.

The most important regulation of secretion of the protein hormones by the pars distalis is by feedback inhibition. One feedback system involves negative feedback inhibition of the tropic pituitary hormone by interaction of the target organ hormone with the hypothalamus, as well as the pituitary; this system is called a *long loop* feedback system (Fig. 32–18). For example, cortisol is produced by the adrenal cortex, as a result of ACTH stimulation, and cortisol, in turn, has a negative feedback effect on ACTH production at the level of the hypothalamus and the anterior pituitary. *Short loop* feedback systems have been described also in which an anterior pituitary hormone,

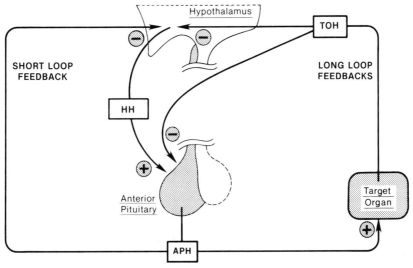

Figure 32–18. Regulation of anterior pituitary hormone (*APH*) secretion by hypophysiotropic hormones (*HH*), short loop negative feedback, and long loop negative feedback by target organ hormones (*TOH*). (From Hedge GA, Colby HD, Goodman RL: Clinical Endocrine Physiology. Philadelphia, WB Saunders, 1987, p 78.)

e.g. ACTH, has a direct negative feedback inhibition of CRH secretion within the hypothalamus.

Even under conditions of negative feedback inhibition, the secretion of anterior pituitary hormones is not constant. For example, even though estrogens exert a continuous, potent negative feedback inhibition on gonadotropin secretion, gonadotropin secretion alternates between secretion and no secretion with *pulses of gonadotropins* released into the blood vascular system. In the case of gonadotropins, the ovarian endocrine status influences the pulse rate and the amplitude of each pulse. Progesterone domination is associated with a decreased pulse rate and increase pulse amplitude, whereas estrogen causes the opposite effect. The work of Irvine and Alexander has provided the best documentation of the precise relationship between secretory activity of hypothalamic regulatory and anterior pituitary hormones. Their data have been obtained through analysis of hormones obtained from the intercavernal sinus, which collects venous blood from the pituitary of the horse.

Circadian patterns of hormone secretion can occur also in conjunction with pulsatile secretion, e.g., ACTH (and cortisol) values are lowest at midnight and highest at 6 A.M. In contrast, GH concentrations are only elevated for a few hours following the onset of deep sleep. Sustained increases in plasma hormone concentrations, as observed daily for ACTH and GH, occur when the pulse secretion of the hormone is faster than the metabolic clearance rate. Veterinarians need to be aware of circadian hormone patterns in order to select the optimal sampling time if the hormone of interest has circadian patterns of secretion.

CLINICAL CORRELATION

EQUINE CUSHING'S DISEASE

HISTORY □ You are called to examine a 15-year-old mare whose owner complains that the mare has been stiff in her legs for the past 9 months. The mare has been used as a broodmare and delivered a foal the past spring (and for the seven previous years). She failed to conceive last spring and now, in the early summer of the next year, she has yet to exhibit normal estrous cycles.

CLINICAL EXAMINATION □ As you gain a general perspective on the mare, you notice that she appears to have been clipped recently. She is not a show mare, and because it is early summer, you inquire why she has been clipped. The owner indicates that the mare has been slow to shed this spring, and she is tired of seeing the mare with a rough hair coat. The finding of a long hair coat out of season prompts you to ask about the water consumption of the mare; the owner indicates that the mare drank more water (and urinated accordingly) than would be expected. You examine the feet and find that the soles appear slightly "dropped"; you find a small abscess in the sole of one of the feet.

COMMENT □ The main clue regarding the nature of the disease is the presence of a long hair coat out of season; this is the *sine qui non* of the disease. The usual complaints of owners of horses with Cushing's disease are related to chronic processes, such as pneumonia, laminitis, or weight loss, the latter often associated with parasitism and an inability to masticate properly because of teeth problems. It is relatively common for broodmares that are progressing into Cushing's disease to have a recent history of infertility following a successful broodmare career. Although the cause of infertility is not known, it is likely that a disturbance of gonadotropin secretion occurs in conjunction with disturbance of the proopiomelanocortin system.

The disease represents a classic case of loss of control of the intermediate lobe of the pituitary by the hypothalamus, in this case the loss of dopaminergic control. Under normal conditions, melanotropes of the intermediate lobe process proopiomelanocortin to α-MSH and acetylated β-endorphin, 1-31, and nonopiate active carboxy-terminally shortened 1-26, or 1-27, endorphin. In the absence of dopamine, the melanotropes produce α-MSH as well as β-endorphin, 1-31 (the active form) and small amounts of ACTH; the latter stimulates glucocorticoid production by the adrenal cortex. The negative feedback control system fails in this situation, because the melanotropes do not have glucocorticoid receptors, even under normal conditions. The result is unchecked synthesis and secretion of melanotrope products, including ACTH and unchecked glucocorticoid secretion. Activity of the corticotropes in the pars distalis is decreased because of negative feedback inhibition by the glucocorticoids. One of the long-term effects of excess glucocorticoid secretion is muscle-wasting, a common finding in these animals. Also, some of the common manifestations of the disease are polydypsia and polyuria, which are due to compression of the pars nervosa by the enlarging pars intermediate and reduction in antidiuretic hormone synthesis.

Although there is hyperplasia of the intermediate lobe in this disease, the chicken and the egg question has not been solved, i.e., is this a disease that occurs because of autonomous hyperplasia of the intermediate lobe, or does the hyperplasia occur because of gradual loss of dopaminergic control by the hypothalamus? One theory is that chronic stress, such as occurs with laminitis, could affect dopamine secretion by the hypothalamus, leading to loss of control of the intermediate lobe and the development of hyperplasia.

TREATMENT ☐ At the present time, the only proven treatment is to provide the affected animals with the best possible husbandry. This care includes parasite control, floating of teeth, providing good nutrition, and taking proper care of the feet.

Bibliography

Dickson WM: Endocrine glands. In Swenson MJ (ed): Dukes' Physiology of Domestic Animals, 10th ed. Ithaca, Cornell University Press, 1984, pp 761–797.

Feldman EC, Nelson RW: Canine and Feline Endocrinology and Reproduction. Philadelphia, WB Saunders, 1987.

Hedge GA, Colby HD, Goodman RL: Clinical Endocrine Physiology. Philadelphia, WB Saunders, 1987.

Martin R: Endocrine Physiology. New York, Oxford University Press, 1985.

McDonald LE, Pineda MH (eds): Veterinary Endocrinology and Reproduction, 4th ed. Philadelphia, Lea and Febiger, 1989.

Tepperman J, Tepperman M: Metabolic and Endocrine Physiology, 5th ed. Chicago, Year Book Medical Publishers, 1987.

Wilson JD, Foster DW: Williams Textbook of Endocrinology, 7th ed. Philadelphia, WB Saunders, 1985.

PRACTICE QUESTIONS FOR CHAPTER 32

1. In general, hormones are classified as proteins, peptides, and steroids. Which one of the following hormones is a peptide?

   a. Growth hormone
   b. Insulin
   c. Vasopressin
   d. Dopamine
   e. Epinephrine
   f. Melatonin

2. In general, steroid hormones are classified as mineralocorticoid, glucocorticoid, and sex steroids. Which one of the following hormones is a glucocorticoid?

   a. Aldosterone
   b. Corticosterone
   c. Cortisol
   d. Testosterone
   e. Estrone

3. Direct feedback control of corticotropin-releasing hormone by ACTH is termed

   a. negative feedback.
   b. positive feedback.
   c. short loop feedback.
   d. long loop feedback.

4. The synthesis of hormones from the family known as proopiomelanocortin depends upon whether the precursor hormone is produced in the pars distalis or the pars intermedia. The two main hormones produced by these two lobes (in respective order) are

   a. α-MSH and endorphin.
   b. ACTH and endorphin.
   c. α-MSH and ACTH.
   d. ACTH and α-MSH.
   e. ACTH and γ-lipotropin.

5. Increased hormonal activity that occurs during daylight hours is termed _____ rhythm.

   a. circadian
   b. diurnal
   c. nocturnal
   d. ultradian

33

Endocrine Glands and Their Function

1. The thyroid hormones are synthesized from two tyrosine molecules that are connected and contain three or four iodine molecules
2. Thyroid hormones are stored outside the cell, attached to thyroglobulin in the form of colloid
3. The release of thyroid hormones involves transport of thyroglobulin with attached thyroid hormones into the cell, cleavage of the thyroid hormones from thyroxine-binding globulin (TBG), and their release into the interstitial tissues
4. Thyroid hormones are transported in the plasma attached to plasma proteins: thyroxine-binding globulin, albumin, and thyroxine-binding pre-albumin; less than 1% of the thyroid hormones are free in plasma
5. The main routes of metabolism of thyroid hormones are through deiodination or the formation of glucuronides and sulfates
6. Thyroid hormones are the primary factors for the control of metabolism
7. The ingestion of compounds that inhibit the uptake or the organic binding of iodine block the ability of the thyroid to secrete thyroid hormones and cause goiter

THE ADRENAL GLANDS

1. The adrenal glands are composed of two organs: the outer gland is called the cortex and secretes corticoids, and the inner gland is called the medulla and secretes catecholamines

THE ADRENAL CORTEX

1. The adrenal cortex has three zones: the zona glomerulosa, which secretes mineralo-corticoids, and the zona fasciculata and the zona reticularis, which secrete gluco-corticoids
2. Adrenal corticoids are synthesized from cholesterol with the critical difference being a hydroxyl group on C-17 of glucocorticoids
3. Adrenocortical hormones are carried in plasma in association with specific-binding globulins (corticosteroid-binding globulin) and less specific-binding albumins—a relatively large amount (10%) of the hormone exists in the free state
4. The metabolism of adrenocortical hormones involves the reduction of double bonds and ketone configurations as well as the conjugation of the steroids to glucuronides and sulfates

5. One of the most important functions of glucocorticoids is control of metabolism and, in particular, the stimulation of hepatic gluconeogenesis
6. Adrenocorticotropic hormone is the main regulator of glucocorticoid synthesis by the adrenal cortex
7. One of the most important clinical uses of glucocorticoids is the suppression of the inflammatory response

HORMONES OF THE PANCREAS

1. The synthesis of insulin is biphasic, an acute phase involving the release of preformed insulin, and a chronic phase involving the synthesis of protein
2. The metabolism of insulin involves splitting the A and B chains, and reducing the chains to amino acids and peptides
3. The main metabolic functions of insulin are to promote the conversion of glucose, fatty acids, and amino acids to their storage form
4. The most important functions of glucagon are to decrease glycogen synthesis, increase glycogenolysis, and increase gluconeogenesis, all at the level of the liver
5. The main factor that stimulates glucagon synthesis is decreased glucose concentrations in the blood
6. The main functions of somatostatin are to regulate (inhibit) the secretion of hormones produced by the pancreas (insulin, glucagon, pancreatic polypeptide) and to inhibit digestive processes

THE ADRENAL MEDULLA

1. The synthesis of catecholamines is from tyrosine; the main catecholamine synthesized by the adrenal medulla is epinephrine
2. The main actions of catecholamines are on metabolism, especially effects that increase the concentration of glucose; catecholamines also enable animals to rapidly adapt to stress
3. The main factors that stimulate catecholamine secretion are hypoglycemia and conditions that produce stress

CALCIUM AND PHOSPHATE METABOLISM

1. Calcium is important for intracellular reactions, including muscle contraction, nerve cell activity, the release of hormones through exocytosis, and the activation of enzymes; extracellular functions include blood coagulation, the maintenance and stability of cell membranes, and the maintenance of structural integrity of bone and teeth
2. Phosphate is important for the structure of bone and teeth; on a cellular basis, organic phosphate serves as part of the cell membrane and as part of a number of intracellular components
3. The most important body pool of calcium involved in homeostasis is the extracellular fluid component; the amorphous (soluble) portion of bone calcium readily contributes calcium for the maintenance of homeostasis.

THE THYROID GLAND

In most mammals, the thyroid gland is located caudal to the trachea at the level of the first, or second, tracheal ring. The thyroid gland is composed of two lobes lying on either side of the trachea and connected by a narrow piece of tissue called the isthmus.

The thyroid gland is the most important endocrine gland for metabolic regulation. The glandular tissue has cells formed in a circular arrangement called a *follicle* (Fig. 33–1). The follicles are filled with a homogenous-staining substance called *colloid*, which is the main storage form of the thyroid hormones. The follicular cells are cuboidal when the secretion is basal, and elongated when stimulated to release hormone. Another important endocrine cell is located outside of the follicles, which is the *parafollicular, or C, cell*. This cell secretes *calcitonin*, a hormone important for the regulation of calcium. The activity of this hormone is discussed under calcium metabolism.

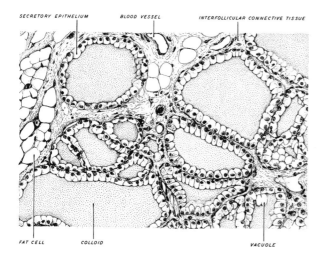

Figure 33–1. Histologic features of the normal thyroid gland of the rat. All normal thyroid glands are structurally similar, though slight variations occur with age, diet, habitation, and sexual status. The normal animals of this colony were maintained on a high protein ration, which probably accounts for the slight hypertrophic condition of the secretory epithelium. (From Turner CD, Bagnara JT: General Endocrinology, 6th ed. Philadelphia, WB Saunders, 1976, p 180.)

The Thyroid Hormones Are Synthesized from Two Tyrosine Molecules That Are Connected and Contain Three or Four Iodine Molecules

The synthesis of thyroid hormone is interesting, because a large amount of the active hormone is stored as a colloid outside of the follicle cells within the lumen, or acinus, created by the circular arrangement of glandular cells. Two molecules are important for thyroid hormone synthesis: *tyrosine* and *iodine*. Tyrosine is a part of a large molecule (MW 660,000) called *thyroglobulin* which is formed within the follicle cell and secreted into the lumen of the follicle. Iodine is converted to iodide in the intestinal tract and then is transported to the thyroid, where the follicle cells effectively trap the iodide through an active transport process. This allows intracellular iodide concentrations to be 25 to 200 times greater than extracellular iodide.

As iodide passes through the apical wall of the cell, it attaches to the ring structures of the tyrosines, which are part of the thyroglobulin amino acid sequence. The tyrosyl ring can accommodate two iodide molecules; if one iodide attaches, it is called *monoiodotyrosine* (MIT), if two, *diiodotyrosine* (DIT). The coupling of two iodinated tyrosines results in the formation of the main thyroid hormones; two DIT molecules form *tetraiodothyronine* (T_4) and one MIT and one DIT molecule form *triiodothyronine* (T_3) (Fig. 33–2). A key enzyme in the biosynthesis of thyroid hormones is *thyroperoxidase* (plus an oxidant, hydrogen peroxide). Thyroperoxidase catalyzes the iodination of the tyrosyl residues of thyroxine-binding globulin (TBG) and the formation of T_3 and T_4. In addition to the unusual storage form of the hormone, thyroid hormones are also unique in that they are the only hormones that contain a halide, i.e., iodine.

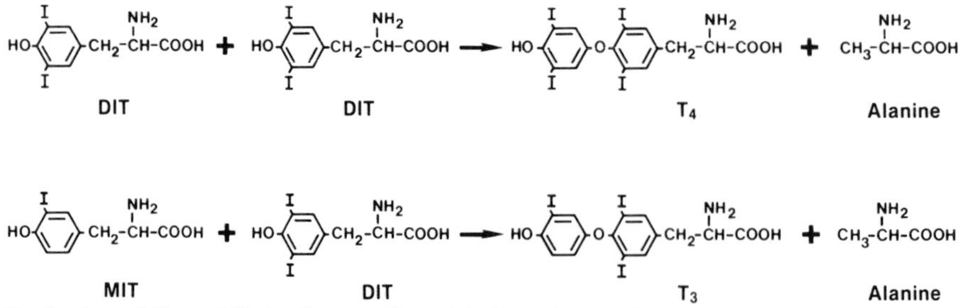

Figure 33–2. Production of T_4 and T_3 by the coupling of iodinated tyrosyl residues with thyroglobulin molecule. (From Hedge GA, Colby HD, Goodman RL: Clinical Endocrine Physiology. Philadelphia, WB Saunders, 1987, p 106.)

Thyroid Hormones Are Stored Outside the Cell, Attached to Thyroglobulin in the Form of Colloid

Once the thyroid hormones are formed, they remain in the extracellular acinar lumen until the cell is called upon to release them. This is an unusual storage arrangement, with hormones stored extracellularly within an endocrine gland. This storage method allows the thyroid gland to have a large reserve of the hormone. It is not clear why this should be important, except thyroid hormone is the most important hormone of metabolism, and it allows mammals to withstand periods of iodine deprivation without an immediate effect on the production of thyroid hormones.

The Release of Thyroid Hormones Involves Transport of Thyroglobulin with Attached Thyroid Hormones into the Cell, Cleavage of the Thyroid Hormones from Thyroxine-binding Globulin (TBG), and Their Release into the Interstitial Tissues

In order for thyroid hormones to be released from the thyroid gland, thyroglobulin with its attached MIT, DIT, T_3, and T_4 molecules must be translocated into the follicle cell, and the hormones have to be cleaved from thyroglobulin (Fig. 33–3). Key enzymes in this transfer are found in the lysosomes. The TBG molecules fuse with lysosomes upon entering the cell, and lysosomal enzymes cleave both the iodinated tyrosines and the iodinated thyronines from the thyroglobulin molecule. The thyronines are released through the basal cell membrane (they freely pass through the cell membrane); MIT and DIT are deiodinated by an enzyme called iodotyrosine dehalogenase; and both the iodide and the remaining tyrosine molecules are recycled to form new hormone in association with thyroglobulin.

The majority of T_3 formation occurs outside of the thyroid gland by the deiodination of T_4. Tissues that have the highest concentration of deiodinating enzymes are the liver and kidneys, although tissues such as muscle are important for the formation of T_3 on the basis of size. The enzyme that is involved in the removal of iodide from the outer phenolic ring of T_4 in the formation of T_3 is called *5'-monodeiodinase* (Fig. 33–4). Another type of T_3 is formed also in which an iodide molecule is removed from the inner phenolic ring of T_4, a compound called *reverse* T_3. rT_3 has little of the biological effects of thyroid hormones. rT_3

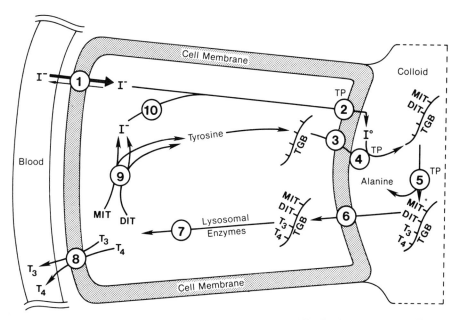

Figure 33–3. Follicular cell showing steps in synthesis and release of T_3 and T_4. *TP*, thyroperoxidase. The numbers identify the major steps: (1) trapping of iodide; (2) oxidation of iodide; (3) exocytosis of thyroglobulin; (4) iodination of thyroglobulin: (5) coupling of iodotyrosines; (6) endocytosis of thyroglobulin; (7) hydrolysis of thyroglobulin; (8) release of T_3 and T_4; (9) deiodination of MIT and DIT; (10) recycling of iodide. (From Hedge GA, Colby HD, Goodman RL: Clinical Endocrine Physiology. Philadelphia, WB Saunders, 1987, p 105.)

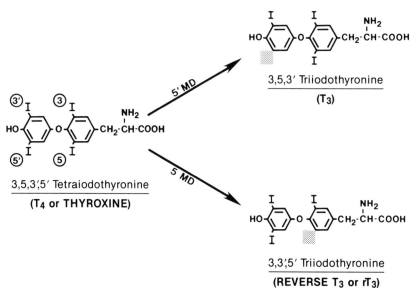

Figure 33–4. Structure and nomenclature of thyroxine, and its conversion to the two triiodothyronines by 5'- and 5-monodeiodinase (*MD*). Shaded squares indicate the sites of deiodination. (From Hedge GA, Colby HD, Goodman RL: Clinical Endocrine Physiology. Philadelphia, WB Saunders, 1987, p 103.)

is formed only by the action of extrathyroidal deiodinating enzymes and not by activity of the thyroid gland.

Thyroid Hormones Are Transported in the Plasma Attached to Plasma Proteins: Thyroxine-Binding Globulin, Albumin, and Thyroxine-Binding Pre-Albumin; Less Than 1% of the Thyroid Hormones Are Free in Plasma

As indicated in Chapter 32, lipid-soluble hormones are transported in the blood vascular system through association with specific binding plasma proteins. There is considerable species variation in the proteins that bind the thyroid hormones. The most important carrier protein is *thyroxine-binding globulin,* which has high affinity for T_4, although low capacity because of its low concentration. TBG also is an important carrier protein for T_3 in spite of the name of the globulin, i.e., thryoxine-binding. TBG has been reported in all domestic animals except the cat. *Albumin* is also involved in the transport of thyroid hormones, with conditions reversed as compared to TBG, i.e., the protein has low affinity, but high capacity because of its high concentration in plasma. In the absence of TBG, albumin is the most important carrier of thyroid hormones.

All species have a third plasma protein, *thyroxine-binding pre-albumin* (TBPA), that is specific for T_4, with a specificity and capacity that is intermediate between TBG and albumin. The term pre-albumin refers to the migration of the protein during electrophoresis, not to synthesis of the molecule.

As for all lipid-soluble hormones that are transported in plasma, most of the T_3 and T_4 is bound; little is free to interact with receptors on the cells of the target tissues. The amount of thyroid hormone that is free in plasma is remarkably low, e.g., in humans, 0.03% for T_4 and 0.3% for T_3. In dogs, the amount of free hormone is somewhat greater, being a little less than 1.0% for T_4 and slightly greater than 1.0% for T_3. This is because of less affinity between plasma-binding proteins and thyroid hormones in canine plasma as compared to humans. The equilibrium between free and bound hormone is easily shifted because of physiological or pharmacological situations, such as increased estrogen concentrations that occur during pregnancy. Estrogens cause increased synthesis of TBG by the liver with a consequent shift toward the bound form. Adjustments to maintain a normal amount of free hormone occur rapidly with a decline in the rate of metabolism, or stimulation of thyroid hormone production through the release of thyroid-stimulating hormone (TSH).

The Main Routes of Metabolism of Thyroid Hormones Are Through Deiodination or the Formation of Glucuronides and Sulfates

The main form of metabolism of thyroid hormones involves the removal of iodide molecules. Except for the formation of T_3 from T_4, none of the deiodinated thyronine derivatives have any significant metabolic activity. The two enzymes involved in T_3 and rT_3 synthesis, *5'-deiodinase* and *5-deiodinase,* are involved also in the catabolism of thyroid hormones. Only these two enzymes are needed for catabolism, because they do not differentiate between the three and five positions of the phenolic rings of the thyronines. Skeletal muscle, liver, and kidneys are important tissues involved in the catabolism of thyroid hormones through deiodination. The formation of thyroid hormone conjugates represents another form of inactivation, with sulfates and glucuronides formed mainly in the liver and kidneys. Conjugation is less important than deiodination as a means of metabolism of thyroid hormones. Another form of metabolism involves modification of the alanine moiety of the thyronines by either transamination or decarboxylation. The deiodinated and conjugated forms of the thyronines are eliminated primarily in the urine, with unmetabolized thyronines excreted into feces through bile secretion. Degradation of the conjugate forms in the feces results in the production of iodide molecules,

which are reabsorbed as part of a cycle called the *enterohepatic cycle.* Humans are more efficient than dogs in recovery of iodide both intrathyroidally and enterohepatically.

One of the striking aspects of thyroid hormones is their long half-life; T_3 has a half-life of 1 day and T_4 of 6–7 days, whereas most other hormones have half-lives of seconds or minutes. One reason for these long half-lives is the large percentage of the circulating thyronines that are bound to the plasma proteins, which protects them from degradation. The difference in half-lives between T_3 and T_4 springs from the tighter T_4 protein binding as compared to T_3 and the resultant reduction in free circulating hormone.

Thyroid Hormones Are the Primary Factors for the Control of Metabolism

The mechanism of action of thyroid hormones at the cell level is based on the fact that they can penetrate the cell membrane even though they are amino acids; in essence, they are lipophilic. While it is thought that thyroid hormones interact directly with the nucleus to initiate the transcription of mRNA (Fig. 33–5), the presence of T_3 receptors has been reported on mitochondria.

It is likely that thyroid hormones are the primary determinants of general metabolism. Having indicated this, it becomes more difficult to define the precise physiological effects

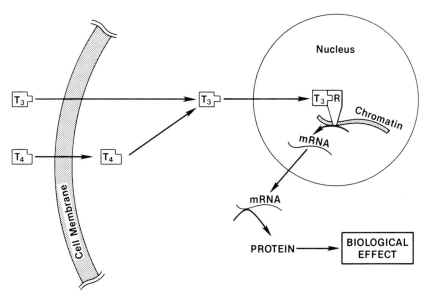

Figure 33–5. Proposed subcellular mechanism of thyroid hormone action. (From Hedge GA, Colby HD, Goodman RL: Clinical Endocrine Physiology. Philadelphia, WB Saunders, 1987, p 113.)

of thyroid hormones. This is because many of the effects of thyroid hormones have been demonstrated through the creation of hypothyroid, or hyperthyroid, states with biphasic responses to the administration of thyroid hormone occurring as a result of the dosage. Nevertheless, it has long been recognized that thyroid hormones increase the oxygen consumption of tissues and, as a result, heat production. This effect is known as the *calorigenic* effect. One site of action of the calorigenic effect of thyroid hormones is the mitochondrion.

Thyroid hormones affect carbohydrate metabolism in several ways. They increase intestinal glucose absorption and facilitate the movement of glucose into both fat and muscle. Further, *thyroid hormones facilitate insulin-mediated glucose uptake* by cells. Glycogen formation is facilitated by small amounts of thyroid hormones with glycogenolysis occurring following larger dosages.

Thyroid hormones are required, together with growth hormone (GH), for *normal growth*. This is accomplished, in part, by the enhancement of amino acid uptake by tissues and enzyme systems that are involved in protein synthesis.

Whereas thyroid hormones affect all aspects of lipid metabolism, the emphasis is placed on *lipolysis*. One particular effect of thyroid hormones is the tendency to reduce plasma cholesterol. This appears to involve both increased cell uptake of low-density lipoproteins (LDL) with associated cholesterol molecules and a tendency for increased degradation of both cholesterol and LDL. These effects on lipid metabolism are usually seen in pathophysiological situations involving hypersecretion of thyroid hormone. In this same context, the effects of thyroid hormones on metabolic processes, including carbohydrate, proteins, and lipids, are often described as catabolic.

Thyroid hormones have effects that are noteworthy concerning the *nervous and cardiovascular* systems. The effects of the *sympathetic nervous system* are enhanced by the presence of thyroid hormones. This is thought to occur through thyroid stimulation of β-*adrenergic receptors* in tissues that are targets for the *catecholamines,* epinephrine and norepinephrine. Concerning the central nervous system (CNS), thyroid hormones are important for normal development of tissues in the fetus and neo-

nate, and retardation of mental activity occurs (in humans) in individuals who have developed without adequate thyroid hormone exposure. Again in humans, individuals with hypothyroid activity are mentally dull and lethargic, which suggests that normal CNS function in the adult is dependent upon the presence of adequate amounts of thyroid hormone.

Concerning the cardiovascular system, thyroid hormones *increase heart rate and force of contraction,* likely through their interaction with the catecholamines. This interaction is thought to be brought about by an increase in tissue responsiveness through the induction of catecholaminergic β-receptors by thryoid hormones. Blood pressure is elevated because of increased systolic pressure, with no change in diastolic pressure, the end result being an increase in cardiac output. Again, it should be emphasized that these responses are most easily observed in situations of increased thyroid activity. Perhaps the conclusion regarding the effect of thyroid hormones on cardiovascular activity is to state that they are important for maintaining normal contractile activity of cardiac muscle, including the transmission of nerve impulses.

The classic experiments involving the *metamorphosis* of amphibian larvae and the role of thyroid should be mentioned. Thyroxine administration causes the differentiation of tadpoles into frogs, whereas thyroidectomy results in the development into large tadpoles. Thyroid-induced metamorphosis is limited to amphibians, yet thyroid hormones are important for many (subtle) aspects of differentiation in other classes of animals.

It is emphasized that thyroid hormone activity is usually defined in terms of tissue, or organ, responses to inadequate, or excessive, amounts of hormone. A more balanced view is that thyroid hormones are important for the normal metabolic activity of all tissues.

Thyrotropin, or thyroid-stimulating hormone (TSH), is the most important regulator of thyroid activity. It acts through the initiation of adenosine $3':5'$-cyclic phosphate (cAMP) formation and the phosphorylation of protein kinases. TSH secretion is regulated by thyroid hormones by way of negative feedback inhibition of the synthesis of thyrotropin-releasing hormone (TRH) at the level of the hypothalamus and by inhibition of the activity of TSH at the level of the pituitary (Fig. 33–6).

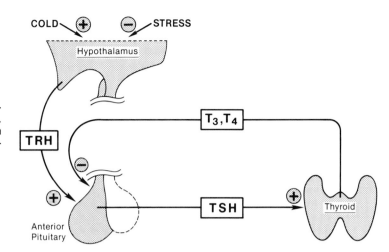

Figure 33–6. Hypothalamo-pituitary-thyroid axis. +, stimulation; −, inhibition. (From Hedge GA, Colby HD, Goodman RL: Clinical Endocrine Physiology. Philadelphia, WB Saunders, 1987, p 116.)

The Ingestion of Compounds That Inhibit the Uptake or the Organic Binding of Iodine Block the Ability of the Thyroid to Secrete Thyroid Hormones and Cause Goiter

An inability to secrete adequate amounts of thyroid hormone often leads to the enlargement of the thyroid gland, a condition called *goiter*. In many places in the world, this condition is, or has been, due to a deficiency in iodine in the diet. This has largely been corrected through the use of iodized salt. Certain plants, e.g., cruciferous plants such as cabbage, kale, rutabaga, turnip, and rapeseed, contain a potent antithyroid compound called *progoitrin*, which is converted into *goitrin* within the digestive tract. Goitrin interferes with the organic binding of iodine. Many of the goitrogenic feeds also contain *thiocyanates*, which interfere with the trapping of iodine by the thyroid gland. The feeding of excess iodine can sometimes overcome the effects of thiocyanate, but has less influence on overcoming the effects of goitrin. From these studies has come the development of compounds for the treatment of hyperthyroidism; the most potent ones are the *thiocarbamides*, thiourea and thiouracil. Other antithyroid drugs include sulfonamides, p-aminosalicylic acid, amphenone, phenylbutazone, and chlorpromazine.

Of the domestic species, dysfunction in terms of *hypothyroidism* is most common in the dog. The cause is not known, just that it is not dietary in origin; the presence of plasma antibodies to thyroglobulin have raised the possibility of the presence of an autoimmune disease. *Hyperthyroidism*, relatively common in older cats, is usually associated with thyroid tumors.

Laboratory test procedures in animals useful as diagnostic aids include TSH stimulation tests and the measurement of plasma T_3, or T_4, concentrations (Table 33–1). Stimulation tests are usually done when hypothyroidism is suspected; if the condition is *primary*, i.e., of thryoid origin, there usually is little response to the TSH. The determination of T_3 and T_4 concentrations in plasma often gives

Table 33–1
SERUM T_4 AND T_3 VALUES BY PLA

	T_4 μg/dL	T_3 ng/dL
Equine	1.63 ± 0.51 (0.95 − 2.38)	77.1 ± 45.75 (31 − 153)
Bovine	6.22 ± 2.03 (3.60 − 8.9)	92.50 ± 53.61 (41 − 170)
Capine	3.45 ± 0.47 (3.0 − 4.23)	145.9 ± 29.32 (88 − 190)
Ovine	4.41 ± 1.13 (2.95 − 6.15)	99.6 ± 27.34 (63 − 150)
Porcine	3.32 ± 0.80 (1.70 − 4.68)	89.8 ± 36.7 (43 − 140)
Canine	1.51 ± 0.38 (0.70 − 2.18)	96.2 ± 21.39 (63 − 130)
Feline	2.02 ± 0.61 (1.18 − 2.95)	64.7 ± 20.62 (39 − 112)

From Reap M, Cass, C and Hightower, D: Thyroxine and triiodo thyronine levels in ten species of animals. Southwestern Vet 31:31, 1978.

N = 10 in all species.

From McDonald LE, Pineda MH (eds): Veterinary Endocrinology and Reproduction, 4th ed. Philadelphia, Lea & Febiger, 1989, p 86.

useful information concerning hyperthyroid activity, a situation wherein randomly-obtained values are usually above the normal range. It should be emphasized, though, that there is considerable variability in T_4 and T_3 concentrations as a function of age, breed, environmental temperature, nutritional status, and health. Thus, values need to be interpreted with some caution. The calculation of a *free thyroxine index*, as done in humans, unfortunately has not been proven to be of value in animals. Because of variability of results concerning thyroid hormone concentrations reported from different laboratories, one should carefully validate assay systems when investigating diseases of thyroid activity.

THE ADRENAL GLANDS

The Adrenal Glands Are Composed of Two Organs: the Outer Gland Is Called the Cortex and Secretes Corticoids, and the Inner Gland Is Called the Medulla and Secretes Catecholamines

The adrenal glands are endocrine organs that consist of two bilaterally symmetrical organs that are located just anterior to the kidneys. Each gland is divided into two separate entities, a medulla and a cortex (Fig. 33–7), each of which produces different types of hormones. As might be surmised, the tissues have different embryonic origins; the medulla comes from the neuroectoderm and produces amines such as norepinephrine and epinephrine. The cortex comes from the mesodermal coelomic epithelium and produces steroid hormones such as cortisol, corticosterone, and aldosterone. The utility of placing two such disparate tissues together is not apparent. The one common factor is that both sets of hormones are important for adaptation to adverse environmental conditions.

Interest in the function of the adrenal cortex was heightened in the 1930s because of the research of Hans Selye. He published a series of papers on the effects of adrenalectomy and the ability of the surgically-treated animal to defend itself against injury. Selye's hypothesis was termed the *general adaptation syndrome*, which he divided into three parts: the *alarm reaction, the stage of resistance,* and the *stage of exhaustion.* The critical aspect of this theory was that, in addition to specific responses to injury, animals responded in nonspecific ways to combat injury, and the adrenal cortex was the most important organ in leading the nonspecific response. One example of the beneficial effects of glucocorticoids in a situation of injury is the mobilization of glucose. The adaptation of animals to stressful environments is often accompanied by enlargement of the adrenal cortex, such as for domestic chickens raised in crowded conditions and wild animals living in relatively high density.

THE ADRENAL CORTEX

The Adrenal Cortex Has Three Zones: the Zona Glomerulosa, Which Secretes Mineralocorticoids, and the Zona Fasciculata and the Zona Reticularis, Which Secrete Glucocorticoids

The adrenal cortex is organized into three zones in mammals (see Fig. 33–7). The outer zone, the *zona glomerulosa,* is relatively narrow and is organized in a whorl-type cell arrangement. The middle zone, the *zona fasciculata,* is relatively wide and is organized with cells in columns. In the cow and sheep, the zona fasciculata is further divided into inner and outer layers. The inner zone of the adrenal cortex, the *zona reticularis,* which is adjacent to the adrenal medulla, is intermediate in size with cells having a more random organization.

All of the cells of the adrenal cortex have intracellular features characteristic of steroid hormone synthesis, i.e., an abundance of lipid droplets (containing cholesterol esters), mitochrondria, and smooth endoplasmic reticulum. Human adrenals have an additional zone that is present during fetal life and for the first year of life, i.e., the *fetal zone*. The fetal zone participates with the placenta in the production of estrogen during gestation. Immature mice and rabbits have an inner X-zone that becomes the zona reticularis at puberty.

The adrenal cortex produces two major types of steroid hormones, namely, the *mineralocorticoids* and the *glucocorticoids;* these are hormones that have distinctly different functions. The mineralocorticoids, produced by the zona glomerulosa, play an important role in *electrolyte* balance and, as a result, are important in the regulation of blood pressure. The major mineralocorticoid is *aldosterone.* The glucocorticoids, produced by the zona fasciculata (most important) and reticularis, are important in the regulation of all aspects of *metabolism,*

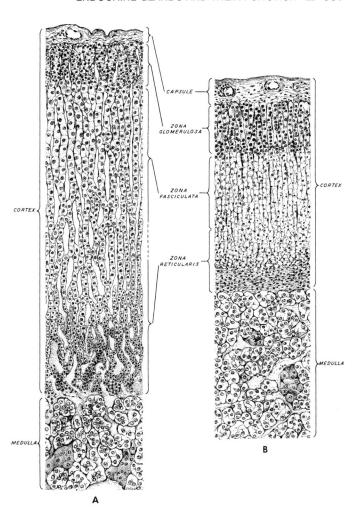

Figure 33–7. Comparable sections through the adrenal glands of normal (A) and hypophysectomized (B) rats. Since the functional capacity of the adrenal cortex is conditioned by the release of ACTH, hypophysectomy results in tremendous shrinkage of the cortex. The medulla is not influenced by hypophysectomy. Both sections are drawn to scale. (From Turner CD, Bagnara JT: General Endocrinology, 6th ed. Philadelphia, WB Saunders, 1976, 293.)

either directly or through an interaction with other hormones. The major glucocorticoid is *cortisol*.

Adrenal Corticoids Are Synthesized from Cholesterol with the Critical Difference Being a Hydroxyl Group on C-17 of Glucocorticoids

The synthesis of adrenal steroids involves the use of the classic pathways for steroid biosynthesis. As indicated previously, cholesterol is the major starting material for the synthesis of steroid hormones. Cholesterol is readily available to the cell for steroid synthesis, because it is stored within steroid-synthesizing cells in large quantities within lipid droplets in ester form. One of the initial steps in steroid formation is the hydrolysis of the ester. The first step in steroid synthesis involves the presence of a side-cleavage enzyme that cleaves the carbon side chain from the steroid molecule, leaving a C-21 steroid known

as *pregnenolone*. This step occurs within the mitochondrion (Fig. 33–8). The synthesis of all steroid hormones, regardless of their form, utilizes pregnenolone in the synthetic pathway.

The critical aspect of adrenal corticoid synthesis, which differentiates adrenal steroids from the progesterone family of steroids, is a hydroxylation step at C-21 (directed by a C-21 hydroxylase). The difference between the mineralocorticoids (aldosterone) and the glucocorticoids (cortisol) is a hydroxyl group on C-17, which is part of the glucocorticoid molecule. As expected, cells of the zona fasciculata and reticularis have the hydroxylating enzyme for C-17 (17α-hydroxylase), whereas cells of the zona glomerulosa do not have this enzyme. Both aldosterone and cortisol have hydroxyl groups on C-11. Because of the marked difference in biological activity of the mineralocorticoids and glucocorticoids, it is useful to view the zona glomerulosa as an endocrine organ

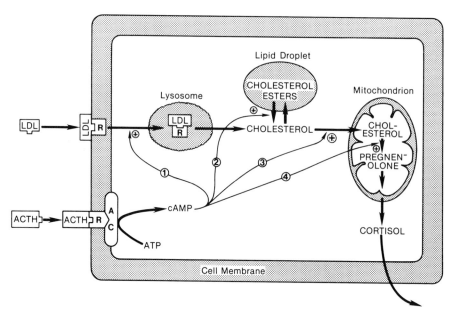

Figure 33–8. Mechanism of action of ACTH on adrenocortical steroidogenesis. The numbers indicate the processes stimulated by ACTH as follows: (1) stimulates the uptake of low-density lipoproteins which are further processed to free cholesterol; (2) stimulates the hydrolysis of stored cholesterol esters to generate free cholesterol; (3) stimulates the transport of cholesterol into mitochondria, where cleavage of the cholesterol side-chain occurs; (4) promotes the binding of cholesterol to the enzyme. (From Hedge GA, Colby HD, Goodman RL: Clinical Endocrine Physiology. Philadelphia, WB Saunders, 1987, p 146.)

that is distinct from the zona fasciculata and zona reticularis.

Two intermediate compounds in the synthesis of aldosterone have significant adrenocortical activity. *11-deoxycorticosterone* (DOC) has significant mineralocorticoid activities, although it is secreted in relatively small amounts. *Corticosterone*, the immediate precursor to aldosterone, is a relatively important glucocorticoid in animals, although its potency is less than for cortisol.

Biosynthetic pathways are present in adrenal cortical cells that allow some synthesis of *androgens* and *estrogens*. Although the amount of sex steroids produced by the adrenal cortex under normal conditions is low, significant amounts can be synthesized under pathological conditions.

Adrenocortical Hormones Are Carried in Plasma in Association with Specific-Binding Globulins (Corticosteroid-Binding Globulin) and Less Specific-Binding Albumins—a Relatively Large Amount (10%) of the Hormone Exists in the Free State

Steroid hormones, as indicated previously, are lipids and depend on binding to plasma proteins for transport in the blood. A specific globulin has been identified that has a high affinity for cortisol, namely, *corticosteroid-binding globulin* (CBG), also known as *transcortin* in humans. Of the cortisol carried in plasma, 75% is bound to CBG and 15% to albumin, leaving 10% in the unbound, or free, state. This large amount of free hormone is in contrast to the thryoid hormones in which less than 0.1% of T_4 is free. The transport of aldosterone is mainly associated with albumin (50%) with only 10% being associated with CBG, leaving a large amount (40%) in the free state.

Changes in physiological or pathophysiological states can influence the amount of binding proteins present in plasma. Estrogen produced in increasing amounts by the fetoplacental unit during pregnancy results in an increase in hepatic synthesis of CBG, whereas liver dysfunction can result in lower concentrations of CBG. The large pool of hormone present in the bound state during pregnancy gives animals a good reserve from which to make appropriate adjustments in the amount of free hormone available for influencing biological activity. Because the total amount of glucocorticoid is determined in the assay of plasma concentrations, the veterinary clinician needs to be aware that total concentrations do not reflect secretion rate only, but also can be influenced by the amount of glucocorticoid-binding plasma proteins.

The Metabolism of Adrenocortical Hormones Involves the Reduction of Double Bonds and Ketone Configurations As Well As the Conjugation of the Steroids to Glucuronides and Sulfates

Regarding the clearance of adrenocortical hormones, the half-life of cortisol is about 60 minutes and aldosterone about 20 minutes. This is attributable to the difference observed for protein binding for these hormones within the plasma. In general, metabolism of minerlo- and glucocorticoid hormones involves the reduction of double bonds and ketone configurations, which reduces the biological activity of the molecules. The liver, an important organ for modification of these hormones, is an important site for the conjugation of these steroids with sulfates and glucuronides, which reduces their biological potency and renders them water-soluble for passage in the urine.

One of the Most Important Functions of Glucocorticoids Is Control of Metabolism and, in Particular, the Stimulation of Hepatic Gluconeogenesis

The mechanism of action of adrenal hormones involves the basic approach for all lipophilic hormones, i.e., they are able to penetrate the cell membrane and interact in the cytoplasm with specific *cytosolic receptors.* This complex is transferred to the nucleus with a resultant transcription of certain genes and the synthesis of specific proteins that effect the biological action of the adrenal hormones.

As emphasized previously, *adrenocortical hormones* are classified as either glucocorticoid or mineralocorticoid in their activity. Before discussing the biological actions of each class, it is important to realize that there is *overlap of activity* (Table 33–2). For example, whereas cortisol is the dominant glucocorticoid hormone, it has mineralocorticoid effects also, although at a reduced potency.

The glucocorticoid hormones are important mediators of intermediary metabolism. One of the important specific effects of glucocorticoids is the stimulation of *hepatic gluconeogenesis,* which involves the conversion of amino acids

Table 33–2
RELATIVE GLUCOCORTICOID AND MINERALOCORTICOID POTENCIES OF VARIOUS STEROIDS

Steroid	Glucocorticoid Potency	Mineralocorticoid Potency
	(Relative to Cortisol)	
Cortisol	1	1
Aldosterone	0.1	400
Corticosterone	0.2	2
11-Deoxycorticosterone	<0.1	20
Dexamethasone	30	2
Fludrocortisone	10	400
Prednisone	4	0.7
Triamcinolone	5	<0.1

From Hedge GA, Colby HD, Goodman RL: Clinical Endocrine Physiology. Philadelphia. WB Saunders, 1987, p 136.

to carbohydrates. The net result is an increase in hepatic glycogen and a tendency to increase blood glucose. These effects on glycogen metabolism are observed mainly in animals that are on low planes of nutrition, or that have an insulin deficiency. The effect of glucocorticoids on carbohydrate metabolism is *permissive,* i.e., their presence is required for the gluconeogenic and glycogenolytic actions of glucagon and epinephrine, respectively.

Whereas glucocorticoids and insulin have similar effects on liver glycogen metabolism, their effects on the peripheral utilization of glucose are different. Glucocorticoids inhibit glucose uptake and metabolism in the peripheral tissues, particularly in muscle and adipose cells. This effect has been termed the *anti-insulin effect.* The chronic administration of glucocorticoids can lead to the development of a syndrome called *steroid diabetes* because of the hyperglycemic effect produced at the level of the liver, with decreased utilization of glucose occurring in the peripheral tissues because of insulin antagonism.

Whereas the actions of glucocorticoids on fat metabolism tend to be complex, the direct effect on adipose tissue is to increase the rate of *lipolysis.*

Protein synthesis is inhibited by glucocorticoids; in fact, *protein catabolism* is enhanced, with an accompanying release of amino acids. This process supports hepatic gluconeogenesis. Two tissues, cardiac and brain, are spared as far as the effect of glucocorticoids on protein catabolism. Chronic administration of glucocorticoids results in muscle wasting and the weakening of bone. The mobilization and incorporation of amino acids into glycogen results in an increase in urinary excretion of nitrogen and a *negative nitrogen balance.*

Glucocorticoids play a role in water *diuresis,* i.e., the enhancement of water excretion. Whereas glucocorticoids inhibit vasopressin activity at the level of the distal tubule, the most important effect is to increase the glomerular filtration rate. A summary of the effects of glucocorticoids is shown in Table 33–3.

Adrenocorticotropic Hormone Is the Main Regulator of Glucocorticoid Synthesis by the Adrenal Cortex

The control of the secretion of the *glucocorticoids* by the zona fasciculata and zona reticularis is by the tropic hormone adrenocorticotropic hormone (ACTH) (Fig. 33–9). A *negative feedback* system exists, whereby glucocorticoids inhibit the release of hypothalamic corticotropin-releasing hormone (CRH) which, in turn, results in decreased ACTH secretion by the pituitary. There is some evidence that glucocorticoids also have a negative feedback effect at the level of the pituitary. The potency of a glucocorticoid regarding negative feedback inhibition of ACTH is directly related to its glucocorticoid potency, e.g., cortisol has more potent negative feedback effects than corticosterone, the former having more potent glucocorticoid effects than the latter.

The negative feedback control system that exists for the secretion of glucocorticoids does not result in the maintenance of uniform hormone concentrations in blood throughout the day. Sleep and activity patterns are superimposed on the negative feedback system so that a predictable circadian rhythm occurs in which concentrations of glucocorticoids are lowest late at night and highest in the early morning hours (Fig. 33–10).

Another factor that can modify the negative feedback control of glucocorticoids is *stress.* Stress can result from physical or psychological inputs that are hurtful to the individual.

Table 33–3
GLUCOCORTICOID EFFECTS AND TARGET TISSUES

Effect	Site of Action
Stimulates gluconeogenesis	Liver
Increases hepatic glycogen	Liver
Increases blood glucose	Liver
Facilitates lipolysis	Adipose tissue
Catabolic (negative nitrogen balance)	Muscle, liver
Inhibits ACTH secretion	Hypothalamus, anterior pituitary
Facilitates water excretion	Kidney
Blocks inflammatory response	Multiple sites
Suppresses immune system	Macrophages, lymphocytes
Stimulates gastric acid secretion	Stomach

From Hedge GA, Colby HD, Goodman RL: Clinical Endocrine Physiology. Philadelphia, WB Saunders, 1987, p 137.

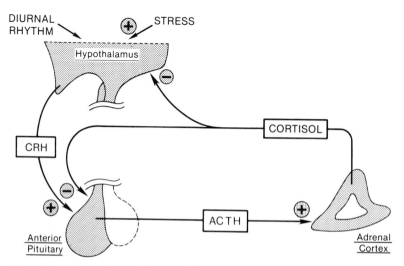

Figure 33–9. Regulation of cortisol secretion by the hypothalamo-pituitary axis. +, stimulation; −, inhibition. (From Hedge GA, Colby HD, Goodman RL: Clinical Endocrine Physiology. Philadelphia, WB Saunders, 1987, p 143.)

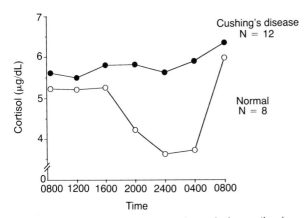

Figure 33–10. Circadian changes in cortisol secretion in normal horses (open circles) compared with no circadian change in horses with equine Cushing's disease. (From Dybdal N: Studies on equine Cushing's disease. PhD thesis. University of California, Davis, CA, 1990.)

The effects of stress are mediated through the CNS, similar to the factors that influence circadian rhythms of glucocorticoid secretion. The glucocorticoid response to stress is immediate, with concentrations of cortisol increasing rapidly to reach values that are several-fold greater than normal within minutes. The glucocorticoid response is proportional to the severity of the stress, i.e., lower levels of stress result in less cortisol production as compared to higher levels of stress.

One of the Most Important Clinical Uses of Glucocorticoids Is the Suppression of the Inflammatory Response

Glucocorticoids have particularly valuable *clinical effects,* particularly concerning the *inhibition of the inflammatory response,* including the prevention of capillary dilatation, extravasation of fluid into tissue spaces, leukocyte migration, fibrin deposition, and connective tissue synthesis. Whereas the process of inflammation is important for the walling off and destruction of systemic noxious agents, the end response is often the replacement of functional tissue with fibrous connective tissue, with a resultant loss of function. For example, inflammatory processes in the mammary gland often result in the isolation of the injurious agent by the laying down of connective tissue as a part of the defense mechanism, yet the gland may lose much of its functional capacity as a result. Administration of glucocorticoids, in conjunction with antibiotic therapy, can help reduce the loss of functional

tissue by inhibiting the development of connective tissue. Some of the synthetic glucocorticoids used in clinical practice are shown in Figure 33–11.

One of the ways that glucocorticoids inhibit the inflammatory response is through the inhibition of the formation of substances that promote inflammation. Glucocorticoids inhibit the synthesis of inflammatory-mediating compounds, such as prostaglandins, thromboxanes, and leukotrienes, that arise as a result of arachidonic acid metabolism. This is done through the stabilization of lysosomal membranes, preventing the activation of phospholipase A_2, an enzyme important for initiating the metabolism of arachidonic acid. Glucocorticoids are used also to inhibit allergic reactions. This action occurs through the inhibition of the release of certain biogenic amines from the granules of mast cells, e.g., histamine.

The *mineralocorticoids,* produced in the outer

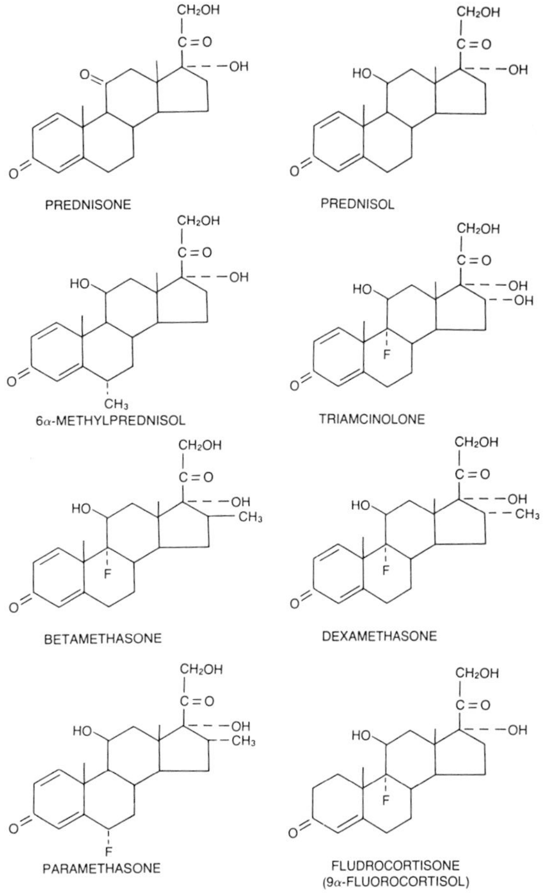

Figure 33–11. Some clinically useful glucocorticoid analogs. (From Martin CR: Endocrine Physiology. London, Oxford University Press, 1985, p 246.)

zone (zona glomerulosa) of the adrenal cortex, have surprisingly different functions compared to glucocorticoids; the functions are surprising because both types of hormones are produced by tissues that are part of the same gland. As indicated previously, *electrolyte balance* and *blood pressure homeostasis* represent the principal physiological effects of mineralocorticoids (Table 33–4). These actions are carried out at the level of the distal tubules in the kidney. The effect of the mineralocorticoids is to promote *sodium retention,* and *potassium and hydrogen secretion.* The cellular response to mineralocorticoids is to synthesize a protein that increases the permeability of the luminal cell surface to sodium influx from the renal filtrate and increases Na⁺, K⁺ ATPase activity in the contraluminal cell surface which allows movement of sodium out of the cell into the interstitial tissue (Fig. 33–12).

The control of secretion of potassium by mineralocorticoids is passive in the sense that potassium is retained in the renal filtrate to maintain the osmolality of urine. There is, however, evidence that mineralocorticoids have an effect on sodium secretion that is independent of sodium retention. The secretion of potassium continues to be influenced by mineralocorticoids following mineralocorticoid administration, whereas sodium retention decreases within a few days.

Table 33–4
MINERALOCORTICOID EFFECTS AND TARGET TISSUES

Effect	Site of Action
Stimulates NA⁺ reabsorption	Kidney, salivary glands, sweat glands
Stimulates K⁺ excretion	Kidney, salivary glands, sweat glands
Stimulates H⁺ excretion	Kidney

From Hedge GA, Colby HD, Goodman RL: Clinical Endocrine Physiology. Philadelphia, WB Saunders, 1987, p 139.

In situations of *excess mineralocorticoid* production, the effect of increased sodium retention is to increase the extracellular fluid volume and to cause *hypertension;* conversely, low blood pressure (hypotension) occurs as a result of inadequate secretion of mineralocorticoids. Hypersecretion of mineralocorticoids can also lead to excess hydrogen ion loss and *metabolic alkalosis,* whereas *hyposecretion* can result in increased retention of hydrogen ion and *metabolic acidosis.*

The regulation of mineralocorticoid secretion, in contrast to the glucocorticoids, is not controlled by tropic hormones from the pituitary (Fig. 33–13). In the case of mineralocorticoids, the main controlling factors are produced in the target organ, the kidney. Cells in the *juxtaglomerular apparatus* of the kidney pro-

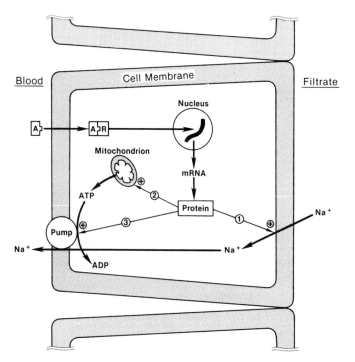

Figure 33–12. Mechanism(s) of action of aldosterone on sodium transport in the renal tubular cell. The numbered arrows indicate the three putative sites of action of aldosterone; (1) increases the permeability of the luminal membrane to sodium; (2) increases mitochondrial ATP production; and (3) increases Na⁺, K⁺ ATPase activity in the contraluminal membrane. *A,* aldosterone; *R,* receptor; +, stimulation. (From Hedge GA, Colby HD, Goodman RL: Clinical Endocrine Physiology. Philadelphia, WB Saunders, 1987, p 140.)

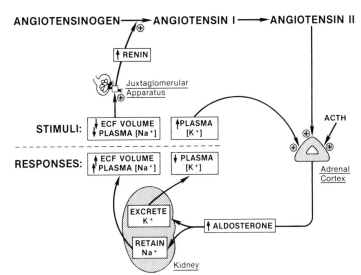

Figure 33–13. Regulation of aldosterone secretion by the zona glomerulosa of the adrenal cortex. +, stimulation; *ECF,* extracellular fluid. (From Hedge GA, Colby HD, Goodman RL: Clinical Endocrine Physiology. Philadelphia, WB Saunders, 1987, p 147.)

duce an enzyme, *renin,* in response to decreases in blood pressure. This enzyme acts on *angiotensinogen,* an α_2 globulin produced by the liver and present in the circulation, which results in the production of *angiotensin I,* a decapeptide. Angiotensin I is further hydrolyzed to *angiotensin II,* an octapeptide, by angiotensin-converting enzyme. Angiotensin II stimulates the zona glomerulosa to produce mineralocorticoids. Angiotensin II also increases peripheral resistance of the blood vascular system by causing vasoconstriction of smooth muscle of the blood vessels. Angiotensin II, if present on a long-term basis, also increases the size of the zona glomerulosa.

There is evidence that cells of the *macula densa,* groups of specialized cells that are located at the origin of the distal tubule of the kidney, exert control on the renin-angiotensin system (Fig. 33–14). This is done through the sensing of changes in sodium concentrations in tissue fluids. Sodium increase results in decreased renin release, and sodium decrease results in increased renin release. In either case, the change produced tends to restore mineralocorticoid concentrations to normal. In addition to the effect of sodium, the macula densa may control changes in the renin-angiotensin system through the sensing of changes in chloride ion concentrations in tissue fluids.

Another major regulatory factor in the control of mineralocorticoid secretion is *blood potassium concentration.* An increase in potassium concentration stimulates the zona glomerulosa to secrete mineralocorticoids, whereas a decline in potassium has the opposite effect. This

stimulation is independent of the renin-angiotensin system.

It has been thought that ACTH has little to do with control of the zona glomerulosa. This concept has come from experimental studies, where hypophysectomy has little effect on the zona glomerulosa. More recently it has been shown that cells of the zona glomerulosa have receptors for ACTH, and it may be that ACTH plays some role, albeit minor, in the control of mineralocorticoid secretion.

In contrast to the sodium-conserving effect of mineralocorticoids, a 28 amino acid peptide called atrial-natriuretic peptide (ANP) has been identified. It reduces sodium retention

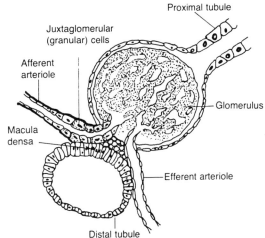

Figure 33–14. Diagrammatic representation of juxtaglomerular apparatus. (From Martin CR: Endocrine Physiology. London, Oxford University Press, 1985, p 338.)

by the kidneys. ANP also causes peripheral vasodilation and, as a consequence, a lowering of blood pressure. ANP may also act to inhibit the production of mineralocorticoids and renin. As indicated in its name, ANP is produced by cells of the atria as well as in other sites, including the brain.

HORMONES OF THE PANCREAS

The pancreas has important *endocrine* and *nonendocrine functions.* The nonendocrine functions occur as a result of activity of the exocrine part of the pancreas and are concerned with gastrointestinal (GI) function. The endocrine portion of the pancreas is organized as discrete islets (*islets of Langerhans*) (Fig. 33–15) that contain four cell types, each of which produces a different hormone. The most numerous of the islet cells are β-cells, which produce *insulin,* whereas α-cells produce *glucagon,* D-cells produce *somatostatin,* and F- or PP-cells produce *pancreatic polypeptide* (Fig. 33–16). Whereas these hormones have different functions, they all are involved in the control of metabolism and, more particularly, in glucose homeostasis.

Insulin

The first studies that associated the pancreas with carbohydrate metabolism were done by von Mering and Minkowski in 1889, when they showed that pancreatectomy of dogs resulted in signs that were similar to those characteristic of diabetes mellitus. Later, Banting and Best were able to show that injection of pancreatic extracts could alleviate the signs of diabetes mellitus in dogs and humans. Able was the first to crystallize insulin, and its structure was elucidated by Sanger in 1960.

Insulin is a protein consisting of two chains, designated A and B, with 21 and 30 amino acids, respectively, that are connected by two disulfide bridges. Whereas the monomer form of the hormone is thought to be the active form, insulin exists also in dimer and hexamer forms, the latter being complexed with two zinc molecules. Although there are some differences in amino acid composition among species, the differences are small, e.g., cattle, sheep, horses, dogs, and whales differ only in positions 8, 9, and 10 of the A-chain. As a result, *the biological activities of insulin are not highly species-specific.*

The Synthesis of Insulin Is Biphasic, an Acute Phase Involving the Release of Preformed Insulin, and a Chronic Phase Involving the Synthesis of Protein

The synthesis of insulin, similar to other peptide hormones, begins with the formation of a linear polypeptide preproinsulin within the rough endoplasmic reticulum. A small peptide fragment is removed to form proinsulin. Proinsulin is coiled, and the end fragments are joined by disulfide bonds. Proin-

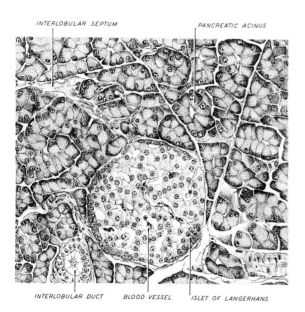

INTERLOBULAR SEPTUM   *PANCREATIC ACINUS*

INTERLOBULAR DUCT   *BLOOD VESSEL*   *ISLET OF LANGERHANS*

Figure 33–15. Section through the pancreas of the rat. The islet of Langerhans is a gland of internal secretion, whereas the surrounding acinar tissue forms an exocrine gland. (From Turner CD, Bagnara JT: General Endocrinology, 6th ed. Philadelphia, WB Saunders, 1976, p 259.)

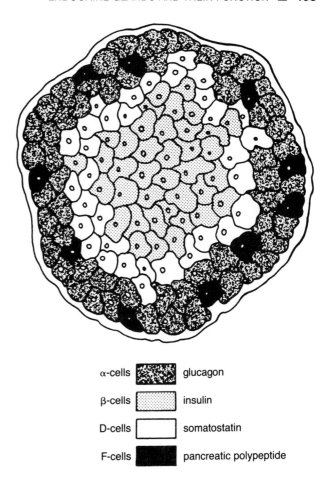

Figure 33-16. The pancreatic islet. (From McDonald LE: Veterinary Endocrinology and Reproduction, 4th ed. Philadelphia, Lea & Febiger, 1989, p 188.)

α-cells		glucagon
β-cells		insulin
D-cells		somatostatin
F-cells		pancreatic polypeptide

sulin is transferred to the Golgi apparatus, where it is further processed and packaged into granules that contain both insulin and the connecting- or *C-peptide* (33 amino acids in length).

The secretion of insulin follows *biphasic kinetics* in response to appropriate stimuli (Fig. 33-17). The initial, acute release of insulin involves the exocytosis of preformed insulin from secretion granules. Following the acute phase, a chronic phase of secretion occurs that involves the synthesis of protein and hence probably the synthesis of insulin.

The Metabolism of Insulin Involves Splitting the A and B Chains, and Reducing the Chains to Amino Acids and Peptides

The *metabolism of insulin* is affected mainly by the liver and kidneys. Enzymes are present that reduce the disulfide bonds that link the A and B chains, and the chains are then subjected to protease activity, which reduces them to peptides and amino acids. The half-life of insulin is about 10 minutes.

The Main Metabolic Functions of Insulin Are to Promote the Conversion of Glucose, Fatty Acids, and Amino Acids to Their Storage Form

Insulin acts at a number of sites within the metabolic pathways of carbohydrates, fats, and proteins (Fig. 33-18). It is important to realize that the *liver is an especially important target organ*, in part because the pancreatic venous effluent passes directly to the liver. The net effect of the actions of insulin is to lower blood concentrations of glucose, fatty acids, and amino acids, and to promote intracellular conversion of these compounds to their storage forms, i.e., glycogen, triglycerides, and protein, respectively (Table 33-5). Glucose does not readily penetrate cell membranes except for a few tissues, such as brain,

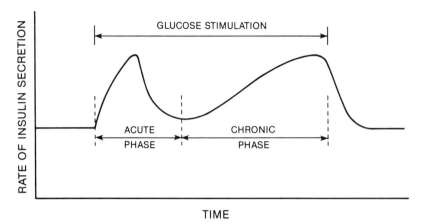

Figure 33–17. Kinetics of insulin secretion by the β cell in response to a continued glucose stimulus. (From Hedge GA, Colby HD, Goodman RL: Clinical Endocrine Physiology. Philadelphia, WB Saunders, 1987, p 270.)

liver, and red and white blood cells, cells that must have continual access to glucose on a continuous basis. The presence of insulin is critical to the movement of glucose through the plasma membrane into the cell.

Insulin has profound effects on carbohydrate metabolism. Insulin facilitates the utilization of glucose, i.e., *glycolysis,* which involves the oxidation of glucose to pyruvate and lactate through the induction of enzymes, such as glucokinase, phosphofructokinase, and pyruvate kinase. Insulin promotes *glycogen production* in liver, adipose tissue, and skeletal muscle by increasing glycogen synthe-

tase activity with a concomitant decrease in glycogen phosphorylase activity. Gluconeogenesis is decreased by insulin because of the promotion of protein synthesis in peripheral tissues, thereby decreasing the amount of amino acids available for gluconeogenesis. In addition, insulin decreases the activities of hepatic enzymes (fructose-1-6, bisphosphate aldolase, pyruvate carboxylase, phosphoenolpyruvate carboxylase, and glucose-6-phosphatase) that are involved in the conversion of amino acids to glucose.

In adipose tissue, insulin promotes the *synthesis of triglycerides.* Insulin facilitates the in-

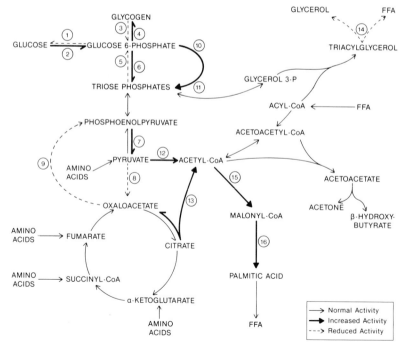

Figure 33–18. Metabolic pathways affected by insulin. The numbers correspond to each of the following enzymes: (1) glucose-6-phosphatase; (2) glucokinase; (3) phosphorylase; (4) glycogen synthase; (5) fructose—1,6-bisphosphate aldolase; (6) 6-phosphofructokinase; (7) pyruvate kinase; (8) pyruvate carboxylase; (9) phosphoenolpyruvate carboxykinase; (10) glucose-6-P-dehydrogenase; (11) 6-phosphogluconate dehydrogenase; (12) pyruvate dehydrogenase; (13) ATP-citrate lyase; (14) hormone-sensitive lipase; (15) acetyl-CoA carboxylase; (16) fatty acid synthase. (From Hedge GA, Colby HD, Goodman RL: Clinical Endocrine Physiology. Philadelphia, WB Saunders, 1987, p 271.)

Table 33–5
SITES OF ACTION AND EFFECTS OF INSULIN ON CARBOHYDRATE, LIPID, AND PROTEIN METABOLISM

Site of Action			Process Affected
Liver	Muscle	Adipose	*Carbohydrate Metabolism*
	×	×	↑ glucose transport
×	×	×	↑ glycogen synthesis
×	×	×	↓ glycogenolysis
×			↓ gluconeogenesis
			Lipid Metabolism
×		×	↑ lipogenesis
×		×	↓ lipolysis
			Protein Metabolism
	×		↑ amino acid uptake
	×		↑ protein synthesis
	×		↓ protein degradation
×			↓ gluconeogenesis

Modified from Hedge GA, Colby HD, Goodman RL: Clinical Endocrine Physiology. Philadelphia, WB Saunders, 1987, p 272.

tracellular utilization of glucose, which results in increased pyruvate, a precursor of acetyl coenzyme A (acetyl CoA) (in turn, a precursor of fatty acids) and increased glycerol 3-phos-

phate for the esterification of fatty acids. Insulin activates the enzymes pyruvate dehydrogenase and acetyl CoA carboxylase, which promote the synthesis of fatty acids from acetyl CoA. Insulin also increases the activity of lipoprotein lipase located in the endothelium of capillaries of extrahepatic tissues, which promotes the movement of fatty acids into adipose tissue. Finally, insulin decreases lipolysis in adipose tissue.

With *protein metabolism,* insulin promotes uptake of amino acids by most tissues, including skeletal muscle, but not liver. Insulin promotes *protein synthesis* and inhibits protein degradation. Therefore, insulin promotes the maintenance of a positive nitrogen balance. With insulin deficiency, protein catabolism increases, with increased amounts of amino acids available for hepatic gluconeogenesis and a resultant increase in blood glucose concentrations.

The most important factor in the control of insulin secretion is the *concentration of blood glucose.* Increased concentrations of blood glucose initiate the synthesis and release of insulin by the β-cells of the pancreatic islets (Fig. 33–19). There are two theories regarding the mechanism of cellular induction of insulin synthesis and release. One is at the level of the plasma membrane, with glucose interacting with a membrane receptor protein that directs intracellular events toward the synthe-

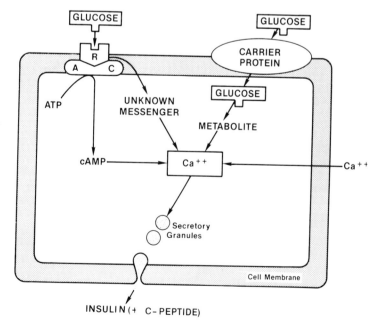

Figure 33–19. Proposed mechanisms of action of glucose on insulin secretion by the β cell. *R,* receptor; *AC,* adenylate cyclase. (From Hedge GA, Colby HD, Goodman RL: Clinical Endocrine Physiology. Philadelphia, WB Saunders, 1987, p 269.)

sis and release of insulin. The other is at the intracellular level, with the metabolism of glucose producing the signal for insulin synthesis and release. It is worth noting that glucose control of insulin secretion is a positive feedback system in which increased concentrations of glucose lead to increased concentrations of insulin.

Because the oral administration of glucose produces a larger insulin response than does systemic administration, factors from the intestinal tract were thought to affect insulin secretion. It is now known that a number of *GI hormones stimulate insulin secretion*, including gastrin, pancreozymin-cholecystokinin, secretin and gastric inhibitory peptide. The presence of amino acids and fatty acids in the intestinal tract also stimulates the release of insulin, although with less potency as compared to glucose (Table 33–6).

Hormones other than those from the GI tract are important for the control of insulin secretion. *Glucagon* from the α-cells of the pancreas has a *direct stimulatory effect* on the β-cells to secrete insulin. Conversely, *somatostatin inhibits* the secretion of insulin. Both hormones work through the adenylate cyclase system, with glucagon being stimulatory and somatostatin being inhibitory. *Catecholamines* tend to decrease insulin secretion through an interaction with the α-adrenergic receptors on the β-cells. Whereas epinephrine is the main circulating catecholamine that affects insulin secretion, norepinephrine also influences insulin secretion, because the pancreas has adrenergic innervation by the *autonomic nervous system (ANS)*. The pancreas also has cholinergic innervation by the ANS and, in contrast to adrenergic stimulation, cholinergic activity increases insulin secretion through the release of acetylcholine.

A lack of insulin produces a syndrome called *diabetes mellitus*. Blood glucose concentrations increase because of a variety of factors: (1) decreased uptake of glucose by body tissues; (2) increased glycogenolysis, and (3) increased gluconeogenesis. The latter occurs as a result of increased hepatic gluconeogenesis due to the increased availability of amino acids, which occurs as a result of increased protein catabolism. Glucose appears in the urine when the capacity of the kidney for reabsorption is exceeded; the resulting osmotic effect leads to diuresis or *polyuria*. As mentioned previously, increased metabolism of triglycerides leads to increased concentrations of fatty acids in the blood and the formation of *ketone bodies* by the liver. Insulin deficiency increases lipolysis and, as a result, increases free fatty acids in blood. The fatty acids are oxidized by the liver to form acetyl CoA, which can be further converted to acetoacetate, β-hydroxybutyrate, and acetone, collectively called ketone bodies (see Fig. 33–17). The ketone bodies are acidic anions, and their presence produces acidosis because of the depletion of bicarbonate ions.

Glucagon

Glucagon is a protein hormone produced by the α-cells of the islets of Langerhans. It has a close relationship with insulin in the control of glucose metabolism.

Glucagon is a polypeptide consisting of a single chain composed of 29 amino acids. There is considerable homology among species as to amino acid composition. There are other sites of production of glucagon besides the pancreas; the stomach produces a molecule that is identical to pancreatic glucagon called *gut glucagon*, and the small intestine produces an immunologically similar molecule called *glicentin*.

Similar to other polypeptide hormones, glucagon is first synthesized in the endoplasmic reticulum as part of a precursor molecule, packaged in the Golgi apparatus, with final processing occurring in the secretory granules. Glucagon is released by exocytosis.

Glucagon is metabolized mainly by the liver and kidneys. It has a half-life in plasma of about 5 minutes.

Table 33–6
FACTORS AFFECTING INSULIN SECRETION

Stimuli	Inhibitors
Glucose	Somatostatin
Amino acids	Epinephrine
Fatty acids	Norepinephrine
Gastrin	
Pancreozymin-cholecystokinin	
Secretin	
Gastric inhibitory polypeptide	
Glucagon	
Acetylcholine	

Modified from Hedge GA, Colby HD, Goodman RL: Clinical Endocrine Physiology. Philadelphia, WB Saunders, 1987, p 276.

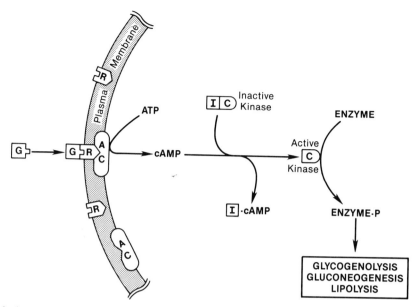

Figure 33–20. Mechanism of action of glucagon *(G)* on its target cells. *R,* receptor; *AC,* adenylate cyclase. (From Hedge GA, Colby HD, Goodman RL: Clinical Endocrine Physiology. Philadelphia, WB Saunders, 1987, p 286.)

The Most Important Functions of Glucagon Are to Decrease Glycogen Synthesis, Increase Glycogenolysis, and Increase Gluconeogenesis, All at the Level of the Liver

The physiological actions of glucagon are opposite those of insulin; most of the effect of glucagon is centered on the liver. Glucagon increases cAMP production in the liver, which leads to *decreased glycogen synthesis, increased glycogenolysis, and increased gluconeogenesis,* the latter being related to the effects of glucagon on protein metabolism (Fig. 33–20). The net result is an increase in glucose concentrations in the blood.

Changes in glucagon secretion counterbalance the effects of insulin in association with the daily ingestion of food and the intervals that occur in between food intake periods. Following the consumption of food, the initial response of the metabolic system is increased insulin secretion, which results in conservation of energy through the formation of storage forms of carbohydrates, fats, and proteins. Glucagon secretion, which begins with the ingestion of food, increases as the interval from food ingestion lengthens and blood glucose concentrations begin to decline. This secretion allows the individual to mobilize energy stores for the maintenance of glucose homeostasis, i.e., to prevent postprandial hypoglycemia (Fig. 33–21).

Figure 33–21. Effects of hyperglycemia and hypoglycemia on the secretion of insulin and glucagon by the pancreatic β cells and α cells, respectively. (From Hedge GA, Colby HD, Goodman RL: Clinical Endocrine Physiology. Philadelphia, WB Saunders, 1987, p 288.)

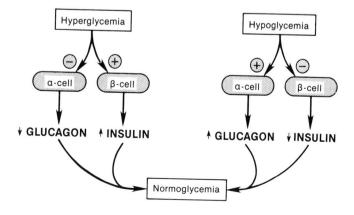

The Main Factor That Stimulates Glucagon Synthesis Is Decreased Glucose Concentrations in the Blood

The main factor that regulates glucagon secretion is *plasma glucose concentration*. In contrast to insulin, decreased glucose concentrations stimulate glucagon synthesis and release, a relationship that represents a *negative feedback system*. It is emphasized that glucagon regulation works in tandem with that of insulin in order to maintain glucose concentrations within the physiological range. In fact, if glucagon were not secreted to maintain blood glucose concentrations, the individual would die in hypoglycemic shock. Because the α-cells require insulin for glucose entry into the cells (as do most cells), in clinical syndromes involving insulin insufficiency (diabetes mellitus), glucose entry into the α-cells is reduced, and plasma glucagon concentrations are paradoxically elevated. Glucagon promotes lipolysis and an increase in fatty acids, which has a negative feedback effect on glucagon secretion.

Protein ingestion represents an exception to the rule of opposite responses of glucagon versus insulin. The release of both insulin and glucagon in response to protein ingestion appears logical; increased insulin secretion, in response to increased plasma amino acids, leads to lower glucose concentrations, and increased glucagon would counteract this through increased hepatic gluconeogenesis, resulting in maintenance of blood glucose within normal limits. The complementary response of insulin and glucagon allows growth to occur in animals fed a diet of protein and fat only.

Intestinal hormones, with the exception of secretin, stimulate both glucagon and insulin secretion. A similar (inhibitory) response to somatostatin is observed for both glucagon and insulin. Both sympathetic and parasympathetic stimulation of the ANS induce secretion of glucagon (Fig. 33–22).

Some birds have a predominance of glucagon in their pancreas, suggesting that glucagon may have a more important role in carbohydrate metabolism of avian species than in mammals.

Somatostatin

As indicated in Chapter 32, somatostatin was first described in the brain as a 14 amino acid peptide that inhibits growth hormone secretion by the pars distalis. The molecule has since been identified in a number of tissues, including other areas of the brain, the GI tract, and the D-cells of the pancreatic islets. Its synthesis and secretion are similar to that observed for other protein hormones. The metabolism of somatostatin is rapid, i.e., about 5 minutes, and occurs mainly in the liver and kidneys.

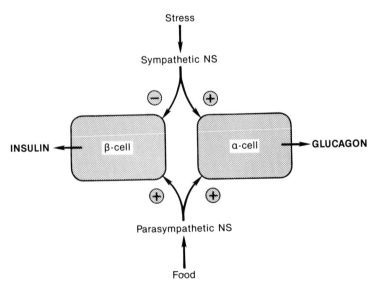

Figure 33–22. Regulation of insulin and glucagon secretion by the autonomic nervous system. +, stimulation; −, inhibition. (From Hedge GA, Colby HD, Goodman RL: Clinical Endocrine Physiology. Philadelphia, WB Saunders, 1987, p 277.)

The Main Functions of Somatostatin Are to Regulate (Inhibit) the Secretion of Hormones Produced by the Pancreas (Insulin, Glucagon, Pancreatic Polypeptide) and to Inhibit Digestive Processes

The actions of somatostatin can be classified as inhibitory. Pancreatic somatostatin inhibits the digestive processes by *decreasing nutritive absorption* and *digestion*. The motility and secretory activity of the GI tract are decreased by somatostatin. One of the most important physiological functions of pancreatic somatostatin is the regulation of the endocrine cells of the pancreas (Fig. 33–23). Somatostatin inhibits secretion of all endocrine cell types of the islets of Langerhans, including the D-cells. The α-cells are more affected by the inhibitory action of somatostatin compared to β-cells; therefore, glucagon secretion is more affected than insulin secretion by somatostatin.

Somatostatin secretion is increased by nutrients, such as glucose and amino acids, and by the neurotransmitters of the ANS, epinephrine, norepinephrine, and acetylcholine. Of the hormones produced by the pancreas, only glucagon stimulates somatostatin secretion.

Pancreatic Polypeptide

Pancreatic polypeptide, a 36 amino acid polypeptide, is produced by the F-cells of the pancreas (see Fig. 33–15). In contrast to somatostatin, pancreatic polypeptide secretion is limited to the pancreas.

The effects of pancreatic polypeptide are directed toward the GI tract. The secretion of pancreatic enzymes and the contraction of the gallbladder are inhibited by the actions of this hormone. Both gut motility and gastric emptying are increased by the action of pancreatic polypeptide.

The *secretion of pancreatic polypeptide is stimulated by intestinal hormones,* including cholecystokinin, secretin, and gastrin. Stimulation of the vagus nerve is also stimulatory for pancreatic polypeptide secretion. The ingestion of protein is stimulatory for secretion, whereas carbohydrates and fats have little effect. As indicated previously, somatostatin inhibits pancreatic polypeptide secretion.

THE ADRENAL MEDULLA

The adrenal medulla, as its name indicates, occupies the central portion of the adrenal gland (see Fig. 33–7). A stimulatory effect of adrenal medullary extracts on cardiac activity was first recognized by Oliver and Schafer in 1894. Thereafter, the main hormone of the adrenal medulla, epinephrine, became the first hormone to be isolated (by Abel in 1898), crystallized (by Takamine and Aldrich in 1901),

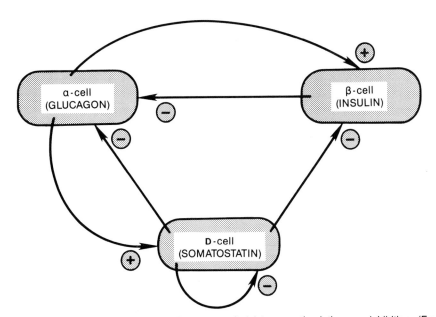

Figure 33–23. Possible cell-to-cell interactions in the pancreatic islets. +, stimulation; −, inhibition. (From Hedge GA, Colby HD, Goodman RL: Clinical Endocrine Physiology. Philadelphia, WB Saunders, 1987, p 292.)

and synthesized (by Stolz in 1904). Theories on the importance of the adrenal medulla include those of Cannon, who in 1932 proposed the *flight-or-fight* hypothesis in which the adrenal medulla was activated to aid in combating situations of extreme stress. Others advocated the *tonus theory*, which stated that cells of the adrenal medulla were constantly in a state of readiness. In fact, the adrenal medulla has a constant output of catecholamines that can be accentuated dramatically if the need arises.

It was recognized early that cells of the adrenal medulla were the equivalent of postganglionic cells of the sympathetic nervous system. Therefore, it was assumed that epinephrine was the mediator of postganglionic activity of the sympathetic nervous system. It was later recognized that another catecholamine, *norepinephrine*, was the neurotransmitter of the sympathetic nervous system. Both epinephrine and norepinephrine are released when preganglionic nerve fibers to the adrenal medulla are stimulated; in fact, most of the norepinephrine found in plasma originates from the adrenal medulla. However, epinephrine is the major catecholamine secreted by the adrenal medulla of most mammals. Exceptions to this generalization include the dominance of norepinephrine over epinephrine in whales and chickens and in the fetal tissues of all species.

The Synthesis of Catecholamines Is from Tyrosine; the Main Catecholamine Synthesized by the Adrenal Medulla Is Epinephrine

The cells of the adrenal medulla that synthesize catecholamines are classified as *chromaffin* cells. This classification has sprung from the histochemical reaction of the cells when exposed to postassium dichromate, i.e., a darkening of the cells due to the formation of colored pigments in conjunction with the oxidation of the catecholamines. The cells that produce epinephrine are different from those that synthesize norepinephrine; accordingly, the type of *chromaffin granule* present in each cell type is different. In cattle, the epinephrine-secreting cells tend to be on the outer edge of the medulla. Acetylcholine release from the preganglionic nerve fibers initiates the synthesis of the catecholamines by the medullary cells (Fig. 33–24). Acetylcholine also stimulates the release of catecholamines from chromaffin granules, a phenomenon called stimulus-secretion coupling.

The synthesis of the catecholamines begins with either of the amino acids, *phenylalanine* or *tyrosine* (Fig. 33–25). However, tyrosine is a naturally occurring amino acid, and most of the synthesis of catecholamines begins with this amino acid. The initial step in the biosynthetic pathway begins with the conversion of tyrosine to *dihydroxyphenylalanine* (DOPA). *Tyrosine hydroxylase (TH)*, the enzyme responsible for the conversion of tyrosine, is the rate-limiting enzyme in the formation of catecholamines. The end products of tyrosine metabolism, including DOPA, dopamine, norepinephrine, and epinephrine, inhibit the activity of TH. DOPA is converted to *dopamine* through the enzymatic activity of *aromatic-L-amino acid decarboxylase* (DOPA decarboxylase). To this point, the biochemical transformations have occurred in the cytosol. The conversion of dopamine to norepinephrine occurs within the chromaffin granule, because the key enzyme, *dopamine-β-hydroxylase*, is localized within the granule (Fig. 33–26).

If the cell secretes norepinephrine, the biochemical pathway is ended, and the hormone remains in the norepinephrine granule, ready

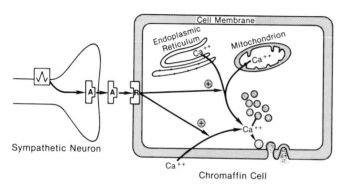

Figure 33–24. Stimulus-secretion coupling in the adrenal chromaffin cell. Note that cytosolic calcium may be derived from intracellular or extracellular sources. *A*, acetylcholine; *R*, receptor. (From Hedge GA, Colby HD, Goodman RL: Clinical Endocrine Physiology. Philadelphia, WB Saunders, 1987, p 303.)

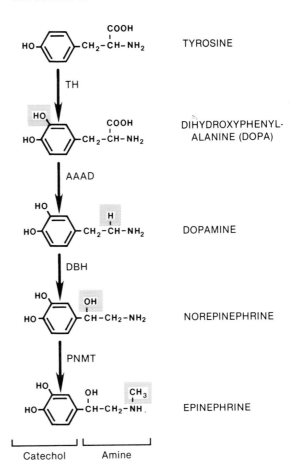

Figure 33–25. Pathway of catecholamine synthesis in the adrenal medulla. Shaded areas denote the structural changes occurring at each step. *TH,* tyrosine hydroxylase; *AAAD,* aromatic-L-amino acid decarboxylase; *DBH,* dopamine-β-hydroxylase; *PNMT,* phenylethanolamine-*N*-methyltransferase. (From Hedge GA, Colby HD, Goodman RL: Clinical Endocrine Physiology. Philadelphia, WB Saunders, 1987, p 298.)

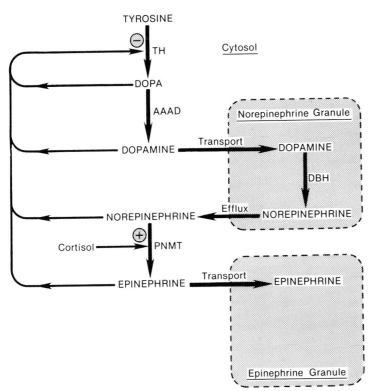

Figure 33–26. Regulation of catecholamine biosynthesis in the adrenal medulla. *TH,* tyrosine hydroxylase; *AAAD,* aromatic-L-amino acid decarboxylase; *DBH,* dopamine-β-hydroxylase; *PNMT,* phenylethanolamine-*N*-methyltransferase +, stimulation; −, inhibition. (From Hedge GA, Colby HD, Goodman RL: Clinical Endocrine Physiology. Philadelphia, WB Saunders, 1987, p 300.)

for secretion. If the cell secretes epinephrine, norepinephrine moves back into the cytosol, where it is converted to epinephrine through the activity of *phenylethanolamine-N-methyltransferase* (PNMT). Epinephrine then moves into an epinephrine granule for storage prior to its release. The metabolism of catecholamines is rapid (2 minutes for norepinephrine, less for epinephrine) and is carried out mainly by the liver and kidneys.

The importance of the anatomical association of the adrenal cortex and medulla may be related to the fact that cortisol is important for the activity of the enzyme PNMT. The chromaffin cells are located close to the venous sinuses that drain the adrenal cortex and, therefore, are exposed to venous effluent that contains high concentrations of cortisol.

The Main Actions of Catecholamines Are on Metabolism, Especially Effects That Increase the Concentration of Glucose; Catecholamines Also Enable Animals to Rapidly Adapt to Stress

The actions of the catecholamines involve the *regulation of intermediary metabolism* as well as responses that allow animals to adjust to situations involving acute stress. The actions of catecholamines are mediated through *adrenergic receptors* located on target tissues (Fig. 33–27). There are two major types of receptors, α and β, which are further divided into α_1, α_2 and β_1, β_2. Alpha receptors control catecholamine release from sympathetic nerve endings, α_1 affecting postsynaptic nerve endings and α_2 affecting presynaptic terminals. Beta$_1$ recep-

tors affect mainly the heart, and β_2 receptors affect smooth muscle contraction and intermediary metabolism. Whereas all adrenergic receptors are responsive to both epinephrine and norepinephrine, there are differential responses of the receptors to the two catecholamines. In addition, the receptor types on various tissues vary in number, which together with the differential response of adrenergic receptors on tissues, results in variable adrenergic responses being produced by a particular catecholamine.

The *metabolic effects* of catecholamines are mediated mainly by β_2 receptors. Because epinephrine is ten times more potent than norepinephrine with β_2 receptors, epinephrine plays a much more important role in the control of intermediary metabolism than norepinephrine. The effects of epinephrine on glucose metabolism are similar to those of glucagon and opposite to insulin. Epinephrine *increases blood glucose concentrations* with the effect mainly at the level of the liver, i.e., epinephrine promotes both hepatic glycogenolysis and gluconeogenesis. Epinephrine also stimulates glycogenolysis in skeletal muscle, which in this situation contrasts with the action of glucagon. Because glucose-6-phosphatase is not present in skeletal muscle, lactate is produced instead of glucose. The liver takes up lactate and converts it to glucose. Additional effects on glucose metabolism include the inhibition of insulin secretion (through α receptors) and stimulation of glucagon secretion by the pancreas; both actions increase blood glucose concentrations.

Epinephrine promotes *lipolysis* through in-

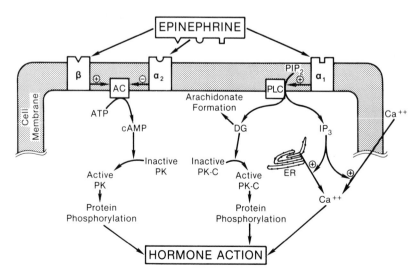

Figure 33–27. Mechanisms of action of epinephrine in target cells mediated by β-, α_2-, and α_1-adrenergic receptors. *PIP$_2$* phosphatidylinositol-4,5-biphosphate; *PLC*, phospholipase C; *DG*, diacylglycerol; *IP$_3$*, inositol-1, 4,5-triphosphate; *AC*, adenylate cyclase; *PK*, protein kinase; *PK-C*, protein kinase C; *ER*, endoplasmic reticulum; +, stimulation; –, inhibition. (From Hedge GA, Colby HD, Goodman RL: Clinical Endocrine Physiology. Philadelphia, WB Saunders, 1987, p 305.)

teraction with β_2 receptors on adipose cells. Activation of a lipase enzyme results in an increase in free fatty acids in the blood. Glucocorticoids potentiate the effect of epinephrine on lipolysis.

Catecholamines stimulate cardiac function. Both epinephrine and norepinephrine interact with β_1 receptors to increase both the force of contraction and the heart rate, the latter due to the promotion of a shorter period of diastolic depolarization. Whereas both catecholamines promote arteriolar constriction through interaction with α receptors, epinephrine through its high affinity for β_2 receptors causes the dilation of blood vessels both in the heart and in skeletal muscle. The end result is that total peripheral resistance is decreased by the action of epinephrine with a concomitant decline in diastolic pressure; however, blood pressure is changed little, and cardiac output increases because of the increase in heart rate. The action of epinephrine to increase cardiac output is an obvious beneficial effect in situations that are described as "flight or fight."

Concerning the effects of catecholamines on smooth muscle, epinephrine causes relaxation of bronchial smooth muscle, particularly in situations where the muscle is in a contracted state. As the action is mediated through β_2 receptors, norepinephrine has little effect on bronchial smooth muscle. Epinephrine causes relaxation of the smooth muscle of the GI tract through interaction with β_2 receptors. Concerning the effects of catecholamines on uterine smooth muscle, stimulation of α receptors results in contraction, and stimulation of β_2 receptors results in relaxation. Because of its dominant effect on β_2 receptors, epinephrine causes relaxation of the uterus, whereas both epinephrine and norepinephrine interact with α receptors to cause contraction. The physiological state of the animal influences the response to catecholamines; the feline nongravid uterus is relaxed (uterine motility inhibited) by epinephrine, whereas the gravid uterus responds by contraction.

The effects of the catecholamines on bladder smooth muscle are dependent on a differential location of α and β receptors; α receptors are located within the neck, and β receptors are located within the body of the bladder. Epinephrine relaxes the body and contracts the neck of the bladder; norepinephrine contracts the neck of the bladder. The net effect is retention of urine.

Although the parasympathetic nervous system is the principal system involved in penile erection, the sympathetic nervous system may play a role also. Epinephrine promotes erection through vasodilation of the blood vasculature mediated by β receptors. Higher concentrations of epinephrine (and norepinephrine) can cause ejaculation through α receptor interaction and vasoconstriction. In the eye, epinephrine causes relaxation of the lens through stimulation of β receptors on the ciliary muscles, and dilation of the pupil through stimulation of α receptors with resultant contraction of the radial muscle of the iris.

The effects of epinephrine on the CNS are excitatory. It is likely that drugs that affect the CNS do so by modulation of catecholamine concentrations with sedation associated with lower values of epinephrine. Other effects of catecholamine include the promotion of sweating and piloerection. Epinephrine also increases renin production by the renal juxtaglomerular cells. A summary of the effects of catecholamines is shown in Table 33–7.

The Main Factors That Stimulate Catecholamine Secretion Are Hypoglycemia and Conditions That Produce Stress

Any factor that increases *sympathetic nervous system* stimulation of the adrenal medulla results in the immediate secretion of catecholamines. The main physiological factor that influences catecholamine secretion is *hypoglycemia*. In this situation, epinephrine secretion is stimulated by decreases in blood glucose concentrations that are within normal physiological limits. In contrast, other parts of the sympathetic nervous system are depressed by decreases in blood glucose. Factors that elicit a massive release of catecholamines fall under the category of *stress*, particularly those that are acute. Catecholamines are particularly important for the maintenance of blood pressure in conjunction with severe blood loss, and *decreased blood pressure* stimulates epinephrine secretion. Catecholamines are also important for adaptation to *cold exposure* in terms of increased heat production, and *decreased temperature* increases epinephrine secretion. The response to acute stress can be particularly marked, because each preganglionic sympathetic neuron that supplies the adrenal medulla affects a number of chromaffin cells, i.e., the signal is greatly amplified.

Table 33–7
RESPONSES OF TARGET TISSUES TO CATECHOLAMINES

Target Tissue	Receptor Type	Response
Liver	β_2	Glycogenolysis, lipolysis, gluconeogenesis
Adipose tissue	β_2	Lipolysis
Skeletal muscle	β_2	Glycogenolysis
Pancreas	α_2	Decreased insulin secretion
	β_2	Increased insulin secretion
Cardiovascular system	β_1	Increased heart rate, increased contractility, increased conduction velocity
	α	Vasoconstriction
	β_2	Vasodilation in skeletal muscle arterioles, coronary arteries, and all veins
Bronchial muscle	β_2	Relaxation
Gastrointestinal tract	β_2	Decreased contractility
	α	Sphincter contraction
Urinary bladder	α	Sphincter contraction
	β_2	Detrusor relaxation
Uterus	α	Contraction
	β_2	Relaxation
Male sex organs	α	Ejaculation, detumescence
	β_2	Erection?
Eye	α_1	Radial muscle contraction
	β_2	Ciliary muscle relaxation
CNS	α	Stimulation
Skin	α	Piloerection, sweat production
Renin secretion	β_1	Stimulation

From Hedge GA, Colby HD, Goodman RL: Clinical Endocrine Physiology. Philadelphia, WB Saunders, 1987, p 305.

CALCIUM AND PHOSPHATE METABOLISM

Calcium Is Important for Intracellular Reactions, Including Muscle Contraction, Nerve Cell Activity, the Release of Hormones Through Exocytosis, and the Activation of Enzymes; Extracellular Functions Include Blood Coagulation, the Maintenance and Stability of Cell Membranes, and the Maintenance of Structural Integrity of Bone and Teeth

The control of calcium and phosphate metabolism is important, because these ions play an important role in physiological process. Calcium homeostasis is tightly controlled; ad-justments are made within a range of $\pm 5\%$ of normal. Calcium is important for a number of intracellular reactions, including muscle contraction, nerve cell activity, the release of hormones through the process of exocytosis, and activation of a number of enzymes. Calcium is important for coagulation of blood and for maintaining the stability of cell membranes and the linkage between cells. On a less acute basis, calcium is important for the structural integrity of bone and teeth.

Phosphate Is Important for the Structure of Bone and Teeth; on a Cellular Basis, Organic Phosphate Serves as Part of the Cell Membrane and as Part of a Number of Intracellular Components

Phosphate concentrations are controlled by the same systems that control calcium. Inorganic phosphate in blood serves as the source of phosphate, which is important for the structure of bone and teeth. Inorganic phosphate also functions as an important hydrogen ion buffering system in blood. Organic phosphate is an important part of the cell, including the plasma membrane and intracellular components, including nucleic acids, ATP, and AMP.

The Most Important Body Pool of Calcium Involved in Homeostasis Is the Extracellular Fluid Component; the Amorphous (Soluble) Portion of Bone Calcium Readily Contributes Calcium for the Maintenance of Homeostasis

The great majority (99%) of calcium in the body is in bone in the form of *hydroxyapatite crystals*, which contain calcium, phosphate, and water. The next largest pool of calcium is *intracellular* calcium. As stated previously, calcium is important for the response of cells in carrying out their physiological activities, including the secretion of hormones. In the inactive cell state, calcium concentrations are relatively low in the cytosol; calcium is bound to proteins or contained within the mitochondria or granules of the endoplasmic reticulum. Increased intracellular calcium concentrations are indicative of increased cell activity.

The smallest pool of calcium, that which resides in the *extracellular fluid*, is the most important pool for physiological control of calcium concentrations in the blood. This component is composed of interstitial calcium, blood calcium, and a small (0.5%) but important part of the bone calcium pool, which exists as amorphous crystals or in solution. The soluble bone calcium pool allows access to the large reserve of calcium that resides in bone.

The regulation of calcium involves control of the movement of calcium between the extracellular fluid and three body organs: bone, GI tract, and kidneys. The exchange of calcium ions between the extracellular and intracellular fluid occurs in conjunction with the control of intracellular metabolism with little effect on plasma concentrations of calcium.

The absorption of calcium from the GI tract is by *passive diffusion* and *active transport*. The passive diffusion of calcium across the intestinal mucosa occurs in the presence of high concentrations and, as such, is not an important aspect of calcium absorption. Active transport involves the movement of calcium into the intestinal cell down a concentration gradient, which is facilitated by carrier proteins located on the lumenal side of the mucosal cell. Calcium is moved through the serosal side of the mucosal cell into the interstitial fluid through a calcium pump system. The active transport system adjusts according to the amount of calcium in the diet, becoming more active when calcium concentrations in the diet are lower and less active when calcium concentrations are higher. Calcium excretion into the GI tract is not affected by calcium uptake, a factor that can exacerbate conditions involving hypocalcemia. The GI tract serves as the source of calcium for the body, even though both absorption and excretion of calcium occur through the tract. As discussed later, vitamin D plays an important role in the absorption of calcium from the GI tract.

The kidney serves as the route of excretion of calcium. Most of the calcium that passes into the kidney is reabsorbed, with a net loss of only about 2%. This amount is matched by net absorption of calcium by the GI tract. Most of the calcium filtered by the kidneys is reabsorbed in the proximal tubules, with the next largest amount absorbed by the distal tubules, and a lesser amount by the ascending loop of Henle. The *distal tubules* are under hormonal control and, therefore, are the *site of regulation* of calcium in the kidneys.

The most important regulation of calcium metabolism between bone and extracellular fluid involves the soluble portion of bone. Amorphous crystals and soluble calcium, which form the source of ready exchange of ions with the blood, are located between the osteoblasts, which line the blood vessel channels, and the osteocytes, which are located deeper in the bone (Fig. 33–28). These two cell types have cytoplasmic projections that interact intimately through the presence of tight cell junctions. In order for labile bone calcium to reach the blood, calcium must cross the membrane barrier created by the *osteoblasts* and *osteocytes*. Movement of calcium from stable bone into the extracellular fluid occurs also, but it has little impact on the acute regulation of calcium concentrations. The process of remodeling bone, which occurs on a continuous basis, involves the breakdown of hydroxyapatite crystals by *osteoclasts*; a laying down of organic matrix by osteoblasts in the tunnels made by the osteoclasts; and finally, the mineralization of the organic matrix by hydroxyapatite crystals. If an animal is subjected to prolonged changes involving calcium metab-

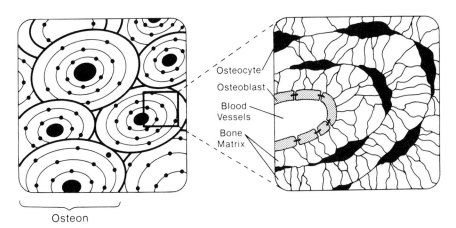

Osteocyte
Osteoblast
Blood Vessels
Bone Matrix

Osteon

Figure 33–28. Structure of the osteon, the functional unit of bone, shown in cross section at two magnifications. (From Hedge GA, Colby HD, Goodman RL: Clinical Endocrine Physiology. Philadelphia, WB Saunders, 1987, p 360.)

olism, the slow aspect of bone calcium exchange can have a significant impact on calcium metabolism.

Parathyroid Hormone

The main organ involved in the control of calcium and phosphate metabolism is the *parathyroid gland* (Fig. 33–29). Most domestic animals have four pairs of parathyroid glands that are generally located at the poles of the two lobes of the thyroid gland; the pig has only one pair of parathyroid glands, and they lie anterior to the thyroid. The cranial pair of glands in dogs and cats are at the craniolateral poles of the thyroid, and those of ruminants and horses are anterior to the thyroid. The caudal pair of parathyroid glands in dogs, cats, and ruminants are located within the medial surface of the thyroid, whereas in the horse they lie near the bifurcation of the carotid trunk. The parathyroid cells that are in the active process of hormone secretion are called *chief cells*, whereas inactive, or degenerate, cells are called *oxyphil cells.*

The synthesis of parathyroid hormone (PTH) is as for other protein hormones; a preproPTH of 115 amino acids is synthesized in the rough endoplasmic reticulum, then cleaved by 25 amino acids to form proPTH. A 6 amino acid pro-portion is removed by the Golgi apparatus; the resulting molecular weight of PTH is 84 amino acids. PTH is secreted by the process of exocytosis. PTH is rapidly metabolized by the liver and kidneys, and has a relatively short half-life of 5–10 minutes in blood.

The effect of PTH is to *increase calcium and decrease phosphate* concentrations in extracellular fluids. PTH has direct effects on bone and kidney metabolism of calcium, and indirect effects on GI metabolism of calcium. The initial effect of PTH on bone is to promote the transfer of calcium across the osteoblast-osteocyte membrane. This level of action occurs without the movement of phosphate and, therefore, has no effect on phosphate concentrations in blood. PTH has additional effects on stable bone, which results in the resorption of the bone. This effect involves increased osteoclast activity and an inhibition of osteoblast activity. The effect of PTH on stable bone results in the release of both calcium and phosphate.

PTH acts on the distal convoluted tubules of the kidneys to increase absorption of calcium and decrease renal phosphate reabsorption through an effect on the proximal tubules. PTH is involved also in the activation of vitamin D at the kidney level. PTH mediates the absorption of calcium from the gut indirectly through its effect on vitamin D.

PTH secretion is controlled by free (ionized) calcium concentrations in blood; decreases in calcium stimulate PTH secretion, and increases in calcium turn off secretion (Fig. 33–30). Both actions are mediated by an effect on cAMP metabolism. Epinephrine stimulates PTH secretion through stimulation of β-adrenergic receptors. Magnesium affects PTH secretion in the same manner as calcium, but its physiological impact is much less. Sleep affects the secretion of PTH, with values highest during early morning.

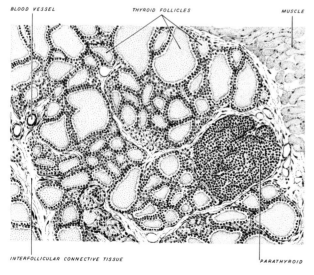

BLOOD VESSEL   THYROID FOLLICLES   MUSCLE

INTERFOLLICULAR CONNECTIVE TISSUE   PARATHYROID

Figure 33–29. A section of the thyroid and parathyroid glands of the rat as seen under low power of the microscope. Notice that the parathyroid gland lies near the surface and is surrounded on three sides by the thyroid follicles. (From Turner CD, Bagnara JT: General Endocrinology, 6th ed. Philadelphia, WB Saunders, 1976, p 226.)

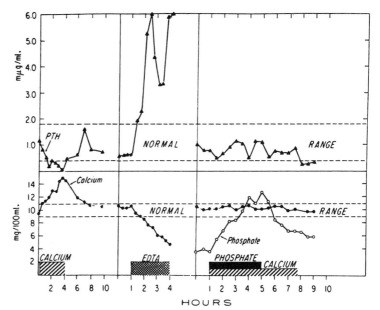

Figure 33–30. Changes of plasma immunoreactive parathyroid hormone in response to hypercalcemia induced by calcium infusion, hypocalcemia produced by EDTA infusion, and hyperphosphatemia with normocalcemia in a cow. (From Capen CC: The calcium regulating hormones: Parathyroid hormone, calcitonin, and cholecalciferol. *In* McDonald LE, Pineda MH (eds): Veterinary Endocrinology and Reproduction. Philadelphia, Lea & Febiger, 1989, p 105.)

Calcitonin

Calcitonin (CT), a hormone produced by cells in the thyroid gland, also affects calcium metabolism. The cell type involved in the synthesis of CT, *parafollicular* or *C cells*, are scattered throughout the thyroid gland and are distinctly different from the cells that synthesize thyroid hormones. It was found during the early studies of CT in animal classes, such as fish, amphibia, reptiles, and birds, that had separate thyroid and ultimobranchial glands, that all of the CT activity was in the ultimobranchial glands. Therefore, the CT cells represent ultimobranchial gland tissue that has been incorporated into the thyroid during embryonic development.

CT, synthesized as a preprohormone, has 32 amino acids; a ring structure at the N-terminus contains a disulfide link that bridges between amino acids 1 and 7. The processing of the molecule is interesting, because CT is located in the middle of proCT, so that an additional enzyme cleavage is required for the formation of the active molecule. The secretion of CT is by exocytosis from granules.

CT acts as a counterbalance to PTH, because it causes hypocalcemia and hypophosphatemia. The effect of CT on mineral metabolism is mainly on bone (Fig. 33–31). CT decreases the movement of calcium from the labile bone calcium pool (behind the osteoblast-osteocyte barrier) to the extracellular fluid, and decreases bone resorption through an inhibitory effect on osteoclasts. Whereas the inhibition of bone resorption explains one aspect of the hypophosphatemic effects of CT, CT also increases movement of phosphate from the extracellular

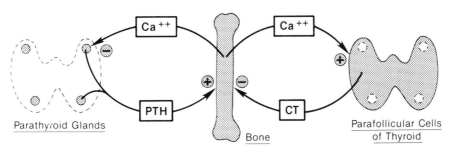

Figure 33–31. Negative feedback loops controlling parathyroid hormone *(PTH)* and calcitonin *(CT)* secretion. (From Hedge GA, Colby HD, Goodman RL: Clinical Endocrine Physiology. Philadelphia, WB Saunders, 1987, p 363.)

fluid into bone. CT decreases GI activity directly by inhibiting gastric acid secretion and indirectly by inhibiting gastrin secretion. The importance of this in a physiological sense is not known. CT also increases renal excretion of calcium and phosphate.

The control of secretion of CT is by calcium; increased concentrations cause increased secretion of CT. The physiological control of calcium metabolism by CT operates in situations of *hypercalcemia* with increased secretion of CT, and concomitant inhibition of PTH secretion. During *hypocalcemic* conditions, CT synthesis is inhibited, and PTH becomes responsible for re-establishing normal calcium concentrations in the extracellular fluids. GI hormones, including gastrin, cholecystokinin, secretin, and glucagon, stimulate the secretion of CT, with gastrin the most potent. These hormones limit postprandial hypercalcemia.

Vitamin D

Vitamin D is important for the absorption of calcium from the gut. It is a steroid-like molecule, and because it is produced in one tissue and transported by the blood to a distant site of action, it should probably be called a hormone instead of a vitamin. All of the vitamin D produced by the body is done so in the skin. Epithelial cells of the skin synthesize the immediate precursor of vitamin D, *7-dehydrocholesterol,* from acetate. Exposure of the skin to ultraviolet light results in cleavage of the C-9 and C-10 bonds of 7-dehydrocholesterol, which results in the formation of vitamin D (Fig. 33–32). The vitamin D molecule, as such, is inactive, and must be transformed by both the liver and kidney before the molecule is biologically activate. The liver first hydroxylates the molecule at C-25, and the kidney subsequently hydroxylates the molecule at C-1 to produce the active compound, *1,25-(OH)2-vitamin D (1,25-vitamin D).*

Control of the C-1 hydroxylase in the kidney by PTH is the most important control linkage for the synthesis of 1,25-vitamin D. Decreases in calcium concentrations stimulate PTH secretion, which in turn favors the synthesis of active vitamin D and increased intestinal absorption of calcium. Phosphate also regulates vitamin D metabolism. Increased serum phosphate concentrations stimulate an enzyme that promotes hydroxylation of C-24 (instead of

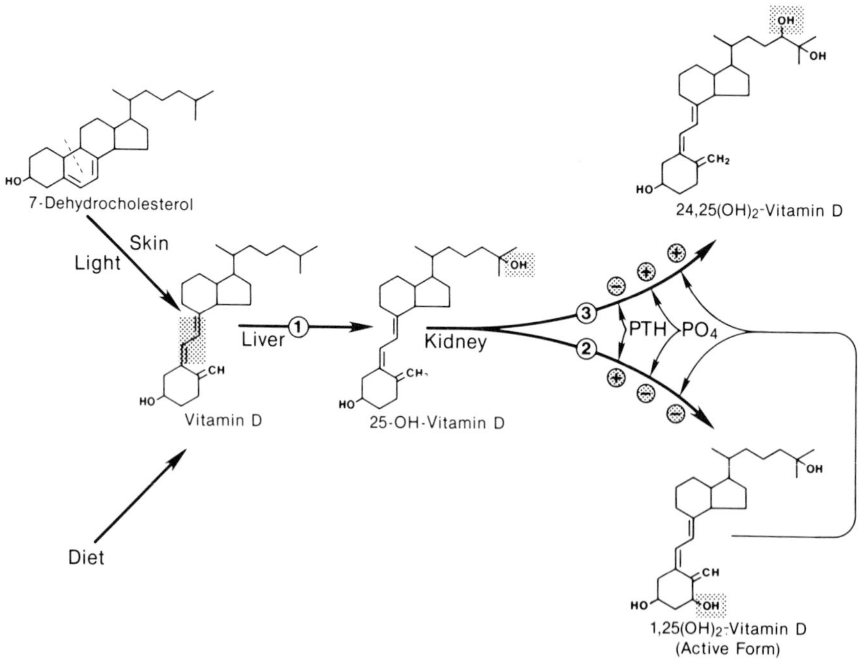

Figure 33–32. Synthesis and metabolism of vitamin D. The position of hydroxylation of 25-OH-vitamin D in the kidney is controlled by PTH, phosphate (PO$_4$), and 1,25-(OH)$_2$-vitamin D. Shading indicates structural change at each step; the dashed line indicates position of cleavage of 7-dehydrocholesterol to produce vitamin D. Enzymes: (1) 25-hydroxylase; (2) 1α-hydroxylase; (3) 24-hydroxylase. (From Hedge GA, Colby HD, Goodman RL: Clinical Endocrine Physiology. Philadelphia, WB Saunders, 1987, p 367.)

C-1) by the kidney, which leads to the formation of *24,25-(OH)2-vitamin D*—an inactive molecule. The active molecule, 1,25-vitamin D, also regulates itself by decreasing C-1 hydroxylase and increasing C-24 hydroxylase activity; decreased active vitamin D is the result.

1,25-Vitamin D, due to its lipid nature, is transported by binding to proteins in the plasma. Most of vitamin D is carried in association with a specific α globulin called *transcalciferin*, a molecule synthesized by the liver.

The most important effects of vitamin D are concerned with increased absorption of calcium by the GI tract. Vitamin D stimulates the synthesis of protein within the mucosal cells, which aids the rate-limiting step in calcium absorption, i.e., movement of calcium into the mucosal cell (Fig. 33–33). Because the intestinal effect of vitamin D depends on the activation of protein synthesis by mucosal cells, the effect on calcium absorption usually requires several hours. Although the stimulation of protein synthesis relates mostly to active transport of calcium, vitamin D also stimulates passive transfer of calcium. Vitamin D has effects also on bone, promoting the movement of calcium ions from the labile pool into extracellular fluids and the resorption of bone, as well as enhancing the effects of PTH on bone metabolism of calcium.

The control of 1,25-vitamin D synthesis is by PTH and phosphate. A decrease in calcium results in increased PTH secretion and increased formation of 1,25-vitamin D through enhancement of C-1 hydroxylation. This action leads to the correction of hypocalcemia by increasing absorption of calcium by the gut. A decline in phosphate concentrations results in decreased inhibition of the C-1 hydroxylation, which indirectly results in increased 1,25-vitamin D production and increased absorption of phosphate. There is some evidence that hormones associated with pregnancy, such as growth hormone (GH) and prolactin (PRL), increase 1,25-vitamin production by stimulating C-1 hydroxylation.

In the overall control of calcium metabolism, PTH is primarily responsible for the maintenance of calcium homeostasis. The primary target tissue for PTH in calcium homeostasis is the labile pool in bone; changes in renal absorption of calcium are also important. In the case of long-term calcium deficit in the diet, both PTH and 1,25-vitamin D are important for correction of the deficit. Decreased dietary calcium leads to decreased concentrations of calcium in the extracellular fluids and the release of PTH. PTH affects resorption of calcium by the kidneys, but most importantly for long-term correction of the problem, it causes increased 1,25-vitamin D secretion with increased absorption of dietary calcium. PTH

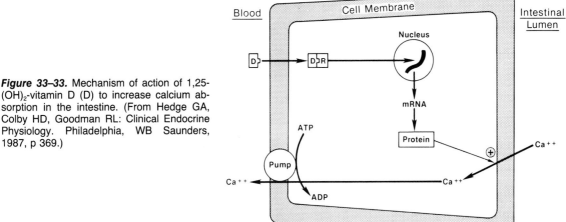

Figure 33–33. Mechanism of action of 1,25-(OH)$_2$-vitamin D (D) to increase calcium absorption in the intestine. (From Hedge GA, Colby HD, Goodman RL: Clinical Endocrine Physiology. Philadelphia, WB Saunders, 1987, p 369.)

also contributes to the overall calcium pool through its effect on stable bone, i.e., the promotion of resorption.

The most common type of acute disorder of calcium metabolism in domestic animals is that of hypocalcemia in association with parturition in the dog and cow (Fig. 33–34). Animals thus affected are usually recumbent with severe neuromuscular dysfunction. Dogs often have involuntary muscle spasms and contractions of groups of muscles, which is known as *tetany* or *eclampsia*. The main manifestation in cows is paralysis. The condition in cows occurs usually at the time of parturition, whereas in the dog the syndrome may not occur until the dog is heavily lactating, a week or two after parturition. The condition arises from the heavy demand that is placed on calcium reserves by the sudden onset of lactation with an inability of the animal to maintain calcium homeostasis. One suggested mechanism for the disease is a temporary lack of responsiveness of tissues to PTH; a decrease in PTH secretion does not appear fundamental to the disease. In order to accustom cows to the heavy parturient drain of calcium, cows are often fed a diet low in calcium late in pregnancy, so that factors that control calcium mobilization are active at delivery.

The most common type of chronic disorder of calcium metabolism in domestic animals is associated with *secondary hyperparathyroidism,* in which there is excess secretion of PTH because of chronically low calcium concentrations. Causes include improper diets that involve inadequate intake of either calcium or vitamin D, or inappropriate diets, such as all-meat diets for carnivores, that are low in calcium, or those for horses that are high in phosphate relative to calcium. Kidney disease, also a cause of secondary hyperparathyroidism, results in increased calcium diuresis with retention of phosphates. The resultant hyperphosphatemia further depresses calcium concentrations through increased formation of hydroxyapatite crystals. This process removes excess phosphate, but also removes calcium from an already marginal extracellular fluid concentration. The syndrome has been called *rubber jaw syndrome* in dogs when skeletal demineralization occurs or *renal osteitis fibrosa cystica* in the case of excessive bone resorption.

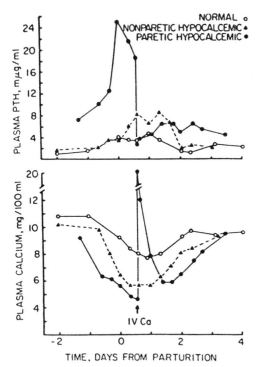

Figure 33–34. Development of varying degrees of hypocalcemia in cows near parturition with corresponding increase in plasma PTH levels. The cow developing severe hypocalcemia (below 5 mg/100 mL) had a considerably greater increase in plasma PTH than the moderate rise detected in nonparetic, hypocalcemic, and normal cows. Note that PTH levels decline rapidly following treatment of the paretic cow with intravenous calcium. (From Mayer, CP: The roles of parathyroid hormone and thyrocalcitonin in parturient paresis. *In* Anderson JJB (ed): Parturient Hypocalcemia. New York, Academic Press, 1970, p 179.)

CLINICAL CORRELATION

DIABETES MELLITUS

HISTORY □ You are presented with a 10-year-old, intact, female poodle whose owner is upset because the dog urinates in the house. In addition, the owner has noticed that the animal drinks larger amounts of water than it has in the past. Although the owner indicates the dog has a good appetite, it appears to have lost weight over the past few months.

CLINICAL EXAMINATION □ During the examination you check the dog's breath and detect a sweet odor. Among the organ systems you check are the eyes, and you find developing cataract formation. Because you have seen this dog many times before, you check its weight and find that it has lost 2 pounds since its last admittance a year ago. You are able to run a blood glucose determination in your hospital and tell the owner that the glucose concentration is 278 mg/dL. Just to be on the safe side, you ask the owner when the dog was last fed; he indicates it has been 8 hours.

COMMENT □ The findings in diabetes mellitus are all attributable to inadequate availability of insulin. Regarding carbohydrate metabolism, glycogen synthesis decreases in tissues, whereas glycogenolysis and gluconeogenesis increase, the latter two contributing to the high concentrations of glucose found in blood. When glucose concentrations exceed the reabsorption capacity in the tubular cells of the kidney, glucose appears in the urine. The loss of glucose in urine causes an osmotic diuresis (polyuria), and the dog compensates for this by drinking additional amounts of water. The sweetness of the breath is due to the presence of ketone bodies. These form as the result of decreased triglyceride synthesis in adipose tissue, which stimulates lipase activity and the release of free fatty acids. These fatty acids are metabolized to ketone bodies (acetoacetate, acetone, β-hydroxybutyrate) by the liver in a situation of excess of fatty acids. The end result is both a ketonemia and a ketonuria. Protein metabolism shifts toward catabolism during diabetes mellitus with decreased protein synthesis and increased protein degradation by muscle cells. This process increases the circulating concentrations of amino acids that are available to the liver for gluconeogenesis. The end result is nitrogen loss and a decrease in the muscle mass of the animal. The changes noted in the lenses of the eyes represent only one of a number of degenerative changes that occur in the presence of diabetes mellitus. Among other deleterious changes noted, atherosclerosis can and does compromise the entire blood vascular system.

Your question about the timing of feeding of the animal prior to the examination concerned normal postprandial increases in glucose concentrations that occur following the ingestion of food. The feeding-to-examination interval of 8 hours ruled out a postprandial effect; admittedly, the glucose concentration was higher than would be expected from this effect.

TREATMENT □ Insulin administration is essential to the treatment of diabetes mellitus. During the initial stages of treatment, considerable care needs to be taken to assure that the dosage is correct. The goal of treatment is to maintain glucose concentrations between a low of 80 mg/dL and a high of 200 mg/dL with one insulin injection every 24 hours. Too much insulin has the potential for producing a hypoglycemic coma. Two other important aspects of treatment include feeding the animal in conjunction with insulin administration and adequate exercise. Finally, the owner needs to be educated and prepared for the necessity of his or her intensive involvement in the management of the disease.

Bibliography

Dickson WM: Endocrine glands. *In* Swenson MJ (ed): Dukes' Physiology of Domestic Animals, 10th ed. Ithaca, NY, Cornell University Press, 1984, pp 761–797.

Feldman EC, Nelson RW: Canine and Feline Endocrinology and Reproduction. Philadelphia, WB Saunders, 1987.

Hedge GA, Colby HD, Goodman RL: Clinical Endocrine Physiology. Philadelphia, WB Saunders, 1987.

Martin R: Endocrine Physiology. New York, Oxford University Press, 1985.

McDonald LE, Pineda MH (eds): Veterinary Endocrinology and Reproduction, 4th ed. Philadelphia, Lea & Febiger, 1989.

Tepperman J, Tepperman HM: Metabolic and Endocrine Physiology, 5th ed. Chicago, Year Book Medical Publishers, 1987.

Wilson JD, Foster DW: Williams Textbook of Endocrinology, 7th ed. Philadelphia, WB Saunders, 1985.

PRACTICE QUESTIONS FOR CHAPTER 33

1. The other main hormone secreted by the thyroid gland, in addition to tetraiodothyronine and triodothyronine, is

   a. calcitonin.
   b. insulin.
   c. parathyroid hormone.
   d. glucagon.
   e. somatostatin.

2. The most important function of mineralocorticoids is

   a. control of carbohydrate metabolism.
   b. control of glucose metabolism.
   c. control of electrolyte metabolism.
   d. control of protein metabolism.

3. The pancreas has four types of cells, each of which produce a specific hormone. For

example, the α cells of the pancreas produce

a. insulin.
b. glucagon.
c. somatostatin.
d. pancreatic polypeptide.

4. Two hormones play an important role in calcium homeostasis. The two hormones, _____ and _____ , cause an increase and a decrease in calcium concentrations, respectively.

a. calcitonin .... glucagon
b. somatostatin ....calcitonin
c. calcitonin .... parathyroid hormone
d. parathyroid hormone ....calcitonin
e. parathyroid hormone .... glucagon

5. The main functions of the catecholamines are to allow rapid body responses to acute stimuli, which include the mobilization of glucose. The catecholamines are secreted by the sympathetic portion of the autonomic nervous system. The hormone _____ is the main neurotransmitter of the sympathetic nervous system, whereas _____ is the main hormone produced by the postganglionic fibers of the adrenal medulla.

a. serotonin ....epinephrine
b. epinephrine ....serotonin
c. epinephrine ....norepinephrine
d. norepinephrine ....epinephrine
e. serotonin .... melatonin

GEORGE H. STABENFELDT

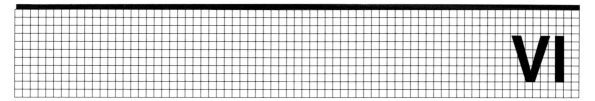

REPRODUCTION/ LACTATION

34

Control of Gonadal and Gamete Development

DEVELOPMENT OF THE REPRODUCTIVE SYSTEM

1. The organization of the gonads is under genetic control
2. The sexual organization of the genitalia and brain depends on the presence (or absence) of testosterone

HYPOTHALAMO-PITUITARY CONTROL OF REPRODUCTION

1. The hypothalamus and anterior pituitary secrete protein and peptide hormones, which control gonadal activity
2. The adenohypophysis (pars distalis) produces FSH, LH and prolactin, all of which control reproductive processes

MODIFICATION OF GONADOTROPIN RELEASE

OVARIAN FOLLICLE DEVELOPMENT

1. Gamete development occurs initially without gonadotropin support, subsequently with pulsatile gonadotropin secretion
2. In the preantral follicle, gonadotropin receptors develop on the theca for LH, which results in androgen synthesis; FSH direction of the granulosa causes it to transform the androgens to estrogens
3. Late in the ovarian follicular phase, LH receptors develop on the granulosa, which allows the preovulatory surge of LH to cause ovulation

DEVELOPMENT OF THE REPRODUCTIVE SYSTEM

The Organization of the Gonads Is Under Genetic Control

The initial development of the embryonic ovary involves the migration of germ cells into the genital ridge from the yolk sac. The primordial germ cells populate sex cords that have formed in the cortical region of the gonad from the proliferation of cells from the *coelomic epithelium* (so-called germinal epithelium) of the *genital ridge* (Fig. 34–1). The sex cords contribute cells, known initially as follicle cells and subsequently as *granulosa cells,* that immediately surround the oocyte. The mesenchyme of the genital ridge contributes cells that will become the theca. The entire structure is called a *follicle,* which includes oocyte, granulosa, and theca cells.

There are no direct connections formed between the oocytes and the tubes destined to become the oviducts, which are derived from *müllerian ducts.* The final result is that oocytes are released through the surface of the ovary by rupture of tissue elements that surround the ovary; this process is called *ovulation.* A specialized end of the oviduct, the fimbria, develops to enable the oocyte to be removed efficiently from the surface of the ovary. Some animals funnel oocytes to the fimbria through the use of a bursa, which tends to encompass the ovary with oocytes directed to a relatively small opening in the bursa.

The development of the embryonic testis has similarities with that of the ovary; germ cells migrate into the genital ridge and populate sex cords that have formed from an invagination of the surface (coelomic) epithelium. *Sertoli cells* (female counterpart: granulosa cells) develop from the sex cords, and *Leydig's cells* (female counterpart: thecal cells) develop from the mesenchyme of the genital ridge. One fundamental difference from ovarian development is that the invagination of the sex cords in the male continues into the medulla of the embryonic gonad, where connections are made with medullary cords from the mesonephros, or primitive kidney. The duct of the mesonephros (wolffian duct) becomes the epididymis, vas deferens, and urethra, which has a direct connection to the seminiferous tubules. Thus, male germ cells pass to the exterior of the animal through a closed tubular system.

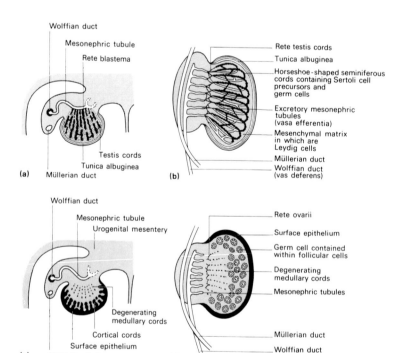

Figure 34–1. Testicular development during (*a*) the eighth and (*b*) the sixteenth to twentieth weeks of human fetal life. (*a*) The primitive sex cords proliferate in the medulla and establish contact with the rete testis. The tunica albuginea (fibrous connective tissue) separates the testis cords from the coelomic epithelium and eventually forms the capsule of the testis. (*b*) Note the horseshoe shape of the seminiferous cords and their continuity with the rete testis cords. The vasa efferentia, derived from the excretory mesonephric tubules, connect the seminiferous cords with the wolffian duct (see text). Comparable diagrams of ovarian development around (*c*) the seventh and (*d*) the twentieth to twenty-fourth weeks of development. (*c*) Any primitive medullary sex cords degenerate and are replaced by the well-vascularized ovarian stroma. The cortex proliferates, and mesenchymal condensations later develop around the arriving primordial germ cells. (*d*) In the absence of medullary cords and a true persistent rete ovarii, no communication is established with the mesonephric tubules. Hence, in the adult, ova are shed from the surface of the ovary and are not transported by tubules to the oviduct. (From Johnson M, Everitt B (eds): Essential Reproduction, 3rd ed. London, Blackwell Scientific Publications, 1988, p 9.)

Labels for figure (a): Wolffian duct; Mesonephric tubule; Rete blastema; Testis cords; Tunica albuginea; Müllerian duct

Labels for figure (b): Rete testis cords; Tunica albuginea; Horseshoe-shaped seminiferous cords containing Sertoli cell precursors and germ cells; Excretory mesonephric tubules (vasa efferentia); Mesenchymal matrix in which are Leydig cells; Müllerian duct; Wolffian duct (vas deferens)

Labels for figure (c): Wolffian duct; Mesonephric tubule; Urogenital mesentery; Degenerating medullary cords; Cortical cords; Surface epithelium; Müllerian duct

Labels for figure (d): Rete ovarii; Surface epithelium; Germ cell contained within follicular cells; Degenerating medullary cords; Mesonephric tubules; Müllerian duct; Wolffian duct

The Sexual Organization of the Genitalia and Brain Depends on the Presence (or Absence) of Testosterone

The development of the genital tubular system and the external genitalia are under control of the developing gonad. If the individual is female, i.e., the developing gonad is an ovary, the müllerian duct develops into oviduct, uterus, cervix, and vagina, whereas the wolffian duct regresses; the absence of testosterone is important for both changes (Fig. 34–2). If the individual is male, müllerian inhibiting factor is produced by the rete testis, which causes regression of the müllerian ducts. The wolffian duct is maintained in the male because of the influence of androgens produced by the testis. To summarize, the müllerian ducts are "permanent" structures,

and the wolffian ducts are "temporary" structures unless acted upon by the presence of male hormones. The presence of an enzyme, 5α-reductase, is important for the effect of the androgens, because testosterone must be converted intracellularly into dihydrotestosterone for masculinization of the tissues to occur.

Development of the external genitalia follows the development and direction of the gonads. If the individual is female in genotype, folds of tissue called *labia* form the *vulva*, and a *clitoris* develops. If the individual is male, androgens from the testis direct formation of the *penis* (female counterpart: clitoris) and the *scrotum* (female counterpart: labia). Again, the absence or presence of androgens is an important factor influencing the formation of external genitalia.

The final organization of the individual re-

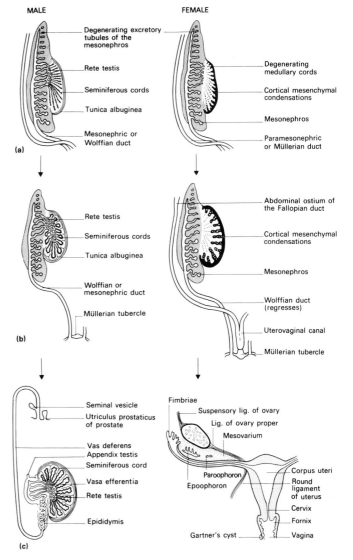

Figure 34–2. Differentiation of the internal genitalia in the human male and female at (*a*) the sixth week, (*b*) the fourth month, and (*c*) the time of descent of testis and ovary. Note that the müllerian and wolffian ducts are present in both sexes early on, the müllerian ducts eventually regressing in the male and persisting in the female, and the wolffian ducts regressing in the female and persisting in the male. The appendix testis and utriculus prostaticus in the male, and epoöphoron, paroöphoron and Gartner's cyst in the female, are remnants of the degenerated müllerian and wolffian ducts, respectively. (From Johnson M, Everitt B (eds): Essential Reproduction, 3rd ed. London, Blackwell Scientific Publications, 1988, p 10.)

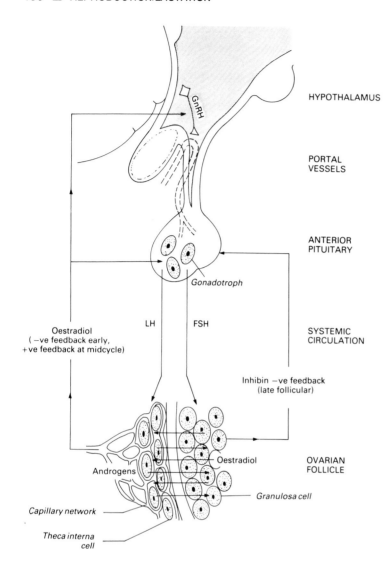

HYPOTHALAMUS

PORTAL VESSELS

ANTERIOR PITUITARY

Gonadotroph

LH   FSH

Oestradiol
(−ve feedback early,
+ve feedback at midcycle)

SYSTEMIC CIRCULATION

Inhibin −ve feedback
(late follicular)

Oestradiol

OVARIAN FOLLICLE

Androgens

Granulosa cell

Capillary network

Theca interna cell

Figure 34–3. Summary of hypothalamo-pituitary-ovarian interactions during the follicular phase of the cycle. (From Johnson M, Everitt B (eds). Essential Reproduction, 3rd ed. London, Blackwell Scientific Publications, 1988, p 151.)

garding gender comes with sexual differentiation of the hypothalamus. Exposure of the hypothalamus to androgens at around the time of birth causes the hypothalamus to be organized as male. A paradoxical finding is that enzymes (aromatases) must be present in neural tissue for masculinization to occur, with conversion (aromatization) of androgens to estrogens an essential biochemical change for maleness. In the absence of androgens, the hypothalamus is organized as female.

The fundamental concept of organization of the reproductive system regarding genotype is that the female system is organized in the absence of a testis. If the individual is to be male, there must be active intervention by the testis through the production of androgens and appropriate tissue enzymes in two circumstances: (1) within the internal genitalia for conversion to more potent androgens, and (2) within the hypothalamus for conversion to estrogens.

HYPOTHALAMO-PITUITARY CONTROL OF REPRODUCTION

The Hypothalamus and Anterior Pituitary Secrete Protein and Peptide Hormones, Which Control Gonadal Activity

Gonadal activity is under the control of both the *hypothalamus* and the *anterior pituitary* (Fig. 34–3). The hypothalamus is a relatively small structure that lies midcentral in the base of the brain. It is divided into halves by the third ventricle and, in actuality, forms the ventral and lateral walls of the third ventricle. The hypothalamus has clusters of neurons, collectively called nuclei, that secrete peptide hormones important for controlling pituitary activity. As described in more detail later, these peptides move to the pituitary either directly by passage through the axons of neurons, or by a blood vascular portal system. The pituitary responds to the hypothalamic peptides to produce hormones that are important for the control of the gonads.

The Adenohypophysis (Pars Distalis) Produces FSH, LH and Prolactin, All of Which Control Reproductive Processes

The pituitary is composed of three parts: an anterior lobe called the *adenohypophysis* or *pars distalis;* an intermediate lobe called the *pars intermedia;* and a posterior lobe called the *neurohypophysis* or *pars nervosa.* The lobes are of different embryological origins; the pars distalis is from the endoectoderm (derived from a small diverticulum off the dorsal pharynx, called Rathke's pouch), and the pars intermedia and pars nervosa are derived from neuroectoderm. The adenohypophysis produces protein hormones that are important for the control of reproduction, namely, two gonadotropins, *follicle-stimulating hormone (FSH)* and *luteinizing hormone (LH),* and a third hormone called *prolactin;* other pituitary hormones include *growth hormone (GH), adrenocorticotropic hormone (ACTH),* and *thyrotropic hormone (TSH).* FSH and LH are synergistic in the development and ovulation of ovarian follicles; FSH plays a more dominant role during the growth of follicles, and LH plays a more dominant role during the final stages of follicle maturation through ovulation. The gonadotropins, as well as TSH, are called *glycoproteins,* because their molecules contain carbohydrate moieties that contribute to their function. *Oxytocin* is the hormone of importance for reproduction, which is produced by the neurohypophysis.

Besides being an important center for control of reproduction, the hypothalamus regulates appetite and temperature, and integrates the activity of the autonomic nervous system. Because of a common embryological origin, the hypothalamus has a direct connection to the neurohypophysis. This connection is by the neural stalk, which contains axons that originate from neuronal cell bodies located in the hypothalamus. Two sets of neurons within

the hypothalamus, the *supraoptic* and *paraventricular nuclei,* are responsible for the synthesis of *vasopressin* and oxytocin, respectively. These small peptide hormones are coupled to larger peptide molecules, called *neurophysins,* and are transported from the site of synthesis in the hypothalamus (neuronal cell bodies) through axons to the site of storage and eventual release, i.e., the neurohypophysis.

The connection of the hypothalamus to the adenohypophysis does not involve the direct passage of axons through the *neural stalk.* A *venous portal system* connects the median eminence within the hypothalamus to the adenohypophysis. Hypothalamic substances that control the adenohypophysis are carried from the median eminence of the hypothalamus to the pituitary by a venous portal system. For example, *GnRH,* a peptide, is produced in the medial preoptic nucleus, and dopamine, an amino acid, is produced in the *arcuate nucleus.* Both substances are transported from the hypothalamus to the *median eminence* by axons, where they are released into the venous portal system. The synthesis of GnRH, like oxytocin and vasopressin, involves the production of a larger precursor molecule with a C-terminal region of 56 amino acids called *GnRH-associated peptide,* or *GAP.* Although GAP can stimulate the release of FSH and LH, GnRH is still thought to be the critical hormone for gonadotropin release. An even more important function of GAP may be its ability to inhibit prolactin secretion.

MODIFICATION OF GONADOTROPIN RELEASE

The main secretory pattern of gonadotropins is *pulsatile* in form; the pattern is driven by pulsatile secretion of GnRH from the hypothalamus (Fig. 34–4). The importance of this mode of delivery is shown by the fact that if GnRH is administered in a continuous (pharmacological) manner, the system can be downregulated. Continual occupancy of GnRH receptors on gonadotrophs by GnRH interrupts the intracellular signal for the synthesis and release of gonadotropins.

In general, the *pulse generator system* for gonadotropin secretion is increased in the *follicular phase* and decreased in the *luteal phase* of the estrous cycle (Fig. 34–5). Estrogen decreases the pulse amplitude, and progesterone decreases the pulse frequency of gonadotropin

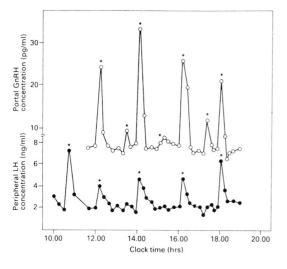

Figure 34–4. Concentrations of GnRH in portal plasma (○ — ○) and LH in jugular venous plasma (● — ●) of four ovariectomized ewes. Asterisks indicate secretory episodes (pulses) of GnRH and LH. (From Johnson M, Everitt B (eds): Essential Reproduction, 3rd ed. London, Blackwell Scientific Publications, 1988, p 110.)

secretion. This means that during the follicular phase, pulse frequency increases because of the absence of progesterone, and pulse amplitude decreases because of the presence of estrogen. This combination of increased pulse frequency and decreased pulse amplitude is important for nurturing the final growth phase of the developing antral follicle.

The hypothalamus and adenohypophysis are capable of responding to a sustained increase in estrogen secretion by increased secretion of gonadotropins, a relationship that is termed *positive feedback*. The sustained increase in estrogen concentrations, which occurs over one to several days during final antral follicle development, causes an increase in gonadotropin secretion by increasing the frequency of pulsatile release of GnRH and, as a result, gonadotropin secretion. In essence, the frequency of pulsatile release of gonadotropins overcomes the metabolic clearance rate. The purpose of the gonadotropin surge is to induce changes within the follicle that lead to its rupture (ovulation). The duration of the gonadotropin surge is relatively short (usually 12–24 hours), possibly because the main factor driving the response, estrogen, declines in concentration as the follicle(s) respond to the preovulatory gonadotropin surge. This particular physiological mechanism for initiating the onset of ovulation is effective, because the follicle is able to signal its stage of maturity to the hypothalamus and adenohypophysis by a product (estrogen) that is produced in increasing amounts with increasing follicle maturity.

The secretion of gonadotropins is modified by the ovarian steroid hormones *estrogen* and *progesterone*. For the most part, the effect of these hormones is suppressive for gonadotropin secretion. Estrogens, in particular, are able to effect *negative feedback inhibition* of gonadotropin secretion, which is characterized by its sensitivity (effective at low concentrations) and its rapid onset (within a few hours). The large increase in gonadotropin concentrations that occurs following ovariectomy is largely due to the removal of estrogens.

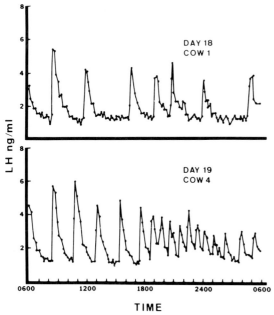

Figure 34–5. Pattern of plasma LH concentration on day 18 or 19 of the estrous cycle in two cows. (From Rahe CH, Ownens RE, Fleeger JL, et al: Pattern of plasma luteinizing hormone in the cyclic cow: Dependence upon the period of the cycle. Endocrinology 107:498, 1980.)

Because progesterone affects gonadotropin pulse frequency, it is thought that its modulatory effect is at the level of the hypothalamus. Estrogens are thought to affect gonadotropin secretion through an effect on both the pituitary and the hypothalamus. Although there are differences in site of action among species, it appears that the hypothalamic site for negative feedback inhibition of gonadotropins by both progesterone and estrogen is in an area immediately above the median eminence, known as the *arcuate nucleus*. The hypothalamic site for positive feedback stimulation of gonadotropin release by estrogen is likely further anterior, i.e., in the *preoptic anterior hypothalamic region*.

The secretion of gonadotropins can be modified by peptide and protein hormones produced by both the hypothalamus and ovary. Beta-Endorphin, an opioid peptide produced from the hypothalamic precursor molecule *proopiomelanocortin*, can inhibit LH secretion when administered systemically. Its role in the physiological modulation of gonadotropin secretion, however, remains to be identified. Another hormone, *inhibin*, a protein produced by the granulosa of the developing follicle, also inhibits gonadotropin secretion, particularly FSH, during the final stages of follicle development. As described under the section on folliculogenesis, this depression of FSH secretion may be important to the animal for controlling the number of follicles that are brought to final maturation.

Control of gonadotropin secretion in the male is similar to the female; pulses of GnRH, arising in the hypothalamus, affect pulsatile secretion of the gonadotropins. This, in turn, causes the secretion of testosterone, also in pulsatile form, from the testis. One major difference between the sexes is that the need for positive feedback release of gonadotropins in males does not exist; gametes are produced and released on a continuous basis within a tubular system that opens to the exterior. This negates any need for a surge release of gonadotropins as is required in the female to rupture the ovarian surface for the release of oocytes.

Prolactin is the third hormone produced by the adenohypophysis that is important in the reproductive process, mainly for its effect on the mammary gland and lactation in mammals. Although the secretion of prolactin is pulsatile, the control of secretion has more emphasis on inhibition than stimulation of secretion. This concept is supported by the finding that prolactin secretion increases if the pituitary is disconnected from the hypothalamus by either cutting the pituitary stalk or transplanting the pituitary to another site (e.g., kidney capsule). Thus, most attention has been given to factors that inhibit prolactin secretion. The catecholamine *dopamine,* which is produced by neurons in the ventral hypothalamus (arcuate nucleus), is a potent inhibitor of prolactin secretion (Fig. 34–6). Other factors that inhibit prolactin secretion are *GABA* (gamma amino butyric acid) and *GAP.* Dopamine agonists, such as the ergot type compound *bromocriptine,* can be used to suppress prolactin secretion in cases of *hyperprolactinemia.* The negative feedback control of prolactin is shown in Figure 34–6.

One of the first known prolactin releasing factors was thyrotropin-releasing hormone (TRH). The physiological relevance of TRH in prolactin secretion is still unknown in spite of the fact that receptors for TRH have been identified on lactotrophs within the adenohypophysis. *Vasoactive intestinal peptide (VIP),* a potent stimulator of prolactin, may play a physiological role in prolactin secretion through inhibition of dopamine synthesis within the hypothalamus. Estrogens can increase prolactin secretion by lactotrophs by decreasing lac-

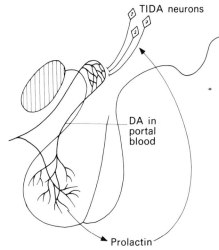

Figure 34–6. Diagrammatic summary of the proposed negative-feedback relationship between prolactin and dopamine. Prolactin is believed to accelerate dopamine (*DA*) turnover in the arcuate nucleus neurons (tuberoinfundibular dopamine or *TIDA* neurons), and the amine is then released into the portal capillaries to gain access to the lactotropes. Hyperprolactinemia could be caused by either a failure of PIF activity at the dopamine receptor level in the anterior pituitary or a reduction of TIDA neuron activity in the hypothalamus. (From Johnson M, Everitt B (eds): Essential Reproduction, 3rd ed. London, Blackwell Scientific Publications, 1988, p 138.)

totroph sensitivity to dopamine and increasing the number of TRH receptors.

OVARIAN FOLLICLE DEVELOPMENT

Gamete Development Occurs Initially Without Gonadotropin Support, Subsequently with Pulsatile Gonadotropin Secretion

Oocyte proliferation, which occurs by *mitotic division* during fetal development, ends at about the time of birth for most mammalian species. Oocytes begin the process of reduction of chromosome numbers to the haploid state by *meiosis* shortly after birth under the influence of *meiosis initiating factor*, thought to be produced by the *rete ovarii*. The process is soon interrupted at *diplotene*, or *dictyate*, stage of meiosis I by the meiosis inhibiting factor, which is likely produced by the developing follicle cells. Oocytes remain in this stage until the follicle begins its final development, an interval that can be as long as 50-plus years in humans. The *follicle*, at this point, is delineated by an outer basement membrane (*membrana propria*), which is secreted by the follicle cells.

The initial development of the follicle involves growth of the *oocyte*. This growth is accompanied by intense synthetic activity with a large amount of RNA being synthesized. At the same time, follicle cells begin to divide and form a granulosa of several cells in thickness. The granulosa cells then secrete another boundary substance, the *zona pellucida*, that is interior to the granulosa and that immediately surrounds the oocyte. Granulosa cells maintain contact with the oocyte through the zona pellucida through the development of cytoplasmic processes. Interaction among granulosa cells is facilitated by the development of *gap junctions*. This form of communication is important, because the granulosa is without blood supply; blood vessels are excluded at the level of the membrana propria. The theca layer of the follicle forms around the membrana propria to complete the layers of the follicle. Follicles at this stage are called primary, or *preantral*, *follicles*.

Factors that control initial follicle growth are not known. External factors, such as gonadotropins, are not required, because hypophysectomized animals can develop preantral follicles. In species such as cattle and horses (perhaps sheep and goats, also) wherein several dominant follicles develop during the estrous cycle, it is likely that a few follicles begin to develop each day. In animals that develop a cohort of follicles synchronously (pigs, cats, dogs), there appears to be less tendency to have competing follicle growth waves during the luteal phase (pig), or only one cohort of follicles during the preovulatory period (cat and dog). Thus, the development of a cohort of follicles may restrain, or limit, follicle development from the primordial state, at least during the period of active follicle development leading to ovulation. It is obvious that initial follicle growth is under genetic control, and the pattern reflects the needs of the particular species.

In the Preantral Follicle, Gonadotropin Receptors Develop on the Theca for LH, Which Results in Androgen Synthesis; FSH Direction of the Granulosa Causes it to Transform the Androgens to Estrogens

In order for follicles to progress beyond the preantral stage, the granulosa and theca need to develop *receptors* for gonadotropins. FSH and LH receptors develop on the granulosa and theca, respectively. The onset of the antral follicle is marked by the appearance of fluid that begins to divide the granulosa. The follicular fluid, a secretory product of the granulosa, coalesces to form an increasingly larger fluid cavity (*antrum*) within the granulosa. In later development of the antral follicle, the oocyte remains surrounded by a layer of granulosa cells called the *cumulus oophorus*, which are attached to the wall of the follicle by a small stalk of granulosa cells.

The presence of different receptors for gonadotropins on the granulosa and thecal cells results in a cooperative effort concerning estrogen synthesis (Fig. 34–7). The *theca* produces *androgens* (testosterone and androstenedione) under the influence of LH, which diffuses across the membrana propria into the *granulosa*, where it is transformed into *estrogen* (estradiol-17β). At this time of development, the granulosa is incapable of forming androgens, the precursors of estrogen biosynthesis, and the theca has limited capacity to produce estrogens. This concept, called the *two-cell mechanism* for estrogen secretion, is generally accepted as being the way most follicular estrogen is produced. These estrogens have a

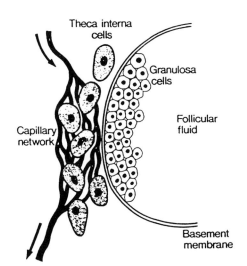

Figure 34–7. The structure of the wall of the graafian follicle, showing how the granulosa cells are deprived of a blood supply by the basement membrane. (From Austin CR, Short RV (eds): Germ cells and fertilization. Reproduction in Mammals, Vol 1. Cambridge, Cambridge University Press, 1982.)

positive feedback effect upon the granulosa; they stimulate the cells to undergo mitotic division and, thus, the follicle grows in size as the granulosa proliferates in response to its own secretory product (estrogen).

One effect of estrogen is the formation of additional receptors for FSH as follicle development proceeds. In this situation, the antral follicle becomes increasingly sensitive to FSH as it develops, and is able to grow under a relatively steady state of FHS secretion.

Late in the Ovarian Follicular Phase, LH Receptors Develop on the Granulosa, Which Allows the Preovulatory Surge of LH to Cause Ovulation

Late in antral follicle development, FSH and estrogens initiate the formation of LH receptors on the granulosa, whereas FSH receptors begin to diminish. Increasing secretion of estrogen by the antral follicle finally results in the initiation of the *preovulatory surge of gonadotropins.* Thus, in the last stages of development, the follicle falls progressively under the control of LH as it makes its last growth spurt to the point of ovulation.

CLINICAL CORRELATION

ANDROGEN INSENSITIVITY

HISTORY □ You are called to examine a mare that has recently been brought to a brood-mare farm after a successful racing career. (The mare's name, Awful Alice, turns out to be prophetic!) It is late spring, yet the mare has shown estrous behavior only on an intermittent basis.

CLINICAL EXAMINATION □ As you approach the mare you notice that she is a large, raw-boned animal. The genital examination reveals a normal vulva, but when you introduce the speculum it can be inserted only about 5–6 inches. Digital examination of the genital tract through the vulva results in a finding of complete blockage at the level of the vestibulo-vaginal conjunction with no evidence for the presence of the external os of the cervix. Upon doing an examination *per rectum,* you find the vagina, cervix, uterus, and oviducts to be absent; the gonads are symmetrical in shape without the usual indentation caused by the ovulation fossa that is characteristic of equine ovaries.

COMMENT □ You tell the shocked owner that you are suspicious that the animal is not, in fact, a mare, but a male masquerading as a female. One of the easiest ways to confirm the diagnosis is to have a testosterone analysis done on plasma. If the gonads are testes, they still will retain the ability to secrete significant amounts of testosterone even though they are retained (cryptorchid, in a sense) within the abdominal cavity. You could also have a chromosomal analysis to verify that the animal has an XY sex chromosome complement. In this case, it is likely that the testes were able to secrete the *müllerian inhibiting factor,* which resulted in regression of the tubular system of the genital tract that forms the female system, i.e., oviducts, uterus, cervix, and vagina. But why, asks the owner, didn't the external genitalia turn out to be male? There is evidence, in cases such as this, that the tissues of the external genitalia lacked critical receptors for androgens; thus, the external genitalia were female in type. The rule of sexual development is that the female state develops in the absence of testicular input, the latter including müllerian inhibiting factor and testosterone. In this case, the lack of sexual differentiation also appeared to involve the hypothalamus, because the "mare" did not exhibit male behavior in spite of relatively high testosterone concentrations.

TREATMENT □ There is obviously no treatment for this syndrome. It would be unethical to take her back to the track and race her once again as a female, when the owner knows that "she" is a he.

Bibliography

Austin CR, Short RV (eds): Reproduction in Mammals, Vols 1–6. Cambridge, Cambridge University Press, 1976, 1982, 1984, 1986.

Cupps PT (ed): Reproduction in Domestic Animals, 4th ed. New York, Academic Press, 1991.

Concannon PW, Morton DB, Weir BJ (eds): Dog and cat reproduction, contraception and artificial insemination. J Reprod Fertil (Suppl) 39, 1989.

Feldman EC, Nelson RW: Canine and Feline Endocrinology and Reproduction. Philadelphia, WB Saunders, 1987.

Hafez EWE (ed): Reproduction in Farm Animals, 5th ed. Philadelphia, Lea and Febiger, 1987.

Johnson M, Everitt B (eds): Essential Reproduction, 3rd ed. London, Blackwell Scientific Publications, 1988.

Knobil E, Neill JD, Ewing LL, et al (eds): The Physiology of Reproduction, Vols 1, 2. New York, Raven Press, 1988.

McDonald LE, Pineda MH (eds): Veterinary Endocrinology and Reproduction, 4th ed. Philadelphia, Lea and Febiger, 1989.

PRACTICE QUESTIONS FOR CHAPTER 34

1. Which of the following statements is true?

   a. Müllerian ducts develop in the female because of the presence of estrogen.
   b. Müllerian ducts develop in the female because of a müllerian stimulating factor.
   c. Wolffian ducts develop in the male because of a wolffian stimulating factor.
   d. Wolffian ducts develop in the male because of the presence of androgen.

2. The most potent factor involved in the organization of the internal and external parts of the genital tract is

   a. müllerian inhibiting factor.
   b. müllerian stimulating factor.
   c. estrogen.
   d. androgen.

3. Which of the following groups of hormones is transported to the anterior pituitary by the hypothalamo-hypophyseal portal system?

   a. Oxytocin, GnRH, and dopamine
   b. GnRH, dopamine, and vasopressin
   c. Dopamine, vasopressin, and oxytocin
   d. Dopamine and GnRH

4. Which of the following groups of hormones controls the synthesis and release of hypophyseal hormones involved in reproductive processes?

   a. Oxytocin, GnRH, VIP, and dopamine
   b. GnRH, dopamine, VIP, and vasopressin
   c. Dopamine, vasopressin, VIP, and oxytocin
   d. GAP, dopamine, VIP, and GnRH
   e. GAP, GnRH, VIP, and oxytocin

5. Which of the following factors is responsible for causing oocytes to remain in an undifferentiated state?

   a. Müllerian inhibiting factor
   b. Müllerian stimulating factor
   c. Meiosis inhibiting factor
   d. Meiosis stimulating factor
   e. Wolffian inhibiting factor
   f. Wolffian stimulating factor

35

Control of Ovulation and the Corpus Luteum

OVULATION

1. Ovulatory follicles are selected at the onset of luteolysis (large domestic animals)
2. Ovulation is caused by an estrogen-induced preovulatory surge of gonadotropins

CORPUS LUTEUM

1. The corpus luteum secretes progesterone, which is essential for pregnancy
2. Luteinizing hormone is important for the maintenance of the corpus luteum
3. Regression of the corpus luteum in nonpregnant large domestic animals is controlled by uterine secretion of prostaglandin F–2α
4. Changes in luteal life span in large domestic animals occur because of changes in prostaglandin F–2α synthesis by the uterus

OVARIAN CYCLES

1. In spontaneously ovulating animals, ovarian cycles have two phases—follicular and luteal; animals that require copulation for ovulation have only a follicular phase
2. The luteal phase is modified by copulation in some species

OVULATION

Ovulatory Follicles Are Selected at the Onset of Luteolysis (Large Domestic Animals)

Until the advent of ultrasonography, it was difficult to identify growth patterns of follicles in domestic animals, especially those that develop during the luteal phase of the cycle. The concept that follicles do develop during the luteal phase was emphasized by the earlier work of the scientist, Rajakowski, who described the midcycle follicle in the cow. With ultrasonography, it has been possible to define follicular growth and regression during the luteal phase of the cycle in the cow and mare. In cattle, the predominant pattern is for several dominant (large) antral follicles to develop sequentially during the cycle (Fig. 35–1). The follicular cycles are distinct to the extent that

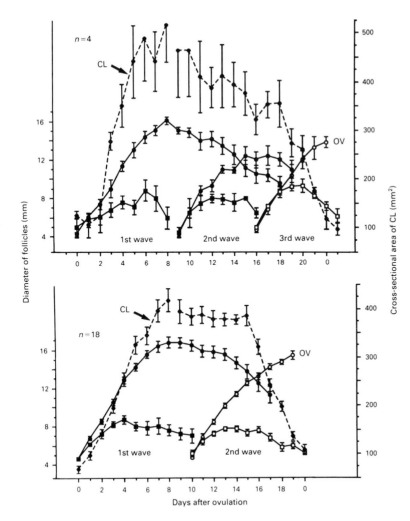

Figure 35–1. Mean (± s.e.m.) profiles of diameters of dominant follicles and the largest subordinate follicle and the cross-sectional luteinized area of the corpus luteum (*CL*) for the interovulatory intervals with 3 and 2 follicular waves in cattle. Regression (*P* < 0.05) of the corpus luteum began between days 18 and 20 for 3-wave intervals and between days 15 and 16 for 2-wave intervals. *OV*, ovulation. (From Ginther OJ, Knopf L, Kastelic JP: Temporal associations among ovarian events in cattle during oestrous cycles with two and three follicular waves. J Reprod Fertil 87:223, 1989.)

follicle regression usually begins (as indicated by follicle size) prior to the onset of the growth of the next follicle. The first dominant follicle regresses about midluteal phase, with a second dominant follicle beginning growth immediately. Whether the second dominant follicle is the ovulatory follicle, or whether a third develops, depends on the stage of the follicle at the time of regression of the *corpus luteum* (*CL*). If the second dominant follicle has begun to regress at the time of CL regression, a third follicle develops. Thus, the selection of the ovulatory follicle is, by chance, the dominant follicle that is still in a developmental stage late at the time regression of the CL is initiated. The duration required for the development of the antral follicle to the point of ovulation has been estimated by various techniques to be about 10 days in domestic animals, perhaps slightly longer in some primates.

From ultrasonographical and endocrinolog-

ical studies, it appears that there are two different phases in final antral follicle development in large domestic animals: a relatively slow one that lasts for 4–5 days, followed by a second phase of accelerated growth, again lasting 4–5 days, that terminates in ovulation (Fig. 35–2). Because the final growth phase of follicle development can be initiated during the luteal phase, it is apparent that the initiation of this phase can occur under the influence of a relatively slow pulse rate of gonadotropin release that occurs during the luteal phase. The rapidly-growing follicle requires exposure to a faster gonadotropin pulse rate by the third, or fourth, day in order for the follicle(s) to complete its normal growth pattern through ovulation. This situation usually occurs in conjunction with the onset of CL regression, which passively allows an increase in pulsatile rate of gonadotropin secretion (see Fig. 34–4).

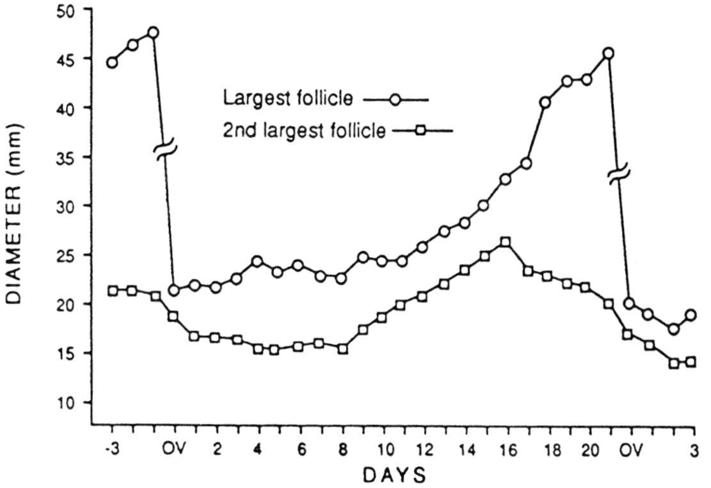

Figure 35–2. Development of the dominant and second largest follicle during the estrous cycle of the mare. Note the divergence in diameter between the largest and second largest follicles 1 day after ovulation. (From Pierson RA, Ginther OJ: Follicular population dynamics during the estrous cycle of the mare. Anim Repro Sci 14:219, 1987.)

One of the ways the dominant follicle maintains its status is to produce substances that inhibit the development of other antral follicles. One of the substances is *inhibin*, a peptide hormone produced by the granulosa, which inhibits the secretion of FSH. The dominant follicle is able to compensate for the lower FSH concentrations and continue to grow because of the numbers of FSH receptors it has compared to competitor follicles. Follicle development is dynamic once the rapid growth phase is achieved; the follicle(s) must be acted upon through proper gonadotropin stimulation within a few days, or the result is death of the follicle. If the rapidly growing antral follicle is not exposed to the proper gonadotropin environment, *atresia* (regression) of the follicle begins almost immediately. Follicles that regress are invaded by inflammatory cells, and the area previously occupied by the antral follicle is eventually filled by connective tissue, i.e., the follicle is replaced by an ovarian scar.

Ovulation Is Caused by an Estrogen-Induced Preovulatory Surge of Gonadotropins

The preovulatory surge of luteinizing hormone (LH), which begins about 24 hours before ovulation in most domestic species, including the cow, dog, goat, pig, and sheep, initiates the critical changes in the follicle that affect its endocrine organ status and result in release of the oocyte (Fig. 35–3). Two important tissues, the oocyte and the granulosa, have been kept under control by the production of inhibitory substances that are probably of granulosa origin. One is an *oocyte inhibiting factor*, which prevents the oocyte from resuming meiosis, and another is a *luteinizing inhibiting factor*, which prevents the granulosa from prematurely being changed into luteal tissue. The impact of the LH surge blocks the production of both of these factors. In most animals, the resumption of meiosis results in the first division of meiosis (meiosis I), or formation of the *first polar body*, which is complete prior to ovulation. In animals with the potential for reasonably long reproductive longevity, e.g., cattle, the initiation of the meiotic process could have begun as long as 10, or more, years prior to its completion.

The effect of the LH surge on the granulosa is to allow the initiation of the process of luteinization, one that transforms the cells from estrogen to progesterone secretion. This process is underway before ovulation occurs. With the advent of the LH surge, estrogen secretion declines concomitantly with the onset of progesterone secretion.

Another function of the preovulatory surge release of LH is to cause the granulosa to produce substances, such as *relaxin* and *prostaglandin F–2α*, which affect the continuity of the connective tissue of the thecal layers of the follicle. These and other unknown substances disrupt the theca through the development of vesicles (within fibrocytes) that contain hydrolytic enzymes capable of breaking down the collagen matrix of connective tissue; the rupture of the follicle is due to the disintegration of the connective tissue.

In summary, estrogen is used by the follicle(s) (1) to stimulate the growth and devel-

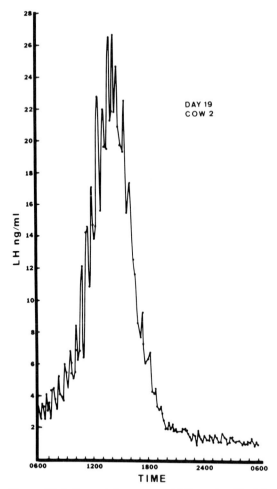

Figure 35–3. Preovulatory surge of LH on day 19 of the estrous cycle in a cow. (From Rahe CH, Owens RE, Fleeger JL, et al. Pattern of plasma luteinizing hormone in the cyclic cow: Dependence upon the period of the cycle. Endocrinology 107:498, 1980.)

opment of the granulosa, and (2) to signal the hypothalamus and anterior pituitary as to the readiness of the follicle(s) for ovulation.

CORPUS LUTEUM

The Corpus Luteum Secretes Progesterone, Which Is Essential for Pregnancy

The main function of the CL is the secretion of progesterone, which prepares the uterus for the initiation and maintenance of pregnancy.

The CL forms from the wall of the follicle, which is collapsed and folded following ovulation. With rupture of the follicle, there is a breakdown of the tissues that surround the

granulosa, particularly the membrana propria, and hemorrhage into the cavity can occur from vessels in the theca. The folds of tissue that protrude inward into the cavity contain granulosa and theca cells and, very importantly, the blood vascular system that will support cell growth and differentiation. Although the granulosa cell is the dominant cell of the CL, theca cells also contribute significantly to the composition of the structure. The process that granulosa cells undergo during the change from estrogen to progesterone secretion, i.e., *luteinization,* begins with the onset of the preovulatory LH surge and accelerates with ovulation. In most domestic species, significant production of progesterone by the CL begins within 24 hours of ovulation. In some species, including the dog and primates, small amounts of progesterone are produced during the preovulatory LH surge; in the dog, this is important for the expression of sexual receptivity.

Luteinizing Hormone Is Important for the Maintenance of the Corpus Luteum

For domestic animals, LH is the important *luteotropin,* with the CL maintained in either nonpregnant or pregnant animals by a relatively slow pulsatile pattern of LH release (one pulse/2–3 hours). In rodents, prolactin is the important luteotrophin; daily biphasic release of prolactin is initiated by copulation, which is essential for the maintenance of CL. Of the domestic species, sheep are the only species for which prolactin has been implicated as a luteotropin.

Normal folliculogenesis, a prerequisite for ovulation, sets the stage, wherein the development of the postovulatory CL is almost always normal. Thus, more attention is paid to factors controlling the regression of the CL than to luteotropic factors.

Regression of the Corpus Luteum in Nonpregnant Large Domestic Animals Is Controlled by Uterine Secretion of Prostaglandin F–2α

Regression of the CL is important in large domestic nonpregnant animals in order that animals re-enter a potentially fertile state as soon as possible. The CL's lifespan following ovulation (in the nonpregnant animal) must be of sufficient duration to allow a newly developing conceptus to synthesize and release factors that allow the CL to be maintained, yet be relatively short so that a non-pregnant animal can return to a potentially fertile state. In large domestic animals, the duration of the luteal phase is about 14 days in the absence of pregnancy. This allows large domestic animals to recycle at relatively frequent intervals, i.e., at about 3-week intervals.

Leo Loeb first showed (in 1923) the importance of the uterus for the regression of the CL through hysterectomy studies that extended the luteal phase in guinea pigs. He concluded that the uterus must produce a substance that terminated luteal activity. This information lay dormant for many years, until hysterectomy studies in cattle, pigs, and sheep in the 1950s produced similar results, i.e., a prolongation of the luteal phase of the estrous cycle. Through these studies, the concept developed that the uterus was responsible for control of the duration of the life span of the CL, at least in large domestic species (and guinea pigs).

It is now accepted that *prostaglandin F(PGF)–2α*, a 20-carbon unsaturated fatty acid, is the uterine substance that causes regression of the CL in large domestic animals, including cattle, goats, horses, pigs, and sheep; PGF–2α has no role in CL regression in cats and dogs, nor in primates. In large domestic species, regression of the CL is initiated by uterine synthesis and release of PGF–2α (likely of endometrial origin) at about 14 days postovulation. The mode of transfer of PGF–2α from the uterus to the ovary is thought to occur either by *local counter-current* or *general systemic transfer*. Counter-current transfer involves the movement of molecules across the blood vascular system from higher concentrations in the venous effluent (utero-ovarian vein) to an area of lower concentration (ovarian artery) (Fig. 35–4). Systemic transfer involves passage of the molecules through the general circulatory system. In some species (cow and ewe), PGF–2α synthesis from a uterine horn only influences the life span of the CL in the ipsilateral ovary. In other species (sow and perhaps mare), PGF–2α synthesis from one horn is sufficient to cause regression of CL in both ovaries. This effect likely occurs because of greater production of PGF–2α by uterine tissue, as well as a difference in the rate of metabolism of PGF–2α. PGF–2α is rapidly metabolized systemically, with more than 90% changed by one passage through the lungs. Thus, the system involving the use of PGF–2α as the luteolytic agent in large domestic species requires that PGF–2α be conserved through a special transfer system, or that it be produced in relatively large amounts.

The pattern of synthesis and release of PGF–

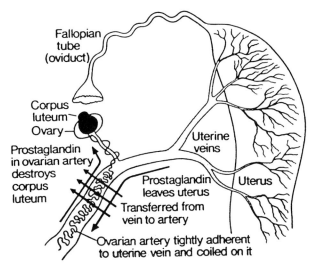

Figure 35–4. Postulated route by which prostaglandin secreted by the progesterone-primed uterus is able to enter the ovarian artery and destroy the corpus luteum in sheep. (From Baird DT: The ovary. *In* Austin CR, Short RV (eds): Hormonal Control of Reproduction. Reproduction in Mammals, Vol 3. Cambridge, Cambridge University Press, 1984.)

2α is essential to its luteolytic effect. For example, PGF-2α must be pulsatile in form, with pulses occurring at about 6-hour intervals, in order for luteolysis to be affected (Fig. 35–5). The concept has developed that a minimum of four to five pulses within 24 hours is required to affect complete luteolysis. If pulse intervals increase significantly prior to complete luteolysis, e.g., to 12 hours, the CL can recover and continue to function, even if at a lower level of steroid synthetic activity. The uterus must be exposed to estrogen and progesterone in order to synthesize and release PGF-2α. While the initiation of PGF-2α synthesis that leads to luteolysis is not completely understood, one possible explanation is that estrogen (from an antral follicle) causes the initial synthesis and release of PGF-2α. In sheep, it is thought that an interplay occurs between the uterus and ovary following the initial PGF-2α pulse, in which PGF-2α affects the corpus luteum to cause both a reduction in progesterone production and the release of *luteal oxytocin.* Oxytocin then interacts with receptors within the uterus to initiate another round of PGF-2α synthesis. PGF-2α synthesis ceases within 6–12 hours after progesterone concentrations have become basal, i.e., with the completion of luteolysis. A system for early recycling is not present in nonpregnant dogs and cats as far as regression of corpora lutea; the luteal phase is about 70 and 35 days, respectively.

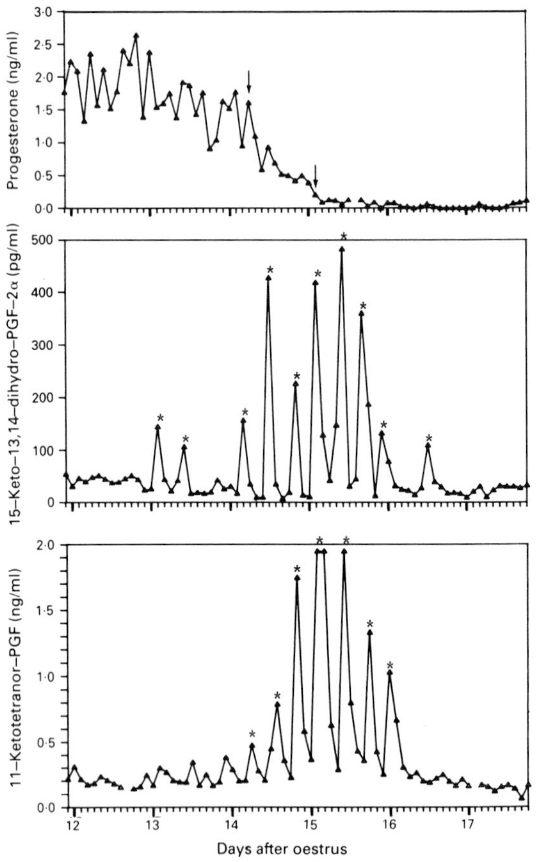

Figure 35–5. Concentrations of progesterone, 15-keto-13,14-dihydro-PGF-2α, and 11-ketotetranor-PGF metabolites in a nonpregnant ewe. Values identified as significant pulses of either PGF-2α metabolite are indicated by an asterisk. The times of initiation and completion of functional luteolysis are indicated by arrows. (From Zarco L, Stabenfeldt GH, Basu S, et al: Modification of prostaglandin F-2α synthesis and release in the ewe during the initial establishment of pregnancy. J Reprod Fertil 83:527, 1988.)

Changes in Luteal Life Span in Large Domestic Animals Occur Because of Changes in Prostaglandin F–2α Synthesis by the Uterus

Significant changes in the length of the lifespan of the CL in nonpregnant large domestic species occur only because of changes within the uterus. As discussed in Chapter 37, the presence of an embryo results in the blockage of PGF-2α synthesis and a continuance in luteal activity. The CL life span can be prolonged also in cases of uterine infection, e.g., in the postpartum cow, where infection is low grade, and PGF-2α synthesis is inhibited, with the CL failing to be regressed. Prolonged luteal phases also commonly occur in mares in the absence of uterine infection. This deficit in mares appears to be a genetic propensity toward inadequate synthesis and release of PGF-2α. The absence of a uterine horn can result also in a lengthened luteal phase in animals in which the ipsilateral horn controls the CL (local control). In this situation, (e.g., cow), if ovulation occurs in the ovary ipsilateral to the missing horn, the luteal phase is prolonged because of the necessity of the ipsilateral uterine horn for controlling the life span of the CL.

In nonpregnant large domestic animals, inflammatory responses of the endometrium owing to bacterial contamination can result in significant synthesis and release of PGF-2α, leading to premature luteolysis and a shortening of the estrous cycle. It should be emphasized that luteal activity is almost always normal in the absence of uterine pathology in large domestic species. Thus, short estrous cycles in large domestic animals are pathog-nomonic for uterine infection.

OVARIAN CYCLES

In Spontaneously Ovulating Animals, Ovarian Cycles Have Two Phases— Follicular and Luteal; Animals That Require Copulation for Ovulation Have Only a Follicular Phase

An *ovarian cycle* in a nonpregnant animal is defined as the interval between successive ovulations. The cycle is composed of two phases, an initial *follicular phase* and a subsequent *luteal phase*, with ovulation separating the phases. In most domestic animals and primates, the ovulatory process is governed by internal mechanisms; estrogen from the antral follicle initiates the ovulatory release of gonadotropins. These animals are called *spontaneous* ovulators.

There are fundamental differences between animals regarding the relationship of the follicular and luteal phases of the cycle. In higher primates, there is complete separation of follicular and luteal phases, with no significant follicle growth occurring until luteolysis is complete. In large domestic animals, significant follicle growth does occur during the luteal phase of the cycle. For example, in the cow a large antral follicle is present at the time of the onset of luteolysis, and in the mare follicle growth can even result in ovulation of follicles during the luteal phase (about 5% of cycles). Thus, in large domestic animals, much of the follicle growth is telescoped into the luteal phase. This situation results in shorter cycles in large domestic animals versus primates (17–21 days versus 28 days); the interval of luteolysis to ovulation is shorter in large domestic animals (5–10 days) than in primates (12–13 days). The period of antral follicle growth leading to ovulation is not appreciably different, however, with the final progression of antral follicle growth requiring about 10 days in large domestic animals and about 12–13 days in primates.

Animals that require copulation for ovulation are known as *induced ovulators.* They include cats, rabbits, ferrets, mink, camels, llamas, and alpacas. Copulation replaces estrogen as the stimulus that induces the ovulatory release of gonadotropins. However, these animals require exposure to elevated estrogen concentrations before they can respond to copulation by the release of gonadotropins.

Induced ovulators have follicle growth patterns (in the absence of coitus) in which cohorts of follicles develop, are maintained in a mature state for a few days, and then regress. Follicle growth patterns can be distinctly separated, as in the cat, wherein follicles develop and regress over a 6–7 day period with a minimum of 8–9 days between follicle growth waves. Follicle waves can also have some overlap, as in llamas and alpacas (Fig. 35–6), or can closely overlap, as in the rabbit.

The Luteal Phase is Modified by Copulation in Some Species

In rodent species, the luteal phase of the ovarian cycle is extended by copulation. The

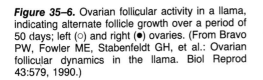

Figure 35–6. Ovarian follicular activity in a llama, indicating alternate follicle growth over a period of 50 days; left (○) and right (●) ovaries. (From Bravo PW, Fowler ME, Stabenfeldt GH, et al.: Ovarian follicular dynamics in the llama. Biol Reprod 43:579, 1990.)

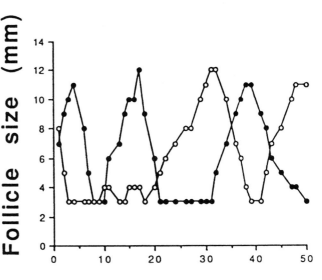

life span of CL is only 1–2 days in the absence of copulation. Copulation initiates the release of prolactin that results in prolongation of luteal activity for up to 10–11 days in the absence of pregnancy. This phenomenon is often called *pseudopregnancy*.

CLINICAL CORRELATION

PERSISTENT LUTEAL PHASE IN THE MARE

HISTORY ☐ You have been called to examine a mare that foaled this spring, but was not bred at the foal "heat" because of a retained placenta. It has been 40 days since the foal "heat," and the owner want to know why the mare has not returned to estrus.

CLINICAL EXAMINATION ☐ The main clinical findings are a cervix that is relatively small and tightly constricted (through speculum examination) and that has considerable tone (through palpation *per rectum*). Rectal palpation also reveals a uterus that has considerable tone. The ovaries are normal in size; in fact, one ovary has a 35 mm follicle present. This prompts you to ask the owner if the mare has been vigorously teased by a stallion for the detection of estrus. The owner brings the teasing stallion to the mare to demonstrate the farm's teasing technique and, as predicted, the mare vigorously rejects the stallion.

COMMENT ☐ A history of a mare that has been previously in estrus, and that has not returned to estrus within 30 days, usually indicates the presence of a persistent corpus luteum. The corpus luteum persists because of inadequate PGF-2α synthesis and release, which normally occurs at about 14 days postovulation and causes regression of the corpus luteum in the absence of pregnancy. The incidence of the syndrome is relatively common, perhaps as high as 15–20%. The corpus luteum can remain active for as long as 3 months before the mare is able to synthesize and release PGF-2α sufficient to cause regression of the corpus luteum. It is difficult to palpate a persistent corpus luteum *per rectum* because it tends to shrink into the interior of the ovary. The structure may be visualized by ultrasonography, but this is not always possible. The appearance of the cervix and the tone of the cervix and uterus suggest that the genital tu-

bular system is under the influence of progesterone, findings that, together with the history, support a tentative diagnosis. A tentative diagnosis can also be made if the mare returns to estrus within a few days following the administration of PGF-2α. A definitive diagnosis can be made by progesterone analysis of blood; values are often 1–2 ng/mL in this syndrome versus 3 ng/mL+ in mares with normal estrous cycle corpora lutea.

The clinical finding that can be confusing in this syndrome is the presence of a large follicle in the absence of estrus. Ovarian follicles develop in this syndrome, and sometimes even ovulation occurs. However, mares do not show sexual receptivity in the presence of large follicles if luteal phase concentrations of progesterone are present. One syndrome that needs to be considered on a differential diagnosis is that the mare has stopped ovarian activity, i.e., has become anestrus. Although this does not occur often in foaling mares, mares that foal early can be deleteriously affected by the relatively short photoperiod that is present. In this case, the clinical signs do not support the diagnosis of anestrus.

TREATMENT ☐ The administration of PGF-2α, or one of its analogs, will usually initiate regression of the persistent corpus luteum and result in the appearance of estrus within a few days. The early return to estrus is based on the fact that ovarian follicles tend to develop on a continuous basis throughout the persistent luteal phase syndrome. Regression of the corpus luteum allows the current dominant follicle to continue to develop and produce estrogen, which brings the mare into estrus. One caveat: If the mare has a large follicle present at the time of treatment, e.g., 40–45 mm, the follicle may ovulate before the mare manifests estrus, and the treatment will be judged as failing. In this case, the animal needs to be monitored daily; if ovulation occurs within a few days of treatment, the animal may need to be inseminated artificially if breed rules allow.

Bibliography

Austin CR, Short RV (eds): Reproduction in Mammals, Vols 1–6. Cambridge, Cambridge University Press, 1976, 1982, 1984, 1986.

Cupps PT (ed): Reproduction in Domestic Animals, 4th ed. New York, Academic Press, 1991.

Concannon PW, Morton DB, Weir BJ (eds): Dog and cat

reproduction, contraception and artificial insemination. J Reprod Fertil (Suppl) 39, 1989.

Feldman EC, Nelson RW (eds): Canine and Feline Endocrinology and Reproduction. Philadelphia, WB Saunders, 1987.

Hafez EWE (ed): Reproduction in Farm Animals, 5th ed. Philadelphia, Lea and Febiger, 1987.

Johnson M, Everitt B (eds): Essential Reproduction, 3rd ed. London, Blackwell Scientific Publications, 1988.

Knobil E, Neill JD, Ewing LL, et al (eds): The Physiology of Reproduction, Vols 1, 2. New York, Raven Press, 1988.

McDonald LE, Pineda MH (eds): Veterinary Endocrinology and Reproduction, 4th ed. Philadelphia, Lea & Febiger, 1989.

PRACTICE QUESTIONS FOR CHAPTER 35

1. The main hormone secreted by the dominant follicle allowing the follicle to maintain its dominant state is

   a. estrogen.
   b. inhibin.
   c. oocyte inhibiting factor.
   d. progesterone.

2. The factor that is most important in deciding whether a luteal-phase dominant follicle will go on to ovulation is

   a. inadequate pituitary stimulation.
   b. presence of the corpus luteum.

   c. atresia of the follicle.

3. The initiation of the preovulatory LH surge that leads to ovulation results from

   a. estrogen.
   b. inhibin.
   c. progesterone.
   d. FSH.
   e. prolactin.

4. The substance responsible for the regression of the corpus luteum in large domestic animals is

   a. estrogen.
   b. inhibin.
   c. oxytocin.
   d. prolactin.
   e. prostaglandin F-2α.

5. Ovarian follicle patterns in animals that are induced ovulators, i.e., those that require copulation for the induction of ovulation, are as follows:

   a. Ovarian follicle waves greatly overlap.
   b. Ovarian follicle waves slightly overlap.
   c. Ovarian follicle waves are distinctly separated.
   d. All of the above

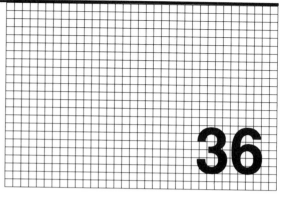

Reproductive Cycles

REPRODUCTIVE CYCLES

1. The two types of reproductive cycles are estrous and menstrual

PUBERTY AND REPRODUCTIVE SENESCENCE

1. Puberty is the time at which animals first release mature germ cells
2. Reproductive senescence in primates occurs because of ovarian inadequacy, not inadequacy of gonadotropin secretion

SEXUAL BEHAVIOR

1. Sexual receptivity is keyed by the hormones estrogen and GnRH in the female and testosterone in the male.

EXTERNAL FACTORS CONTROLLING REPRODUCTIVE CYCLES

1. Photoperiod, lactation, nutrition, and animal interaction are important factors that affect reproduction
2. Inadequate nutrition results in ovarian inactivity, especially in cattle

REPRODUCTIVE CYCLES

The Two Types of Reproductive Cycles Are Estrous and Menstrual

Two types of reproductive cycles are recognized, *estrous* and *menstrual*, with the term *ovarian cycle* representing the interval between two successive ovulations. These terminologies have developed in order to utilize certain external characteristics for the purpose of ac-

curately identifying a particular stage of the reproductive cycle, and most importantly, relating it to the time of ovulation.

In domestic animals, which have limited periods of *estrus* (*sexual receptivity*), the term *estrous cycle* is used, and the onset of estrus defines the start of the cycle (Fig. 36–1). In primates, which are sexually receptive during most of the reproductive cycle, the term *menstrual cycle* is used, with the onset of *menstruation* (vaginal discharge of blood-tinged fluids

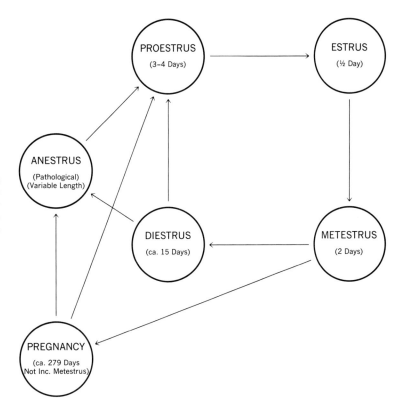

Figure 36–1. Various stages of the ovarian cycle of the cow. (From McDonald LE, Pineda MH (eds): Veterinary Endocrinology and Reproduction, 4th ed. Philadelphia, Lea & Febiger, 1989.)

and tissues) designated as the start of the cycle (Fig. 36–2). The first day of the cycle for both estrous and menstrual cycles begins shortly after the end of the luteal phase.

In domestic animals, estrus usually begins within 48 hours after the end of the luteal phase; the pig is an exception, with estrus not occurring for 5–6 days later. In primates, menstruation usually begins within 24 hours of the end of the luteal phase. Even though both cycles begin at the same time in relation to the luteal phase (shortly after), the time of ovula-

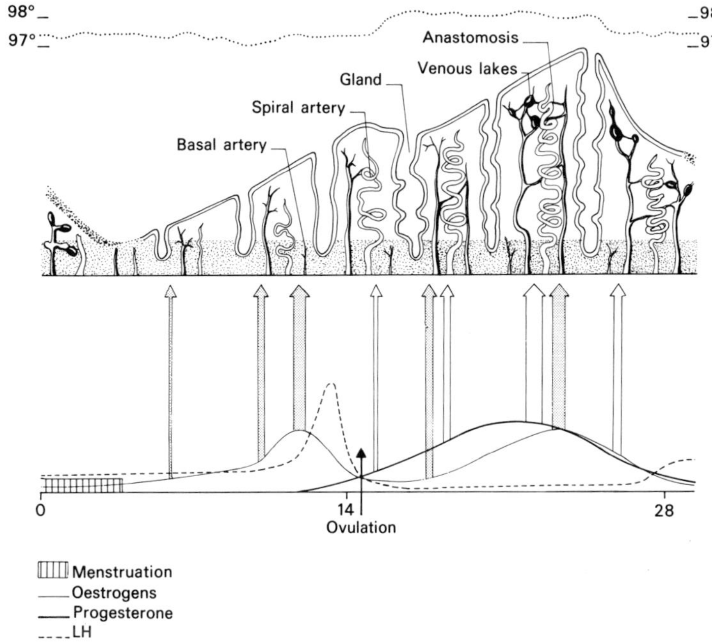

Figure 36–2. Changes in human endometrium during the menstrual cycle. Underlying steroid changes are indicated below, and basal body temperature is indicated above. Thickness of arrows (estrogens stippled; progestogens white) indicates strength of action. (From Johnson M, Everitt B (eds): Essential Reproduction, 3rd ed. London, Blackwell Scientific Publications, 1988, p 176.)

tion differs. This is because, as previously discussed, luteal and follicular phases are separated in primates, with ovulation occurring at a minimum of 12–13 days after the onset of menses. In domestic animals, the follicular phase overlaps the luteal phase and, as a result, ovulation occurs relatively earlier in the estrous cycle. Ovulation is easier to predict in domestic animals (versus primates), because estrus is usually tightly coupled to the preovulatory release of gonadotropins and ovulation. The onset of follicular development in primates can be delayed for a variety of reasons, including stress, making the time of ovulation less predictable for primates than for domestic animals.

The estrous cycle has been classically divided into stages that represent either behavioral or gonadal events. The terminology, originally developed for the guinea pig, rat, and mouse, is as follows: *estrus*—period of sexual receptivity; *metestrus*—period of initial development of the corpus luteum (CL); *diestrus*—period of mature phase of the CL; *proestrus*—period of follicle development, which occurs subsequent to luteal regression and ends at estrus (see Fig. 36–1).

The classic terminology *per se* is not particularly useful for domestic animals. The common terminologies used for domestic animals involve either *behavioral* or *gonadal* activity. The cycle can be described in a behavioral manner by indicating whether animals are in *estrus* (*sexually receptive*) or in *diestrus* (*sexually nonreceptive*). In this case, diestrus includes the stages of metestrus, diestrus, and proestrus. The cycle can also be described with reference to the activity of the gonads if differentiation of follicles and CL is possible. Animals can be in the *follicular phase* (proestrus and estrus) or the *luteal phase* (metestrus and diestrus).

In horses, because the CL is relatively difficult to identify by palpation per rectum, horses are usually classified as to sexual behavior, estrus or diestrus. The behavioral classification is used also in other domestic species, including the cat, dog, goat, pig, and sheep, because of the difficulty of determining ovarian status. The ovarian status of cattle can be determined accurately by palpation per rectum, and cows are usually classified by ovarian status, follicular or luteal. If a CL can be identified, the judgment can be made that ovarian activity is normal in the particular animal, because the CL represents the culmination of follicle growth and ovulation.

PUBERTY AND REPRODUCTIVE SENESCENCE

Puberty Is the Time at Which Animals First Release Mature Germ Cells

In order for females to begin reproductive cycles, they must undergo a process called *puberty*. The term puberty is used to define the onset of reproductive life. For the female, although the onset of sexual activity (in domestic animals) or first menstrual bleeding (in primates) is often used as the onset of puberty, the most precise definition is the time of first ovulation. For all species there is a critical requirement for the attainment of a certain size in order for puberty to be initiated, e.g., in cattle about 275 kg, and in sheep about 40 kg (Fig. 36–3). If this critical requirement is not met because of inadequate nutrition, puberty is delayed. The age at puberty for domestic animals is as follows: cats, 6–12 months; cows, 8–12 months; dogs, 6–12 months; goats, 7–8 months; horses, 12–18 months; sheep, 7–8 months.

The physiological mechanisms involving control of puberty in domestic animals are best known in sheep. One of the fundamental concepts of the onset of puberty involves an increase in the synthesis and release of GnRH from the hypothalamus, which drives gonadotropin secretion (in pulsatile form) and follicle growth. Before puberty, GnRH and gonadotropin secretion is kept in check, because

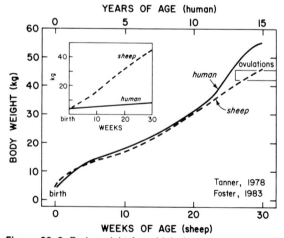

Figure 36–3. Body weight from birth through the initiation of ovulation for sheep (mean) and human beings (50th percentile). Inset shows absolute growth during the first 30 weeks. (From Foster DL, Karsch FJ, Olster DH, et al: Determinants of puberty in a seasonal breeder. Rec Prog Horm Res 42:331, 1986.)

the hypothalamus is highly sensitive to *negative feedback inhibition by estrogens*. One of the keys to puberty in lambs is a maturation of the hypothalamus, which results in reduced sensitivity to negative feedback by estrogen. Puberty onset is not held back because of lack of responsiveness of the prepubertal gonads, because ovarian follicle development can be elicited by gonadotropin administration.

Changes in *photoperiod* are important for allowing lambs to enter puberty. It has been shown that lambs must have some exposure to a long photoperiod during their prepubertal development; the period can be as short as 1–2 weeks (under experimental conditions). Termination of the long photoperiod, which occurs with the summer solstice, allows the sensitivity of the hypothalamus to decrease in response to negative estrogen feedback. The minimal interval from the end of the long photoperiod exposure to the onset of puberty is 10 weeks under experimental conditions. This aspect agrees well with the timing of spontaneous puberty, in which the first ovulation often occurs in the latter part of September, or about 13 weeks from the occurrence of the summer solstice. Note that this concept of the initiation of puberty does not involve decreasing photoperiod *per se*; the emphasis is on a turning point that involves the cessation of exposure to a long photoperiod.

With appropriate growth and photoperiod exposure, the secretion of gonadotropins in lambs causes significant follicle growth. This growth is maintained because of decreased sensitivity of the hypothalamus to estrogens produced by growing follicles. The first endocrine event of puberty in the ewe lamb is the appearance of a preovulatory-type surge of gonadotropins, presumably induced by estrogens produced by developing follicles (Fig. 36–4). The gonadotropin surge results in the production of a luteal structure, through lu-

teinization of a follicle(s), that has a short life span, 3–4 days. Following the demise of the initial luteal structure, another gonadotropin surge occurs, which leads to ovulation and the formation of a CL, usually of a normal life span. At this time, cyclic ovarian activity is finally initiated in the ewe lamb.

Photoperiod can have a suppressive effect on the timing of puberty in animals whose ovarian cyclicity is controlled by light. Kittens born in the spring may be large enough to enter puberty by late autumn, but puberty could be delayed a few months if the kittens are under the natural photoperiod.

Photoperiod influences the timing of puberty onset in macaque monkeys, depending on the physiological maturity of the individual. The first ovulation, or puberty onset, can occur during the late autumn, or early winter, at about 30 months of age (20% of animals) or 12 months later at about 42 months of age (80% of animals). The animals undergoing puberty at about 30 months have an earlier maturation of the neuroendocrine system, wherein significant gonadotropin secretion begins during the previous spring. Thus, there is a window of opportunity for the onset of puberty in macaques that must be entered within the favorable photoperiod of decreasing light if puberty is to occur at an earlier time; nutrition and growth are likely determinants of the earlier time of onset of puberty.

The onset of puberty usually results in the establishment of cyclic ovarian activity within a relatively short period, i.e., within a few weeks to a month in lambs. Ewe lambs can initiate normal ovarian activity at the onset of puberty, which can lead to pregnancy (if mated) at the first estrus, or they can have false starts with the establishment of limited luteal phases and cessation of ovarian activity for several weeks to a month before they resume ovarian activity. In general, the onset

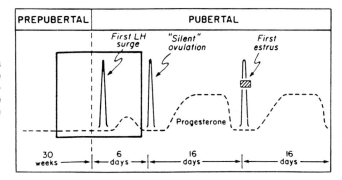

Figure 36–4. Schematic overview of major events during the transition into adulthood in the female sheep. (From Foster D, Ryan K: Mechanisms governing onset of ovarian cyclicity at puberty in the lamb. Ann Biol Anim Bioch Biophys 19:1369, 1979.)

of ovarian cyclicity starts later and ends earlier for ewe lambs compared to adults of the same breed. The earlier cessation of ovarian activity is due to an earlier response to negative estrogen feedback.

The initiation of cyclic ovarian activity in pubertal primates takes longer; the first significant follicle growth usually ends in ovulatory failure. In macaque monkeys, 3–6 months is usually required following the onset of menarche, or first vaginal bleeding, before the occurrence of the first ovulation of puberty. In humans, follicle growth without ovulation can occur for up to a year prior to the establishment of normal ovarian cyclicity, including ovulation and CL formation.

For male lambs, the onset of puberty is first keyed when lambs begin to lose their sensitivity to estrogen feedback inhibition, usually by about 15 weeks of age. For many males, this occurs during the period of increasing, or long, photoperiod, which is in contrast to the ewe lamb. Spermatogenesis (process of sperm production resulting in the presence of mature sperm) usually begins at this time, but because of the length of the process, lambs are usually not capable of successful breeding until about 30-plus weeks of age, or in concert with the onset of puberty in ewe lambs. Thus, puberty is a relatively gradual phenomenon in male sheep compared to the abrupt process in females.

Because adult ewes experience the same double gonadotropin surge at the onset of the breeding season, it has been suggested that adult animals recapitulate puberty each year as they enter the breeding season. Recent studies in adult ewes, however, indicate that *refractoriness* to the long photoperiod experienced by animals during the spring and summer is the most critical aspect for the establishment of ovarian activity. Thus, the concept that the renewal of ovarian activity in sheep recapitulates puberty appears not to be accurate, at least in some aspects.

Reproductive Senescence in Primates Occurs Because of Ovarian Inadequacy, Not Inadequacy of Gonadotropin Secretion

The end to ovarian activity that occurs in primates is called *menopause*. In humans, for example, it usually occurs between 45 and 50 years of age. Menopause occurs because of the depletion of oocytes, which has occurred throughout the reproductive life of the individual; in essence, it represents ovarian failure. It is not clear whether follicles fail to develop from their primordial state because of an absolute, or relative, reduction in follicle numbers, or whether the absence of gonadotropin receptors prohibits follicles entering the gonadotropin-dependent stage of growth. The initiation of menopause often involves cyclic irregularity due to failure of follicle development and ovulation. Gonadotropin secretion can be increased, or be normal, because of the lack of estrogen and, therefore, lack of negative feedback on gonadotropin secretion. In the end, ovarian follicle activity ceases, estrogen concentrations decline, and in the absence of negative feedback inhibition, gonadotropin concentrations increase dramatically.

Reproductive senescence is not recognized in domestic animals. This may be, in part, because most domestic species have lives that are shortened for economic or humane reasons. Nevertheless, it seems clear that a phenomenon such as menopause does not occur in domestic animals. One effect of age that can be noted is in the dog, where estrous cycle intervals gradually increase from the norm of 7½ months to 12–15 months toward the end of the life span.

SEXUAL BEHAVIOR

Sexual Receptivity Is Keyed by the Hormones Estrogen and GnRH in the Female and Testosterone in the Male

As indicated previously, the establishment of sexual behavior is dependent upon exposure, or lack of exposure, of the hypothalamus to testosterone during the early neonatal period. In essence, testosterone (aromatized to estrogen) causes masculinization of the sexual centers in the hypothalamus; in the absence of testosterone, the hypothalamus becomes feminized. An area within the hypothalamus, the *medial preoptic area,* has been identified in the rat as an area that is modified structurally by exposure to testosterone.

Several principles exist regarding the effects of hormones on sexual behavior of domestic animals. First, the magnitude of change in hormone concentration that affects sexual behavior is small, e.g., in the cat, an increase in estradiol-17β concentrations from 10–20 pg/mL plasma results in signs of proestrus. Second, synergism between hormones is often important for sexual receptiveness, e.g., in the dog, estrogen priming followed by progesterone is important. Third, the sequence of exposure to hormones can be important, e.g., progesterone priming is required prior to estrogen exposure for manifestation of estrus in the ewe.

Estrogen, from the developing antral follicle, is the one hormone required for sexual receptivity in all domestic animals. Progesterone derived from either the granulosa of the preovulatory follicle, or the CL, is also important for estrus in some animals.

In sheep, estrus occurs in response to estrogen only if the animal has been exposed previously to progesterone (through the presence of a previous CL). Estrus usually begins within a short period after the end of the luteal phase, i.e., 24–36 hours, due to the presence of large antral follicles at luteolysis; thus, the period from last exposure to progesterone and the onset of estrus is short (Fig. 36–5). The requirement for progesterone for sexual receptivity means that the first follicular phase of the breeding season, which leads to ovulation in the ewe, is not accompanied by estrus. Most adult ewes show estrus after the first luteal phase. Ewe lambs often require the exposure of two or more luteal phases before they express estrus.

Of the domestic species, dogs are unusual in that sexual receptivity is keyed by progesterone, initially produced by the granulosa during the preovulatory LH surge and, subsequently, by developing CL. Prior exposure to estrogen makes the female attractive to males, but does not produce sexual receptivity; estrus requires the additional exposure to progesterone. Estrus is often maintained for up to a week in the presence of a developing luteal phase. In other domestic species, progesterone is inhibitory for estrous activity.

The importance of prior progesterone priming for estrus manifestation has been suggested for dairy cattle by the finding of a reduced incidence of estrus at the first postpartum ovulation (days 15–20). Complete progesterone withdrawal occurs in the cow immediately prior to delivery, and animals would not have been exposed to progesterone for 2–3 weeks in this situation. Sows also have a reduced incidence of estrus at the first ovulation, which usually does not occur until after weaning, usually not until at least 45 days after parturition. Other domestic species, i.e., cats, goats, and horses, all show estrus with the first ovulation of the season with no apparent requirement for progesterone priming.

Testosterone is important for *libido* in female primates. The theca layer from degenerating follicles forms an active interstitium that secretes the androgens, androstenedione, and testosterone. Androgens are also essential for the maintenance of libido in males. Occasionally, castrated males, particularly horses, are able to maintain libido in spite of the lower concentrations of androgens (of adrenal origin) that are present postcastration. These animals can be differentiated from those with retained testicles (*cryptorchid*) by testosterone analysis of plasma.

There is both experimental and circumstantial evidence to indicate that GnRH plays a role in sexual receptivity. The administration of GnRH to ovariectomized rats produced sexual (lordotic) responses, and in prepubertal gilts, GnRH administration resulted in the occurrence of estrus within 24 hours. The circumstantial evidence is that the onset of sexual receptivity in animals is tightly coupled to the onset of the preovulatory gonadotropin surge (Fig. 36–6). Because the preovulatory gonadotropin surge is the result of an increased rate of pulsatile release of gonadotropins driven by increased GnRH synthesis and release, it is likely that this increased GnRH secretory activity affects sexual centers within the hypothalamus for the promotion of sexual

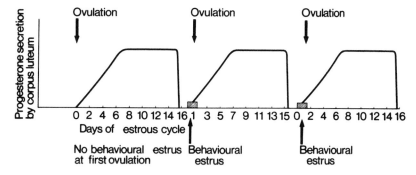

Figure 36–5. The estrous cycle of the ewe, showing how the first ovulation of the season is unaccompanied by estrus. Note the short time interval between regression of the corpus luteum and the next ovulation. (From Short RV: Oestrous and menstrual cycles. *In* Austin CR, Short RV (eds): Hormonal Control of Reproduction. Reproduction in Mammals, Vol 3. Cambridge, Cambridge University Press, 1984.)

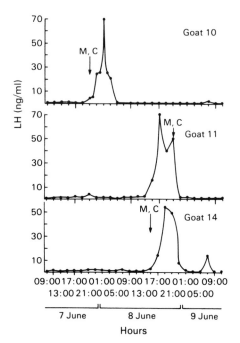

Figure 36–6. Plasma LH levels in three nannies exhibiting an ovulatory surge during the 50-hour period of intensive sampling (7–9 June). *M,* marked; *C,* copulation. (From BonDurant RH, Darien BJ, Munro CJ, et al.: Photoperiod induction of fertile oestrus and changes in LH and progesterone concentrations in yearling goats *(Capra hircus)*. J Reprod Fertil 63:1, 1981.)

receptivity. This allows the onset of the ovulatory process, triggered by the gonadotropin surge, to be tightly coupled with sexual receptivity.

EXTERNAL FACTORS CONTROLLING REPRODUCTIVE CYCLES

Photoperiod, Lactation, Nutrition, and Animal Interaction Are Important Factors That Affect Reproduction

Photoperiod

Photoperiod controls the occurrence of reproductive cycles in a number of domestic species, including cats, goats, horses, and sheep. The result is that these animals have an annual period in which they have continuous (cyclic) ovarian activity, and another period of no ovarian activity, the latter termed *anestrus.* The response to photoperiod is different among these species; cats and horses are positively affected with increasing light,

and goats and sheep are positively affected by decreasing photoperiod (Fig. 36–7).

The response to a positive change in photoperiod usually occurs relatively soon after the occurrence of the summer, or winter, solstice, i.e., within 1–2 months. A change to a negative photoperiod usually requires a longer duration to cause an effect, i.e., 2–4 months to suppress ovarian activity following the occurrence of the particular solstice. The net result is that cyclic ovarian activity, in the absence of pregnancy, usually occupies more than half of the year for these four seasonally breeding species.

In cats, cyclic ovarian activity can range from late January through October (Northern Hemisphere). In horses, the usual range of ovarian activity is from March through October. Conversely, sheep and goats have ovarian activity from late July through February or March (depending upon the breed). As indicated previously, progesterone priming immediately prior to follicle development is required for sexual receptivity in sheep. The full length of the reproductive season of sheep is not manifested externally because, first, the first ovulation is not preceded by the presence of a CL, and second, the last follicle phase may be delayed because of a negative photoperiod, with the priming effects of progesterone lost prior to follicle growth.

The main translator of photoperiod is the *pineal gland,* which produces *melatonin* in response to darkness. The central nervous system (CNS) pathway involved with the translation of light includes the *retina,* the *suprachiasmatic nucleus,* the *superior cervical ganglion,* and the *pineal gland.* Whereas melatonin has been previously described as antigonadal, this is obviously not true, because both short and long phases of darkness, with resultant short and long durations of melatonin secretion, can have a positive effect on reproductive cycles. In sheep, though, exposure to increasing darkness may be only important for maintaining ovarian activity. The onset of ovarian activity is thought to occur in response to the development of refractoriness to the long photoperiod. The development of *photorefractoriness* to a long photoperiod as a requisite to ovarian cyclicity is consonant with the fact that sheep can begin cyclic ovarian activity even before the onset of the summer solstice.

Of the seasonal breeders, the cat is the most sensitive to photoperiod change; estrus, in conjunction with the presence of mature, antral follicles, can occur as early as January 15.

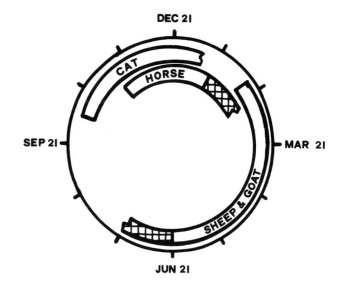

Figure 36–7. A diagrammatic representation of the effect of photoperiod on ovarian activity in the cat, horse, sheep, and goat. The bars represent periods of ovarian inactivity (anestrum). The transitional period for the horse, sheep, and goat is shown by the hatched portion of the bar. (From Stabenfeldt GH, Edqvist L-E: Female Reproductive Processes. *In* Swenson MJ (ed): Dukes' Physiology of Domestic Animals, 10th ed. Ithaca, Cornell University Press, 1984.)

It is likely that initial follicle activity begins at least 10 days before the first expression of estrus, or 15 days after the winter solstice. Thus, a total photoperiod change of as little as 15 minutes can be perceived and translated by the cat into ovarian activity.

The suppressive effects of photoperiod can be overcome by exposure to artificial lighting regimens. This is relatively easy in the case of cats and horses, in which environments with photoperiods are compatible with ovarian activity, i.e., at least 12 hours of light per day. If the photoperiod is established before the end of ovarian activity in the autumn, cyclic ovarian activity continues through the time associated with anestrum. If mares are allowed to become anestrus in the autumn, it can take a minimum of 2 months exposure of mares to increased light to re-establish ovarian activity. The usual time for placing mares under lights is December 1 (Northern Hemisphere), with cyclic ovarian activity expected by early February.

It is usually not possible to place sheep and goats in light-tight barns to increase their exposure to dark in order to overcome the suppressive effects of increasing light. One recent development in this regard has been the administration of melatonin to sheep during the spring by oral, or systemic (implant), administration. This exposure to melatonin has resulted in an early onset of ovarian activity and increased the number of multiple ovulations above that normally observed at the beginning of the breeding season.

Lactation

Lactation can have suppressive effects on ovarian activity. In pigs, suppression of ovarian activity is complete; sows do not come into estrus until after piglets are weaned. Cats often have ovarian activity suppressed throughout lactation, although they occasionally come into estrus during the latter part of lactation. Ovarian activity tends to be suppressed in lactating beef cows, with the first estrus and ovulation not occurring before day 45 postpartum. The suckling process appears important to ovarian suppression; dairy cows are not suppressed by lactation unless it involves a large nutritional deficit.

Goats and sheep usually begin lactation during a photoperiod that is increasingly suppressive for ovarian activity and, therefore, the re-establishment of ovarian activity in these species is confounded by the photoperiod. We have found, however, that ewes delivering in the autumn ovulated as early as postpartum day 12 (average, postpartum day 23), thus indicating that lactation has little suppressive effect on ovarian activity in sheep. Mares usually ovulate by postpartum days 10–15, with lactation having no suppressive effect on ovarian activity concerning this ovulatory interval.

One of the concepts of *lactational suppression of ovarian activity* involves the importance of suckling with its related stimulation of prolactin synthesis. Inhibiting factors for prolactin synthesis, including dopamine and the GnRH-associated peptide (GAP), need to be suppressed in order for prolactin synthesis to proceed. The sensory input from suckling suppresses the production of these prolactin-inhibiting factors. As both dopamine and GAP are essential links in the synthesis of gonadotropins, their reduced output results in reduced ovarian activity through decreased gonadotropin synthesis and release.

Pheromones

Pheromones are chemical compounds that allow communication among animals through the olfactory system. When sexual behavior is affected, the compounds are called *sex pheromones*. Pheromones arise from several tissue sources: the most prominent ones for animals are sebaceous glands, the reproductive tract, and the urinary tract.

Some of the first experiments that demonstrated the potency of male odors to influence reproductive behavior was done in mice. One syndrome, called the *Whitten effect*, involved the synchronization of female mice through the sudden introduction of a male. The introduction of a male (or male odor through bedding) causes estrus to be synchronized with a large number of animals, cycling within 3 days of introduction of the male. The effect of the pheromones in this case is to stimulate the synthesis and release of gonadotropins. Another syndrome, called the *Bruce effect*, involves the blockage of pregnancy development by the introduction of a different (strange) male into proximity with a recently bred female. The effect of the odor of the strange male is to block the release of prolactin, the hormone responsible for the maintenance of CL in association with pregnancy in rodents. Regression of CL, in this case, produces fetal loss. Thus, it is possible for pheromones to strongly affect reproductive cycles.

Pheromones are important for the attraction of the male to the female at the time of sexual receptivity. Sexual attractiveness of the female evolves from the pheromones that she elicits on a limited, cyclic basis in association with estrus. For example, methyl-p-hydroxybenzoate, isolated from the vaginal secretions of dogs in proestrus and estrus, has produced intense anogenital interest by males when applied to anestrous females. Females are also influenced by male odors, e.g., sows in estrus will assume a breeding (*rigidity*) stance when exposed to the urine of males. Androgens can serve as pheromones, or they can influence the production of substances within the kidney that influence female sexual behavior. The attractiveness of the female to the male involves a change in perception of the male by the female due to a changing physiological state within the female, not because of changes that are occurring in the male.

The classic way for males to delineate their territory has been for them to mark the area with urine. In general, pheromones that affect sexual behavior tend to have a musk type of odor. The classic pheromone used by humans is perfume, which is derived from civetone, a cyclic 17 carbon compound obtained from the civet cat.

The Whitten effect has been used to manipulate the estrous cycles of animals. In sheep, males are introduced into a flock of ewes prior to the breeding season to either advance, or ensure, ovarian cyclicity at the beginning of the breeding season. Whereas it was previously thought the effect of the introduction of a male was short-lived, i.e., a gonadotropin response could only be obtained within the first few days from ewes that had antral follicles, it is now clear that the interaction of rams with ewes over extended periods of the anestrum results in earlier ovarian activity.

As discussed under the Whitten effect, pheromones can account for some of the effect of the male. More recent studies, however, have shown that *sight* of the male by the female as well as *physical contact* are important factors that influence gonadotropin secretion and, thus, ovarian activity. The Whitten effect has been used also to influence the onset of puberty in pigs. The introduction of males into groups of gilts beginning several weeks before the expected time of puberty (180–200 days) has been used to ensure, or advance, the onset of puberty.

Nutrition

Inadequate Nutrition Results in Ovarian Inactivity, Especially in Cattle

In dairy cattle, genetically selected for high productivity, the ability to produce up to 100 pounds of milk per day is a remarkable achievement. It is almost impossible for dairy cows to consume enough feed during the first part of the lactation cycle to maintain their body weight, and they are often in a negative nutrition balance for up to 100 days postpartum. As animals must have an adequate level of nutrition to initiate ovarian inactivity, ovarian activity is suppressed until a positive energy balance is established. If one wants a dairy cow to produce large quantities of milk, one must be willing to wait for nutrition to catch up with milk production.

Inadequate nutrition can affect ovarian activity in the postpartum period. A management practice that is sometimes used to enhance production efficiency is to maintain beef cows on a marginal plane of nutrition during the winter. This approach is for the purpose of forcing animals to use fat that has been developed and stored during the grazing season. If pregnant beef cows are not returned to a positive nutritional balance by the last month of gestation, the re-establishment of ovarian cyclicity, which usually occurs between Days 45 and 60 postpartum, will be delayed. Another situation that can affect ovarian activity involves pregnant beef heifers. These animals often need extra nutrition in the postpartum period in order to re-establish ovarian activity, because they have requirements for growth as well as for lactation.

CLINICAL CORRELATION

SEXUAL ATTRACTIVENESS IN THE SPAYED BITCH

HISTORY □ You are called by a veterinary colleague who has seen a bitch owned by one of her best clients. The client is upset because the dog is attracting males in spite of recently undergoing an overiohysterectomy. You inquire if the dog allows intromission by males. Although the answer is no, the owner is sure that a portion of an ovary was left *in situ*. Your colleague is sure she removed the ovaries during the surgical procedure. You are asked to examine the dog as a favor to your colleague.

CLINICAL EXAMINATION □ The dog has a vulva that is slightly swollen with a small amount of discharge present. An examination of a vaginal smear reveals some cornified epithelial cells but mainly an increased number of neutrophils. You indicate to the owner that you believe the male dogs are being attracted by the presence of an infection in the vagina; the owner needs more convincing. You decide to do a

reproductive endocrine panel on the dog (estrogen and progesterone) to satisfy the owner. The values for both estrogen and progesterone are low and thus are not supportive of the presence of ovarian tissue.

COMMENT □ It is common for bitches with vaginal infections to attract male dogs, presumably because of the odors generated by the infection. One of the most important points of differentiation as to cause, i.e., vaginal infection versus presence of an ovarian remnant, is to know about the sexual behavior of the animal. The bitch will allow intromission by a male only if she has been exposed to progesterone following priming with estrogen. This situation only occurs if an ovarian follicle is present that has begun to luteinize following the preovulatory LH surge. If the animal in question had allowed intromission, the possibility of an ovarian remnant being present would be likely. Because of the failure of the bitch to allow intromission, you indicate that the animal is almost certainly without the presence of ovarian tissue. Regarding the endocrine analysis, if the animal was completely ovariectomized, both values will be low. This finding *per se* does not rule out the presence of ovarian tissue, but if the sample is obtained when the animal is showing the "sexual behavior," one can state with assurance that the behavior is not due to hormones and, by extension, activity of ovarian tissue.

TREATMENT □ Treat the vaginal infection and keep the female away from males until the infection is cleared.

Bibliography

Austin CR, Short RV (eds): Reproduction in Mammals, Vols 1–6. Cambridge, Cambridge University Press, 1976, 1982, 1984, 1986.
Cupps PT (ed): Reproduction in Domestic Animals, 4th ed. New York, Academic Press, 1991.
Concannon PW, Morton DB, Weir BJ (eds): Dog and cat reproduction, contraception and artificial insemination. J Reprod Fertil (Suppl)39, 1989.
Feldman EC, Nelson RW: Canine and Feline Endocrinology and Reproduction. Philadelphia, WB Saunders, 1987.
Hafez EWE (ed): Reproduction in Farm Animals, 5th ed. Philadelphia, Lea & Febiger, 1987.
Johnson M, Everitt B (eds): Essential Reproduction, 3rd ed. London, Blackwell Scientific Publications, 1988.
Knobil E, Neill JD, Ewing LL, et al (eds): The Physiology of Reproduction, Vols 1, 2. New York, Raven Press, 1988.

McDonald LE, Pineda MH (eds): Veterinary Endocrinology and Reproduction, 4th ed. Philadelphia, Lea & Febiger, 1989.

PRACTICE QUESTIONS FOR CHAPTER 36

1. The first estrous cycle of the cow subsequent to parturition follows which sequence?

    a. Anestrus, diestrus, estrus, metestrus, proestrus
    b. Anestrus, estrus, diestrus, metestrus, proestrus
    c. Anestrus, metestrus, diestrus, estrus, proestrus
    d. Anestrus, proestrus, estrus, diestrus, proestrus
    e. Anestrus, proestrus, estrus, metestrus, diestrus

2. The usual situation in large domestic animals is for a dominant follicle or dominant follicles to be present at the time of luteal regression, with sexual receptivity being manifested within 1–2 days following luteal regression; the one large animal species that is the exception to this generalization is the

    a. cow.
    b. doe.
    c. ewe.
    d. mare.
    e. sow.

3. The hormones that form the foundation for sexual receptivity are

    a. estrogen and PGF-2α.
    b. progesterone and estrogen.
    c. estrogen and GnRH.
    d. progesterone and PGF-2α.
    e. PGF-2α and GnRH.

4. The following description—decreasing light turns off cyclic ovarian activity after a number of months, while increasing light reverses the process after a number of months, including the development of a transitional period—fits which domestic species?

    a. Cat
    b. Cow
    c. Dog
    d. Goat
    e. Horse
    f. Pig
    g. Sheep

5. What response occurs as a result of the Whitten effect in animals, a situation in which the introduction of a male into a group of noncyclic animals results in the re-establishment of ovarian activity?

    a. Increased estrogen secretion
    b. Increased progesterone secretion
    c. Increased prolactin secretion
    d. Increased FSH secretion
    e. Increased LH secretion
    f. Increased FSH and LH secretion

6. One of the domestic species requires progesterone priming, in addition to estrogen, to manifest estrus. Hence, this species does not manifest estrus with the first ovarian cycle in the postpartum period. The animal is the

    a. cat.
    b. dog.
    c. goat.
    d. horse.
    e. pig.
    f. sheep.

37

Pregnancy and Parturition

PREGNANCY

1. The development of an embryo involves fusion of an oocyte and spermatozoan within the oviduct
2. Extension of the life span of the corpus luteum in large domestic species and cats is essential for pregnancy maintenance
3. The placenta acts as an endocrine organ

PARTURITION

1. Fetal cortisol initiates delivery through increased secretion of estrogen and, as a result, prostaglandin F-2α

PREGNANCY

The Development of an Embryo Involves Fusion of an Oocyte and Spermatozoan Within the Oviduct

The development of a new individual requires the transfer of male gametes to the female genital tract for fertilization of the female gamete(s). *Spermatozoa,* which have been concentrated and stored in the epididymis, gradually change from *oxidative* (aerobic) to *glycolytic* (anaerobic) *metabolism* as they progress through the epididymis. In this state, spermatozoa are in a situation of reduced metabolism. Mature sperm are only able to metabolize a special sugar, *fructose,* within the reproductive tract.

Sperm are ejaculated usually into the vagina, although some domestic species (dog, horse, and pig) ejaculate directly into the cervix and uterus. The movement of sperm through the cervix is aided by estrogen-induced changes in cervical mucus, which result in the formation of channels that facilitate movement of sperm. This has been particularly emphasized in primates, wherein the thinning of mucus occurs just prior to ovulation, a factor that can be used to predict the time of ovulation.

The environment of the female genital system is generally inhospitable to the survival of sperm, e.g., white blood cells are quickly attracted to the uterine lumen because sperm cells are foreign to the female genital tract. Special reservoirs have evolved in the female

457

tract to aid in the survival of sperm during transport; these include the cervix and oviduct, the latter involving areas at the uterotubule junction and within the ampulla. The reservoirs are progressively filled (from posterior to anterior in the tract), requiring hours before the oviductal reservoirs are full. Finally, the reservoir within the ampulla is able to release a few sperm on a continuous basis, so that fertilization can occur shortly after the arrival of oocytes within the oviduct.

The first studies in *sperm transport* emphasized the rapidity of the process, with sperm reported passing from the vagina to the fimbriated end of the oviduct within minutes. It is now known that sperm undergoing so-called fast transport are not involved in fertilization; in fact, they are damaged by the rapid transport.

Sperm need to undergo changes within the female genital tract that are a prerequisite for fertilization; the process is called *capacitation*. One of the effects of capacitation is the removal of glycoproteins from the cell surface. The glycoproteins, perhaps added for protective purposes, interfere with fertilization. This change allows sperm to undergo the *acrosome reaction* when they come in contact with oocytes. The acrosome reaction involves the release of hydrolytic enzymes from the acrosomal cap, which may be important for penetration of the sperm through the granulosa and zona pellucida to the oocyte plasm membrane. *Hyaluronidase* causes breakdown of hyaluronic acid, an important component of the intercellular matrix of granulosa cells that surround the oocyte. *Acrosin,* a proteolytic enzyme, digests the acellular coating around the oocyte. Both enzymatic events allow the sperm to penetrate to the oocyte. The acrosome reaction also changes the surface of the sperm, which allows it to fuse with the oocyte. The acrosomal reaction results in tail movements that feature a flagellar beat that tends to drive sperm in a forward direction.

Because of the changes that spermatozoa must undergo within the female reproductive tract prior to fertilization, the deposition of sperm prior to ovulation is the preferred timing for producing maximal fertility. Females are usually sexually receptive for at least 24 hours before ovulation and, in the natural setting (free interaction between sexes), insemination usually occurs a number of hours before the occurrence of ovulation. Even in induced ovulators, such as cats, the interval from copulation to ovulation is usually 24

hours or more. In essence, the system has evolved to have ready-to-fertilize sperm at the fertilization site when oocytes arrive. This is in concert with the finding that the life span of male gametes tend to be twice that of female gametes.

The presentation of male gametes before female gametes in the oviduct implies that oocytes are ready for fertilization upon arrival in the ampulla; this is likely true for a majority of animals. A prerequisite for fertilization of the oocyte is that it must undergo the first meiotic division before fertilization. Although this occurs in a number of species before ovulation, in the horse and dog the first meiotic division does not occur until after ovulation (in the dog, not for at least 48 hours). In this situation, spermatozoa often wait for oocytes to mature in the oviduct before fertilization can occur. One means of adaptation to delayed completion of meiosis is that spermatozoa have a longer life span in the dog and horse compared to other domestic species.

Once fertilization has occurred, the *embryo* usually develops to the *morula,* or early *blastocyst* stage, within the oviduct before moving into the uterus. This period, usually 4–5 days, affords the uterus time to finish its inflammatory response concerning the removal of spermatozoa and allows the endometrial glands time to secrete nutrients under the influence of progesterone from developing corpus luteum, which are essential for development of embryos during their preimplantation stage.

An interesting finding in the mare is her ability to distinguish fertilized from unfertilized oocytes; unfertilized oocytes from previous cycles are retained within the oviduct, whereas recently fertilized oocytes (embryos) move through the oviduct to the uterus. It is likely that all animals recognize pregnancy by the presence of an embryo(s) at the early oviductal stage. However, this recognition does not necessarily result in prolongation of the corpus luteum (CL) and the continued production of progesterone, which is essential for the maintenance of pregnancy.

Extension of the Life Span of the Corpus Luteum in Large Domestic Species and Cats Is Essential for Pregnancy Maintenance

For those domestic animals (cattle, goats, horses, pigs, sheep) whose luteal activity is controlled by the uterus, modification of *uter-*

ine prostaglandin F(PGF)-2α synthesis and release is critical for the establishment of pregnancy. It seems clear that the embryo produces substances that modify uterine production of PGF-2α. *Estrogen synthesis* by the embryo is one way the endometrium may be informed regarding the presence of an embryo. A specific protein of embryonic origin called *trophoblastin*, produced prior to day 14 of pregnancy (or postovulation) in both sheep and cattle, is of interest for the establishment of pregnancy from an immunological point of view; it has a close structural relationship to the molecule *interferon*. Movement of the embryo(s) in the tract is also important for pregnancy recognition. In the mare, the embryo moves throughout both horns before being fixed at day 16. In pigs, a minimal number of embryos need to be present, i.e., about 4, presumably to occupy a sufficiently large area of the endometrium. Litter-bearing animals also use transuterine migration to maximize the opportunity for fetal development, a procedure that aids the recognition of pregnancy process. The end result is either suppression of PGF-2α synthesis as seen in the cow (Fig. 37–1), or modification of the secretion mode in sheep, i.e., continuous instead of pulsatile. It seems clear that the absence of pulsatile secretion of PGF-2α is critical for the extension of the life span of the CL and the establishment of pregnancy in large domestic species.

In the cat, CL lasts for 35–40 days following ovulation regardless of the presence of pregnancy, and thus the need for early modification of luteal activity is not essential for the establishment of pregnancy. Implantation occurs at about day 13, which allows the fetoplacental unit to influence and extend luteal activity that is compatible with pregnancy maintenance. The luteotropic hormone that is responsible for luteal maintenance in the cat is not known. One hormone that likely synergizes with progesterone for the support of pregnancy is *relaxin,* a placental hormone that is produced in the cat beginning at about day 20 of gestation (Fig. 37–2).

The dog does not extend its luteal phase during pregnancy; the luteal phase in the nonpregnant animal is often longer (70 days) than in pregnant animals. Nevertheless, enhancement of luteal activity occurs through a placental luteotropin of unknown origin, with progesterone secretion enhanced beginning at about day 20 of gestation or a few days after implantation.

The rescue of the CL at the onset of pregnancy in primates involves the production of a luteotrophin called *chorionic gonadotropin* (for humans, *hCG*), which is produced by trophoblastic cells *(syncytiotrophblasts)* of the embryo (Fig. 37–3). In order for trophoblast tissue to produce CG, it must have intimate contact with the interstitium of the endometrium. This contact occurs by a type of implantation called *interstitial,* in which the embryo penetrates the endometrium at about 8–9 days following fertilization in humans and nonhuman primates. Secretion of CG begins 24–48 hours after implantation with immediate enhancement of luteal progesterone production. Rescue of the CL in human pregnancy occurs as late as 4–5 days before the end of the luteal phase.

As indicated for primates, the type of implantation (interstitial) is essential to the development of pregnancy. *Implantation* is less invasive in the dog and cat, with the type termed *eccentric.* In the large domestic species,

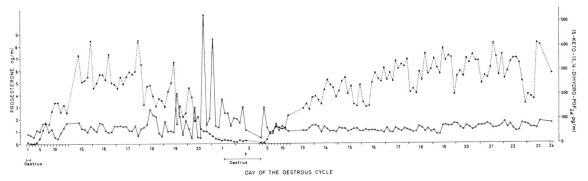

Figure 37–1. The relationship of prostaglandin release, as indicated by the measurement of 15-keto-13,14-dihydroprostaglandin F-2α, and progesterone production by the corpus luteum during a nonfertile cycle and following a fertile insemination in the same cow. (From Kindahl H, Edqvist L-E, Bane A: Blood levels of progesterone and 15-keto-13,14-dihydroprostaglandin F-2α during the normal oestrous cycle and early pregnancy of heifers. Acta Endocrinol 82:134, 1976.)

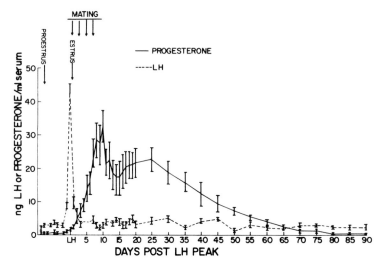

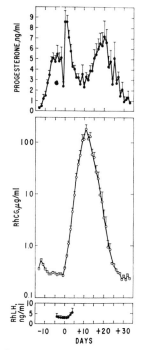

Figure 37–2. LH and progesterone concentrations during pregnancy in nine dogs. Vertical bars represent the standard error of the mean. (From Smith MS, McDonald LE: Serum levels of luteinizing hormone and progesterone during the estrous cycle, pseudopregnancy and pregnancy in the dog. Endocrinology 94:404, 1974. © by The Endocrine Society)

Figure 37–3. Composite of 15 normal rhesus monkey early pregnancies normalized to the day of corpus luteum rescue (day 0). Points are means ± SE. Note the temporal relationship between luteal progesterone production (prior to day + 10) and chorionic gonadotropin output. (From Knobil E: On the regulation of the primate corpus luteum. Biol Reprod 8:246, 1973.)

there is little invasion of the endometrium *per se*, with implantation occurring within special endometrial protrusions called *caruncles* in ruminants and by relatively minor *villus* invasion of the endometrium in horses and pigs. Concerning the time of implantation, domestic animals are more dependent on uterine secretions for the support of pregnancy than are primates. For cattle and horses, the first indications of implantation begin about days 25–

30, and it is likely that another week to 10 days passes before a significant amount of embryonic nutrition is obtained through the implantation site. Subclinical uterine infections, or an inadequate number of endometrial glands, can interfere with the establishment of pregnancy in the species in which a long interval exists from fertilization to implantation. The cervix forms an important barrier to contamination of the uterine lumen, both in the nonpregnant as well as the pregnant animal; in the latter, the cervix becomes sealed.

The Placenta Acts as an Endocrine Organ

Besides the essential role of providing nutrients and oxygen for their metabolism, the placenta functions as an endocrine organ. One of the most important functions of the placenta is the *production of progesterone*. In primates, this function is established early in gestation, and it is likely that the placenta can maintain pregnancy within 2–3 weeks following implantation in primates. Placental production of progesterone, which is sufficient to maintain pregnancy, occurs later in domestic animals (sheep, day 50 of a 150-day gestation; horse, day 70 of a 340-day gestation; cat, day 45 of a 65-day gestation), or the placenta never produces enough progesterone to support pregnancy (cattle, goats, pigs).

The *production of estrogen* requires, in contrast to progesterone, interaction between the fetus and placenta. This interaction has been best described in primates, in particularly by the experiments of the Hungarian immigrant to Sweden, Dycfaluszy. He and his co-workers found that the placenta was unable to produce estrogen from progesterone even though the steroids were only separated by androgens in the steroid biochemical synthetic pathway. The placenta simply does not possess the enzymes necessary for the movement of progesterone to androgens. Therefore, a system has evolved in which the placenta supplies *pregnenolone*, the immediate precursor of progesterone, to the fetus, wherein the *fetal zone of the adrenal cortex* transforms pregnenolone to a C-19 androgen, *dehydroepiandrostrone (DHEA)*. This is returned to the placenta, which is able to convert DHEA to an estrogen. In humans, the primary estrogen of pregnancy is *estriol*. Because the fetus is involved in the production of estriol, well-being of the fetus can be judged by determining estriol concentrations in the plasma of the mother.

The production of estrogen in the mare also involves an interaction between the placenta and fetus (Fig. 37–4). From the work of Pashen and Allen we know that the fetal gonads replace the fetal adrenals in primates as the key fetal endocrine organ involved in the cooperative synthesis of estrogen. The interstitial cells of the gonads appear to be the interactive cells, with fetal gonads enlarging to a size greater than the maternal gonads during the latter part of gestation. The production of estrogens during pregnancy in other domestic species, occurring relatively late in gestation, may involve the development of placental enzymes that allow progesterone to be metabolized to estrogens without the direct intervention of a fetal endocrine organ (fetal cortisol, though, is important for the induction of these placental enzymes, particularly in sheep; see Parturition).

The protein hormones that are produced during pregnancy tend to be of placental origin. For example, *relaxin* is a hormone produced by the placenta in the cat, dog, and horse beginning at about days 20, 20, and 70, respectively (see Fig. 37–2). Besides its importance for preparing the soft tissues of the pelvic canal for passage of the fetus at birth (see Parturition), relaxin may be important for the support of pregnancy through a synergistic action with progesterone. In exception to the general rule of protein hormone production by the placenta, relaxin is produced by CL in the pig, cow, and primates during pregnancy, with prepartum release occurring in conjunction with luteolysis.

The only CG identified in domestic animals to date is equine CG (formerly called pregnant mares' serum gonadotropin by its discoverer, Harold Cole) (see Fig. 37–4). eCG is produced by trophoblast cells that initially form as a band on the chorion (*chorionic girdle*), which detach themselves around day 35 of pregnancy, penetrate the endometrium, and form associations of cells called *endometrial cups*. eCG enhances progesterone production by the primary CL of pregnancy and aids in the formation of additional (secondary) CL through the luteinization, or ovulation, of preformed follicles. The essentiality of eCG for pregnancy maintenance is not known, because the primary CL is adequate for maintaining pregnancy.

Placental lactogen is another placental protein hormone. Its production increases in primates as CG secretion wanes during pregnancy. Placental lactogen has been reported in goats and sheep, with secretion increasing during the latter part of gestation. The hormone appears to have both *somatotropic* and *lactogenic effects* on the basis of growth hormone and prolactin-

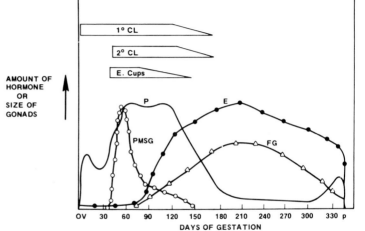

Figure 37–4. Summary of the temporal relationships among changes in hormonal concentrations and morphological changes throughout the gestation period of the mare. *FG*, fetal gonads; *E. Cups*, endometrial cups; *1° CL*, primary corpus luteum; *2° CL*, secondary corpora lutea. (From Daels PF, Hughes JP, Stabenfeldt GH: Reproduction in horses. *In* Reproduction in Domestic Animals, 4th ed. Cupps PT (ed): New York, Academic Press 1991, p 423.)

like properties. In dairy cattle, for example, placental lactogen may be important for setting the stage for the next lactation concerning mammary gland alveolar development. Another hormone whose production is increased during pregnancy, *prolactin,* also is important for alveolar development during the prepartum period. Prolactin is not a hormone of placental origin; prolactin increases during the latter part of gestation due to the effect of estrogen on its release from the adenohypophysis.

PARTURITION

Fetal Cortisol Initiates Delivery Through Increased Secretion of Estrogen and, as a Result, Prostaglandin F-2α

During pregnancy, the uterus progressively enlarges and stretches because of the growing fetus. Progesterone plays an important role in maintaining the quiescence of the myometrium as well as promoting a tightly contracted cervix. During the latter part of gestation, estrogen begins to influence uterine muscle by stimulating the production of *contractile protein* and the formation of *gap junctions;* the former increases the contractile potential of the uterus, and the latter facilitates the contractile process through increased communication among smooth muscle cells. Thus, important changes that set the stage for parturition begin weeks before the actual process begins. In the end, the uterus is converted from a quiescent to a contractile organ and, importantly, the cervix relaxes and opens to allow the fetus to be delivered.

The most important question about parturition concerns what initiates the process. In domestic animals, it is clear that maturation of the fetus eventually brings about changes that initiate the delivery process. The key organ system of the fetus responsible for initiating the process is the *fetal adrenal cortex,* with the hypothalamus and adenohypophysis playing important supporting roles. This concept came from the work at the University of California by Liggins and Kennedy, who showed destruction of the anterior pituitary of the sheep fetus resulted in prolongation of gestation; Drost subsequently found the same results following fetal adrenalectomy. Critical changes in *cortisol secretion* by the fetus eventually result in the synthesis and release of PGF-2α from

the uterus, which produces muscle contraction and relaxation of the cervix. The details of the initiation of parturition that follow emphasize ruminants.

The maturation of the fetal adrenal cortex is of critical importance in the initiation of parturition. It is likely that the adrenal cortex becomes progressively sensitive to fetal ACTH (Fig. 37–5). The time of adrenal maturation is under fetal genetic control as shown by studies conducted at Davis on fetal lambs of different breed in the same uterus (produced by embryo transfer) in which the prepartum initiation of cortisol production occurred at times that were characteristic (and different) for the breed. Fetal cortisol induces placental enzymes (*17α-hydroxylase* and *C17–20 lyase*) that direct steroid synthesis away from progesterone to estrogen. This process occurs at different times prepartum in domestic species, e.g., beginning at prepartum days 25–30 in cattle, 7–10 in pigs, and 2–3 in sheep. The end result of increased estrogen secretion is the secretion of *prostaglandins,* particularly PGF-2α. PGF-2α is the pivotal hormone for the initiation of parturition; once its secretion begins, the acute phase of delivery is activated. The role of oxytocin in the initiation of delivery is not certain; it likely complements PGF-2α once the delivery process has started (Fig. 37–5).

The synthesis of PGF-2α is thought to come about through increased availability of the substrate *arachidonic acid,* which is the main rate-limiting step in the synthesis of PGF-2α. Estrogens are proposed to influence the system by making available the enzyme *phospholipase A,* a membrane-bound lysosomal enzyme that initiates the subsequent hydrolysis of phospholipids and release of arachidonic acid. This likely results from an increasing estrogen:progesterone ratio, with progesterone initially stabilizing, and then estrogens destabilizing, lysosomal membranes. The end result is increased availability of arachidonic acid for the synthesis of PGF-2α. The onset of PGF-2α synthesis results in the immediate release of the hormone, because PGF-2α is not synthesized and stored. The critical effect of PGF-2α on the myometrium is to release intracellular Ca^{2+}, which binds to *actin* and *myosin* to initiate the contractile process. Prostaglandins, both PGE-2 and PGF-2α, also have important effects on the *cervix,* which allow it to relax and dilate, allowing the passage of the fetus. The end result is a direct effect of PGF-2α on the intracellular matrix of the cervix in which there is a loss of collagen with a con-

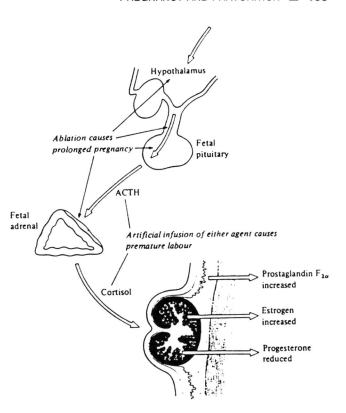

Figure 37–5. Diagrammatic summary explaining how the fetal lamb controls the onset of labor. Experimental procedures that lengthen or shorten pregnancy are shown. (Redrawn from Liggins CG: The foetal role in the initiation of parturition in the ewe. *In* Foetal Autonomy. Wolstenholme GEW, O'Connor M (eds). London, Churchill Livingstone, 1969.)

comitant increase in *glycosaminoglycans*, the latter affecting the aggregation of collagen fibers.

In some animals, such as the cow, goat, dog, and cat, PGF-2α synthesis and release initiates regression of the CL beginning 24–36 hours before delivery, with complete withdrawal of progesterone occurring 12–24 hours before delivery. Although the withdrawal of progesterone in these species is essential for delivery, it should be pointed out that progesterone withdrawal *per se* does not initiate delivery; it is the release of PGF-2α that both causes luteolysis and drives myometrial contractions.

In the mare, as in primates, delivery occurs even though progesterone concentrations remain elevated during the process. In this situation, PGF-2α is able to overcome the suppressive effects of progesterone on myometrial activity. For animals dependent on placental production of progesterone for pregnancy maintenance, it is not possible to turn off one function, i.e., steroid synthesis, and still continue with other functions that are necessary for the support of the fetus through the time of delivery.

Oxytocin is also important to the delivery process (Fig. 37–6). Estrogen induces *oxytocin*

receptor formation in the myometrium. Recent information indicates that significant amounts of oxytocin are released only with the entry of the fetus into the birth canal. Oxytocin release occurs through the so-called *Ferguson reflex.* The afferent arm of the reflex is by passage of impulses through sensory nerves in the spinal cord to the appropriate nuclei in the hypothalamus; the efferent arm involves transport of oxytocin from the neurohypophysis by the blood vascular system. Oxytocin is synergistic with PGF-2α in promoting contraction of the uterus.

One hormone important for the preparation of parturition is relaxin. This hormone was first identified as responsible for the separation of the pubic symphysis through relaxation of the interpubic ligament. Relaxin causes the ligaments and associated muscles surrounding the pelvic canal to relax, which allows the fetus to expand the pelvic canal to its fullest potential. In the mare, a well-defined area of muscle softening can be discerned on the midline from the top of the croup through the ventral commissure of the vulva. In the cow, muscles posterior to the hip become relaxed to the point that they undulate as the animal walks in the final 24 hours before parturition. In the cow and pig, the CL is the source of

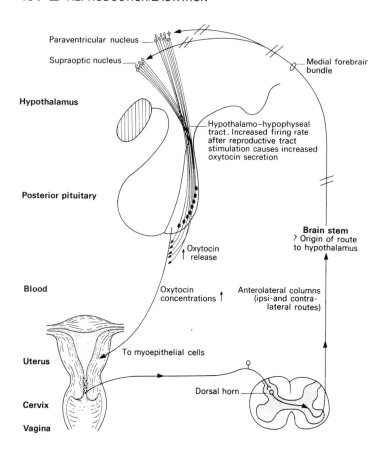

Paraventricular nucleus

Supraoptic nucleus

Medial forebrain bundle

Hypothalamus

Hypothalamo–hypophyseal tract. Increased firing rate after reproductive tract stimulation causes increased oxytocin secretion

Posterior pituitary

Brain stem
? Origin of route to hypothalamus

Oxytocin release

Blood

Oxytocin concentrations ↑

Anterolateral columns (ipsi-and contra-lateral routes)

Uterus

To myoepithelial cells

Dorsal horn

Cervix

Vagina

Figure 37–6. The neuroendocrine reflex (Ferguson reflex) underlying oxytocin synthesis and secretion. (From Johnson M, Everitt B (eds): Essential Reproduction, 3rd ed. London, Blackwell Scientific Publications, 1988, p 299.)

relaxin. In both of these species, the prepartum release of PGF-2α causes luteolysis with a concomitant decline in progesterone production and the release of preformed relaxin. In other domestic species, such as cats, dogs, and horses, the source of relaxin is the placenta. In these species, significant relaxin production begins during the first part of gestation, with values sustained through parturition. It may be that relaxin is important in these species for the maintenance of pregnancy in synergism with progesterone (see Fig. 37–2).

The first stage of parturition involves presentation of the fetus at the internal os of the cervix. This likely comes about because of increased myometrial activity due to PGF-2α release. Once the cervix opens and the fetus passes into the pelvic canal, myometrial contractions become less important for delivery of the fetus; abdominal press, accomplished by closure of the epiglottis and contraction of maternal abdominal muscles, becomes the main force involved in the delivery process. The actual delivery process is called the *second stage of parturition.*

The *third stage of parturition* involves the delivery of the fetal membranes. In litter-bearing animals, such as the cat, dog, and pig, the placental membranes are delivered often with, or immediately after, the appearance of each fetus. In single-bearing species, the placenta may be delivered immediately or within a few hours. From studies done on the mare at the University of California, Davis, we know that major, sustained surges of PGF-2α occur in the immediate postpartum period that are important for expulsion of placental membranes and reduction of uterine size through myometrial contraction. PGF-2α is likely the most important component of uterine size reduction in the immediate postpartum period for all domestic species. This can be inferred from the episodes of discomfort that parturient animals undergo during the hours immediately following delivery.

The neonate must make a major physiological adjustment to life on the outside. The major change involves the blood vascular system, in particular, the respiratory system. During fetal life, blood bypasses the lungs (except for the perfusion of lung tissue in support of development) by two routes: through the ventricles by way of the *foramen ovale*, and from the pulmonary artery to the aorta by the *ductus arteriosus*. The foramen ovale is closed functionally at birth by a flap of tissue in the left ventricle through the development of higher pressures within the left versus the right ventricle. Although the ductus arteriosus immediately constricts at birth, it requires months before it is completely closed. This course of closure is also true for the *ductus venosus*, which serves as a hepatic shunt during fetal life. The rapid conversion from a fluid to a gaseous environment, as occurs at birth, is a truly remarkable adaptation.

CLINICAL CORRELATION

PROLONGED GESTATION

HISTORY □ You are called to examine a purebred Holstein cow that is 12 days overdue compared with the herd gestation average of 280 days. She was artificially inseminated, was diagnosed pregnant 35 days later, and has not been observed in estrus since insemination. You inquire about the presence of bulls on the dairy, but there are none.

CLINICAL EXAMINATION □ The cow has a greatly enlarged abdomen. Upon palpation of the uterus *per rectum*, you find the presence of a large calf. The cow certainly appears to be term as far as the size of the calf. You are puzzled, though, by the lack of colostrum in the udder.

COMMENT □ The history and physical examination findings are compatible with an animal that has a defective fetus concerning the initiation of parturition. A normal fetal hypothalamo-pituitary-adrenocortical system is essential for the production of cortisol, which initiates the delivery process. In the cow, this can begin 3–4 weeks prepartum, with fetal cortisol directing the increased production of estrogen; this, in turn, eventually initiates PGF-2α synthesis and release. The deficit could be due to a malformed adrenal gland, pituitary, or hypothalamus. In one syndrome described for Holsteins, the critical defect was a lack of ACTH-producing cells in the pituitary, which led to inadequate stimulation of the adrenal cortex and inadequate fetal cortisol production. The lack of lactogenesis reflects the fact that the endocrine changes that begin 3–4 weeks prepartum as a prelude to delivery are also important for lactogenesis and, in their absence, colostral formation is delayed.

TREATMENT □ The animal can respond to glucocorticoids, with delivery usually occurring 2–3 days later. The placenta is normal in this situation, and the systemic administration of glucocorticoids substitutes for fetal cortisol in initiating the endocrine events that lead to parturition. Lactogenesis is usually initiated by glucocorticoid treatment, although the process is usually less advanced than that expected at normal delivery. Because the calf continues to grow *in utero* in this syndrome, it is often too large to be delivered *per vaginum*, and a cesarean section may have to be performed 2–3 days after treatment in concert with dilation of the cervix.

You need to tell the owner that the calf will likely not survive because of inadequate adrenal secretion. If the calf were an extremely valuable bull prospect, one could admininster both glucocorticoids and mineralocorticoids for a number of months with the hope the animal would eventually be able to take over its own adrenal support (this actually occurred in one case at the University of California, Davis). It would be questionable, though, to initiate treatment of the calf on the basis that the disease is an autosomal recessive inherited condition.

Bibliography

Austin CR, Short RV (eds): Reproduction in Mammals, Vols 1–6. Cambridge, Cambridge University Press, 1976, 1982, 1984, 1986.

Cupps PT (ed): Reproduction in Domestic Animals, 4th ed. New York, Academic Press, 1991.

Concannon PW, Morton DB, Weir BJ (eds): Dog and cat reproduction, contraception and artificial insemination. J Reprod Fertil (Suppl)39, 1989.

Feldman EC, Nelson RW: Canine and Feline Endocrinology and Reproduction. Philadelphia, WB Saunders, 1987.

Hafez EWE (ed): Reproduction in Farm Animals, 5th ed. Philadelphia, Lea & Febiger, 1987.

Johnson M, Everitt B (eds): Essential Reproduction, 3rd ed. London, Blackwell Scientific Publications, 1988.

Knobil E, Neill JD, Ewing LL, et al (eds): The Physiology of Reproduction, Vols 1, 2. New York, Raven Press, 1988.

McDonald LE, Pineda MH (eds): Veterinary Endocrinology and Reproduction, 4th ed. Philadelphia, Lea & Febiger, 1989.

PRACTICE QUESTIONS FOR CHAPTER 37

1. Active rescue of luteal activity by means of suppression of pulsatile prostaglandin synthesis and release by the production of embryonic signals must occur in which of the following species in order for a developing pregnancy to have the early progestational support that is essentail for pregnancy maintenance? (Select more than one letter.)

   a. Cat
   b. Dog
   c. Goat
   d. Horse
   e. Pig
   f. Sheep

2. In primates, it has been established that estrogen production during much of pregnancy is a cooperative venture between fetal adrenals and the placenta. The domestic species most extensively studied in this regard is the horse. In this species, the main two interactive organs involved in the synthesis of estrogen during pregnancy are

   a. the placenta and the fetal adrenals.
   b. the placenta and the fetal gonads.
   c. the placenta and the fetal liver.
   d. the placenta and the fetal hypothalamus.
   e. the placenta and the fetal pituitary.

3. Which of the following hormones initiates the final process that eventually leads to parturition?

   a. Maternal estrogen
   b. Maternal progesterone
   c. Fetal cortisol
   d. Maternal relaxin
   e. Maternal prostaglandin
   f. Maternal oxytocin

4. The hormone that initiates the myometrial contractile process that acutely initiates parturition is

   a. maternal estrogen.
   b. maternal progesterone.
   c. fetal cortisol.
   d. maternal relaxin.
   e. maternal prostaglandin.
   f. maternal oxytocin.

5. The hormone released by the passage of the fetus into the pelvic canal through the cervix is

   a. maternal estrogen.
   b. maternal progesterone.
   c. fetal cortisol.
   d. maternal relaxin.
   e. maternal prostaglandin.
   f. maternal oxytocin.

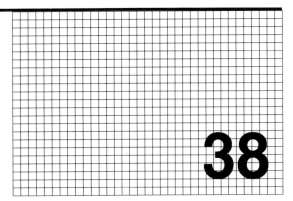

38

The Mammary Gland

ANATOMICAL ASPECTS OF THE MAMMARY GLAND

1. The milk-secreting cells of the mammary gland develop through the proliferation of epithelium into hollow structures called alveoli
2. Most of the milk that accumulates prior to suckling or milking is stored in the alveoli even though animals have enlarged areas for the storage of milk called cisterns
3. A suspensory system involving the udder of the cow allows the animal to carry a large amount of milk

CONTROL OF MAMMOGENESIS

1. The initial development of the mammary gland is programmed by embryonic mesenchyme
2. Proliferation of the mammary duct system begins at puberty with ducts under the control of estrogens, growth hormone, and adrenal steroids, and alveoli under the control of progesterone and prolactin

COLOSTRUM

1. Prepartum milk secretion (without removal) results in the formation of colostrum
2. The ingestion of colostrum is important because of the passive immunity it confers through the presence of high concentrations of immunoglobulins
3. The time immunoglobulins can be absorbed through the gut is limited to the first 24–36 hours of life
4. Lipids (particularly vitamin A) and proteins (caseins and albumins) are high in concentration in colostrum; carbohydrates (lactose) are low

LACTOGENESIS

1. Prolactin, inhibited by dopamine and stimulated by vasoactive intestinal peptide, is the most important hormone involved in the process of milk synthesis, or lactogenesis; growth hormone is also important for lactogenesis
2. The release of fat into milk from the alveolar cell involves constriction of the plasma membrane around the fat droplet; fats are dispersed in milk in droplet form
3. Milk proteins and lactose are released from alveolar cells by the process of exocytosis

MILK REMOVAL

1. Efficient milk removal requires the release of oxytocin, which causes contraction of

muscle cells that surround the alveoli (myoepithelial cells), and movement of milk into the ducts and cisterns

2. Milk removed during suckling or hand milking is trapped in the teat and forced out, whereas milk removed by milking machines moves by suction
3. Carbohydrate stores are good in neonates born as singles or twins, whereas carbohydrate stores are low in neonates born in litters; the former can stand a longer interval to first suckling than can the latter

COMPOSITION OF MILK

1. Fats are the most important energy source in milk
2. Lactose, composed of glucose and galactose, is the main carbohydrate of mammalian milk
3. The main proteins in milk are called caseins and are found in curd

THE LACTATION CYCLE

1. Milk production peaks at 1 month postpartum in dairy cattle, followed by a slow decline in production; milking usually stops at 305 days of lactation, so that the animal can prepare the mammary gland for the next lactation
2. Lactation can be induced by hormone administration (estrogen and progesterone) and enhanced by growth hormone and increased photoperiod exposure

DISEASES ASSOCIATED WITH THE MAMMARY GLAND

1. The main diseases that affect the mammary gland directly are mastitis (prevalent in dairy cattle) and neoplasia (prevalent in intact dogs)
2. The main conditions that involve the mammary gland, although indirectly, are the passive transfer of red blood cell–agglutinating antibodies by the ingestion of colostrum (mare), and hypocalcemia due to the transient drain of calcium that occurs with the initiation of lactation (dairy cattle) or during lactation (dog)

Animals that belong to the class *Mammalia* are characterized as having bodies that are basically covered with hair, delivering live young instead of eggs (the monotremes are an exception), and pertinent to this chapter, nurturing their young through the use of structures called mammary glands. The ability of mammals to nurture their young through milk secretion by mammary glands during the early part of postfetal life has given these animals survival advantages. Because the reproductive strategy of mammals involves the production of far fewer young, compared to reptiles, amphibians, and birds, mammary glands have allowed mammals to be much more efficient in the nurture of their young. Egg-laying classes of animals, such as fish, reptiles, and amphibians, depend upon favorable environmental factors for the nurture of their young; the offspring are often vulnerable to the vagaries of nature. Mammalian young do not require teeth for the *suckling* process and thus can be delivered in a relatively mature state, although with immature maxillae and mandi-

bles, which facilitates the delivery of the head. The development of teeth coincides with the need to consume food other than milk.

ANATOMICAL ASPECTS OF THE MAMMARY GLAND

The Milk-Secreting Cells of the Mammary Gland Develop Through the Proliferation of Epithelium into Hollow Structures Called Alveoli

Embryonic ectoderm is the source of the mammary glands. The mammary ectoderm is first represented by parallel linear thickenings on the ventral belly wall. The continuity of the ridge that is formed is broken into the appropriate number of *mammary buds* from which the functional part of the mammary gland will be derived.

The *parenchyma*, or milk-secreting cells, of the mammary gland develops through the proliferation of epithelial cells that arise from

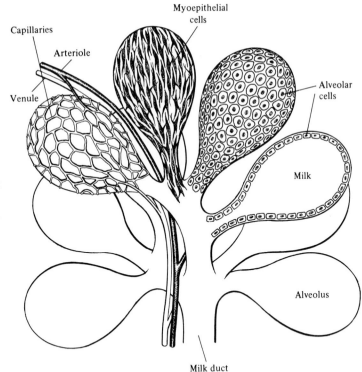

Figure 38–1. Diagram of a cluster of alveoli in the mammary gland of a goat. (From Cowie AT: Lactation. *In* Austin CR, Short RV (eds): Hormonal Control of Reproduction. Reproduction in Mammals, Vol 3, 2nd ed. Cambridge, Cambridge University Press, 1984.)

the primary mammary cord. The epithelial cells eventually form hollow, circular structures called *alveoli,* which are the fundamental milk-secreting units of the mammary gland (Fig. 38–1). In concert with this development, an enlarged area of epithelium develops on the surface, i.e., the *nipple,* which is the external connection to the internal milk-secreting system. In males, while nipples often develop, the underlying primary mammary cord does not develop into glandular tissue.

Most of the Milk That Accumulates Prior to Suckling or Milking Is Stored in the Alveoli Even Though Animals Have Enlarged Areas for the Storage of Milk Called Cisterns

Duct systems connect alveoli with the nipple, or teat, enabling milk to pass from the area of formation to the area of delivery (nipple). The ducts may come together so that there is only one final duct per gland, which has one opening through the nipple, or teat, such as occurs in cattle, goats, and sheep. Two main ducts and associated openings occur in the mare and sow, whereas the cat and dog

can have 10, or more, openings in the nipple, with each opening representing separate glands (Fig. 38–2). Both the cow and doe (goat) have specialized areas for holding milk, called cisterns, which are located in the ventral part of the gland and into which all main ducts empty (Fig. 38–3). This has enabled the cow, for example, to synthesize and store larger amounts of milk than would otherwise be possible. In spite of this adaptation, it is important to realize that a majority of the milk present at the time of milking is stored in the duct system of the mammary glands.

Mammary glands develop typically as paired structures. The number of pairs in domestic animals vary from one in goats, horses, and sheep; two in cattle; and seven to nine in the sow. The position of mammary glands varies in animals, being thoracic in primates; extending the length of the thorax and abdomen in cats, dogs, and pigs; and being inguinal in cattle, goats, and horses. In domestic species, such as cattle, goats, horses, and sheep, pairs of mammary glands are closely opposed to each other; the resulting structure is called an *udder.* In the cow, for example, two pairs of glands (four quarters) compose the udder.

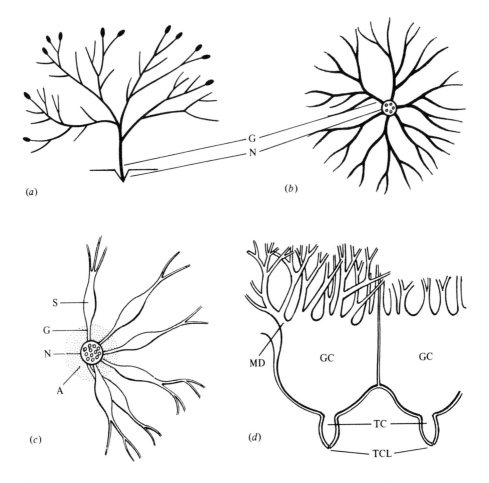

Figure 38–2. Diagram showing four different arrangements of the mammary duct system. (From Cowie AT: Lactation. *In* Austin CR, Short RV (eds): Hormonal Control of Reproduction. Reproduction in Mammals, Vol 3, 2nd ed. Cambridge, Cambridge University Press, 1984.)

A Suspensory System Involving the Udder of the Cow Allows the Animal to Carry a Large Amount of Milk

One of the important anatomical adaptations of the udder that allows dairy cows to carry large amounts of milk is the development of a suspension system for the udder. This system is formed by the median suspensory ligament (formed between pairs of mammary glands) composed of elastic connective tissue that originates from the abdominal tunic. The lateral (nonelastic) suspensory ligament, which originates from prepubic and subpubic ligaments, enters the glands laterally at various levels to become part of the interstitial connective tissue framework of the udder. It is not unusual for heavy-producing dairy cows to have 50 pounds of milk in their udder

immediately prior to milking. If the suspensory support system were not in place, the mammary gland system would soon break down because of the weight of the milk.

CONTROL OF MAMMOGENESIS

The Initial Development of the Mammary Gland Is Programmed by Embryonic Mesenchyme

The fetal development of the mammary gland is under both genetic and endocrine control. The initial development of the mammary bud is under control of embryonic mesenchyme (connective tissue). If mammary mesenchyme is transplanted to another area, mammary bud formation will occur at the site

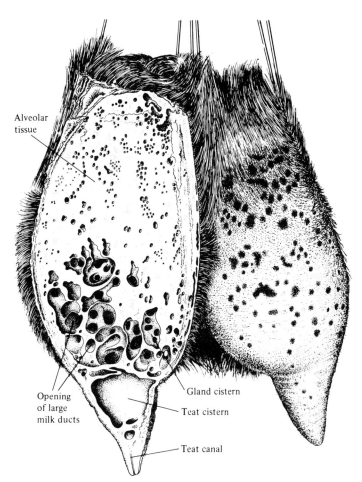

Figure 38–3. Udder of a goat in which part of the left mammary gland has been cut away to show the dense alveolar tissues, the gland cistern with the large ducts opening into it, the teat cistern, and the teat canal. (From Cowie AT: Lactation. *In* Austin CR, Short RV (eds): Hormonal Control of Reproduction. Reproduction in Mammals, Vol 3, 2nd ed. Cambridge, Cambridge University Press, 1984.)

Alveolar tissue

Opening of large milk ducts

Gland cistern

Teat cistern

Teat canal

of transplantation. Although little is known about fetal mammary development, it is not thought to be driven by hormones. It is possible, though, to have actively secreting mammary glands at birth that have been caused by exogenous administration of certain hormones to the mother.

Proliferation of the Mammary Duct System Begins at Puberty with Ducts Under the Control of Estrogens, Growth Hormone, and Adrenal Steroids, and Alveoli Under the Control of Progesterone and Prolactin

Development of the mammary gland in postfetal life usually starts in concert with puberty. Cyclic ovarian activity results in the production of estrogen and progesterone. Estrogen, plus growth hormone and adrenal steroids, are responsible for proliferation of the duct system. The development of alveoli from the terminal ends of the ducts requires the addition of progesterone and prolactin (Fig. 38–4).

Although the development of the mammary gland begins with the onset of puberty, the gland remains relatively undeveloped until the occurrence of pregnancy. Udder development usually becomes evident by the middle of gestation in most domestic animals. In domestic species, the secretion of milk often begins during the latter part of gestation (mainly due to increasing prolactin secretion), which results in the formation of colostrum (colostrum is discussed later). By the end of pregnancy, the mammary gland has been transformed from a structure involving mostly stromal (connective tissue) elements to a structure that is filled with alveolar cells that are actively synthesizing and secreting milk. Groups of adjacent alveoli form lobules that are further associated into larger structures called lobes. Connective tissue bands delineate the lobules and the lobes (Fig. 38–5).

COLOSTRUM

Prepartum Milk Secretion (Without Removal) Results in the Formation of Colostrum

The milk formed before parturition is called *colostrum*. Its formation represents a secretory

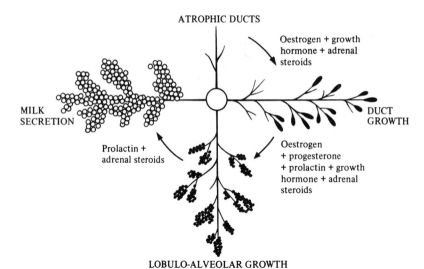

ATROPHIC DUCTS

Oestrogen + growth
hormone + adrenal
steroids

MILK
SECRETION

DUCT
GROWTH

Prolactin +
adrenal steroids

Oestrogen
+ progesterone
+ prolactin + growth
hormone + adrenal
steroids

LOBULO-ALVEOLAR GROWTH

Figure 38–4. The hormones concerned in the growth of the mammary gland and in the initiation of milk secretion in the hypophysectomized-ovariectomized-adrenalectomized rat. (Lyons WR: Proc R Soc Lond [Biol] 149:303–325, 1958.) (From Cowie AT: Lactation. *In* Austin CR, Short RV (eds): Hormonal Control of Reproduction. Reproduction in Mammals, Vol 3, 2nd ed. Cambridge, Cambridge University Press, 1984.)

process in which lactogenesis occurs in the absence of milk removal. *Lactation,* however, cannot fully blossom until pregnancy is terminated. This is due to the inhibitory effects of progesterone and estrogen on milk secretion, inhibitory factors that are removed at or just before delivery.

The Ingestion of Colostrum Is Important Because of the Passive Immunity It Confers Through the Presence of High Concentrations of Immunoglobulins

As indicated previously, colostrum is the milk that is formed prior to parturition, with certain substances concentrated in the process. Ingestion of colostrum is important for the well-being of the neonate. In addition to nutrition, colostrum has an important function concerning temporary, or passive, protection against infectious agents. *Immunoglobulins* (IgA) are produced in the mammary gland by plasma cells (derived from B-lymphocytes originating in the gut) as a result of exposure of the mother to certain microorganisms. The immunoglobulins gain access to the milk system through the migration of the plasma cells from adjacent tissue sites. The immunoglobulins are highly concentrated in colostrum, and through the consumption of colostrum the neonate can receive passive immunity against pathogens experienced by the mother. This allows the young to receive immediate protection from environmental organisms. The neonates of all domestic animals acquire antibodies through the ingestion of colostrum. The absorption of antibodies through milk in do-

mestic animals contrasts with other species, including humans, rabbits, and guinea pigs, in which a significant amount of antibody is passed to the fetus through the placenta.

The Time Immunoglobulins Can Be Absorbed Through the Gut Is Limited to the First 24–36 Hours of Life

Neonates usually have a limited time (24–36 hours) in which immunoglobulins (proteins) can be absorbed through the gut. Thus, the feeding of colostrum within this time period is important to ensure the presence of immunoglobulins in the newborn. Other antimicrobial factors found in milk that are important for protection against the development of enteric bacterial flora include lysozymes, lactoferrin, and the lactoperoxidase system.

Lipids (Particularly Vitamin A) and Proteins (Caseins and Albumins) Are High in Concentration in Colostrum; Carbohydrates (Lactose) Are Low

In addition to immunoglobulins, colostrum is a rich source of nutrients, especially *vitamin A*. Placental transfer of vitamin A is limited in domestic animals, with calves and piglets being particularly low in vitamin A at birth. This deficiency is corrected by the ingestion of colostrum. Lipids and proteins, including *caseins* and *albumins*, are also relatively high in colostrum. One exception concerning the concentration of milk products is *lactose*, whose synthesis is significantly inhibited by progesterone until about the time of delivery. Nev-

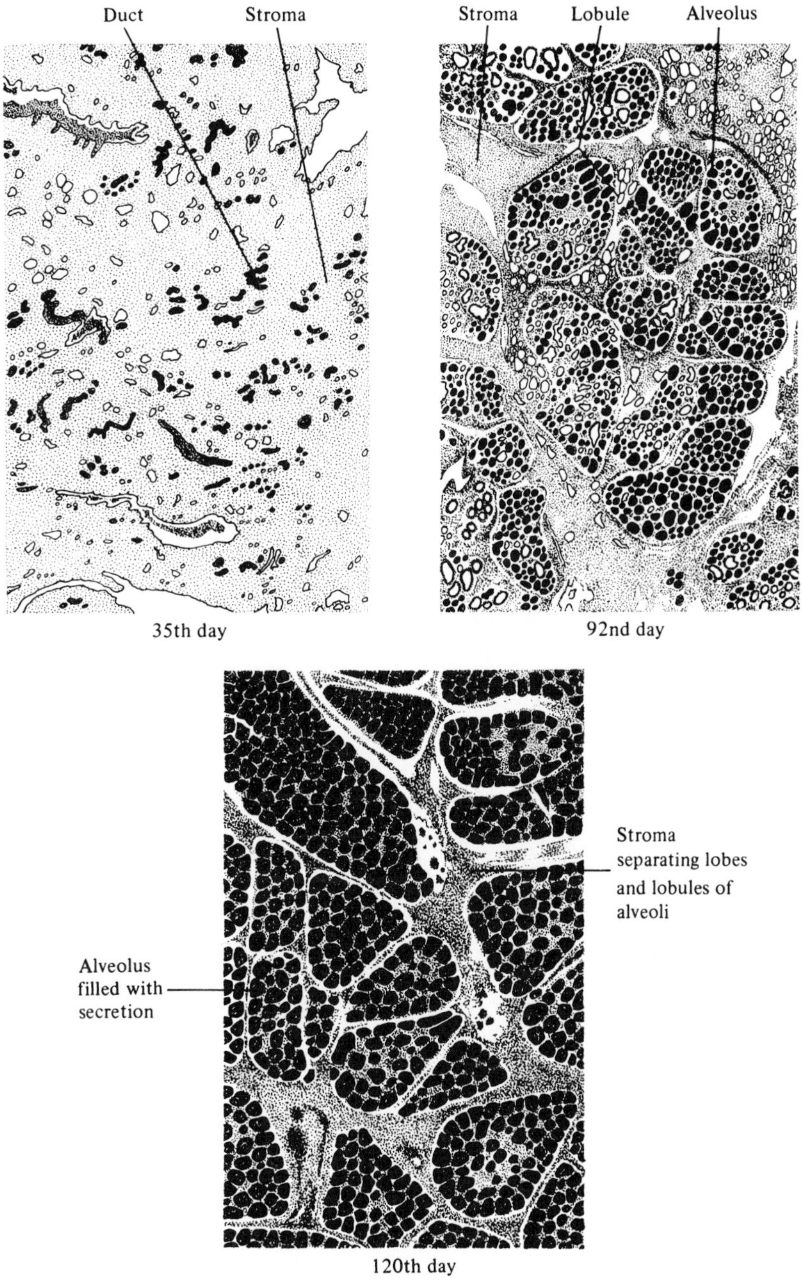

Duct   Stroma

35th day

Stroma   Lobule   Alveolus

92nd day

Alveolus
filled with
secretion

Stroma
separating lobes
and lobules of
alveoli

120th day

Figure 38–5. Sections of the mammary gland of the goat at three different times during pregnancy (gestation is about 150 days). 35th day of pregnancy—note the small collections of ducts scattered throughout the stroma; 92nd day of pregnancy—the lobules of alveoli are now forming in groups known as lobes; secretion is present in some of the alveolar lumina and there is still considerable stromal tissue; 120th day of pregnancy—the lobules of alveoli are almost fully developed; the alveoli are full of secretion and the stromal tissue is reduced to thin bands separating lobules and thicker strands between lobes. (A and C from Falconer IR (ed): Lactation. London, Butterworths, 1970; D—unpublished data.) (From Cowie AT: Lactation. *In* Austin CR, Short RV (eds). Hormonal Control of Reproduction. Reproduction in Mammals, Vol 3, 2nd ed. Cambridge, Cambridge University Press, 1984.)

ertheless, at the moment of delivery, the newborn's milk supply is nutritive (high protein, fat, and vitamin A content) and protective (immunoglobulins) (Table 38–1).

LACTOGENESIS

Prolactin, Inhibited by Dopamine and Stimulated by Vasoactive Intestinal Peptide, Is the Most Important Hormone Involved in the Process of Milk Synthesis, or Lactogenesis; Growth Hormone Is Also Important for Lactogenesis

Prolactin plays an important role in the secretion of milk, or *lactogenesis*. Prolactin is released in conjunction with manipulation of the teat through either the milking or suckling process. Sensory stimuli are carried into the hypothalamus, wherein the synthesis of *dopamine*, a major inhibitor of prolactin secretion, is blocked while neurons in the *paraventricular nucleus* are stimulated to produce *vasoactive intestinal peptide* (VIP), a stimulator of prolactin release (Fig. 38–6). A short-lived surge of prolactin secretion occurs immediately following the onset of milk removal; peak values are reached usually within 30 minutes following the initial stimulus. It is apparent that major

surges of prolactin do not have to be elicited on an hourly basis to maintain lactation, because 12-hour release intervals, as occur in association with the milking of dairy cows, are sufficient to maintain lactogenesis. Prolactin responses, as judged by the amount of hormone release following mammary gland stimulation, decrease as the lactation period progresses.

Another major hormone required for milk production in ruminants is *growth hormone* (GH). As discussed later, there is now considerable interest in the use of GH to promote additional milk production from cows through exogenous administration of the hormone.

The Release of Fat into Milk from the Alveolar Cell Involves Constriction of the Plasma Membrane Around the Fat Droplet; Fats Are Dispersed in Milk in Droplet Form

The synthesis and release of milk by alveolar epithelial cells is a remarkable physiological process (Fig. 38–7). Alveolar cells synthesize fats, proteins, and carbohydrates and extrude the products into the lumen of the alveolus. Fat droplets first accumulate in the basal cytoplasm of the cell, then move to the apex, where the droplet protrudes into alveolar lumen. The cell membrane constricts about the base of the fat droplet, so that fat is dispersed in milk in small droplets, surrounded by cell membranes; the droplet often contains portions of cell cytoplasm.

Table 38–1
AMOUNTS OF SELECTED COMPONENTS OF BOVINE COLOSTRUM AS PERCENTAGE OF LEVEL IN NORMAL MILK

Constituent	Days After Parturition		
	0	*3*	*5*
Dry matter	220	100	100
Lactose	45	90	100
Lipids	150	90	100
Minerals	120	100	100
Proteins			
Casein	210	110	110
Albumin	500	120	105
Globulin	3500	300	200
Vitamins			
A	600	120	100
Carotene	1200	250	125
E	500	200	125
Thiamin	150	150	150
Riboflavin	320	130	110
Pantothenic acid	45	110	105

From Jacobson NL, McGilland AD: The mammary gland and lactation. *In* Swenson MJ (ed): Dukes' Physiology of Domestic Animals, 10th ed. Ithaca, Cornell University Press, 1984.

Milk Proteins and Lactose Are Released from Alveolar Cells by the Process of Exocytosis

Milk proteins are synthesized on the endoplasmic reticulum; the casein molecules pass to the Golgi apparatus, where they are phosphorylated and formed into micelles within the Golgi vesicles. Lactose is synthesized also within the Golgi vesicles and is released in conjunction with milk proteins. The process of extrusion for proteins and carbohydrates is different from fat; the Golgi vesicles fuse with the cell membrane, and the release of proteins and carbohydrates occurs by *exocytosis*. Al-

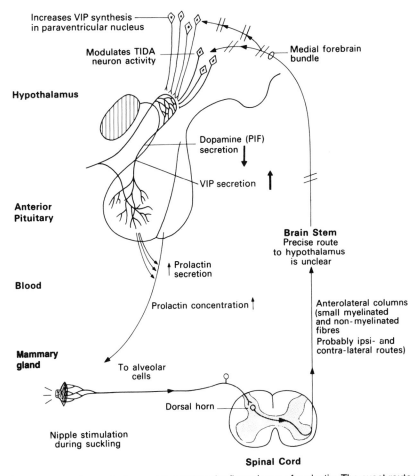

Figure 38–6. Somatosensory pathways in the suckling-induced reflex release of prolactin. The exact route taken by sensory information between brainstem and hypothalamus is speculative. Although tubero-infundibular dopamine neuron (TIDA) activity is modulated as a result of the arrival of this somatosensory derived input, the increased secretory activity of VIP-containing neurons in the paraventricular nucleus is probably also crucial in driving prolactin secretion during suckling. (Adapted from Johnson M, Everitt B: Essential Reproduction, 3rd ed. London, Blackwell Scientific Publications, 1988.)

though it is not certain how often cells go through a synthesis and extrusion cycle, it may occur twice daily, particularly in dairy cows that are milked two times per day.

MILK REMOVAL

In order for lactogenesis to be maintained, milk must be removed from the mammary gland by suckling or milking. If milk is not removed within about 16 hours in dairy cows, the synthesis of milk begins to be suppressed. As indicated previously, most of the milk in the udder of a dairy cow at the time of milking is located in the ducts and alveoli. The movement of milk into the gland cistern at suckling or milking would be slow, and less milk would be obtained during the milking of a cow if the drainage of milk were a passive process.

Efficient Milk Removal Requires the Release of Oxytocin, Which Causes Contraction of Muscle Cells That Surround the Alveoli (Myoepithelial Cells), and Movement of Milk into the Ducts and Cisterns

To facilitate the process of milk removal, *myoepithelial cells* surround the alveoli and ducts (see Figs. 38–1, 38–7). The myoepithelial cells are particularly responsive to *oxytocin* and, in fact, contract when exposed to the hormone. The synthesis and release of oxytocin from the posterior pituitary is elicited by a neuroendocrine reflex involving tactile stimulation of the udder by oral stimulation by the

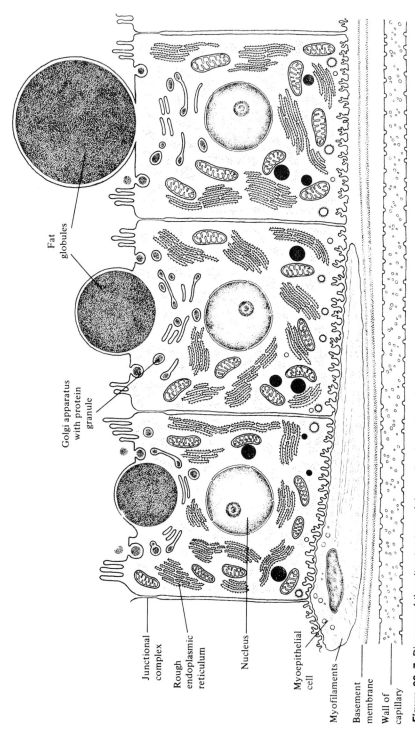

Figure 38–7. Diagram of the ultrastructure of three alveolar cells and a myoepithelial cell. (*From* Cowie AT: Lactation. *In* Austin CR, Short RV (eds): Hormonal Control of Reproduction. Reproduction in Mammals, Vol 3, 2nd ed. Cambridge, Cambridge University Press, 1984.)

Fat globules

Golgi apparatus with protein granule

Junctional complex

Rough endoplasmic reticulum

Nucleus

Myoepithelial cell

Myofilaments

Basement membrane

Wall of capillary

young or by the manual stimulation of washing prior to milking. The sensory stimuli from the udder are carried through the spinal cord into the hypothalamus. Neurons in the paraventricular and supraoptic nuclei are stimulated to synthesize oxytocin and release it from nerve terminals that impinge on the median eminence (Fig. 38–8). Other sensory stimuli that elicit oxytocin release include auditory, visual, or olfactory stimuli that occur near or within the milking parlor. Earlier societies used various deceptions to get earlier breeds of cattle to release their milk. They often allowed the calf to suckle one teat while they milked the other glands. They also knew about the *Ferguson reflex*, if not in name, wherein stimulation of the cervix (and release of oxytocin) was effected by blowing air into the vagina by the use of hollow tubes.

The release of oxytocin occurs within seconds after the stimulus arrives in the hypothalamus; increased pressure within the mammary gland is evident within a minute of stimulation as milk is forced out of the alveoli and ducts due to contraction of the myoepithelial cells. The term used in cattle to describe this phenomenon is *let-down* of milk. Increased pressure within the udder is often obvious within a minute of the stimulation. The release of oxytocin lasts only a few minutes, and it is important that the milking process begin soon after the let-down of milk is complete (Fig. 38–9). The milking process, as done by machine or by hand in earlier times, is completed often within 4–5 minutes.

It is interesting to compare stimuli that release oxytocin, which initiates the passive part of lactogenesis, with stimuli that release prolactin, which directly influences lactogenesis. Any sensory stimulus that a cow associates with milking has the potential for releasing oxytocin. The neuroendocrine reflex is elicited in the expectation of milk removal because of the environment (milking parlor) to which the animal is exposed. Prolactin, on the other hand, is released only by tactile stimulation of the udder. The latter makes sense, because there is no need to stimulate milk synthesis and release unless the evidence for milk removal (udder stimulation) is strong.

Milk Removed During Suckling or Hand Milking is Trapped in the Teat and Forced Out, Whereas Milk Removed by Milking Machines Moves by Suction

Milk is removed in essentially the same manner in both suckling and hand milking.

The base of the teat containing milk is compressed between either the tongue and hard palate of the young, or between the thumb and index finger of the hand. Then the milk is expressed from the teat through the teat orifice by applying pressure to the teat. The constriction around the base of the teat is released, the teat refills with milk, and the process is repeated. Milking machines, on the other hand, work by suction (Fig. 38–10). The teat-cup is formed by an outer metal shell with a rubber liner inside with an opening from the liner into the milk collection system. Pressure outside the rubber liner is controlled by a vacuum pump, which allows atmospheric pressure to enter and then evacuates air. When a vaccum is applied, the liner is pulled away from the teat, and milk is sucked through the teat orifice. When atmospheric pressure is present, the end of the teat collapses, shutting off the flow of milk. Thus, the system allows the teat to recover from the effects of being compressed against the rubber liner during the milk suction phase in a rhythmic, repeating fashion. This tends to ameliorate the damage that is done to the teat by the pressure that is exerted upon it. Cows that have good teat sphincters around the opening of the teat (streak canal) are better able to maintain the integrity of the mammary gland against invasion by microorganisms.

Carbohydrate Stores Are Good in Neonates Born as Singles or Twins, Whereas Carbohydrate Stores Are Low in Neonates Born in Litters; the Former Can Stand a Longer Interval to First Suckling Than Can the Latter

In domestic animals that have one or two offspring, such as cattle, horses, sheep, and goats, the young have to be able to stand in order to suckle. Neonates, in this situation, have reasonably good carbohydrate stores, and suckling may not occur for 1–2 hours without adverse effect as the young gain the ability to stand and locate the mammary gland. Young that are part of litters (cats, dogs, and pigs) are usually immediately nestled toward the mammary glands and often will be sucking within 30 minutes. This is important for animals born in litters, because they tend to be immature at birth and susceptible to hypoglycemia, especially piglets, and suckling delays are often detrimental to their survival.

The suckling interval varies considerably

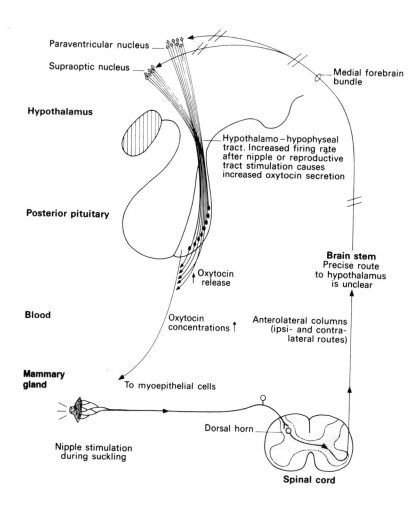

Figure 38–8. Somatosensory pathways in the suckling-induced reflex release of oxytocin. Doubts exist about the brainstem-hypothalamic route taken by the sensory information, but it probably involves the medial forebrain bundle. (Adapted from Johnson M, Everitt B: Essential Reproduction, 3rd ed. London, Blackwell Scientific Publications, 1988.)

Figure 38–9. Oxytocin in the blood of cows before, during, and after milking. *PM,* preparation for milking; *MA,* application of teat cups; *S,* stripping; *EM,* end of machine milking; *C,* control level. Abscissae show time in minutes. (Schams, et al: Acta Endocrinol 92:258–270, 1979.) (From Cowie AT: Lactation. *In* Austin CR, Short RV (eds): Hormonal Control of Reproduction. Reproduction in Mammals, Vol 3, 2nd ed. Cambridge, Cambridge University Press, 1984.)

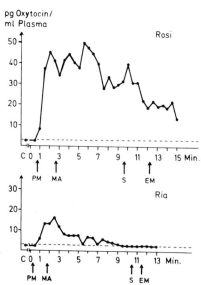

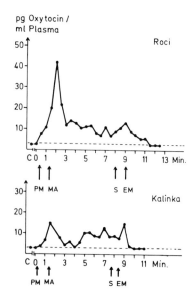

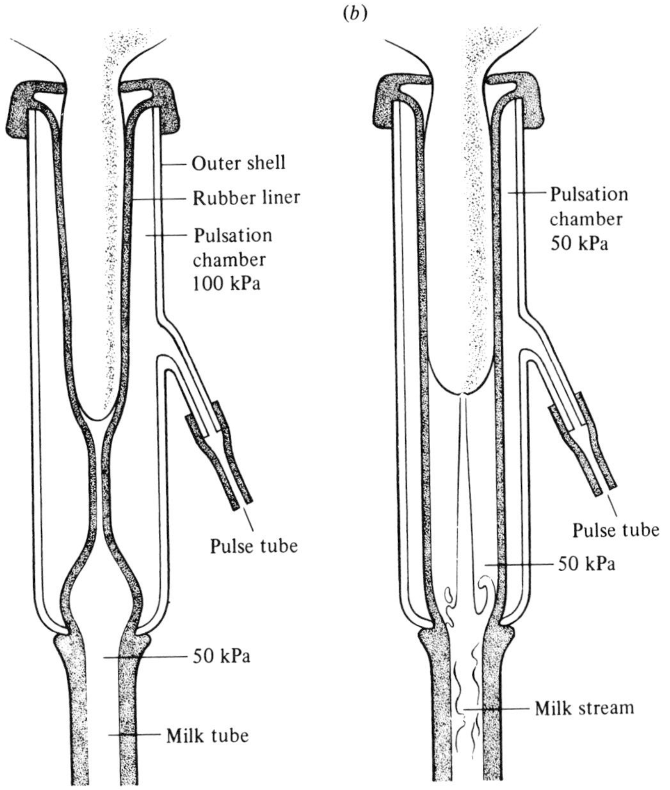

(a)

(b)

Figure 38–10. A double-chambered teat cup. (a) Pulsation chamber is open to the atmosphere, i.e., a pressure of about 100 kilopascals (760 mmHg); within the liner and milk tube there is a relatively constant vacuum of 50 kilopascals (380 mmHg), so that the rubber liner collapses in onto itself below the tip of the teat, occluding the milk tube and hence the flow of milk. (b) Pulsation chamber connected to vacuum system, i.e., 50 kilopascals; the rubber liner is now fully dilated, the vacuum is restored to the tip of the teat, and milk flows into the milk tube. (By courtesy of Mr. D. N. Akam.) (From Cowie AT: Lactation. *In* Austin CR, Short RV (eds): Hormonal Control of Rreproduction. Reproduction in Mammals, Vol 3, 2nd ed. Cambridge, Cambridge University Press, 1984.)

among domestic animals. Species nursing litters, such as cats, dogs, and pigs, often nurse at intervals of 1 hour or less. Goats, horses, and sheep nurse at slightly longer intervals, often up to 2 hours. Rabbits are an exception regarding the time interval between suckling periods; their young nurse at 24-hour intervals. As can be imagined, baby rabbits are engorged following each suckling period.

COMPOSITION OF MILK

Fats Are the Most Important Energy Source in Milk

Of the components of milk, fat is the most important energy source. Milk fat is composed of a number of lipids, including mono-, di-, and triglycerides, free fatty acids, phospholipids, and steroids; *triglycerides* are the main component of milk fat. The types of lipid synthesized are complex, with great variations in both chain length and saturation of fatty acids observed on the basis of species. The amount of fat produced varies greatly both within and among species (Table 38–2). Marine mammals have high fat content in milk, with values of about 40–50% in seals, 40% in

dolphins, and 30% in whales. In this situation, the high energy content of the milk through fat helps offset the heat loss of the young.

In domestic animals, sheep, swine, dogs, and cats have milk fat content that ranges from 7–10%. Dairy cattle have values that range from 3.5–5.5%; goats are similar to cows (3.5%), and mares have lower values (1.6%). During earlier times, milk was sold on a butterfat basis, and breeds that had a relatively high butterfat content of milk, e.g., the Jersey with 5% butterfat, found more acceptance in dairy operations than is currently the case. Small farms produced mainly cream (for butter manufacture); the fat-concentrated portion of

Table 38–2
COMPOSITION OF MILK FROM VARIOUS SPECIES (%)

Species	Fat	Protein	Lactose	Ash
Cat	7.1	10.1	4.2	0.5
Holstein	3.5	3.1	4.9	0.7
Dog	9.5	9.3	3.1	1.2
Goat	3.5	3.1	4.6	0.8
Horse	1.6	2.4	6.1	0.5

Adapted from Jacobson NL, McGilland AD. The mammary gland and lactation. *In* Swenson MJ (ed): Dukes' Physiology of Domestic Animals, 10th ed. Ithaca, Cornell University Press, 1984.

milk was produced by use of a separator that separated cream on the basis of specific gravity and centrifugal force. Because milk is now sold on a solids, not fat, basis, breeds that produce more milk (and protein) are favored, even though the fat content of the favored breed, Holstein Friesian, is lower (3.5%).

Lactose, Composed of Glucose and Galactose, Is the Main Carbohydrate of Mammalian Milk

Lactose is the main carbohydrate of eutherian mammals. It is composed of glucose and galactose. Blood glucose is the main precursor molecule for lactose, with propionate an important precursor for glucose in ruminants. Lactose is formed under the direction of *lactose synthetase*, an enzyme comprised of α-*lactalbumin* (a milk protein) and *galactosyl transferase*. Lactose synthesis is held in abeyance until immediately before term, because progesterone is inhibitory for the formation of α-lactalbumin. Prolactin, on the other hand, is stimulatory for the formation of lactose synthetase. Animals must have the enzyme *lactase* present in the jejunum in order for lactose to be cleaved (to glucose and galactose) and utilized. Lactase is present in most mammalian young, but is usually not present in adult animals, including humans. In the absence of lactase, lactose can have an osmotic effect in the gastrointestinal (GI) tract, which can lead to diarrhea.

The Main Proteins in Milk Are Called Caseins and Are Found in Curd

The main proteins produced by the alveolar cells are called *caseins*. Caseins can be removed (as a curd) from milk through a process called curdling or coagulation, with other milk proteins, such as albumins and globulins, remaining in the fluid part of the milk (whey).

THE LACTATION CYCLE

The time required for change over from colostrum to normal milk secretion varies with each species. In cattle, *colostral milk* tends to be stringy and yellow for several days postpartum. The complex bovine udder needs time for all areas to be flushed of colostrum. The milk of cattle is withheld from the milk supply for several days because of its unacceptable

asthetic quality, not because of the basic quality of the milk.

Milk Production Peaks at 1 Month Postpartum in Dairy Cattle, Followed by a Slow Decline in Production; Milking Usually Stops at 305 Days of Lactation, So That the Animal Can Prepare the Mammary Gland for the Next Lactation

Milk production tends to increase for the first 3–4 weeks of lactation and then begins to slowly decline through the end of lactation (Fig. 38–11). Animals are usually "dried up" after 305-day lactational periods; production rates concerning pounds of milk and butterfat are calculated on this basis. Animals are forced to stop lactating in order to prepare for the next lactation. The usual procedure is to stop milking the animals. The back pressure of milk within the alveoli gradually inhibits the secretion of milk by the alveolar epithelial cells, with a resultant regression of the alveolar cells and small ducts. The process, called *involution*, often requires at least a month, with a 6-week period usually desired as the minimal interval from drying off to the onset of the next lactational period. Within a period of 1–2 months, the secretory (alveoli) and excretory (duct) systems regress and are once again replaced. The process by which epithelial structures regress, yet retain coding for the renewal of duct and alveolar systems, is truly remarkable.

Lactation Can Be Induced by Hormone Administration (Estrogen and Progesterone) and Enhanced by Growth Hormone and Increased Photoperiod Exposure

The *induction of lactation* by hormone treatment is sometimes desired, especially in animals with high lactation records but poor reproductive performance. The use of a combined treatment of estrogen and progesterone over a relatively short period of time (1 week) has induced alveolar development sufficiently to result in milk production. Although the amount of milk produced is less than normal, the cows can be maintained in the milking string while efforts to get them pregnant continue. In order to induce lactogenesis by hormonal means, animals should not be lactating

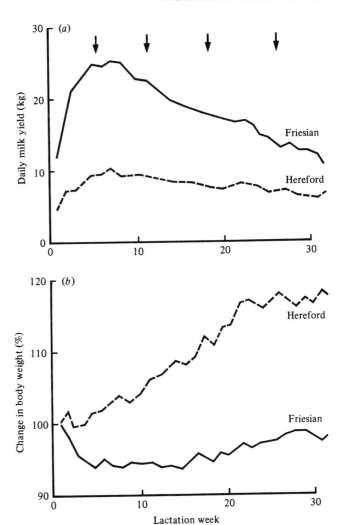

Figure 38–11. (a) Average daily milk yield, and (b) average percentage change in body weight, in seven low-yielding cows (broken line) and eight high-yielding cows (solid line). Arrows indicate blood sampling. (By courtesy of Dr. I. C. Hart.) (From Cowie AT: Lactation. *In* Austin CR, Short RV (eds): Hormonal Control of Reproduction. Reproduction in Mammals, Vol 3, 2nd ed. Cambridge, Cambridge University Press, 1984.)

at the time of treatment and should have mammary glands that are free of infection.

GH, which is important to the normal lactational process, can be used for the *enhancement of lactation* when administered over a rather wide range of concentrations (Fig. 38–12). With the relatively recent ability to synthesize the hormone, its availability has increased interest in its use for increasing the amount of milk produced by dairy cows. In general, GH acts on the postabsorptive use of nutrients so that protein, fat, and carbohydrate metabolism in the whole body are changed, and the nutrients are directed toward milk synthesis. If cows are in early lactation and in a negative energy balance, GH administration results in the mobilization of body fats that are used for milk formation. If cows are in

positive energy balance, GH has no effect on the metabolism of body fat. Initially, GH treatment decreases the energy balance of cows; however, this is adjusted by voluntary increase in feed consumption. In spite of the increased feed consumption, GH administration increases the gross efficiency of lactation by as much as 19%. In essence, the effects of exogenous GH do not depend upon gross alterations in nutrient digestibility or on body maintenance requirements. The use of GH may be economically viable, with the increased milk production justifying the expense of the hormone.

An interesting controversy has arisen from the fact that cows treated with GH do not produce "organically" derived milk, in spite of the fact that synthetic GH is almost identical

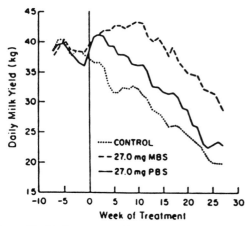

Figure 38–12. Average weekly milk yield of cows injected daily with diluent (control), 27 mg of methionyl bovine somatotropin (MBS), or 27 mg of pituitary bovine somatotropin (PBS). Treatments began at week 0 at an average of 84 ± 10 days post partum. (From Tucker HA: Lactation and its hormonal control. *In* Knobil E, Neill J, Ewing LL, et al (eds): The Physiology of Reproduction, Vol 2. New York, Raven Press, 1988.)

DISEASES ASSOCIATED WITH THE MAMMARY GLAND

The Main Diseases That Affect the Mammary Gland Directly Are Mastitis (Prevalent in Dairy Cattle) and Neoplasia (Prevalent in Intact Dogs)

The most important problems involved in the production of milk are those caused by inflammation of the gland, i.e., *mastitis*. One fundamental cause of mastitis is injury to the teat canal from the repeated stretching that occurs with the milking process. Organisms that ordinarily would be excluded from the gland are able to make their way past the

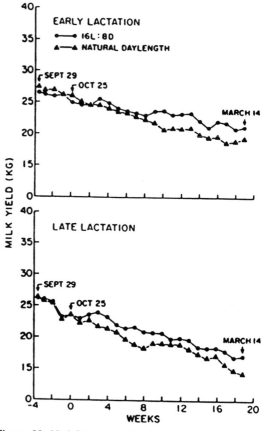

Figure 38–13. Influence of day length on milk production of Holstein cows. Between 9/29 and 10/24, cows 37 to 74 days (early lactation) or 94 to 204 days (late lactation) post partum were exposed to natural photoperiods of 12 hours of light per day and standardized diets. Between 10/25 and 3/14, cows were exposed to natural photoperiod (9–12 hours of light daily) or to 16 hours of fluorescent lighting superimposed on the natural photoperiod. (From Tucker HA: Lactation and its hormonal control. *In* Knobil E, Neill J, Ewing LL, et al (eds): The Physiology of Reproduction, Vol 2. New York, Raven Press, 1988.)

to endogenously derived GH. Although there is no evidence that increased concentrations of GH occur in the milk as a result of its administration, some consider the resultant milk to be abnormal.

The results with GH are in contrast to the studies in which thyroid hormone administration, in the form of *iodinated casein* (thyroprotein), was used to increase lactation in cows. Although the administration of thyroprotein increased lactation, extra feed was necessary to prevent excessive body weight loss, and milk production declined abruptly when thyroprotein was removed from the diet. In essence, the use of thyroprotein does not affect the efficiency of the lactational process as GH does.

Another interesting finding of the 1980s concerning the manipulation of lactation has been that the milk yield in cows can be increased by exposing them to increased light. Cows under a *photoperiod regimen* of 16 hours of light (8 hours of dark) produced 6–10% more milk than animals under the reverse photoperiod (8 hours of light and 16 hours of dark) (Fig. 38–13). Although the mechanism by which light affects lactation is not known, it likely involves prolactin secretion, at least to some extent, in that increased light exposure results in increased prolactin secretion.

barrier located within the teat canal, and with repeated microorganism exposure, an infection is established.

One of the adverse consequences of mastitis is the formation of connective tissue within the udder as a result of the attempt of the gland to wall off the infection. The presence of connective tissue limits the area into which ducts and alveoli can proliferate, thus reducing the milk-producing potential of the gland. The mammary gland is an example of an organ (the eye is another example) where the elicitation of an inflammatory response is often detrimental to the function of the organ. Thus, therapies directed toward the treatment of mastitis often combine *anti-inflammatory* and *antibacterial* agents.

Another process that disturbs the structure of the mammary gland is *neoplasia*. In domestic animals, the dog is most susceptible to the occurrence of mammary tumors. The exposure of the mammae to the ovarian hormones, estrogen and progesterone, greatly increases the chance for neoplasia. The incidence of mammary tumors is relatively low if the dog is ovariectomized prior to the first estrous cycle, but it increases progressively through exposure to two ovarian cycles; ovariectomy has little effect on neoplasia if done after the third or fourth cycle. It has not been uncommon for owners to want their dogs to have one or two cycles before they are ovariectomized. It is important for veterinarians to point out the beneficial aspects of ovariectomy prior to the onset of puberty because of incidence of mammary neoplasia, as well as the usual benefits of fertility and behavioral control.

The Main Conditions That Involve the Mammary Gland, Although Indirectly, Are the Passive Transfer of Red Blood Cell–Agglutinating Antibodies by the Ingestion of Colostrum (Mare), and Hypocalcemia Due to the Transient Drain of Calcium That Occurs with the Initiation of Lactation (Dairy Cattle) or During Lactation (Dog)

An immunological disease associated with the mammary gland involves the transfer of *red blood cell–agglutinating antibodies* to the fetus through the milk. The situation is most common in the horse in which fetal red blood cells pass into the maternal system and elicit antibody formation against the fetal red blood cells. These antibodies tend to be concentrated in the colostrum along with other immunoglobulins. At birth, the foal is able to absorb the red blood cell–agglutinating antibodies (as well as other beneficial immunoglobulins) for up to 48 hours. Foals often go into a hemolytic crisis between 24 and 48 hours after delivery and can die unless given vigorous therapy, including blood transfusions. If fetal red blood cell antibody formation is suspected in a mare, the disease can be handled by muzzling the foal at birth through 48 hours and feeding with colostrum saved (frozen) from other preparturient mares.

A disease that is associated with the mammary gland and that is life-threatening to the dam is *hypocalcemia*. At parturition, the acceleration of lactogenesis causes a great increase in the movement of calcium from the blood into the milk. Both cows and dogs are particularly susceptible, with some dams unable to respond immediately to the calcium drain from the blood by the mobilization of calcium. As a result, the animals lose their ability to maintain normal muscle activity, are often unable to stand, and become prostrate with the appearance of being comatose. The syndrome occurs in cows at parturition and in dogs several weeks postpartum, when lactation reaches its peak. The systemic administration of calcium to hypocalcemic cows often produces a dramatic recovery within 10–20 minutes.

CLINICAL CORRELATION

NEONATAL ISOERYTHROLYSIS

HISTORY □ You are called to examine a mare in foal at 7 months of gestation that has a previous history of having conceived and delivered a normal foal during her first pregnancy; the foal was subsequently suckled and was sold as a weanling. The mare had no trouble conceiving and carrying the next two pregnancies, but the foals died within 2 days of birth even though they were healthy and vigorous at birth. The previous owner became discouraged because of these deaths and, as a result, sold the mare to the current owner at a bargain price.

CLINICAL EXAMINATION □ You do a general physical examination of the mare and find all organ systems to be normal. Palpation of the uterus *per rectum* reveals the presence of a viable fetus that appears to be of the correct size for a pregnancy of the purported duration. Both the external genitalia and the mammary glands are normal in appearance.

COMMENT ☐ From the history, and from the fact that the mare appears to be undergoing a normal pregnancy, you conclude that there is nothing wrong with the reproductive process *per se*. The fact that the previous two foals were healthy at birth, yet weakened rapidly and died within 2 days, indicates that something likely happened to them following delivery. In mares, the most likely cause of this syndrome is *neonatal isoerythrolysis*. In this situation, the mare becomes exposed to the red blood cells of the fetus during the initial pregnancy (or could occur initially at subsequent pregnancies). If fetal red blood cells enter the circulation of the dam, she will respond by making antibodies to the red blood cells because of the presence of foreign antigen on the fetal red blood cells that were inherited from the sire. In the mare, these antibodies do not pass through the placental barrier, so the fetus is protected from these antibodies during pregnancy. The antibodies do pass into the colostrum and are concentrated during the process of colostrum formation.

TREATMENT ☐ The foal needs to be prevented from suckling the mare for the first 2–3 days of life. During the first 1–2 days, the foal is able to absorb large protein molecules, including the important immunoglobulins which enable the foal to ward off infections, as well as, in this case, antibodies against fetal red cell antigens. The gut epithelium closes to the passage of large protein molecules by 36–48 hours of life; at this time, or shortly thereafter, the foal can be allowed to suckle without fear of antibodies' being absorbed by the foal. The key is to prevent the foal from suckling during the first 2–3 days of life. The mare needs to be monitored closely prepartum so that the foal can be muzzled shortly after delivery. The foal does need nourishment during the first 2–3 days of life; thus, it is important that the foal be fed colostrum obtained from other mares (usually maintained frozen).

Bibliography

Cowie T: Lactation. *In* Austin CR, Short RV (eds): Reproduction in Mammals: Hormonal Control of Reproduction, Vol 3. Cambridge, Cambridge University Press, 1984, p 195–231.

Jacobson NL, McGilliard AD: The mammary gland and lactation. *In* Swenson MJ (ed): Dukes' Physiology of Domestic Animals, 10th ed. Ithaca, NY, Cornell University Press, 1984, p 863–880.

McNeilly AS: Suckling and the control of gonadotropin secretion. *In* Knobil E, Neill J, Ewing LL, et al (eds). The Physiology of Reproduction, Vol 2. New York, Raven Press, 1988, p 2323–2340.

Wakerley JB, Clarke G, Summerlee AJS: Milk ejection and its control. *In* Knobil E, Neill J, Ewing LL, et al (eds). The Physiology of Reproduction, Vol 2. New York, Raven Press, 1988, p 2283–2321.

Tucker HA: Lactation and its hormonal control. *In* Knobil E, Neill J, Ewing LL, et al (eds). The Physiology of Reproduction, Vol 2. New York, Raven Press, 1988, p 2235–2263.

PRACTICE QUESTIONS FOR CHAPTER 38

1. The development of the duct system in the mammary gland is under the control of estrogens, growth hormone, and adrenal steroids. If the duct system is to develop functional milk-secreting units called alveoli, which of the following hormone(s) are essential to this development?

   a. Progesterone
   b. Prolactin
   c. Relaxin
   d. Prolactin and progesterone
   e. Prolactin and relaxin
   f. Progesterone and relaxin

2. The hormone that is most important for the maintenance of lactation (lactogenesis) is

   a. estrogen.
   b. oxytocin.
   c. progesterone.
   d. prolactin.
   e. relaxin.

3. Sensory inputs, including sound, sight, and smell, but not necessarily touch, elicit the release of what important hormone required for the lactation process in the cow?

   a. Estrogen
   b. Oxytocin
   c. Progesterone
   d. Prolactin
   e. Relaxin

4. The contraction of what anatomical structure is of fundamental importance for the
release of milk from the udder of the cow?

    a. Alveoli
    b. Duct
    c. Myoepithelial cell
    d. Duct cistern

    e. Teat cistern

5. The most important energy source in milk
is

    a. carbohydrates.
    b. lactose.
    c. lipids.
    d. proteins.

JILL W. VERLANDER

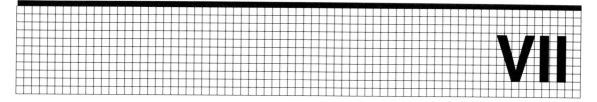

VII

RENAL PHYSIOLOGY

39

Glomerular Filtration

INTRODUCTION TO THE PHYSIOLOGY OF THE MAMMALIAN KIDNEY

1. The glomerulus filters the blood
2. The structure of the glomerulus provides for its filtration properties
3. The glomerular filtration rate is determined by the mean net filtration pressure, the permeability of the filtration barrier, and the area available for filtration
4. The filtration barrier is selectively permeable
5. Changes in the glomerular filtration rate are moderated by systemic and intrinsic factors
6. The glomerular filtration rate is measured by determining the rate of clearance of the plasma

INTRODUCTION TO THE PHYSIOLOGY OF THE MAMMALIAN KIDNEY

The mammalian kidney is a remarkable organ charged with a diverse set of responsibilities in maintaining the homeostasis of the body. The two kidneys receive approximately 25% of the cardiac output. Not only must the kidney filter this blood in order to excrete metabolic waste, but also it must retrieve those filtered materials that are needed by the body, including low molecular weight proteins, water, and a variety of electrolytes. It must recognize when water and specific electrolytes are present in excess and respond by failing to reabsorb or by secreting these substances. It contributes substantially to the maintenance of acid-base homeostasis. In addition, the production and release of hormones by the kidney play a vital role in the control of systemic

blood pressure and red blood cell production. In order to accomplish these tasks, the kidney is composed of an extensive variety of cell types, each endowed with an individual set of functions and designed to respond as needed to a complex battery of direct and indirect signals. These cells are arranged in a particular pattern to form the functional unit of the kidney, the nephron. The nephron is composed of the glomerulus, where the blood is filtered, and various distinct segments of the renal tubule, where filtered substances are absorbed from and plasma components are secreted into the tubular fluid. In the cortex the nephrons join with the collecting duct system, which traverses the kidney and ends with the inner medullary collecting duct, where the final alterations of the tubular fluid take place in the formation of urine. Figure 39–1 provides an overview of the anatomical arrangement of nephrons within the kidney,

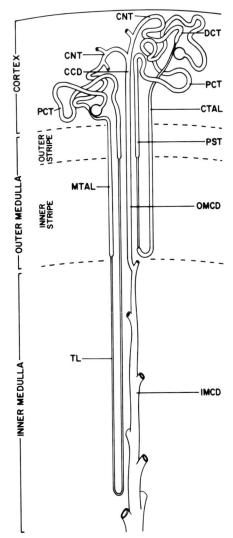

Figure 39–1. Schematic illustration of juxtamedullary and superficial nephrons. The glomerulus of a juxtamedullary nephron is located deep in the cortex near the corticomedullary junction. The thin limb (*TL*) of Henle's loop extends deep into the inner medulla. The glomerulus of a superficial nephron is located in the outer cortex, and Henle's loop extends only into the outer medulla. *PCT*, proximal convoluted tubule; *PST*, proximal straight tubule; *MTAL*, medullary thick ascending limb; *CTAL*, cortical thick ascending limb; *DCT*, distal convoluted tubule, *CNT*, connecting segment, *CCD*, cortical collecting duct; *OMCD*, outer medullary collecting duct, *IMCD*, inner medullary collecting duct. (Reprinted with permission from Madsen KM: Anatomy of the kidney. *In* Tisher CC, Wilcox CS (eds): Nephrology for the House Officer. Baltimore, Williams & Wilkins, 1989.)

and a brief outline of the major functions of the various segments of the nephron is given in Table 39–1.

The specific functions of the kidney and the methods by which they are accomplished are discussed in the following pages. Most of the

experimental evidence for what we believe about renal physiology has been obtained in the rat or the rabbit. Much of what is currently believed about renal physiology remains subject to revision and reinterpretation as more information is gathered.

The Glomerulus Filters the Blood

The first step in the complex series of processes performed by the kidney is the filtration of the blood. This initial step takes place in the glomerulus, which is a network of capillaries with a structure specifically designed to retain cellular components and medium to high molecular weight proteins within the vascular system while providing a tubular fluid that initially has an electrolyte and water composition nearly identical to that of the plasma. This initial tubular fluid is called the *glomerular filtrate*, and the process of formation is called *glomerular filtration*.

The rate of glomerular filtration is undoubtedly the parameter of renal function that is most frequently assessed in clinical practice. The *glomerular filtration rate (GFR)* is expressed as milliliters of glomerular filtrate formed per minute for every kilogram of body weight. It may help your understanding of GFR to think of these numbers in more tangible terms. An average size beagle of 10 kg body weight with a GFR of 3.7 mL/minute/kg would produce approximately 37 mL of glomerular filtrate per minute, or 53.3 L (a little more than 14 gallons) of glomerular filtrate per day, nearly 18 times its blood volume.

Table 39–1
SUMMARY OF NEPHRON SEGMENT FUNCTIONS

Structure	Function
Glomerulus	Filtration of the blood
Proximal tubule	Bulk reabsorption of filtered water and solutes
Thin limbs of Henle's loop	Maintenance of medullary hypertonicity by countercurrent exchange
Thick ascending limb of Henle's loop	NaCl reabsorption, generation of medullary hypertonicity, dilution of the tubule fluid, reabsorption of divalent cations
Distal convoluted tubule	NaCl reabsorption, dilution of the tubule fluid, reabsorption of divalent cations
Collecting duct system	Final control of the excretion rates of electrolytes, acid-base, and water

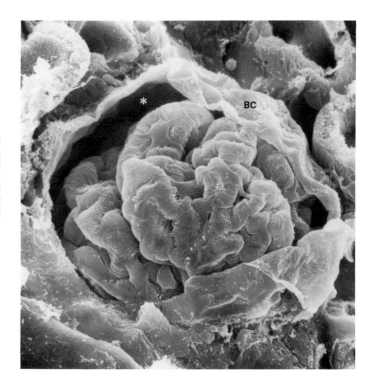

Figure 39–2. Scanning electron micrograph of rat glomerulus. The glomerular tuft is a complex network of capillaries that is encased in visceral epithelial cells and Bowman's capsule (*BC*). Between the visceral epithelial cells and BC is Bowman's space (*), where the glomerular filtrate is collected and delivered to the proximal tubule. Magnification 1000×.

The Structure of the Glomerulus Provides for its Filtration Properties

In order to understand the factors that determine the GFR, it is necessary to be familiar with the ultrastructure of the glomerulus. The glomerular tuft (Figs. 39–2 and 39–3) is composed of a network of capillaries. Blood from the renal artery is delivered to the afferent arteriole, which divides into numerous glomerular capillaries. The capillaries coalesce to form the efferent arteriole, which conducts the

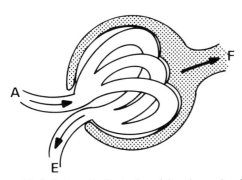

Figure 39–3. Schematic illustration of the glomerulus. The afferent arteriole (*A*) carries blood to the glomerulus and subdivides into numerous glomerular capillaries. Water and solutes cross the glomerular capillary wall into Bowman's space, forming the glomerular filtrate (*F*, stippled area), which flows into the proximal tubule. The glomerular capillaries coalesce and the filtered blood leaves the glomerulus through the efferent arteriole (*E*).

blood away from the glomerulus to be returned eventually to the systemic circulation through the renal vein. The glomerular tuft is encased within a layer of epithelial cells known as *Bowman's capsule.* The area between the glomerular tuft and Bowman's capsule is known as *Bowman's space,* and is the site of collection of the glomerular filtrate, which is funneled directly into the first segment of the proximal tubule.

The structure of the glomerular capillaries is important in determining the rate and selectivity of glomerular filtration. The wall of the capillary consists of three layers: the capillary endothelium, the basement membrane, and the visceral epithelium (Fig. 39–4). The capillary endothelium is composed of a single layer of cells whose cytoplasmic extensions are pierced by numerous fenestrae (windows). The endothelial fenestrae provide channels for the passage of water and noncellular components from the blood to the second layer of the glomerular capillary wall, the glomerular basement membrane. The *glomerular basement membrane (GBM)* is an acellular structure composed of various glycoproteins, including type IV and type V collagens, proteoglycans, laminin, fibronectin, and entactin. The GBM is arranged in three layers presumably created during development by the fusion of the basement membranes of the endothelial and epi-

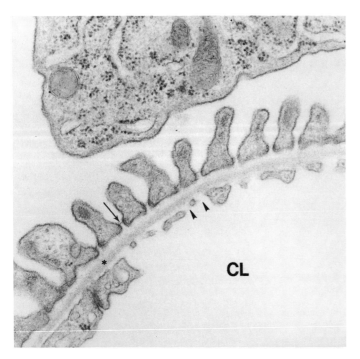

Figure 39–4. Transmission electron micrograph of rat glomerular capillary wall. The three main layers of the capillary wall are viewed in cross section. A single layer of glomerular capillary endothelial cells line the capillary lumen (*CL*). Numerous fenestrae (*arrowheads*) pierce the endothelial cells. On the outside of the capillary is a single layer of visceral epithelial cells. At the top of the micrograph is a portion of the cell body of a visceral epithelial cell. The secondary foot processes are aligned along the capillary wall and the spaces between them are spanned by the slit diaphragm (*arrow*). Between the endothelial and epithelial cell layers is the glomerular basement membrane, consisting of the electron-lucent lamina rara interna adjacent to the endothelial cells, the lamina densa (*), and the lamina rara externa adjacent to the visceral epithelial cells. Magnification 32500×.

thelial cell layers. The three layers are named according to their density to an electron beam and their relative position. As shown in Figure 39–4, the lamina densa (dense layer) is dark, because it is relatively resistant to the passage of electrons when viewed with a transmission electron microscope. The lamina densa is composed of tightly packed glycoprotein fibrils. It is sandwiched between the lamina rara interna (inside thin layer) on the endothelial side of the GBM and the lamina rara externa (outside thin layer) on the epithelial side of the GBM. The laminae rarae are composed of a loose network of glycoprotein fibrils.

The third compartment of the glomerular capillary wall is the visceral epithelium, which is a layer of intricate, interlocking cells called *podocytes*. Numerous long, narrow extensions, called *primary* and *secondary foot processes*, interdigitate with foot processes from other podocytes and wrap around the individual capillaries (Fig. 39–5). Spanning the space between adjacent foot processes is the epithelial slit diaphragm (see Fig. 39–4), which is made up of subunits arranged in a zipper pattern when viewed in a tangential plane.

The Glomerular Filtration Rate Is Determined by the Mean Net Filtration Pressure, the Permeability of the Filtration Barrier, and the Area Available for Filtration

The glomerular capillary wall creates a barrier to the forces favoring and opposing filtra-

tion of the blood. The forces favoring filtration, or movement of water and solutes, across the glomerular capillary wall are the hydrostatic pressure of the blood within the capillary and the oncotic pressure of the fluid within Bowman's space (the ultrafiltrate). Normally, the oncotic pressure of the ultrafiltrate is inconsequential, because medium to high molecular weight proteins are not filtered. Therefore, the main driving force for filtration is the glomerular capillary hydrostatic pressure (P_{gc}). In opposition to filtration are the plasma oncotic pressure within the glomerular capillary (π_b) and the hydrostatic pressure in Bowman's space (P_t). The direction and magnitude of these forces are illustrated in Figure 39–6.

The net filtration pressure (P_f) at any point along the glomerular capillary is the difference between the capillary hydrostatic pressure favoring filtration and the capillary oncotic pressure and hydrostatic pressure of the ultrafiltrate opposing filtration. This relationship is expressed mathematically by the following equation:

$$P_f = P_{gc} - (\pi_b + P_t)$$

As blood travels through the glomerular capillary, a large proportion of the fluid component of the plasma is forced across the capillary wall while the plasma proteins are retained in the capillary lumen. Therefore, the plasma oncotic pressure increases significantly

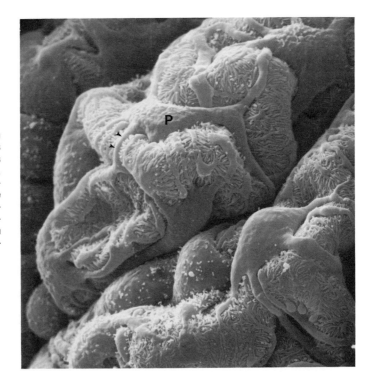

Figure 39–5. Scanning electron micrograph of the surface of rat glomerular capillaries viewed from Bowman's space. The cell bodies (*P*) of visceral epithelial cells, or podocytes, nestle between the capillary loops. The primary foot processes (*arrowheads*) radiate outward and wrap around the capillaries. Secondary foot processes extend from the primary foot processes and interdigitate with secondary foot processes from other podocytes. Magnification 2600 ×.

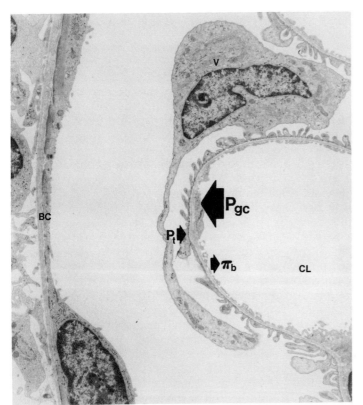

Figure 39–6. Transmission electron micrograph of a rat glomerular capillary and Bowman's capsule (*BC*) illustrating the forces favoring and opposing filtration. The main force favoring filtration is the hydrostatic pressure of the glomerular capillary (*Pgc*). The forces opposing filtration are the hydrostatic pressure of Bowman's space (P_t) and the oncotic pressure of the blood (π_b). *CL,* capillary lumen; V, visceral epithelial cell. Magnification 4000 ×.

along the capillary bed. At the same time, the loss of plasma volume along the capillary bed causes a decrease in the hydrostatic pressure in the capillary, although this change is small because of the resistance created by the efferent arteriole. The result is that the net filtration pressure tends to decrease along the capillary bed.

The GFR is the product of the mean net filtration pressure ($\overline{P_f}$), the permeability of the filtration barrier, and the surface area available for filtration. The permeability of the filtration barrier is determined by the structural and chemical characteristics of the glomerular capillary wall. The product of the filtration barrier permeability and its surface area is the ultrafiltration coefficient (K_f). Thus, the combined effects of the determinants of GFR are mathematically represented by the following equation:

$$GFR = \overline{P_f} \cdot K_f$$

The Filtration Barrier Is Selectively Permeable

In addition to determining the hydraulic permeability of the filtration barrier, the structural and chemical characteristics of the glomerular capillary wall are in large part responsible for the selective permeability (permselectivity) of the filtration barrier. The permselectivity of the filtration barrier is responsible for differences in the rate of filtration of blood components. Normally, all cellular components and plasma proteins the size of albumin or larger are retained within the blood stream, whereas water and solutes are freely filtered. In general, substances with a molecular radius of 4 nm or greater are not filtered, whereas molecules with a radius of 2 nm or less are filtered without restriction. However, characteristics other than size affect the ability of blood components to cross the filtration barrier. The net electrical charge of a molecule has a dramatic effect on its rate of filtration. It has been demonstrated that the cationic (positively charged) form of a variety of substances is more freely filtered than the neutral form, which is more freely filtered than the anionic (negatively charged) form of the same molecule. For example, the cationic form of albumin is excreted at a rate approximately 300 times that of native albumin, which has a net negative charge. These differences are thought to be due to the presence of a charge-selective

barrier in the glomerular capillary wall created by negatively charged residues of glycoproteins incorporated in the glomerular basement membrane and coating the endothelial and epithelial cells. These fixed negative charges are thought to repel negatively charged plasma proteins and, thus, reduce their passage across the filtration barrier. The shape and deformability of the molecule also play a role in its ability to cross the filtration barrier. Neutral dextran, a long, flexible molecule, crosses the filtration barrier approximately seven times as easily as horseradish peroxidase, a globular protein with a similar molecular radius and net charge.

Changes in the Glomerular Filtration Rate Are Moderated by Systemic and Intrinsic Factors

The kidney has the ability to maintain GFR at a relatively constant level despite changes in systemic blood pressure and renal blood flow. The GFR is maintained within the physiological range by both renal modulation of systemic blood pressure and intravascular volume, and by intrinsic control of renal blood flow, glomerular capillary pressure, and the K_f. Renal effects on systemic blood pressure and volume are mediated primarily through humoral factors, the most important being the renin-angiotensin-aldosterone system. Intrinsic control of glomerular capillary perfusion is mediated also by systems controlling the resistance to flow in the afferent and efferent arterioles. These two autoregulatory systems are the *myogenic reflex* and *tubuloglomerular feedback*.

The renin-angiotensin-aldosterone system is an important mechanism of control of GFR and renal blood flow (RBF). Renin is a hormone produced by specialized cells of the wall of the afferent arteriole, the *granular extraglomerular mesangial cells*, which are specialized *juxtaglomerular cells*. Renin release is stimulated by a decrease in renal perfusion pressure, most commonly due to systemic hypotension. Renin catalyzes the transformation of angiotensinogen produced by the liver to angiotensin I. Angiotensin I is converted to the more active angiotensin II by angiotensin-converting enzyme, which is widely distributed throughout the body. Although early research suggested that angiotensin-converting enzyme (ACE) was located exclusively in the vascular endothelium of the lung, it is now known that

ACE is present in the vascular endothelium of numerous other organs as well as a wide variety of body fluids and epithelial cells, including renal proximal tubule cells.

Angiotensin II is a potent vasoconstrictor, acting directly to increase systemic blood pressure and renal perfusion pressure. In addition, angiotensin II stimulates the release of the mineralocorticoid, aldosterone. Aldosterone enhances sodium and water reabsorption by the collecting duct, increasing intravascular volume and thereby improving renal perfusion. Renin release is suppressed by both the improvement in renal perfusion and the elevated plasma angiotensin II, creating a negative feedback system that maintains renal perfusion and GFR within the physiological range (Fig. 39–7).

Increased levels of angiotensin II also stimulate production and release of the vasodilatory renal prostaglandins, PGE_2 and PGI_2. This is an important moderator of the renin-angiotensin-aldosterone system. The intrarenal production of these vasodilators counteracts the vasoconstrictive effect of angiotensin II on the intrarenal vasculature and helps to maintain renal vascular resistance at normal or near normal levels. Without this protective effect, generalized vasoconstriction would result in reduced RBF and GFR, despite an elevation of blood pressure.

Within the kidney itself, there appears to be direct control of glomerular capillary perfusion by two systems previously mentioned, the myogenic reflex and tubuloglomerular feedback.

A mechanism of autoregulation of RBF and GFR was proposed following the observation that glomerular arterioles respond to changes in arteriolar wall tension. This response is called the *myogenic reflex,* and the result is almost immediate arteriolar constriction following an increase in arteriolar wall tension. Conversely, a decrease in arteriolar wall tension results in virtually immediate arteriolar dilation. The arteriolar vasodilation and vasoconstriction result in alterations in the resistance to blood flow provided by the afferent arteriole. The changes in resistance in the afferent arteriole serve to maintain GFR and RBF at a constant level despite marked alterations in the blood pressure in the renal artery. Although there may be chemical mediators of this reflex, it has been shown to be independent of renal innervation and known renal vasoactive agents.

The second intrinsic control mechanism to consider is a poorly understood system known as tubuloglomerular feedback. In order to grasp this concept it is important to review the anatomical arrangement of an individual nephron (see Fig. 39–1). Specifically, recall that the distal tubule is closely associated with the glomerulus of the same nephron. An anatomically distinct cluster of epithelial cells, known as the *macula densa,* is located in the wall of the distal portion of the thick ascending limb of the loop of Henle. The macula densa is situated between the afferent and efferent arterioles and adjacent to the extraglomerular mesangial region. These four structures together are known as the *juxtaglomerular appa-*

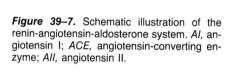

Figure 39–7. Schematic illustration of the renin-angiotensin-aldosterone system. *AI,* angiotensin I; *ACE,* angiotensin-converting enzyme; *AII,* angiotensin II.

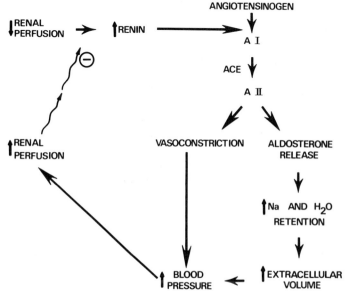

ratus, and they appear to be closely related functionally as well as structurally. The basic observation supporting the concept of a tubuloglomerular feedback mechanism was made using micropuncture of individual nephrons. These experiments demonstrated that an increase in the rate of flow of tubular fluid at the level of the macula densa results in a decrease in the filtration rate of the glomerulus of that nephron. In theory, such a system would check the single nephron glomerular filtration rate (SNGFR) in order to avoid exceeding the capacity of the tubule to reabsorb fluid or solute and thus would prevent excessive fluid and solute loss. Although it is generally accepted that this tubuloglomerular feedback mechanism exists, the actual signal that precipitates the negative feedback is controversial. Increased delivery of fluid, solute, and chloride to the macula densa each have their supporters. Whatever the signal, the result is increased resistance to flow in the afferent and efferent arterioles, reduced K_f, and reduced SNGFR. The mechanism by which the signal at the macula densa is translated into arteriolar constriction and reduced K_f is unknown, but it has been suggested that mesangial cell contraction may be responsible for both effects.

In addition to controls exerted by the kidney itself on GFR, various systemic factors can alter GFR. These include systemic control of blood volume and vessel tone. Blood volume is regulated by numerous hormones. In addition to aldosterone, vasopressin (antidiuretic hormone) secretion enhances water reabsorption by the kidney and increases blood volume. Glucocorticoids and progesterone also increase blood volume. More recently, a hormone produced in the cardiac atria has been shown to cause both a natriuresis (sodium-wasting) and diuresis (water-wasting). This hormone is known by various names, including atrial natriuretic peptide (ANP), atrial natriuretic hormone, and atriopeptin. The role of ANP in volume regulation in physiological and pathological conditions remains to be determined.

Systemic factors that affect vessel tone also affect systemic blood pressure, renal perfusion, and ultrafiltration. Vasopressin and circulating catecholamines can cause vasoconstriction and increase blood pressure. Beta-adrenergic stimulation can activate the renin-angiotensin system, and α-adrenergic stimulation can cause renal vasoconstriction, causing both a reduction and a redistribution of renal blood flow. In addition to altering renal perfusion, vasoconstrictors can affect the other determinant of GFR, the ultrafiltration coefficient (K_f). Vasoconstrictors cause contraction of the mesangial cells within the glomerulus, which reduces the area available for filtration. Because K_f is the product of the area available for filtration and the hydraulic permeability, if mesangial cell contraction occurs *in vivo,* K_f is reduced, which in turn reduces GFR.

GFR can also be enhanced by systemic factors. Recently there has been considerable interest in the effect of dietary protein on renal function. It has been demonstrated that high levels of dietary protein cause increases in RBF and GFR. These parameters are also transiently elevated following a single high-protein meal. The mechanisms and long-term effects of a high protein diet on renal function are under intense investigation at this time.

The Glomerular Filtration Rate Is Measured by Determining the Rate of Clearance of the Plasma

Both in an experimental setting and in clinical practice, the GFR is one of the most important parameters of renal function. Determination of the GFR relies on the concept of clearance, that is, the rate at which the plasma is cleared of a substance. The rate of clearance of a substance is measured by the rate of elimination divided by the plasma concentration of the substance. The measurement of clearance is mathematically expressed by

$$C_x = \frac{U_x \dot{V}}{P_x}$$

where C_x is the volume of plasma cleared of substance X per unit time, U_x is the urine concentration of substance X, $\dot{V}$ is the volume of urine collected divided by the time period of the collection, and P_x is the plasma concentration of substance X.

The total rate of clearance of a substance is the sum of the rates of filtration and secretion minus the rate of reabsorption of the substance. In order to determine the filtration rate accurately, it is necessary to exclude the effects of secretion and reabsorption from the equation. This requirement is neatly satisfied by selecting inulin as the substance for the measurement of clearance. Inulin is a substance that is freely filtered by the glomerulus, but is neither reabsorbed nor secreted by the renal tubular cells. Because of these properties, and because inulin is not produced by the body, after intravascular injection of inulin the rate of its disappearance from the blood is strictly related to the rate of glomerular filtration. Therefore, measurement of GFR can be expressed mathematically by the clearance equation when substance X is inulin

$$GFR = C_{inulin} = \frac{U_{inulin} \dot{V}}{P_{inulin}}$$

where GFR is the GFR in mL/minute, C_{inulin} is the rate of clearance of inulin from the plasma in mL/minute, U_{inulin} is the inulin concentration in a urine sample collected over a period of time (T) in minutes, $\dot{V}$ is the volume of the urine collected over T, and P_{inulin} is the mean plasma inulin concentration during T. Although the standard method of determination of GFR is by the rate of clearance of inulin from the blood, GFR can be measured in a variety of ways. In clinical situations the most widely used measure of glomerular filtration is endogenous creatinine clearance. Creatinine is a byproduct of muscle metabolism that is handled by the kidney in a manner similar to inulin. It is freely filtered, and it is not reabsorbed by the tubule. However, approximately 10% of the excreted creatinine is secreted by the tubule. Depending on the accuracy of the assay used for creatinine (colorimetric assays overestimate the concentration of creatinine in the blood, but not that in the urine), the endogenous creatinine clearance test provides a rough estimate of GFR. Practically, the measurement of endogenous creatinine clearance requires collecting the urine produced by a patient over a 24-hour period, either by using a metabolic cage, "catching" voided urine, or collecting the urine by catheterization if necessary. The volume of urine produced over 24 hours is recorded, and the creatinine concentration is measured. The mean plasma concentration of creatinine is represented by either the plasma concentration measured at the midpoint of the collection period, or by the mean of the plasma concentration measured at the beginning and end of the collection period. These values are used in the clearance equation

$$C_{creatinine} = \frac{U_{creatinine} \dot{V}}{P_{creatinine}}$$

resulting in an approximation of GFR in mL/minute. In veterinary medicine, the GFR is better expressed on a body weight or body surface area basis, that is, as mL/minute/kg or mL/minute/M^2, because of the large variation in size within individual species.

CLINICAL CORRELATIONS

CHRONIC RENAL FAILURE

HISTORY □ You examine a 15-year-old male Siamese cat. The owner reports that her cat is listless, inappetent, and thin. The cat has been drinking more water than usual lately, urinating large volumes, and vomiting frequently.

CLINICAL EXAMINATION □ The cat is very thin and moderately dehydrated. The mucous membranes are pale, and the kidneys feel small and slightly irregular. Her hematocrit is 22% (normal 30–42%), serum creatinine is 8.7 mg/dL (normal 0.5–1.2 mg/dL), and urine specific gravity is 1.012.

COMMENT □ The cat has chronic renal failure, which is seen frequently among geriatric patients in small animal practice. The serum creatinine is elevated because progressive loss of glomerular function has severely reduced the GFR, and creatinine as well as other waste products are not cleared from the plasma. The urine is not concentrated in response to dehydration, because tubular function is also compromised. The small kidney size is an indication of chronicity and is a result of gradual nephron loss and scarring. Anemia is seen commonly in chronic renal failure and is a result of many factors, one of which is decreased production of erythropoietin by the kidney.

In veterinary medicine, the treatment of chronic renal failure is usually supportive and symptomatic. This cat would probably benefit from rehydration with intravenous fluids, correction of electrolyte and acid-base disturbances as dictated by the serum chemistries, and feeding a low protein diet supplemented with the water-soluble vitamins. Anabolic steroids may help improve the anemia. Exogenous erythropoietin has become available more recently for the treatment of humans with anemia due to chronic renal failure and may become an alternative for use in veterinary medicine as well.

GLOMERULONEPHRITIS

HISTORY □ A client presents his 3-year-old spayed female springer spaniel. He reports that the dog has not been eating well for several days and seems to tire easily.

CLINICAL EXAMINATION □ The dog seems bright and alert and is in good flesh. The only abnormality detected by physical examination is slight pitting edema in the distal extremities. The left kidney is palpable, and feels smooth and of normal size. A urinalysis is normal except for 3 + protein and the presence of a few red blood cell casts. A complete blood count is normal, and the only abnormality on a serum chemistry profile is a serum albumin of 1.5 g/dL (normal 2.3–4.3 g/dL).

COMMENT □ This dog has acute glomerulonephritis. Proteinuria is indicative of glomerular disease, because normally the filtration barrier provided by the glomerular capillary wall prevents the passage of proteins into the tubular fluid. When the glomerulus is damaged, it becomes leaky, and protein appears in the urine. The loss of albumin in this case appears to be marked, because the serum albumin has dropped below normal levels. The peripheral edema is probably due to the hypoalbuminemia.

In this case, acute glomerulonephritis is suspected because of the recent onset of clinical signs, the absence of renal failure, and the presence of red blood cell casts in the urine. Additional tests that are helpful in guiding and assessing therapy include a 24-hour urine collection to measure the severity of the protein loss and an endogenous creatinine clearance done at the same time to determine if the GFR has been altered. A renal biopsy is necessary to verify the type and severity of glomerular injury.

The treatment of glomerulonephritis varies. Occasionally, the precipitating cause can be determined and removed. Some cases resolve spontaneously. At other times, various combinations of immunosuppressive and anti-inflammatory agents are used to combat ongoing damage from immune complex deposition in glomerular inflammation. If either renal failure or pulmonary edema secondary to hypoalbuminemia are present, these problems must be treated to sustain the animal until the glomerular lesion is resolved or controlled if possible.

Bibliography

Bovee KC (ed): Canine Nephrology. Media, PA, Harwal Publishing, 1984, p 1–217.
Brenner BM, Rector FC Jr (eds): The Kidney, 3rd ed. Philadelphia, WB Saunders, 1986, p 3–700.
Kanwar YS: Biophysiology of glomerular filtration and proteinuria. Lab Invest 51:7–21, 1984.
Seldin SW, Giebish G (eds): The Kidney: Physiology and Pathophysiology. New York, Raven Press, 1985, p 3–2162.
Sullivan LP, Grantham JJ (eds): Physiology of the Kidney, 2nd ed. Philadelphia, Lea & Febiger, 1982, p 1–224.

PRACTICE QUESTIONS FOR CHAPTER 39

1. The major force favoring filtration across the glomerular capillary wall is

    a. the oncotic pressure of the plasma.
    b. the oncotic pressure of the glomerular filtrate.
    c. the hydrostatic pressure of the blood.
    d. the hydrostatic pressure of the glomerular filtrate.
    e. the ultrafiltration coefficient.

2. The glomerular filtration rate is

    a. the volume of blood filtered by the kidneys/minute/kg of body weight.
    b. the volume of plasma filtered by the kidneys/minute/kg of body weight.
    c. the volume of urine produced by the kidneys/minute/kg of body weight.
    d. the volume of glomerular filtrate formed by the kidneys/minute/kg of body weight.
    e. the volume of blood cleared of creatinine by the kidneys/minute/kg of body weight.

3. In clinical practice, the GFR is estimated often by determining the rate of creatinine clearance. The rate of creatinine clearance is

    a. the volume of plasma cleared of creatinine/minute/kg of body weight.
    b. the volume of glomerular filtrate formed/minute/kg of body weight.
    c. the weight of creatinine filtered from the blood/minute/kg of body weight.
    d. the weight of creatinine/volume of urine formed/minute/kg of body weight.

e. the difference between the rate of plasma flow in the afferent and efferent arterioles.

4. The two major characteristics that determine whether a blood component is filtered or retained in the capillary lumen are its

   a. molecular radius and molecular weight.
   b. molecular radius and membrane permeability.
   c. molecular radius and plasma concentration.
   d. molecular radius and electrical charge.
   e. molecular weight and length.

5. The GFR is increased by

   a. a low protein meal.
   b. autoregulation.
   c. tubuloglomerular feedback.
   d. release of atrial natriuretic peptide.
   e. activation of the renin-angiotensin-aldosterone system.

40

Solute Reabsorption

1. The renal tubule reabsorbs filtered substances
2. Renal tubule function may be assessed by determining fractional excretion and fractional reabsorption rates
3. The proximal tubule is responsible for the reabsorption of the bulk of filtered solutes
4. The proximal tubule secretes organic ions
5. The distal tubule and collecting duct segments are specialized to reabsorb or secrete solutes as required by systemic factors
6. The distal tubule segments reabsorb salts and dilute the tubule fluid
7. The collecting duct reabsorbs NaCl and can secrete or reabsorb K$^+$
8. The distal tubule and collecting duct respond to systemic signals to alter salt excretion as required
9. Aldosterone enhances Na$^+$ reabsorption and K$^+$secretion
10. Parathyroid hormone enhances Ca^{2+} reabsorption

The Renal Tubule Reabsorbs Filtered Substances

It is of vital importance that the bulk of the ultrafiltrate formed be reabsorbed by the remainder of the nephron rather than excreted in the urine. To illustrate the importance of reabsorption of the components of the ultrafiltrate, consider the 10-kg beagle that forms 53.3 L of glomerular filtrate each day. Because the ultrafiltrate contains virtually the same concentration of salts and glucose as does the plasma, in the absence of tubular reabsorption the urinary loss of sodium, chloride, potassium, bicarbonate, and glucose alone would total more than 500 g of solute. In the absence of tubular reabsorption, the

beagle would need to constantly replace these chemicals throughout the day by eating more than a pound of salts as well as drinking more than 50 L of water at the same rate as the urinary loss in order to stay in fluid and salt balance.

Happily, the renal tubule efficiently retrieves these and other constituents of the ultrafiltrate. Figure 40–1 illustrates the percentages of various filtered substances that remain in the tubule fluid at various points along the tubule. One hundred percent of the filtered glucose is rapidly reabsorbed by the proximal tubule; by the time the final urine is formed in the terminal collecting duct, approximately 99% of the filtered water and sodium has been retrieved.

Renal Tubule Function May Be Assessed by Determining Fractional Excretion and Fractional Reabsorption Rates

The percentage of a filtered substance that is ultimately excreted in the urine is called the *fractional excretion rate*. It is the net result of the tubular reabsorption and secretion of the filtered substance. Mathematically, this is determined by relating the urinary concentration of a substance, X, to its plasma concentration, and dividing this ratio by the urinary to plasma ratio of a reference substance in order to eliminate the effect of water reabsorption on the urinary concentration of X. In experimental situations, the urinary and plasma concentrations of inulin during a constant inulin infusion may be used for reference. However, it is more practical in clinical situations to use creatinine as the reference substance. Therefore, the fractional excretion rate of X (FE_x) is determined by the following equation:

$$FE_x = \frac{U_x/P_x}{U_{creatinine}/P_{creatinine}}$$

where U_x is the urinary concentration of X, P_x is the plasma concentration of X, and $U_{creatinine}$ and $P_{creatinine}$ are the urinary and plasma concentrations of creatinine, respectively. By multiplying FE_x by 100, the fractional excretion rate may be expressed as the percent of filtered X that is excreted.

The fractional reabsorption rate of X (FR_x) represents the proportion of filtered X that is reabsorbed by the tubule. FR_x is mathematically determined by the following equation:

$$FR_x = 1 - FE_x$$

and can be expressed as a percentage by multiplying the FR_x by 100.

The Proximal Tubule Is Responsible for the Reabsorption of the Bulk of Filtered Solutes

The rate of reabsorption and secretion of filtered substances varies among segments of the renal tubule. In general, the proximal tubule is responsible for reabsorption of the ultrafiltrate to a greater extent than the remainder of the tubule. At least 60% of most filtered substances are reabsorbed before the tubular fluid leaves the proximal tubule.

The anatomical arrangement of the proximal

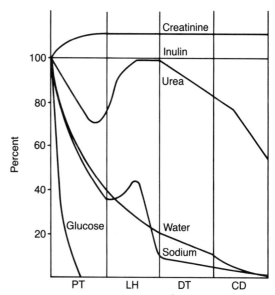

Figure 40–1. Illustration of the per cent of filtered substances $[(U_x/P_x) \times 100/(U_{inulin}/P_{inulin})]$ remaining in the tubule fluid in various tubule segments. Creatinine is secreted by the proximal tubule and is excreted at a greater rate than the reference substance, inulin. *PT*, proximal tubule; *LH*, loop of Henle; *DT*, distal tubule; *CD*, collecting duct. (Modified from Sullivan LP, Grantham JJ (eds): Physiology of the Kidney, 2nd ed. Philadelphia, Lea & Febiger, 1982.)

tubule and its relationship to the peritubular capillary facilitate the movement of tubule fluid components into the blood through two pathways: the transcellular pathway and the paracellular pathway. The tubule fluid flows past the apical surface of the tubular epithelial cell. Substances transported through the transcellular pathway are taken up by the cell from the tubule fluid and are discharged into the interstitial fluid on the blood side of the cell. Transport through the transcellular pathway largely occurs by carrier-mediated transport. The surface area available for transport of tubule fluid components into the cell is vast, owing to extensive infoldings of the apical plasma membrane. As a result, the apical surface of proximal tubule cells is covered with numerous projections called *microvilli*, creating a beautiful membranous structure known as the *brush border* (Figs. 40–2, 40–3). On the blood side of the cell, there are also numerous infoldings of the basolateral plasma membrane, which enhance the surface area available for transport from the cell into the interstitial fluid, where it becomes available for uptake by the peritubular capillary.

The second route of transport in the proximal tubule is the paracellular pathway. This pathway traverses the zonula occludens, a

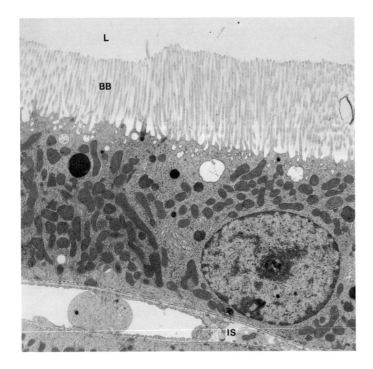

Figure 40–2. Transmission electron micrograph of cross section of rat proximal tubule. The brush border (*BB*) of the apical plasma membrane extends from the epithelial cells into the tubule lumen (*L*), where it is bathed by the tubule fluid. On the basal side of the cell is the interstitial space (*IS*). Magnification 5600×.

highly permeable structure that attaches the proximal tubule cells to each other and creates a boundary between the apical and basolateral plasma membrane domains (Fig. 40–4). Substances reabsorbed through the paracellular pathway move from the tubule fluid by passive diffusion across the zonula occludens into the lateral intercellular space. The fluid in the lateral intercellular space is thought to communicate freely with the interstitial fluid, where it can be taken up by the peritubular capillary.

Movement of water and solute from the interstitial fluid into the blood stream is favored by the location of the peritubular capillary and by Starling's forces. The peritubular

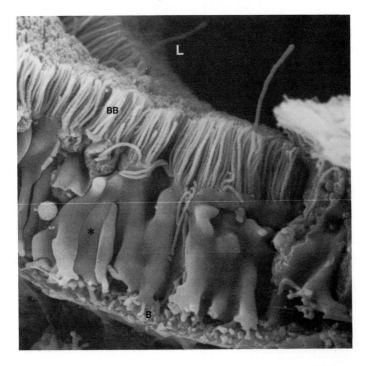

Figure 40–3. Scanning electron micrograph of rat proximal tubule viewed from the lateral intercellular space. The lush brush border (*BB*) carpets the luminal aspect (*L*). Lateral cellular processes (*) interdigitate with those of neighboring cells. The surface of the basal plasma membrane (*B*) is amplified by extensive membrane infoldings, creating numerous processes called micropedici (tiny feet). Magnification 7200×.

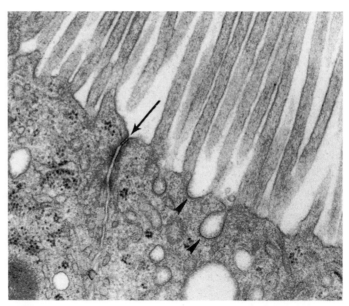

Figure 40–4. Transmission electron micrograph of apical region of rat proximal tubule viewed in cross section. The zonula occludens (*arrow*) joins adjacent proximal tubule cells. The zonula occludens divides the apical plasma membrane compartment and separates the tubule fluid from the fluid of the lateral intercellular space. Also seen are coated pits (*arrowheads*) that contain the binding sites for substances reabsorbed by receptor-mediated endocytosis. Magnification 32,000 X.

capillary originates at the glomerular efferent arteriole, subdivides, and wraps closely around the basal aspect of the proximal tubule (Fig. 40–5). The plasma leaving the glomerulus has a high oncotic pressure due to the selective filtration of water and salts and the retention of proteins within the capillary lumen. Because of the low resistance created by the peritubular capillary, the hydrostatic pressure in the capillary is low. Both of these conditions, high peritubular plasma oncotic pressure and low peritubular capillary hydrostatic pressure, favor the movement of fluid and solute into the blood stream.

Reabsorption of solutes takes place by a number of transport mechanisms, ranging from passive diffusion to primary active transport. (Please review the transport mechanisms described in Chapter 1.) In the proximal tubule, much of the transport of substances from the tubular fluid to the blood is driven by the active transport of sodium (Na^+) by a sodium-potassium-adenosinetriphosphatase (ATPase) pump (Na^+, K^+ ATPase) located in the basolateral plasma membrane (Fig. 40–6). The Na^+, K^+ ATPase exchanges three Na^+ molecules from the cell for two K^+ molecules from the interstitial fluid.

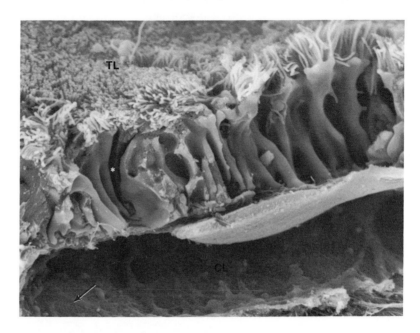

Figure 40–5. Scanning electron micrograph of rat proximal tubule and peritubular capillary. The peritubular capillary wraps around the basal aspect of the proximal tubule cells. Substances retrieved from the tubule lumen (*TL*) are delivered through either the transcellular pathway or the paracellular pathway into the fluid bathing the basolateral aspect of the epithelial cells. Water and solutes enter the interstitial space and diffuse into the peritubular capillary lumen (*CL*). *, lateral intercellular space; *arrow*, fenestrae of peritubular capillary endothelium. Magnification 7000 X.

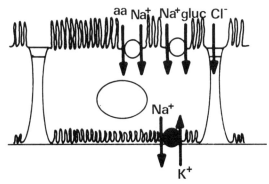

Figure 40–6. Schematic illustration of transport processes in the proximal tubule epithelial cell. Virtually all transport is believed to be driven by active reabsorption of Na^+ by the Na^+, K^+ ATPase located in the basolateral plasma membrane. Glucose (*gluc*) and amino acids (*aa*) as well as many other solutes enter the cell by secondary active transport with Na^+, driven by the low intracellular Na^+ concentration resulting from the active transport of Na^+ out of the cell. Cl^- diffuses across the zonula occludens into the lateral intercellular spaces down its electrochemical gradient.

The transport of Na^+ out of the cell into the interstitial fluid lowers the concentration of Na^+ within the cell. The asymmetrical transport of electrical charge (three Na^+ for two K^+) polarizes the cell, so that the interior of the cell is negative relative to the exterior. Thus, an electrochemical gradient for Na^+ across the apical plasma membrane is established, encouraging the movement of Na^+ from the tubular fluid into the cell. The movement of Na^+ across the apical cell membrane is facilitated by a variety of specific transporters located in the membrane. The movement of Na^+ through most of these transporters is coupled to the movement of other solutes in the same direction as Na^+ (cotransport) or in the opposite direction (countertransport). Substances that are taken up from the proximal tubular fluid into the cells by this mechanism (called *secondary active transport*) include glucose, amino acids, phosphate, sulfate, and organic anions. The active uptake of these substances increases their intracellular concentration and allows them to move across the basolateral plasma membrane and into the blood by passive diffusion.

The reabsorption of bicarbonate (HCO_3^-) by the proximal tubule is also driven by the chemical gradient for Na^+, although indirectly. Na^+ and proton (H^+) countertransport across the apical plasma membrane is driven by the chemical gradient for Na^+. The secreted H^+ combines in the tubular fluid with filtered

HCO_3^- to form carbonic acid (H_2CO_3), which dissociates to form water (H_2O) and carbon dioxide (CO_2). The dissociation is catalyzed by carbonic anhydrase in the apical plasma membrane of proximal tubule cells. The CO_2 diffuses passively across the apical plasma membrane into the cell, where it combines with H_2O to form H_2CO_3. The intracellular hydration of CO_2 is catalyzed by cytoplasmic carbonic anhydrase. The H_2CO_3 dissociates to form H^+ and HCO_3^- within the cell. The HCO_3^- moves across the basolateral plasma membrane and back into the blood through a $Na^+/3\ HCO_3^-$ cotransporter and possibly a HCO_3^-/Cl^- antiporter. The H^+ is transported into the tubular fluid through the Na^+/H^+ antiporter, which completes the cycle. By this complex mechanism, illustrated in Figure 40–7, the proximal tubule reabsorbs 80–90% of the filtered HCO_3^-.

The passive reabsorption of Cl^- in the proximal tubule is also indirectly powered by the Na^+, K^+ ATPase. As Na^+, HCO_3^-, glucose,

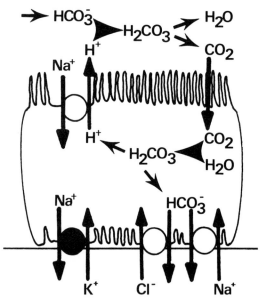

Figure 40–7. Schematic illustration of HCO_3^- reabsorption and acid secretion in the proximal tubule. The active reabsorption of Na^+ by the basolateral Na^+, K^+ ATPase drives the secretion of H^+ through the Na^+/H^+ antiporter in the apical plasma membrane. In the lumen, the secreted H^+ and filtered HCO_3^- form H_2CO_3, which dissociates rapidly under the influence of apical membrane–associated carbonic anhydrase to form H_2O and CO_2. CO_2 readily diffuses across the apical plasma membrane into the cell, where cytoplasmic carbonic anhydrase catalyzes the intracellular formation of H_2CO_3, which dissociates to H^+ and HCO_3^-. The H^+ is secreted into the tubule fluid and the HCO_3^- is transported to the blood side of the cell through countertransport with Na^+ or possibly Cl^-.

amino acids, and other solutes are selectively reabsorbed and water is taken up along with these solutes, the concentration of Cl^- in the tubular fluid rises, establishing a large chemical gradient for Cl^- in the direction of the blood side of the tubule. In addition, the selective uptake of Na^+ exceeds that of HCO_3^- and other anions, resulting in a net transfer of positive charge to the blood side of the epithelium. This creates an electrical gradient for anions in the direction of the blood, although the magnitude of the electrical gradient is small. Thus, a large chemical gradient and a small electrical gradient favoring the reabsorption of Cl^- is established. Because the zonula occludens is highly permeable to Cl^-, passive transfer of Cl^- from the tubule lumen to the interstitial fluid takes place down this electrochemical gradient, primarily through the paracellular pathway.

As the glomerular filtrate passes through the proximal tubule, it is rapidly depleted of many of the substances necessary for Na^+ reabsorption by cotransport. In the latter part of the proximal tubule, Na^+, K^+ ATPase continues to move Na^+ from the cell into the interstitial fluid, but other mechanisms of Na^+ transport across the apical cell membrane predominate. These mechanisms include active, electrogenic uptake of Na^+ and some form of electroneutral Na^+ uptake, where chloride (Cl^-) is transported into the cell in an equivalent amount. In addition to the active, transcellular reabsorption of Na^+, passive reabsorption through the paracellular pathway also occurs in the late proximal tubule. This is made possible by the large chemical gradient for Cl^- established by the selective reabsorption of other solutes. As Cl^- moves passively down its chemical gradient from the urine side to the blood side of the tubule epithelium, its electrostatic attraction for Na^+ carries Na^+ along with it. The passage of Cl^- down its chemical gradient also abolishes the small lumen-negative charge and in fact establishes a small lumen-positive charge, which further favors the passive transfer of Na^+ to the blood side of the epithelium.

Other filtered solutes, such as potassium (K^+) and calcium (Ca^{2+}), are present in the tubule fluid in low concentrations. Nevertheless, they are reabsorbed by the proximal tubule epithelium. The reabsorption of K^+ and Ca^{2+} in the proximal tubule appears to take place by passive mechanisms driven by the tubular lumen-to-blood electrical gradient. The tubular reabsorption of these solutes is dis-

cussed in more detail in the section on reabsorption and secretion in more distal segments of the nephron and in the collecting duct, where K^+ and Ca^{2+} transport is active and is influenced by systemic factors in order to maintain electrolyte balance.

The proximal tubule is also responsible for the reabsorption of filtered peptides and low molecular weight proteins. A large proportion of filtered peptides are degraded to amino acids by peptidases present in the proximal tubule brush border, and are reabsorbed by cotransport with Na^+ across the apical plasma membrane, as previously discussed. There is also evidence that small peptides are themselves transported across the apical plasma membrane through cotransport with H^+, driven by the tubular fluid-to-blood proton gradient.

Low molecular weight proteins are also avidly reabsorbed by the proximal tubule, but by a different mechanism. These filtered proteins, such as insulin, glucagon, parathyroid hormone, and Bence Jones protein, are taken up from the tubule fluid into proximal tubule cells by carrier-mediated endocytosis along the apical plasma membrane (see Fig. 40–4). The proteins are delivered by the endocytic vesicles to a system of intracellular organelles called *lysosomes* (Fig. 40–8). The reabsorbed proteins are degraded by proteolytic enzymes within the lysosomes, and the resultant amino acids are transported into the interstitial fluid and returned to the blood.

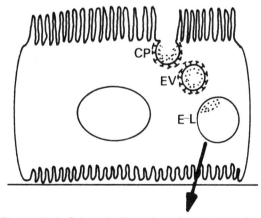

Figure 40–8. Schematic illustration of receptor-mediated endocytosis of filtered proteins in the proximal tubule. Filtered proteins bind with their receptors in the membrane of coated pits (*CP*) in the apical plasma membrane. The CP invaginate and form endocytic vesicles (*EV*) that transport the proteins to the endosomal-lysosomal system (*E-L*) from which the reabsorbed proteins or their degradation products are returned to the circulatory system.

The Proximal Tubule Secretes Organic Ions

Another important function of the proximal tubule is the removal of a wide variety of organic ions from the blood and their secretion into the tubule fluid. This group of organic ions includes both endogenous waste products and exogenous drugs or toxins. Because many of these substances are protein-bound in the plasma, they are poorly filtered by the glomerulus, and tubular secretion plays a vital role in the clearance of these substances from the blood. The mechanism of secretion is not well defined, but is basically composed of active uptake of these substances from the blood into the tubule cell followed by passive diffusion of the substance into the tubule fluid. Endogenous organic compounds secreted by the proximal tubule include bile salts, oxalate, urate, creatinine, prostaglandins, epinephrine, and hippurates. (One of these, para-amino hippurate, can be used as a measure of tubular function.) Also secreted by the proximal tubule are antibiotics, such as penicillin G and trimethoprim; diuretics, such as chlorothiazide and furosemide; the analgesic, morphine, and many of its derivatives; and the potent herbicide, paraquat. The practical applications of this aspect of proximal tubule function are broad. Tubular secretion of endogenous organic ions, drugs, and toxins provides the basis for urine testing for hormones and foreign substances as a reflection of blood levels that may be only transiently elevated. Tubular secretion of certain antibiotics is important in determining which antibiotics can reach high concentrations in the urine for more effective treatment of urinary tract infections. Similarly, secretion of furosemide and other diuretics by the proximal tubule enhances delivery of these drugs to their site of action downstream. Finally, tubular secretion of drugs determines in part their excretion rate and affects the appropriate dosage of renally excreted drugs, particularly in patients with compromised renal function.

The Distal Tubule and Collecting Duct Segments Are Specialized to Reabsorb or Secrete Solutes as Required by Systemic Factors

The structure of the tubule cells changes abruptly and dramatically at the end of the proximal tubule. The proximal tubule, with its large numbers of mitochondria, luxuriant brush border, and pronounced infoldings of the basolateral plasma membrane, is built for high volume transport of a large variety of substances by both active and passive mechanisms. The segments that follow the proximal tubule each have a unique and highly specific cell structure, reflecting their specialized functions. Immediately following the S_3 segment of the proximal tubule is the thin limb of the loop of Henle, which is a low epithelium with few mitochondria and few membranous infoldings (Fig. 40–9). As one might expect, physiologic studies suggest that active transport of solutes in this segment is virtually nonexistent. The function of the thin limb is determined by its passive permeability properties and its orientation. These characteristics are essential to its role in water reabsorption and are discussed in a later section.

In the ascending limb of the loop of Henle, the low epithelium of the thin ascending limb abruptly changes to the tall epithelium of the thick ascending limb. The thick ascending limb is endowed with numerous mitochondria and basolateral plasma membrane infoldings, reflecting its high capacity for active solute transport (Fig. 40–10). The distal convoluted tubule follows with an even taller epithelium and a dense array of mitochondria, and leads into the connecting segment, which makes the transition from the distal nephron to the collecting duct system. Depending on the species, the connecting segment is composed of several cell types, including distal convoluted tubule cells, connecting segment cells, which are similar to distal convoluted tubule cells, intercalated cells, which have large numbers of intracytoplasmic vesicles as well as mitochondria, and principal cells, which have fewer mitochondria but extensive basolateral plasma membrane infoldings. It appears that each of these structurally distinct cell types have distinct physiological functions as well. In the collecting duct system, the principal cell persists as the major cell type through the initial collecting duct, the cortical collecting duct, and the outer medullary collecting duct, accounting for approximately two thirds of the cells in most regions. The intercalated cell accounts for the remainder of the cortical and outer medullary collecting duct cells, and in some species (rat and human, at least) persists even in the inner medullary collecting duct. Structural differences in the cells of the inner medullary collecting duct as it approaches the papillary tip have been described also, but the

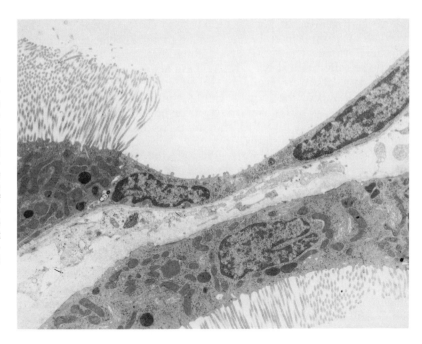

Figure 40–9. Transmission electron micrograph of rat kidney illustrating the transition from the proximal tubule to the thin descending limb of the loop of Henle. The tall epithelium of the proximal tubule with the extensive brush border and abundant mitochondria abruptly changes to the low epithelium of the thin limb of the loop of Henle. Epithelial cells of the thin limb have a smooth, simple plasma membrane surface and few mitochondria, consistent with the absence of active transport functions. Magnification 5900×.

physiological correlates remain to be determined.

The Distal Tubule Segments Reabsorb Salts and Dilute the Tubule Fluid

The distal tubule segments, consisting of the thick ascending limb of the loop of Henle and the distal convoluted tubule, reabsorb Na^+, K^+, Cl^-, and the divalent cations, Ca^{2+} and Mg^{2+}. Although these two segments do not have the capacity for reabsorption of the proximal tubule, by the time the tubule fluid leaves the distal convoluted tubule, more than 90% of the filtered salts has been reabsorbed, and the osmolality of the tubule fluid is typically 100 mosm/L.

Salt reabsorption in the distal tubule seg-

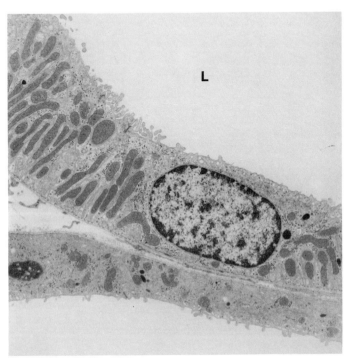

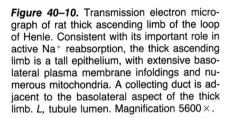

Figure 40–10. Transmission electron micrograph of rat thick ascending limb of the loop of Henle. Consistent with its important role in active Na^+ reabsorption, the thick ascending limb is a tall epithelium, with extensive basolateral plasma membrane infoldings and numerous mitochondria. A collecting duct is adjacent to the basolateral aspect of the thick limb. *L*, tubule lumen. Magnification 5600×.

ments is driven by the Na⁺, K⁺ ATPase in the basolateral plasma membrane, similar to the proximal tubule, and the distal convoluted tubule has the highest Na⁺, K⁺ ATPase activity of any nephron segment. In the thick ascending limb of the loop of Henle, the basolateral Na⁺, K⁺ ATPase actively transports Na⁺ from the cell into the interstitial fluid, creating a chemical gradient for Na⁺ across the apical plasma membrane. This gradient drives a Na⁺, K⁺, 2 Cl⁻ cotransporter in the apical plasma membrane, and these ions move from the tubule fluid into the cell by secondary active transport (Fig. 40–11). The Cl⁻ diffuses down its chemical gradient into the interstitial fluid. The K⁺ rapidly moves extracellularly down its concentration gradient through diffusion channels across not only the basolateral plasma membrane, but also across the apical plasma membrane back into the tubule fluid. The result of the diffusion of K⁺ back into the tubule fluid is a net transport of negative electrical charge into the cell (2 Cl⁻, 1 Na⁺). This leaves a net positive charge in the tubule fluid, creating a lumen-to-blood electrical gradient for cations that then diffuse into the interstitial fluid through the paracellular pathway.

The distal convoluted tubule continues to reabsorb Na⁺ from the tubule fluid through active transport of Na⁺ by the basolateral Na⁺, K⁺ ATPase. A lumen-negative electrical gradient is created, and Cl⁻ moves from the

tubule fluid to the interstitial fluid down its electrical gradient.

Both the thick ascending limb and the distal convoluted tubule are impermeable to water. The reabsorption of salts without concurrent water reabsorption results in a hypotonic tubule fluid, and these segments are sometimes called the *diluting segments*. Dilution of the tubule fluid takes place irrespective of the volume status of the animal, although in some species antidiuretic hormone, which is released when an animal is volume-depleted, enhances salt reabsorption from the thick ascending limb, thereby enhancing the dilution of the tubule fluid. The dilution of the tubule fluid in these segments is an important component of the fluid volume regulation provided by the kidney, allowing the kidney to excrete excess water without salt, thereby preventing water overload and plasma hypotonicity. The role of the thick ascending limb and the distal convoluted tubule in water balance is discussed further in Chapter 41.

The Collecting Duct Reabsorbs NaCl and Can Secrete or Reabsorb K⁺

The collecting duct system begins with the connecting segment, which is a transition region from the distal convoluted tubule to the initial collecting tubule. The initial collecting tubules converge and empty into the collecting duct, which descends through the cortex and medulla to the papillary tip, where the tubule fluid (urine) discharges into the renal pelvis. Throughout much of the collecting duct system, there exist two main cell types: the intercalated cell and the principal cell (Fig. 40–12). The principal cell is responsible for NaCl reabsorption in the collecting duct. It has extensive basolateral plasma membrane infoldings, which have been shown to contain the Na⁺, K⁺ ATPase. As in other tubule segments already discussed, Na⁺ is actively transported from the cell into the interstitial fluid, and a gradient is established for Na⁺ from the tubular fluid into the principal cell. Cl⁻ diffuses passively from lumen-to-blood down the electrical gradient established by Na⁺ reabsorption. At the same time, K⁺ is pumped actively from the interstitial fluid into the cell, raising the intracellular K⁺ concentration above that of the interstitial fluid and the tubule fluid. Because the apical plasma membrane of the principal cell is more permeable to K⁺ than the basolateral plasma membrane, K⁺ diffuses

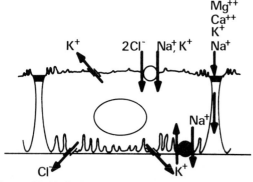

Figure 40–11. Schematic illustration of transport functions of the thick ascending limb. Na⁺ is actively reabsorbed through the basolateral Na⁺, K⁺ ATPase. Na⁺, K⁺, and Cl⁻ enter the cell from the luminal fluid through secondary active cotransport. Cl⁻ diffuses down its concentration gradient across the basolateral plasma membrane through a Cl⁻ channel. K⁺ leaves the cell through both an apical and basolateral K⁺ channel. A lumen-to-blood gradient for cations is present in this segment, which drives reabsorption of Na⁺, K⁺, Ca²⁺, and Mg²⁺ through the cation-selective paracellular pathway.

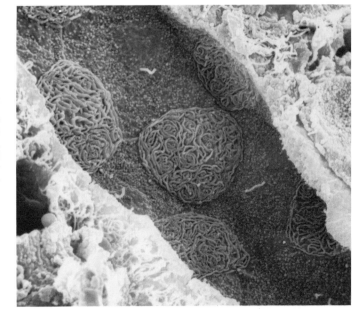

Figure 40–12. Scanning electron micrograph of rat outer medullary collecting duct viewed from the luminal surface. Two cell types are evident, the principal cell with short, small projections over the apical surface and a single central cilium, and the intercalated cell with extensive, complex membrane folds (microplicae) over the apical surface. Magnification 3300×.

preferentially across the apical plasma membrane, and thus K⁺ is secreted (Fig. 40–13).

The collecting duct is also capable of K⁺ reabsorption, and the intercalated cell appears to be responsible for this function. There is recent evidence that K⁺ is actively transported across the apical plasma membrane of the intercalated cell by an H⁺, K⁺ ATPase antiporter similar to that in the parietal cell of the stomach. This antiporter has an additional role in contributing to the acidification of the urine, which is discussed later.

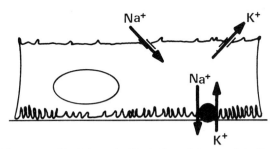

Figure 40–13. Schematic illustration of transport in the principal cell of the collecting duct. The extensive basal plasma membrane infoldings contain large amounts of Na⁺, K⁺ ATPase. Active transport of Na⁺ by this pump drives passive diffusion of Na⁺ from the tubule lumen into the cell through a Na⁺-selective channel in the apical plasma membrane. A K⁺-selective channel in the apical plasma membrane provides a route for passive diffusion of intracellular K⁺ into the tubule fluid. The hormone aldosterone enhances Na⁺, K⁺ ATPase activity and increases the K⁺ permeability of the apical plasma membrane, thus enhancing Na⁺ reabsorption and K⁺ secretion in this segment.

The Distal Tubule and Collecting Duct Respond to Systemic Signals to Alter Salt Excretion as Required

In the proximal tubule, filtered solutes and water are generally reabsorbed regardless of the animal's physiological state. In contrast, the distal tubule and collecting duct control the ultimate rate of excretion of electrolytes and water in order to maintain homeostasis despite variations in dietary intake and extrarenal losses of salts and water. The specific responses of these segments to markedly alter the rate of reabsorption or secretion of Na⁺, K⁺, Ca²⁺, and water are due in large part to the action of several hormones.

Aldosterone Enhances Na⁺ Reabsorption and K⁺ Secretion

One of the most important of these hormones is aldosterone, a mineralocorticoid hormone secreted by the adrenal cortex. Aldosterone release is stimulated by systemic hypotension through the renin/angiotensin system and acts on the connecting segment cells and the principal cells of the collecting duct to enhance Na⁺ reabsorption, which in turn enhances water reabsorption in order to correct perceived volume depletion. At the cellular level, aldosterone increases the permeability of the apical plasma membrane and stimulates Na⁺, K⁺ ATPase activity, thereby enhancing Na⁺ reabsorption. Chronic aldosterone stimulation even causes a structural adaptation in these cells, the proliferation of the basolateral plasma membrane where the Na$^+$, K$^+$ ATPase resides.

Aldosterone release is stimulated also by hyperkalemia (elevated plasma K$^+$). The response of the connecting segment and collecting duct is to enhance K$^+$ secretion not only through stimulation of the Na$^+$, K$^+$ ATPase, but also by a direct effect of aldosterone to increase the apical membrane permeability to K$^+$. Therefore, regardless of the stimulus for its release, aldosterone increases Na$^+$ reabsorption and K$^+$ secretion in the connecting segment and collecting duct.

Although aldosterone appears to be necessary for a rapid response to an increased demand for Na$^+$ reabsorption or K$^+$ secretion, it has been shown that an adaptive response by the distal tubule and collecting duct is possible even in the absence of aldosterone. Chronic administration of a low Na$^+$/high K$^+$ diet to adrenalectomized (mineralocorticoid deficient) rabbits causes proliferation of the basolateral plasma membrane of connecting segment cells and principal cells of the collecting duct, as well as an increase in Na$^+$, K$^+$ ATPase activity in these segments. The mechanism of this response is not known. It is also not known if other species are capable of a similar response in the absence of mineralocorticoids.

Another hormone, vasopressin or antidiuretic hormone, also appears to enhance Na$^+$ reabsorption in distal segments in response to volume depletion, at least in some species. Antidiuretic hormone is best known for its effect on the collecting duct to enhance water reabsorption. However, there is evidence in the rat and the mouse that antidiuretic hormone stimulates NaCl reabsorption in the medullary thick ascending limb of the loop of Henle through stimulation of adenylate cyclase activity in this segment.

Parathyroid Hormone Enhances Ca^{2+} Reabsorption

Hypocalcemia (low plasma calcium) stimulates parathyroid hormone (PTH) release, which has an effect on bone, intestine, and the kidney to raise the plasma calcium level. The response of the kidney occurs in the cortical thick ascending limb, the distal convoluted tubule, and the connecting segment. Experiments using either *in vivo* micropunc-

ture or *in vitro* microperfusion of tubule segments have shown that PTH causes an increase in the rate of production of adenosine 3',5'-cyclic phosphate (cAMP) in these segments, which is thought to mediate the enhanced Ca^{2+} and Mg^{2+} reabsorption also observed in these segments when PTH is present. PTH is also one of the few hormones that have been shown to have an effect on transport in the proximal tubule. However, in this segment, adenylate cyclase activation diminishes Na$^+$-dependent phosphate and fluid reabsorption rather than enhancing Ca^{2+} reabsorption.

In vitro experiments suggest that in the rabbit, the hormone calcitonin also enhances Ca^{2+} reabsorption in the medullary thick ascending limb. The advantage of segmental specificity for two hormones that both enhance Ca^{2+} reabsorption is not known. However, in most species the main effect of calcitonin is to inhibit phosphate reabsorption. Calcitonin may also enhance renal calcium excretion, an apparent contradiction of the *in vitro* evidence in the rabbit.

CLINICAL CORRELATIONS

GLUCOSURIA

HISTORY □ A client presents her 10-year-old female miniature schnauzer with the complaint of a dramatic increase in water consumption and urine volume over the previous 2 weeks.

CLINICAL EXAMINATION □ No major abnormalities are found by physical examination. The dog appears alert and is moderately overweight. The urinalysis reveals 4+ glucose, and the urine specific gravity is 1.030. The plasma glucose is tested immediately and is 275 mg/dL (normal 80–120 mg/dL).

COMMENT □ The dog is suffering from diabetes mellitus, which results from a relative or absolute deficiency of insulin secreted from the β cells of the pancreas. The insulin deficiency results in elevated plasma glucose levels. Glucose is freely filtered by the glomerulus and normally is entirely reabsorbed by the proximal tubule. As the plasma glucose level rises, the glucose concentration in the glomerular filtrate rises. When it exceeds the reabsorptive capacity of the proximal tubule (the renal threshold) of approximately 180 mg/dL, glucose appears in the urine. Glucose acts as an osmotic agent and increases the volume of urine excreted. The dog then drinks more water to replace the excessive fluid loss.

Treatment of diabetes mellitus in veterinary patients usually involves the administration of insulin injections two to three times each day, with adjustments of the dose in accordance with frequent evaluations of the plasma or urine glucose values. When the insulin dosage is appropriate, the plasma glucose is normalized, the glucosuria disappears, and the urine volume and water consumption decrease.

HYPOADRENOCORTICISM

HISTORY □ A concerned client presents her 1-year-old spayed female Samoyed with the complaint of severe weakness, inappetence, and vomiting since the previous day.

CLINICAL EXAMINATION □ You find the dog to be depressed, weak, and markedly dehydrated. The heart rate is normal, but pulses are weak. No other abnormalities are detected by physical examination. You immediately collect samples of blood and urine for a complete blood count, serum chemistries, and a urinalysis, before placing an intravenous catheter to start volume replacement therapy with a balanced electrolyte solution. The urinalysis is normal with a specific gravity of 1.025. Abdominal radiographs are normal, but the thoracic radiographs demonstrate a small cardiac silhouette and small thoracic vessels. You expedite the serum chemistries and find the serum creatinine is 2.5 mg/dL, the serum potassium is 6.5 mEq/L (normal 3.6–5.6 mEq/L), the serum sodium is 129 mEq/L (normal 141–155 mEq/L), the serum chloride is 97 mEq/L (normal 103–115 mEq/L), and the serum bicarbonate is 12 mEq/L (normal 18–24 mEq/L).

COMMENT □ The dog has hypoadrenocorticism. The metabolic disturbances result from a deficiency of the mineralocorticoid hormone, aldosterone. In a normal animal, aldosterone stimulates Na^+, K^+ ATPase activity and enhances the apical plasma membrane K^+ permeability in the connecting segment and the collecting duct, thereby enhancing Na^+ reabsorption and K^+ secretion. In the absence of aldosterone, these segments waste Na^+, and K^+ is inappropriately retained. Cl^- and water follow the path of Na^+ and also are excreted excessively by the kidney. Hyperkalemia (high serum K^+) has profound effects on excitable tissue, including nerve and muscle cells, and results in muscle weakness, decreased cardiac output, hypotension, and cardiac arrhythmias. The loss of Na^+ and water results in volume depletion and the decreased size of the heart and thoracic blood vessels, and exacerbates the hypotension and poor tissue perfusion. Poor perfusion of the kidneys is probably the major cause of the elevated serum creatinine (azotemia), because inadequate renal blood flow and reduced glomerular capillary hydrostatic pressure prevent adequate glomerular filtration. This is called *prerenal* azotemia. In most cases of prerenal azotemia, the urine will be maximally concentrated in an attempt to retain fluid and restore blood volume, but in hypoadrenocorticism, this response is often blunted, possibly by the hyponatremia (reduced serum Na^+) or by the absence of glucocorticoids which have been shown to have a permissive effect on maximal urine concentration (see Chapter 41). The decreased serum bicarbonate indicates metabolic acidosis, which is the result of both the diminished renal ability to secrete H^+ and reabsorb HCO_3^- (see Chapter 42) and the increased production of acid from poorly perfused tissue.

Prompt treatment is important for the survival of the animal, because the hyperkalemia and acidosis can cause fatal cardiac arrhythmias. Volume repletion with normal saline and correction of the *base deficit* (low serum HCO_3^-) often stabilizes the animal. Replacement therapy with mineralocorticoid hormones such as desoxycorticosterone acetate, desoxycorticosterone pivalate, or fludrocortisone acetate restores Na^+, K^+ ATPase activity and should be started as soon as possible. Frequently, glucocorticoid hormones are given early to treat shock even before the electrolyte status is known; they are beneficial for two reasons. Hypoadrenocorticism usually results in glucocorticoid deficiency, sometimes manifested by hypoglycemia, and replacement therapy is indicated. In addition, the mineralocorticoid activity in many of these preparations is beneficial in correcting the hyperkalemia and hypokalemia.

A definitive diagnosis may be obtained by an adrenocorticotropic hormone (ACTH) challenge test, which maximally stimulates the release of cortisol from the adrenal gland and shows little or no response in animals with hypoadrenocorticism.

Chronic maintenance usually involves oral therapy with fludrocortisone acetate, with the proper dosage determined by periodic evaluations of the serum K^+ and Na^+. Chronic replacement of glucocorticoids is recommended also.

Bibliography

Bovee KC (ed): Canine Nephrology. Media, PA, Harwal Publishing, 1984, pp 1–217.

Brenner BM, Rector FC Jr (eds): The Kidney, 3rd ed. Philadelphia, WB Saunders, 1986, pp 3–700.

Madsen KM, Verlander JW, Tisher CC: Relationship between structure and function in distal tubule and collecting duct. J Electron Microsc Tech 9:187–208, 1988.

Rector FC Jr: Sodium, bicarbonate, and chloride absorption by the proximal tubule. Am J Physiol 244:F461–F471, 1983.

Seldin SW, Giebish G (eds): The Kidney: Physiology and Pathophysiology. New York, Raven Press, 1985, pp 3–2162.

Sullivan LP, Grantham JJ (eds): Physiology of the Kidney, 2nd ed. Philadelphia, Lea & Febiger, 1982, pp 1–224.

PRACTICE QUESTIONS FOR CHAPTER 40

1. Which segment of the renal tubule is responsible for the reabsorption of the bulk of filtered solutes?

   a. Proximal tubule
   b. Thin limbs of the loop of Henle
   c. Thick ascending limb of the loop of Henle
   d. Distal convoluted tubule
   e. Collecting duct

2. The main driving force for the reabsorption of solutes from the tubule fluid is

   a. active transport of solutes across the apical plasma membrane.
   b. secondary active transport of solutes across the apical plasma membrane.
   c. active transport of sodium from the tubule epithelial cell across the basolateral plasma membrane by the electrogenic Na^+ pump.
   d. active transport of sodium from the tubule epithelial cell across the basolateral plasma membrane by the Na^+, K^+ ATPase.

   e. passive diffusion of solutes through the paracellular pathway.

3. The net rate of reabsorption of a solute in the proximal tubule fluid is determined by

   a. the rate of active transport of the solute.
   b. the rates of tubular reabsorption and secretion of the solute.
   c. the systemic requirements of the animal for the solute.
   d. the lipid permeability of the solute.
   e. the glomerular filtration rate.

4. The ultimate rate of excretion of K^+ in the urine is determined by

   a. the concentration of K^+ in the glomerular filtrate.
   b. the proximal tubule, which reabsorbs or secretes K^+ to meet the physiological requirements of the animals.
   c. the thick ascending limb, where K^+ secretion is enhanced by high plasma K^+ concentrations.
   d. the distal convoluted tubule, which has K^+ pumps that are inserted in the apical or basolateral plasma membranes, depending on the need for reabsorption or secretion of K^+.
   e. the collecting duct, in which the principal cells are capable of K^+ secretion, and the intercalated cells are capable of K^+ reabsorption.

5. One effect of aldosterone on the connecting segment and collecting duct is to

   a. enhance the Na^+ permeability of the apical plasma membrane, thereby enhancing Na^+ and water reabsorption.
   b. stimulate Na^+, K^+ ATPase activity in the basolateral plasma membrane, thereby enhancing Na^+ and water reabsorption.
   c. reduce the Na^+ permeability of the apical plasma membrane, thereby inhibiting Na^+ and water reabsorption.
   d. reduce Na^+, K^+ ATPase activity in the basolateral plasma membrane, thereby inhibiting Na^+ and water reabsorption.
   e. reduce the K^+ permeability of the apical plasma membrane, thereby inhibiting K^+ reabsorption.

41

Water Balance

1. The renal tubules maintain water balance
2. The proximal tubule reabsorbs over 60% of filtered water
3. The mammalian kidney can produce either a concentrated or diluted urine
4. The hypertonic medullary interstitium permits the formation of concentrated urine
5. The juxtamedullary nephrons extend deep into the inner medulla
6. Medullary hypertonicity depends on solute reabsorption by the medullary thick ascending limb and collecting duct
7. The countercurrent mechanism increases medullary interstitial osmolality with little energy expenditure
8. Countercurrent exchange in the vasa recta results in the removal of water from the medullary interstitium
9. Active NaCl reabsorption in the thick ascending limb and the distal convoluted tubule permits the formation of a dilute urine
10. The collecting duct responds to antidiuretic hormone to determine the final urine osmolality

The Renal Tubules Maintain Water Balance

One of the most important functions of the kidney is the maintenance of the water content of the body and the tonicity of the plasma. Terrestrial animals must be guarded against desiccation, and the kidney is designed to reabsorb the majority of the water in the glomerular filtrate. However, the kidney also is able to respond to a water overload by excreting a hypotonic urine. Under normal conditions, the 10-kg beagle that produces 53.3 L of glomerular filtrate every day may reabsorb over 99% of the water contained in the glomerular filtrate, excreting only 0.2–0.25 L of urine. During water deprivation, a normal dog is able to produce urine that is seven to eight times the osmolality of plasma, well over 2,000

mosm/L. Following a water load, the same dog responds by excreting urine with an osmolality as low as 100 mosm/L, approximately one third that of plasma. The means by which the kidney accomplishes these feats are discussed in this section.

The Proximal Tubule Reabsorbs Over 60% of Filtered Water

As discussed in the section on solute reabsorption, the proximal tubule is responsible for the reabsorption of the majority of the ultrafiltrate. Solutes are retrieved in this segment by both active and passive means, but the energy driving the solute reabsorption is generated by the Na^+, K^+ adenosinephosphatase (ATPase) pump in the basolateral plasma membrane. Water reabsorption is similarly driven by this pump. As Na^+ is actively transported from the cell into the interstitial fluid, Na^+ and other solutes are removed from the tubule fluid by secondary active transport, and Cl^- diffuses passively from the tubule fluid into the lateral intercellular spaces. The reabsorption of these solutes dilutes the tubule fluid, creating a slight gradient favoring the movement of water into the cells and the intercellular spaces. Because the brush border of the proximal tubule provides a large surface area for reabsorption and the epithelium is highly permeable to water, the small gradient results in rapid movement of large volumes of water from the tubule fluid to the interstitial fluid. As discussed previously, the high oncotic pressure and low hydrostatic pressure of the peritubular capillaries favor the movement of reabsorbed water and solute from the interstitial fluid, and the reabsorbate is returned quickly to the systemic blood stream. Considering the 10-kg beagle once again, during the course of a day between 32 and 37 L of water will be reabsorbed by the proximal tubules. However, because the water is reabsorbed nearly isotonically with salt, there is little change in the osmolality of the tubule fluid between Bowman's space and the beginning of the thin descending limb of the loop of Henle.

The Mammalian Kidney Can Produce Either a Concentrated or a Diluted Urine

An ingenious system has evolved in the mammalian kidney to allow the excretion of urine that is either concentrated or diluted relative to plasma as circumstances warrant. This system can be divided into three main components. The first is the generation of a hypertonic medullary interstitium, which permits the formation of a concentrated urine. The second component is the dilution of the tubule fluid by the thick ascending limb and the distal convoluted tubule, which permits the formation of a dilute urine. The third component is the variability in water permeability of the collecting duct in response to antidiuretic hormone (ADH), which determines the final concentration of the urine. The beauty of this system is that all the factors necessary for urine concentration and dilution are operative at any given time, so that the kidney can respond immediately to changes

in ADH levels with corresponding changes in urine osmolality and water excretion.

The Hypertonic Medullary Interstitium Permits the Formation of Concentrated Urine

The urine of terrestrial mammals is usually concentrated well above the osmolality of plasma. The excretion of concentrated wastes conserves water and, therefore, reduces the volume of water that must be consumed each day to prevent dehydration. Two of the three factors mentioned earlier are responsible for the formation of concentrated urine: the generation of a hypertonic medullary interstitium, and enhanced water permeability in the collecting duct in the presence of ADH.

Two main factors are responsible for the hypertonicity of the medullary interstitium. The first is the reabsorption of osmotically active substances by tubules in the medulla. The second is the removal of water from the interstitium by the vasa recta.

The Juxtamedullary Nephrons Extend Deep into the Inner Medulla

The anatomical arrangement of the renal tubules in the medulla is crucial for the function of the urine concentrating mechanism. The nephrons of the mammalian kidney may be subdivided into two populations, called *superficial* and *juxtamedullary nephrons*, based on the location of their respective glomeruli (see Fig. 39–1). Superficial nephrons have short loops of Henle that extend only into the inner stripe of the outer medulla. Juxtamedullary nephrons have long loops of Henle that extend deep into the inner medulla. The juxtamedullary nephrons are particularly responsible for the kidney's ability to concentrate urine far above the osmolality of plasma.

Medullary Hypertonicity Depends on Solute Reabsorption by the Medullary Thick Ascending Limb and Collecting Duct

The thick ascending limb of Henle's loop actively reabsorbs NaCl, but is impermeable to water. Therefore, as discussed in the section on solute reabsorption, this segment contributes salt relatively free of water to the interstitial fluid and raises its osmolality.

The inner medullary collecting ducts also

actively reabsorb NaCl, but their more important contribution to the medullary hypertonicity is the reabsorption of urea (Fig. 41–1). Although the cortical and outer medullary collecting ducts are impermeable to urea, the terminal portion of the inner medullary collecting duct (IMCD) is highly permeable to urea. Urea permeability in the terminal IMCD is enhanced by ADH. This enhanced urea

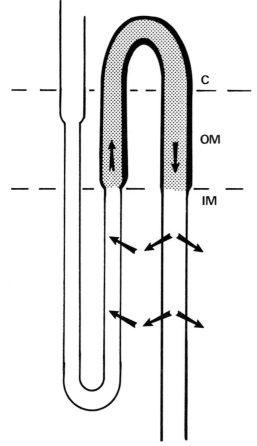

Figure 41–1. Schematic illustration of urea recycling in Henle's loop, the distal tubule, and the collecting duct. The thin limbs of Henle's loop are permeable to urea. Urea diffuses down its concentration gradient into the tubule fluid in the thin ascending limb. The thick ascending limb, the distal convoluted tubule, and the cortical and outer medullary collecting ducts are impermeable to urea (indicated by a broad line). Thus, urea remains in the tubule fluid in these segments (stippled area) rather than diffusing into the urea-poor cortical and outer medullary interstitia. The urea concentration in the tubule fluid increases because of water abstraction. The urea then enters the urea-permeable inner medullary collecting duct (IMCD) and diffuses into the interstitium. There is evidence that the urea permeability of the IMCD may be enhanced by antidiuretic hormone, thus enhancing the contribution of urea to the medullary interstitial hypertonicity during times of maximal water reabsorption.

permeability is probably mediated by stimulation of adenylate cyclase activity. Thus, urea is conserved in the tubule fluid until it reaches the terminal IMCD deep in the medulla. There, urea reabsorption into the interstitial fluid is moderated by ADH, so that when conditions demand enhanced conservation of water (increased concentration of urine), urea reabsorption is enhanced. Because the thin ascending limb is permeable to urea, whereas the tubule segments that intervene between the thin ascending limb and the terminal IMCD are impermeable to urea, the urea that is reabsorbed from the terminal IMCD is recycled back to the IMCD. This system of urea recycling enhances the efficiency of the urine concentrating mechanism.

The Countercurrent Mechanism Increases Medullary Interstitial Osmolality with Little Energy Expenditure

The countercurrent mechanism is responsible for the amplification of the medullary hypertonicity initiated by the active reabsorption of solutes by the thick ascending limb and the medullary collecting duct. This function is accomplished with a minimal expenditure of energy on account of two characteristics: the anatomical arrangement of the thin limbs of the loop of Henle and the vasa recta, and the differential water and salt permeabilities of the descending and ascending thin limbs.

The thin limbs of Henle's loop in juxtamedullary nephrons extend deep into the inner medulla. The descending and ascending thin limbs are joined by a sharp, "hairpin" turn. The result is that the descending and ascending thin limbs are parallel and juxtaposed, with the tubule fluid flow in opposite directions (Fig. 41–2). A similar arrangement exists for the vasa recta. This arrangement of parallel, adjacent conduits with opposite directions of flow enables an energy-efficient conservation of solute in the region. First, consider the contribution of the thin limbs of Henle's loop to solute and water reabsorption (Fig. 41–3). The descending thin limb originates from the S_3 segment of the proximal tubule. It is aligned with the water-impermeable thick ascending limb, where NaCl is actively transported from the tubule fluid, resulting in a local increase in the osmolality of the interstitial fluid. The tubule fluid entering the thin limb is essentially isosmotic to plasma and, therefore, has

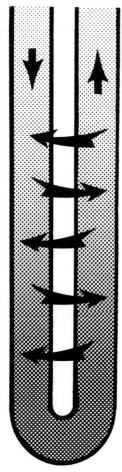

Figure 41–2. Schematic illustration of the effect of countercurrent flow. The amount of energy required to maintain a gradient along a conduit is reduced by arranging the conduit so that the flow is antiparallel and the two arms of the conduit are adjacent. In this way the incoming fluid equilibrates with the exiting fluid at every level in the gradient so that a steep gradient is maintained. This system is used commonly to minimize energy consumption and maximize efficiency in heating or cooling devices. The kidney, the thin limbs of the loop of Henle, and the vasa recta are arranged in this fashion. The gradient is a solute concentration gradient, and the antiparallel conduits are connected by a hairpin turn deep in the medulla where the solute concentration is highest.

a lower osmolality than the surrounding interstitial fluid because of its proximity to the thick ascending limb. Therefore, a gradient for water and solutes is established between the tubule and interstitial fluids. Because the descending thin limb is highly permeable to water, but not to salt, the tubule fluid rapidly equilibrates with the interstitial fluid by the movement of water into the interstitium, and the osmolality of the tubule fluid increases.

Accept for the moment that the osmolality of the medullary interstitial fluid is progressively higher in the deeper regions of the medulla. As the water-permeable descending thin limb reaches regions of higher and higher interstitial osmolality, the tubule fluid continues to equilibrate by the diffusion of H_2O into the interstitium, and the osmolality of the tubule fluid progressively rises until it reaches its maximal concentration at the hairpin turn.

At this point, the thin limb begins to ascend through regions of progressively lower interstitial osmolality, and once again the tubule fluid equilibrates with the interstitial fluid. However, the ascending thin limb is impermeable to water and permeable to NaCl, so the equilibration occurs not by movement of water into the tubule fluid, but by diffusion of NaCl from the tubule fluid into the interstitial fluid. The osmolality of the tubule fluid decreases, and the osmolality of the interstitium increases. This process continues until the ascending thin limb leaves the inner medulla and merges with the thick ascending limb. At the transition to the thick ascending limb, the tubule fluid osmolality is only moderately hypertonic.

At this point, what has been accomplished? By passive means, the thin limbs have reabsorbed both water and salt. The water was reabsorbed from the descending thin limb, and the salt was reabsorbed from the ascending thin limb. At the same time, the countercurrent flow in these two segments has helped to amplify the medullary hypertonicity.

Countercurrent Exchange in the Vasa Recta Results in the Removal of Water from the Medullary Interstitium

The diffusion of water from the descending thin limb into the interstitium would tend to dilute the effect of salt transport into the interstitium if it were not for the ability of the vasa recta to remove the reabsorbed fluid from the medullary interstitium. The walls of the vasa recta are permeable to water and salts. As the vessels descend in the inner medulla, the plasma equilibrates with the interstitial fluid. The plasma osmolality rises as it nears the hairpin turn, then falls as it ascends out of the medulla through passive diffusion of water and salt (Fig. 41–4).

In addition to changes in the composition of the plasma in the vasa recta brought about by equilibration with the interstitial fluid, the relatively high plasma oncotic pressure in the

Figure 41–3. Schematic illustration of the selective permeability of the segments of the loop of Henle. The thick ascending limb of the loop of Henle actively transports Na$^+$ into the interstitium of the outer medulla but is impermeable to H$_2$O. The result is the generation of a hypertonic medullary interstitium. The tubule fluid that enters the thin descending limb is nearly isotonic. Because the thin descending limb is permeable to H$_2$O but impermeable to Na$^+$, equilibration with the progressively higher solute concentration of the medullary interstitium occurs by diffusion of H$_2$O from the tubule fluid into the interstitium (*arrowheads*), and the osmolality of the tubule fluid rises as it approaches the hairpin turn. Conversely, the ascending limb of Henle's loop (*stippled area*) is permeable to Na$^+$ and other solutes but is impermeable to H$_2$O. Therefore, as the highly concentrated tubule fluid leaves the medulla it equilibrates with the progressively lower osmolality of the interstitium by passive diffusion of salt across the epithelium of the thin ascending limb into the interstitium. The osmolality of the tubule fluid in the thin ascending limb progressively falls by passive means until it reaches the thick ascending limb, where active transport of Na$^+$ further dilutes the tubule fluid. The net result is the generation and maintenance of the medullary concentration gradient and the passive reabsorption of water and salt.

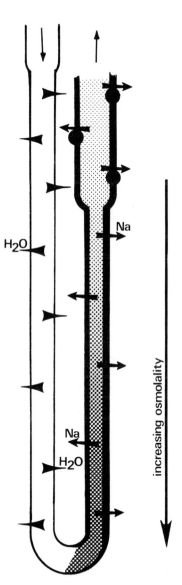

vasa recta entering the medulla favors the movement of water into the capillary lumen, and NaCl is retained with the water. By the time the plasma leaves the medulla, its oncotic pressure has fallen, indicating the net movement of fluid into the capillary. Thus, the vasa recta, by virtue of their countercurrent flow and high initial plasma oncotic pressure, effectively remove solute and water from the medullary interstitium and maintain the medullary hypertonicity.

Active NaCl Reabsorption in the Thick Ascending Limb and the Distal Convoluted Tubule Permits the Formation of a Dilute Urine

As discussed in the section on solute reabsorption, the thick ascending limb and the distal convoluted tubule actively reabsorb Na^+, which drives Cl^- reabsorption secondarily. Because these segments are impermeable to water, active solute reabsorption results in a progressive decline in the osmolality of the tubule fluid. Thus, the thick ascending limb and distal convoluted tubule are often called the *diluting segments*. The result is that the tubule fluid delivered into the collecting duct system is hypotonic regardless of the physiological state of the animal.

The Collecting Duct Responds to Antidiuretic Hormone to Determine the Final Urine Osmolality

The generation of medullary hypertonicity and the dilution of the tubule fluid in the distal nephron segments set the stage for the elimination of either a concentrated or dilute urine as warranted by the fluid volume status of the animal. The permeability characteristics of the collecting duct under the influence of ADH determine the osmolality of the excreted urine.

Under conditions of water overload, ADH is absent, and the collecting duct is relatively impermeable to water. The tubule fluid delivered by the distal convoluted tubule remains hypotonic, because the water is confined within the collecting duct. Thus, in the absence of ADH a dilute urine is formed, and water is excreted in excess of salt (Fig. 41–5). The water load is eliminated, and normal plasma osmolality is maintained.

Under conditions perceived as dehydration or volume depletion, ADH is released from

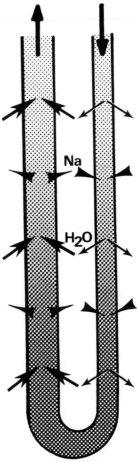

Figure 41–4. Schematic illustration of the removal of water and salt from the medullary interstitium by the vasa recta. Both the descending and ascending arms of the vasa recta are permeable to salt and water. As blood flows through the progressively increasing and then decreasing osmolality of the medullary interstitium, equilibration with the plasma osmolality occurs by passive diffusion of both salt and water across the capillary wall. While the high oncotic pressure of the plasma entering the vasa recta drives the net removal of water and thus solute, the countercurrent exchange prevents the dissipation of the medullary concentration gradient.

the pituitary. These conditions include factors that raise the plasma osmolality, such as dehydration or salt overload. In addition to dehydration, other factors that lower the blood pressure stimulate ADH release; these include isosmotic volume depletion from vomiting, diarrhea, or hemorrhage; systemic vasodilation; or heart failure. In these circumstances, the goal is to reduce the plasma osmolality to normal or to restore fluid volume. The effect of ADH is to markedly enhance the water permeability of the collecting duct. Thus, when ADH is present, water rapidly flows

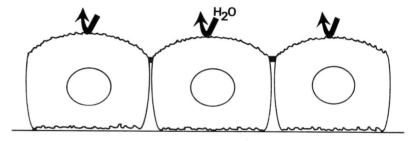

Figure 41–5. Schematic illustration of the collecting duct epithelium in the absence of ADH. When ADH is absent, the apical plasma membrane is impermeable to water, and a dilute urine is excreted.

from the dilute tubule fluid into the interstitium down the concentration gradient (Fig. 41–6). The means by which ADH affects this permeability change is not clear, but it is believed to be mediated by adenylate cyclase; structural alterations in the collecting duct, namely, cell swelling and dilation of the intercellular spaces, have been observed. Nevertheless, as the now water-permeable collecting duct traverses the inner medulla through regions of progressively higher interstitial fluid osmolality, the tubule fluid equilibrates by diffusion of water into the interstitium, and a highly concentrated tubule fluid, now urine, is eliminated.

CLINICAL CORRELATIONS

DIABETES INSIPIDUS

HISTORY □ A client presents her 6-month-old female Boston terrier with the complaint of excessive water consumption and urination.

CLINICAL EXAMINATION □ The physical examination reveals no abnormalities. The dog is alert and active. A urinalysis is normal, and the urine specific gravity is 1.002 (osmolality 152 mosm/L). Serum chemistries and a complete blood count are normal.

You admit the dog to your clinic for a modified water deprivation test. The dog fails to concentrate her urine despite a 5% loss of body weight. You administer vasopressin, and the urine specific gravity is 1.029 (osmolality 852 mosm/L) 1 hour later.

COMMENT □ The dog has central diabetes insipidus, which is a deficiency of ADH. The urine is normally diluted by the thick ascending limb of the loop of Henle and the distal convoluted tubule. Solute-free water absorption in the collecting duct is dependent on the action of ADH. In the absence of ADH, excessive volumes of water are excreted, and the dog drinks voraciously to prevent dehydration.

Other causes of excretion of a dilute urine (urine osmolality markedly lower than serum osmolality) are psychogenic polydipsia, hyperadrenocorticism, glucocorticoid administration, hypercalcemia, hypokalemia, and nephrogenic diabetes insipidus. Most of these can be detected by a good history, physical examination, complete blood count, and serum chemistry profile. When only psychogenic polydipsia, central diabetes insipidus, and nephrogenic diabetes insipidus remain in the differential, the diagnosis usually can be made by using the modified water deprivation test. Animals with psychogenic polydipsia can secrete ADH and have normal kidneys; therefore, they concentrate their urine after water deprivation. Dogs with diabetes insipidus can concentrate their

Figure 41–6. Schematic illustration of the water permeability of the apical plasma membrane of the collecting duct epithelium in the presence of ADH. ADH stimulates the formation of water channels in the apical plasma membrane, which enhances its water permeability. Water rushes into the cells and across the water-permeable basolateral plasma membrane into the lateral intercellular spaces, where solute concentrations are high relative to the tubule fluid. Morphological changes that have been observed include cell swelling into the tubule lumen and dilation of the lateral intercellular spaces.

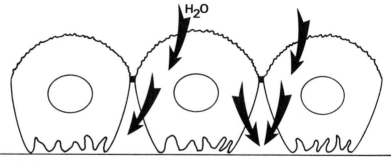

urine minimally or not at all following water deprivation. If the problem is insufficient ADH release (central diabetes insipidus), the urine concentration increases in response to exogenous ADH. If the kidney is unresponsive to ADH (nephrogenic diabetes insipidus), the urine concentration does not increase further in response to additional ADH.

Treatment of central diabetes insipidus includes free access to water and daily administration of exogenous vasopressin by parenteral or intranasal routes.

CHRONIC RENAL INSUFFICIENCY

HISTORY ☐ You recommend routine dentistry for a 15-year-old male miniature schnauzer that appears to be in good health. Before general anesthesia, you obtain a complete blood count, serum chemistry profile, and urinalysis to detect any subclinical organ dysfunction.

CLINICAL EXAMINATION ☐ The complete blood count and serum chemistry profile are normal. The urinalysis is normal with a specific gravity of 1.010 (osmolality 352 mosm/L). You ask the owner to submit a sample of the dog's urine from the first void of the day. The specific gravity of this sample is 1.012 (osmolality 401 mosm/L).

COMMENT ☐ Chronic renal insufficiency is common in geriatric patients and is probably responsible for the two urine specific gravity values in the "fixed range" of 1.008–1.012. These values correspond to osmolalities similar to or slightly higher than normal plasma osmolality. Although additional evaluation would have to be done to verify that this animal could neither dilute nor concentrate his urine significantly, in an animal of advanced age and in the absence of other clinical abnormalities, further evaluation is probably not indicated.

In chronic renal insufficiency, the loss of functional nephrons is first manifested by the inability to significantly alter the urine concentration in response to a water load or water deprivation. The residual nephrons are able initially to sustain adequate filtration rates to prevent azotemia (elevated serum creatinine and urea nitrogen), but the compensatory increase in flow rates in individual nephrons probably exceeds the capacity of the thick ascending limb and distal convoluted tubule to significantly dilute the tubule fluid. The residual nephrons are unable also to generate a steep medullary concentration gradient and, thus, the tubule fluid cannot be concentrated well above the level of the plasma osmolality. If there is progressive nephron loss, the glomerular filtration rate will continue to decline, and renal failure will ensue.

It is important to be aware that your patient has chronic renal insufficiency and is unable to respond efficiently to changes in fluid and salt intake. Water should not be withheld except briefly, and caution should be exercised to support the animal with intravenous fluids during anesthesia while avoiding fluid overload.

There is evidence that a low protein diet may retard the progression of chronic renal disease and delay the onset of renal failure, at least in some species. This question is the point of considerable controversy and is under intense study.

Bibliography

Bovee KC (ed): Canine Nephrology. Media, PA, Harwal Publishing, 1984, pp 1–217.

Brenner BM, Rector FC Jr (eds): The Kidney, 3rd ed. Philadelphia, WB Saunders, 1986, pp 3–700.

Jamison RJ: The renal concentration mechanism. Kidney Int 32 (Suppl) 21:S43–S50, 1987.

Madsen KM, Verlander JW, Tisher CC: Relationship between structure and function in distal tubule and collecting duct. J Electron Microsc Tech 9:187–208, 1988.

Seldin SW, Giebish G (eds): The Kidney: Physiology and Pathophysiology. New York, Raven Press, 1985, pp 3–2162.

Sullivan LP, Grantham JJ (eds): Physiology of the Kidney, 2nd ed. Philadelphia, Lea & Febiger, 1982, pp 1–224.

PRACTICE QUESTIONS FOR CHAPTER 41

1. The bulk of filtered water is reabsorbed by which renal tubule segment?

   a. Proximal tubule
   b. Thin limbs of the loop of Henle
   c. Thick ascending limb of the loop of Henle
   d. Cortical collecting duct
   e. Inner medullary collecting duct

2. The kidney is designed to respond rapidly to changing water requirements. The ability

to efficiently alter the rate of water excretion by markedly concentrating or diluting the urine is the result of several factors. Which of the following does NOT contribute to this ability?

a. Generation of hypertonic medullary interstitium
b. Countercurrent flow and differential salt and water permeabilities in the thin limbs of Henle's loop
c. Dilution of the tubule fluid by the thick ascending limb and the distal convoluted tubule
d. Responsiveness of the collecting duct to ADH
e. Countercurrent flow and enhanced water permeability in the vasa recta under the influence of ADH

3. The hypertonic medullary interstitium (necessary for producing urine that is more concentrated than plasma) is generated in large part by

a. active transport of Na^+ by the S_3 segment of the proximal tubule.
b. active reabsorption of Na^+ by the water-impermeable ascending thin limb of Henle's loop.
c. active reabsorption of Na^+ by the water-impermeable thick ascending limb of Henle's loop.
d. enhanced formation of water channels in the apical plasma membrane of collecting duct cells under the influence of vasopressin.
e. enhanced urea permeability of the ascending thin limb of Henle's loop under the influence of vasopressin.

4. In volume depletion, ADH is released, which reduces water excretion by

a. enhancing water reabsorption in the proximal tubules by stimulating Na^+, K^+ ATPase.
b. enhancing water reabsorption in the thick ascending limb by stimulating the formation of water channels in the apical plasma membrane.
c. enhancing water reabsorption in the collecting duct by stimulating Na^+, K^+ ATPase activity.
d. enhancing water reabsorption in the collecting duct by stimulating the formation of water channels in the apical plasma membrane.
e. reducing the glomerular filtration rate by activation of tubuloglomerular feedback.

5. In clinical situations, the excretion of a dilute urine may be due to all but which of the following?

a. Chronic renal disease
b. Glucocorticoid administration
c. ADH deficiency
d. Hypoadrenocorticism
e. Acute renal hypoperfusion

42

Acid-Base Balance

1. Buffers, lungs, and kidneys collaborate to maintain acid-base balance
2. The kidneys excrete nonvolatile acids
3. Acid excretion by the renal tubules is achieved by H^+ secretion and buffering in the tubule fluid
4. The proximal tubule has a high capacity for H^+ secretion and HCO_3^- reabsorption
5. The collecting duct determines the final urine pH
6. The collecting duct can secrete protons and generate an acid urine
7. The collecting duct is capable of net bicarbonate secretion

Buffers, Lungs, and Kidneys Collaborate to Maintain Acid-Base Balance

The normal blood pH is approximately 7.4, and it is necessary for normal function of cellular processes to maintain the pH close to this value. Three systems are at work to maintain acid-base homeostasis: intracellular and extracellular buffers, the respiratory system, and the kidneys. The first two of these are responsible for rapid correction of pH changes, whereas the kidneys are responsible for long-term acid-base homeostasis and the excretion of excess hydrogen ion.

The usual condition that must be corrected is the addition of excess acid, or hydrogen ion, to body fluids. Acid is constantly produced in the body as a byproduct of metabolism and catabolism. The amount of acid produced varies, depending on changes in the diet, level of exercise, or function of other physiological processes; therefore, the systems designed to maintain acid-base homeostasis must be able to adapt to changes in the acid load. Less often, certain disturbances result in

an excess base load, which also must be eliminated.

Several intracellular and extracellular buffers act to titrate H^+ to maintain the pH within physiological limits. These include hemoglobin and other proteins, carbonates in bone, phosphates, and bicarbonate. These buffers rapidly normalize the pH after acute alterations in the acid load, unless the buffering capacity is exceeded.

The respiratory system also can respond rapidly to maintain the blood pH within the normal range by altering the rate of removal of carbon dioxide (CO_2) and, thus, lowering the concentration of carbonic acid (H_2CO_3) in the blood. You may remember that the enzyme carbonic anhydrase, present in red blood cells as well as in many other cells, catalyzes the dehydration of carbonic acid in the reaction:

$$H^+ + HCO_3^- \rightleftharpoons H_2CO_3 \rightleftharpoons CO_2 + H_2O$$

Removal of CO_2 from the blood by respiration shifts this reaction to the right, ultimately

Figure 42–1. Schematic illustration of the buffer mechanisms at work in the tubule fluid of the proximal tubule and the collecting duct. In the proximal tubule, buffering by filtered HCO_3 predominates because of the relatively high concentration of HCO_3^-. NH_3, generated in proximal tubule cells by the hydrolysis of glutamine, is the buffer second in importance in the proximal tubule. In

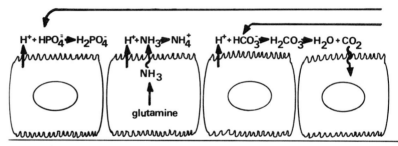

the cortical collecting duct, buffering by HCO_3^- and filtered, nonbicarbonate buffers, such as $HPO_4^=$, predominates. The predominant buffer in the medullary collecting duct is NH_3 because of the high concentration of NH_3 in the medullary interstitium.

reducing the concentration of H^+ (raising the pH). The lung provides an important avenue for stabilization of the blood pH, particularly in response to rapid changes in the acid load.

The kidney provides the third arm of defense of acid-base balance. Although the buffering and respiratory systems are able to modulate alterations in blood pH, the kidneys are responsible for the actual excretion of the majority of excess H^+.

The Kidneys Excrete Nonvolatile Acids

Whereas the lungs alter blood pH by the removal of CO_2 and reducing the concentration of H_2CO_3 (a volatile acid), the kidneys are capable of excretion of nonvolatile acid by tubular secretion of H^+. Large amounts of H^+ can be removed from the body by tubular secretion, primarily in the proximal tubule and the collecting duct. These two segments operate by different mechanisms to excrete excess acid and to precisely control blood pH. The proximal tubule is primarily responsible for the bulk of acid secretion, whereas the collecting duct is primarily responsible for the control of net acid excretion and the final urine pH.

Acid Excretion by the Renal Tubules Is Achieved by H^+ Secretion and Buffering in the Tubule Fluid

Efficient acid excretion is achieved in the kidney by the activity of an array of enzymes and transporters that specifically promote the transport of H^+ from the epithelial cells into the tubule fluid, combined with the presence of buffers that prevent large increases in H^+ concentration in the tubule fluid.

The majority of H^+ transported across the apical plasma membrane is handled by two transporters, an Na^+/H^+ antiporter and an H^+

adenosinetriphosphatase (H^+ ATPase). The Na^+/H^+ antiporter exchanges intraluminal Na^+ for intracellular H^+ and is driven by the lumen-to-blood gradient for Na^+ provided by Na^+, K^+ ATPase (secondary active transport). This Na^+/H^+ exchange is the primary route of H^+ secretion in the proximal tubule. The H^+ ATPase is an electrogenic proton pump (active transport), transporting only intracellular H^+ across the apical plasma membrane and contributing a net positive charge to the tubule fluid. The H^+ ATPase is believed to be responsible for the majority of H^+ secretion by the intercalated cells of the collecting duct.

The presence of buffering systems in the tubule fluid is vital for efficient acid excretion. The buffers accept secreted H^+ and minimize the lowering of the tubule fluid pH that would otherwise result from rapid rates of H^+ secretion by the epithelial cells. The three most important buffers are HCO_3^-, ammonia, and phosphate. (Although ammonia technically is not a buffer because it will only release H^+ from the protonated form at a very alkaline pH, it nevertheless serves to remove free protons from solution and is loosely included as a "buffer" in this discussion.) The mechanisms of removal of acid by these buffers are illustrated in Figure 42–1. In the proximal tubule, HCO_3^- is the most important intraluminal buffer for two main reasons. The first is that the concentration of HCO_3^- in the tubule fluid is high. Although large amounts of HCO_3^- are reabsorbed in the proximal tubule, roughly proportional amounts of H_2O are reabsorbed, and the HCO_3^- concentration remains similar to that of the glomerular filtrate. Secondly, after titration of HCO_3^-, the H_2CO_3 is dispersed as H_2O and CO_2, and accumulation of the acid form is averted. The removal of the volatile component of carbonic acid by respiratory loss essentially creates a sink for the secreted acid.

Ammonia (NH_3) is generated in proximal tubule cells by hydrolysis of the amino acid glutamine. Ammonia freely diffuses across plasma membranes, and when it diffuses into the luminal fluid, it combines with H^+ to form ammonium ion (NH_4^+). Also, NH_4^+ that is formed intracellularly can enter the tubule fluid through secondary active transport by substitution for H^+ on the Na^+/H^+ antiporter. However, because ammonium ion is lipid-insoluble, it cannot diffuse back across the apical plasma membrane and is trapped within the tubule fluid.

The formation of NH_4^+ from intraluminal NH_3 and H^+ lowers the concentration of NH_3 in the tubule fluid and thus contributes to the maintenance of a favorable gradient for the diffusion of NH_3 into the tubule fluid as well as for the secretion of H^+. The formation of NH_3 from glutamine (ammoniagenesis) is enhanced by acidosis and provides one avenue of increased H^+ excretion in response to an increase in the acid load.

Filtered phosphate also contributes to the buffering capacity of the tubule fluid. Secreted H^+ titrates HPO_4^{2-} to form $H_2PO_4^-$. As with ammonia, the titrated form is a charged molecule and is lipid-insoluble; therefore, it does not diffuse readily across the epithelium, and the secreted acid is retained in the tubule fluid in segments where phosphate transporters are absent.

The Proximal Tubule Has a High Capacity for H^+ Secretion and HCO_3^- Reabsorption

You may remember from the section on tubular reabsorption of solutes that the proximal tubule normally reabsorbs 80–90% of the filtered HCO_3^-. The mechanism of bicarbonate reabsorption in the proximal tubule is described in that section and is illustrated in Figure 40–7). Briefly, filtered HCO_3^- combines with H^+ to form H_2CO_3, which is dehydrated rapidly under the influence of apical membrane–bound carbonic anhydrase to form H_2O and CO_2. The CO_2 diffuses into the epithelial cell and is hydrated under the influence of cytoplasmic carbonic anhydrase to form H_2CO_3, which dissociates into H^+ and HCO_3^-. The HCO_3^- is transported across the basolateral plasma membrane and is reabsorbed into the blood, whereas the H^+ is transported into the lumen, primarily by the Na^+/H^+ antiporter. There is also evidence that significant electrogenic H^+ secretion occurs across the apical plasma membrane of proximal tubule cells. The contribution of the H^+ ATPase to acid secretion in this segment may be as much as 35% of the total. It should be evident that HCO_3^- reabsorption and H^+ secretion are essentially equivalent terms in this system and are used interchangeably by renal physiologists.

Although the proximal tubule has a great capacity for HCO_3^- reabsorption (H^+ secretion), it is incapable of maintaining a large pH gradient across the apical plasma membrane. The net secretion of H^+ in this segment is particularly dependent on the presence of the intraluminal buffers discussed earlier to combine with secreted H^+ and maintain the concentration of H^+ in the tubule fluid at a relatively constant level. As a result, although the majority of renal acid secretion (HCO_3^- reabsorption) occurs in the proximal tubule, the pH of the tubule fluid when it leaves this segment is similar to that of the glomerular filtrate. As mentioned, the buffer that is most important in the proximal tubule is HCO_3^-, primarily because of its high concentration in the glomerular filtrate and the rapid dispersion of the acid form through respiratory loss of CO_2.

The Collecting Duct Determines the Final Urine pH

The rate of acid secretion by the collecting duct determines the final urine pH and the net acid excretion by the kidney. Although the proximal tubule has a large capacity for H^+ secretion (HCO_3^- reabsorption) and reabsorbs 80–90% of the filtered HCO_3^-, the pH of the tubule fluid is virtually unchanged when it leaves the proximal tubules. The segments intervening between the proximal tubule and the connecting segment have little acid-secreting ability, so the tubule fluid that reaches the connecting segment has a H^+ concentration similar to that of the glomerular filtrate. Yet, the normal urine pH of carnivores ranges from 5.5 to 7.5, and that of ruminants ranges from 6 to 9, with even greater extremes of pH being possible in response to acidosis and alkalosis. The collecting duct is responsible for this ability to excrete urine with a pH markedly different from that of plasma.

The Collecting Duct Can Secrete Protons and Generate an Acid Urine

In contrast to the proximal tubule, which is a high capacity, low gradient system of H^+

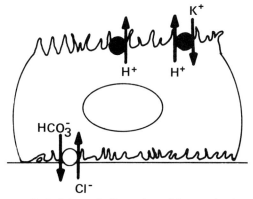

Figure 42–2. Schematic illustration of the mechanism of H^+ secretion/HCO_3^- reabsorption in the acid-secreting intercalated cells of the collecting duct. Two means of active transport of H^+ across the apical plasma membrane are present: the electrogenic proton pump, H^+ATPase, and the H^+K^+ATPase. The basolateral plasma membrane contains a Cl^-/HCO_3^- exchanger that allows HCO_3^- reabsorption.

secretion, the collecting duct has a lower capacity for H^+ secretion, but can generate a steep H^+ concentration gradient.

Acid secretion in the collecting duct system is a function of a specialized group of cells, the intercalated cells (see Fig. 40–12). The intercalated cells, which are rich in carbonic anhydrase, first appear in the connecting segment and persist as far as the terminal inner medullary collecting duct in some species. H^+ generated from H_2CO_3 is secreted into the tubule fluid by the electrogenic proton pump, H^+ ATPase, present in the apical plasma membrane. The HCO_3^- that remains is transported across the basolateral plasma membrane to the blood side of the cell by a Cl^-/HCO_3^- exchan-

ger similar to the Cl^-/HCO_3^- exchanger in red blood cell membranes (Fig. 42–2). The acid-secreting intercalated cells are capable of altering the rate of H^+ secretion by altering the numbers of proton pumps in the apical plasma membrane. This is accomplished by the insertion or removal of proton pump–containing membrane vesicles and results in structural changes that mirror the physiological response (Figs. 42–3, 42–4). In this way, the acid-secreting intercalated cells are able to respond to changes in the acid load and alter acid secretion accordingly.

There is recent evidence that the acid-secreting intercalated cells also actively secrete H^+ in exchange for K^+ by means of an apical H^+, K^+ ATPase similar to that of the parietal cells of the stomach (see Fig. 42–2). The magnitude of the contribution of the H^+, K^+ ATPase to net acid secretion under normal conditions is unknown, but the activity of this transporter is enhanced by hypokalemia (low serum K^+) and appears to be an important contributor to renal acidification in this condition. Mineralocorticoid hormones, such as aldosterone, are also known to enhance acidification in the collecting duct. It has been postulated that this increase in H^+ secretion is due to an increase in the numbers of proton transporters, either H^+ATPase or H^+, K^+ ATPase or both, in the apical plasma membrane of the acid-secreting intercalated cells, similar to the adaptive response seen in acidosis.

There is also evidence that the terminal segments of the collecting duct, where few or no intercalated cells exist, are capable of acid

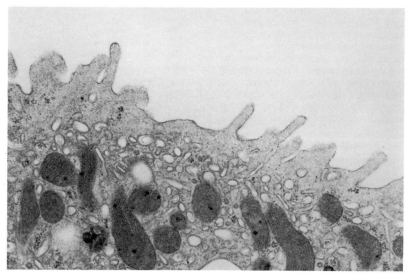

Figure 42–3. Transmission electron micrograph of an acid-secreting (type A) intercalated cell from the cortical collecting duct of a control rat. The apical plasma membrane contains few small membranous projections, and the apical cytoplasm is filled with numerous membrane vesicles. *L*, tubule lumen. Magnification 11,300 ×.

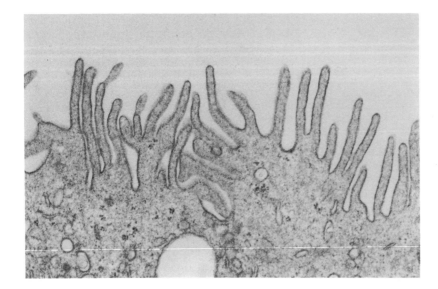

Figure 42–4. Transmission electron micrograph of an acid-secreting intercalated cell from the cortical collecting duct of a rat with acute respiratory acidosis. The apical surface is covered with numerous long membranous projections, and the number of apical cytoplasmic vesicular profiles is markedly reduced. This is the result of the insertion of membrane vesicles containing H^+ transporters into the apical plasma membrane in response to acidosis, thus enhancing the acid-secreting capacity of the cell. Magnification 11,300 ×.

Figure 42–5. Scanning electron micrograph of rat cortical collecting duct viewed from the tubule lumen. Three cell types are evident. The principal cells (*P*) are large with a single central cilium and few apical surface microprojections. The type A (acid-secreting) intercalated cells (*arrows*) have a large apical surface covered with extensive membrane folds (microplicae). The type B (bicarbonate-secreting?) intercalated cells (*arrowheads*) have a small apical surface area covered with sparse microprojections, either microvilli or a mixture of microvilli and microplicae. Magnification 4000 ×.

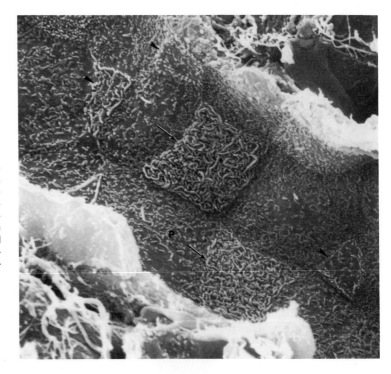

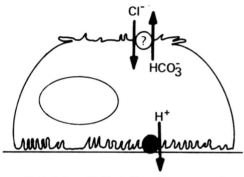

Figure 42–6. Schematic illustration of the proposed mechanism of HCO_3^- secretion (H^+ reabsorption) in the type B intercalated cell of the cortical collecting duct. These cells are known to contain H^+ ATPase in the basolateral plasma membrane and to be rich in carbonic anhydrase. Although there is no direct evidence for it, a Cl^-/HCO_3^- exchanger is thought to be present in the apical plasma membrane.

secretion. Both an electrogenic proton pump and a Na^+/H^+ exchanger have been suggested as routes of H^+ transport in this region, but the question of the importance and mechanism of acid secretion in these segments is currently unresolved.

The Collecting Duct Is Capable of Net Bicarbonate Secretion

The proximal tubule reabsorbs HCO_3^- and secretes H^+ regardless of the plasma HCO_3^- concentration and the blood pH. In fact, as the plasma HCO_3^- concentration increases, the concentration of HCO_3^- in the glomerular filtrate increases, and the amount of HCO_3^- reabsorption by the proximal tubule epithelium also increases. Although the HCO_3^- reabsorptive capacity of the proximal tubule can be saturated, in general the amount of H^+ secretion and HCO_3^- reabsorption in this segment is determined by the concentration of intraluminal buffers rather than by the need for conserving or excreting acid or base.

However, the collecting duct is capable of net HCO_3^- secretion in response to alkalosis. Net HCO_3^- secretion has been shown to be a function of the cortical collecting duct in rats and rabbits (Fig. 42–5). A distinct subset of intercalated cells (type B intercalated cells) is present in the cortical collecting duct in many species, and it has been postulated that these cells are capable of HCO_3^- secretion. The type B intercalated cells are known to be rich in carbonic anhydrase and to contain a basolateral electrogenic proton pump. Although it has not been demonstrated, it is suspected

that the type B intercalated cell contains an apical Cl^-/HCO_3^- exchanger. If this is the case, bicarbonate-secreting cells would represent essentially a mirror image of acid-secreting cells, with active H^+ reabsorption and exchange of Cl^- in the tubule fluid for intracellular HCO_3^- (Fig. 42–6).

Although information about these mechanisms is accumulating rapidly, little is known about the comparative physiology of renal control of acid-base balance. It is likely that considerable anatomical and functional differences exist among species, particularly among carnivores, which usually excrete acid urine, and ruminants, which usually excrete neutral or alkaline urine.

CLINICAL CORRELATIONS

RESPIRATORY ACIDOSIS WITH RENAL COMPENSATION

HISTORY □ A 6-year-old male German shepherd is presented to you with the complaints of weakness, exercise intolerance, and inappetence that have become progressively worse over the previous 6 weeks.

CLINICAL EXAMINATION □ The dog is recumbent and anxious. Respiration is labored, and the heart rate is rapid, but pulses are strong and regular. Crackles are heard over all lung fields. Thoracic radiographs reveal a diffuse, severe pulmonary interstitial and alveolar infiltrate with enlargement of the hilar lymph nodes. You obtain samples of blood and urine for a complete blood count, serum chemistry panel, urinalysis, and arterial blood gases. The urine pH is 5.0, and the arterial blood gas results are pH 7.37 (normal 7.45), P_{O_2} 38 mmHg (normal 80–100 mmHg), P_{CO_2} 70 mmHg (normal 31–35 mmHg), and HCO_3^- 37 mEq/L (normal 18–24 mEq/L).

COMMENT □ The dog has chronic respiratory acidosis due to severe pulmonary infiltrates. The lung is unable to ventilate adequately, and the blood level of CO_2 rises, increasing the concentration of carbonic acid and lowering the blood pH. Although the increased level of CO_2 will contribute slightly to an increase in blood HCO_3^-, the marked increase in the blood HCO_3^- in this case is largely due to enhanced renal retention of HCO_3^- and secretion of H⁺. Acidemia enhances ammoni-agenesis in the proximal tubule, thereby increasing the buffering capacity in the tubule fluid and favoring H^+ excretion. Respiratory acidosis activates the acid-secreting intercalated cells in the collecting duct, where HCO_3^- is reabsorbed, and H^+ is secreted. The blood HCO_3^- concentration rises and helps return the blood pH toward normal. A steep H^+ gradient is established in the collecting ducts, and an acid urine is excreted.

Treatment requires diagnosis and correction of the pulmonary disease if possible. Bicarbonate therapy is not indicated, because the blood bicarbonate is elevated already, and the blood pH is partially corrected. Oxygen therapy may be beneficial to support the animal until specific treatment is instituted.

METABOLIC ALKALOSIS WITH PARADOXIC ACIDURIA

HISTORY □ You are asked to examine a 3-year-old Holstein-Friesian cow that has been inappetent for 2–3 days. The cow recently calved and freshened normally, but milk production has dropped in the last 2 days, and the feces are loose.

CLINICAL EXAMINATION □ Physical examination reveals dehydration and an elevated heart rate. Percussion of the abdomen reveals an area of high-pitched resonance on the right side. A distended abomasum is palpable on rectal examination. You diagnose a right displaced abomasum and suspect abomasal torsion. Attempts to correct the displacement by rolling the cow fail. The cow is transported to your clinic for surgery, and samples are obtained for a complete blood count, serum chemistries, and urinalysis. The serum K^+ is 2.7 mEq/L (normal 4.0–5.1 mEq/L), serum Cl^- is 77 mEq/L (normal 85–103 mEq/L), and total CO_2 ($\approx$ serum HCO_3^- concentration) is 35 mEq/L (normal 24–27 mEq/L). The urine pH is 6.0.

COMMENT □ The cow has hypokalemic, hypochloremic, metabolic alkalosis secondary to abomasal displacement, which is the result of continued secretion of HCl by the abomasum and blunted HCO_3^- secretion by the intestine following the gastrointestinal obstruction. The hypokalemia is largely due to intracellular movement of K^+ secondary to alkalosis and may not reflect a decrease in total body K^+.

The expected renal response to alkalosis is the excretion of an alkaline urine. However, in this case the volume contraction and hypochloremia prevent the formation of alkaline urine, and the result is *paradoxic aciduria.* Remember that the proximal tubule reabsorbs the filtered HCO_3^- regardless of the plasma pH or serum HCO_3^- concentration. The volume depletion enhances Na^+ reabsorption primarily through the action of aldosterone, and Cl^- and H_2O reabsorption are enhanced secondary to the increased Na^+ uptake.

Renal secretion of HCO_3^- is believed to result from apical exchange of Cl^- in the tubule fluid for intracellular HCO_3^-, probably in type B intercalated cells in the collecting duct. Because NaCl is avidly reabsorbed to combat volume depletion, little Cl^- remains for exchange with HCO_3^-, and net HCO_3^- secretion does not occur. Acid secretion in the collecting duct is known to increase in response to aldosterone and may be enhanced in this volume-depleted animal. Hypokalemia may contribute also to the excretion of acid urine in this case. Hypokalemia activates the acid-secreting intercalated cells in the collecting duct. It is possible that the activity of the apical H^+, K^+ ATPase, which exchanges luminal K^+ for intracellular H^+, is enhanced in these cells and, thus, net acid secretion is favored by this mechanism as well.

Treatment involves vigorous volume replacement with intravenous normal saline with KCl added and surgical correction of the abomasal displacement.

Bibliography

Bovee KC (ed): Canine Nephrology. Media, PA, Harwal Publishing, 1984, pp 1–217.

Brenner BM, Rector FC Jr (eds): The Kidney, 3rd ed. Philadelphia, WB Saunders, 1986, pp 3–700.

Hamm LL, Simon EE: Roles and mechanisms of urinary buffer excretion. Am J Physiol 253:F595–F605, 1987.

Rector FC Jr: Sodium, bicarbonate, and chloride absorption by the proximal tubule. Am J Physiol 244:F461–F471, 1983.

Seldin SW, Giebish G (eds): The Kidney: Physiology and Pathophysiology. New York, Raven Press, 1985, pp 3–2162.

Sullivan LP, Grantham JJ (eds): Physiology of the Kidney, 2nd ed. Philadelphia, Lea & Febiger, 1982, pp 1–224.

PRACTICE QUESTIONS FOR CHAPTER 42

1. In carnivores, the usual role of the kidney in maintaining acid-base homeostasis is to

a. secrete excess bicarbonate.
b. secrete excess ammonia.
c. secrete excess nonvolatile acid.
d. secrete excess carbon dioxide.
e. secrete excess phosphate buffer.

2. The bulk of acid secretion (bicarbonate reabsorption) is accomplished by which renal tubule segment?

a. Proximal tubule
b. Thin limbs of the loop of Henle
c. Thick ascending limb of the loop of Henle
d. Distal convoluted tubule
e. Collecting duct

3. Which of the following factors does NOT contribute to efficient acid excretion (bicarbonate reabsorption) by the renal tubules?

a. Vasopressin-responsive bicarbonate reabsorption
b. Intraluminal buffering by bicarbonate
c. Intraluminal buffering by ammonia and phosphate
d. Intracellular and membrane-associated carbonic anhydrase
e. Transmembrane proton transport by the Na^+/H^+ antiporter and the electrogenic Na^+ pump

4. Which of the following statements regarding mechanisms of acid-base regulation by the collecting duct is false?

a. The cortical collecting duct responds to acidosis by increasing the net rate of acid secretion.
b. The cortical collecting duct responds to alkalosis with net bicarbonate secretion.
c. Proton and bicarbonate transport in the collecting duct are only slightly altered in response to systemic acid-base disturbances.
d. The collecting duct ultimately determines the pH of the urine.
e. The intercalated cells are largely responsible for acid secretion by the collecting duct.

5. Which of the following statements is correct?

a. Aldosterone affects acid excretion by enhancing proton secretion by the proximal tubule.
b. Aldosterone affects acid excretion by enhancing proton secretion by the collecting duct.
c. Aldosterone affects acid excretion by enhancing bicarbonate secretion by the collecting duct.
d. Aldosterone affects acid excretion by inhibiting bicarbonate reabsorption by the proximal tubule.
e. Aldosterone has no effect on acid excretion.

N. EDWARD ROBINSON

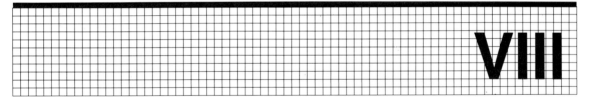

RESPIRATORY FUNCTION

43

Overview of Respiratory Function: Ventilation of the Lung

INTRODUCTION TO RESPIRATORY FUNCTION

1. The respiratory system's primary function is the transport of oxygen and carbon dioxide between the environment and the tissues

VENTILATION OF THE LUNG

1. Ventilation is the movement of gas in and out of the alveoli through the anatomical dead-space
2. Ventilation requires muscular energy
3. The respiratory muscles generate work to stretch the lung and overcome the frictional resistance to air flow
4. Lung elasticity is due to tissue and surface tension forces
5. Differences between air and saline pressure-volume curves are due to surface tension
6. The lung mechanically interacts with the thoracic cage
7. Airflow is opposed by frictional resistance in the airways
8. A major factor affecting the diameter of the tracheobronchial tree is smooth muscle contraction
9. Dynamic airway compression occurs when the pressure surrounding the airway exceeds the pressure within the airway lumen
10. The distribution of air depends on the local mechanical properties of the lung and the local changes in pleural pressure
11. Collateral ventilation and interdependence tend to maintain uniform ventilation distribution

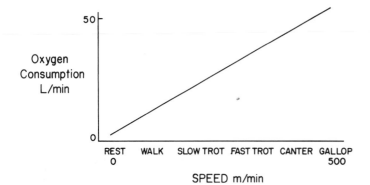

Figure 43–1. The effect of exercise on oxygen consumption in the horse. Oxygen consumption increases in a linear fashion as the horse increases speed; the total increase is approximately 30-fold. (Modified from Hörnicke H, Meixner R, Pollman U: Equine Exercise Physiology. Cambridge, Granta Editions, 1983, p 7.)

INTRODUCTION TO RESPIRATORY FUNCTION

The Respiratory System's Primary Function Is the Transport of Oxygen and Carbon Dioxide Between the Environment and the Tissues

Although *gas exchange* requirements vary with metabolism and may increase up to 30-fold during strenuous exercise (Fig. 43–1), they are normally accomplished with a small energy cost. When animals have respiratory disease, the energy cost of breathing increases, so there is less energy available for exercise or for weight gain. The owner then notices poor performance of the animal. The respiratory system is also important in thermoregulation; metabolism of endogenous and exogenous substances; and protection of the animal against inhaled dusts, gases, and infectious agents.

Figure 43–2 shows the processes involved in gas exchange including *ventilation, distribution* of gas within the lung, *diffusion* at the alveolocapillary membrane, transport of oxygen in the blood from the lungs to the tissue capillaries and transport of carbon dioxide in the reverse direction, and diffusion of gases between blood and tissues. *Oxygen consumption* and *carbon dioxide production* vary with metabolic rate, which is dependent on activity. Basal metabolism is a function of metabolic body weight ($M^{0.75}$), so smaller species have a higher oxygen consumption per kilogram of body weight than larger species. When animals exercise, oxygen consumption increases up to a maximum known as V_{O_2max}. Although V_{O_2max} generally increases with body size, there are some interesting deviations from this general relationship. Maximal oxygen consumption in the horse is threefold greater than maximal oxygen consumption in a cow of similar body weight, and dogs have higher maximal oxygen consumption than similarly sized goats. The more aerobic species, such as the dog and horse, have a higher V_{O_2max}/kg, because the skeletal muscle mitochondrial density is greater than in the less aerobic species.

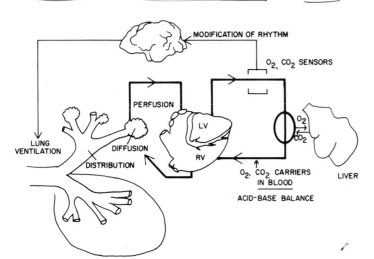

Figure 43–2. Diagrammatic representation of the processes involved in gas exchange. The lung is shown on the left, the heart in the center, and tissues on the right. The brain is shown at the top.

VENTILATION OF THE LUNG

Ventilation Is the Movement of Gas In and Out of the Alveoli Through the Anatomical Dead-Space

The volume of air breathed per minute, *minute ventilation* ($\dot{V}E$), is determined by the volume of each breath, *tidal volume* (VT), and the number of breaths per minute, *respiratory frequency* (f). The changes in minute ventilation that occur with changes in metabolic rate can be brought about through changes in either tidal volume or respiratory rate, or both.

Air flows into the *alveoli* through the *nares, nasal cavity, pharynx, larynx, trachea, bronchi,* and *bronchioles*. These structures comprise the *conducting airways,* and because gas exchange does not occur in these airways, they are also called the *anatomical dead-space* (Fig. 43–3). A portion of each tidal volume and, therefore, of minute ventilation, ventilates the anatomical dead-space, and a portion known as *alveolar ventilation* participates in gas exchange. Alveolar ventilation is regulated by control mechanisms to match the oxygen uptake and carbon dioxide elimination necessitated by metabolism.

Dead-space ventilation can occur within the alveoli also. This *alveolar dead-space* is a result of alveoli poorly perfused with blood, where gas exchange cannot occur optimally (see the section on ventilation perfusion matching). *Physiological dead-space* is a term used to describe the sum of the anatomical and the alveolar dead-space. The ratio of the ventilation to the physiological dead-space to minute ventilation, known as the *dead-space/tidal volume ratio* (VD/VT), varies considerably between species. In smaller species, such as dogs, it approximates 33%, whereas in some larger species, such as cattle and horses, it approximates 50–75%.

Because the volume of the anatomical dead-space is relatively constant, changes in the combination of tidal volume and respiratory frequency such as occur during exercise and thermoregulation can alter VD/VT. The small tidal volume and rapid respiratory frequency characteristic of *panting* in dogs increase VD/VT. Cattle, pigs, and mules subjected to heat stress also increase respiratory rate, minute ventilation, and VD/VT when trying to lose heat. In contrast to the effects of heat stress, cold-stressed animals increase alveolar ventilation and decrease dead-space ventilation by reducing f and increasing VT. The increase in alveolar ventilation is required, because oxygen consumption and carbon dioxide production increase due to the higher metabolic rate necessary to maintain body temperature.

The veterinarian should ensure that equipment used for anesthesia or respiratory therapy does not increase the dead-space. Excessively long endotracheal tubes or overly large face masks should be avoided.

Ventilation Requires Muscular Energy

During *inhalation,* energy provided by muscles causes air to enter the lungs. During *exhalation,* much of the energy causing air to leave the lungs is provided by the *elastic force* stored in the stretched lung and thorax. Therefore, in most animals at rest, inhalation is an active process, whereas exhalation is passive. Horses are an exception to this general rule and have an active phase to exhalation even at rest. During exercise or in the presence of respiratory disease, exhalation may be assisted by muscle contraction in most species.

The *diaphragm,* a domed musculotendinous sheet separating the abdomen and thorax and innervated by the *phrenic nerve,* is the primary inspiratory muscle. It consists of a costal portion arising from the xiphoid process and the

Figure 43–3. Types of dead-space. The volume of the trachea and bronchi comprises the anatomical dead-space, equipment dead-space is created by an endotracheal tube, and alveolar dead-space is the volume of air ventilating poorly perfused alveoli. At the top of the diagram an unperfused alveolus is shown, at the bottom a normally perfused alveolus, and in the middle an alveolus with less than optimal perfusion for the amount of ventilation received.

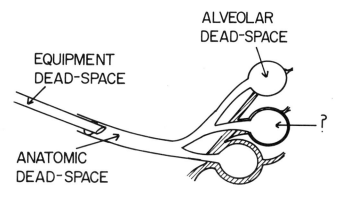

ALVEOLAR DEAD-SPACE

EQUIPMENT DEAD-SPACE

ANATOMIC DEAD-SPACE

costochondral junctions of the eighth to twelfth ribs (eighth to fourteenth ribs in equidae), and a crural portion arising from the ventral surface of the first three to four lumbar vertebrae and extending toward the tendinous center of the diaphragm. The apex of the dome of the diaphragm extends rostrally to the seventh or eighth intercostal space at the level of the base of the heart. During contraction, the dome of the diaphragm is pulled caudally and thereby enlarges the thoracic cavity. The tendinous center pushes against the abdominal contents, elevating intra-abdominal pressure, which displaces the caudal ribs outwards.

The *external intercostal muscles*, which join the ribs, are also active during inhalation. The fibers of this muscle are directed caudoventrally from the caudal border of one rib to the cranial border of the next, so contraction moves the ribs rostrally and outwards. The relative contributions of diaphragmatic and costal movement to ventilation under different metabolic demands are not well defined. Because the cranial ribs support the forelimbs, they probably participate less in ventilation than the more caudal ribs. Other inspiratory muscles include those connecting the sternum and head. These muscles contract during strenuous breathing and move the sternum rostrally.

The subatmospheric pressures generated within the respiratory tract during inhalation tend to collapse the external nares, pharynx, and larynx. Contraction of *abductor muscles* attached to these structures is essential to prevent collapse. Abductor muscle contraction during inhalation can be observed as dilation of the external nares. Failure of contraction of the abductor muscles of the larynx is responsible for "roaring" in horses. The roaring sound is caused by turbulent air flow as the vocal fold on the paralyzed side of the larynx is sucked into the lumen.

The *abdominal muscles* and *internal intercostals* are the expiratory muscles. Contraction of the abdominal muscles increases abdominal pressure, which forces the relaxed diaphragm forward and reduces the size of the thorax. Because of a continued accentuated expiratory effort, hypertrophy of the external abdominal oblique muscle occurs in horses with chronic airway disease and can be observed as a "heave line" extending from the tuber coxae to the costochondral junctions. The fibers of the internal intercostal muscles are directed cranioventrally from the cranial border of one rib to the caudal border of the next cranial rib,

so that contraction decreases the size of the thorax by moving the ribs caudally and downwards.

During exercise, respiratory muscle activity increases. To supply the necessary metabolic substrates, the blood flow to the diaphragm increases over 20-fold in exercising ponies. In cursorial (running) mammals at the canter and gallop, but not at the trot, ventilation is assisted also by synchronizing gait and respiration (Fig. 43–4). Inhalation occurs as the forelimbs are extended and the hind limbs are accelerating the animal forward. Exhalation occurs when the forelimbs are in contact with the ground. The piston-like action of the abdominal contents against the diaphragm probably facilitates breathing.

The Respiratory Muscles Generate Work to Stretch the Lung and Overcome the Frictional Resistance to Air Flow

At the end of a tidal exhalation, a volume of air (approximately 45 mL/kg) remains in the lung. This air volume is known as *functional residual capacity* (FRC). The *pressure in the pleural cavity* (Ppl) at FRC is approximately 5 cm H_2O subatmospheric (-5 cm H_2O). During inhalation, Ppl decreases as the thorax enlarges and the respiratory muscles perform work to stretch the *elastic lung* and thorax, generate air flow through *resistive airways*, overcome the *viscous resistance* of tissues, and overcome the *inertia* provided by the air and tissues (Fig. 43–5). The change in pleural pressure during each breath is determined by the change in lung volume (ΔV), lung compliance (C), airflow rate ($\dot{V}$), respiratory resistance (R), acceleration ($\ddot{V}$), and inertance (I) of the respiratory system:

$$\Delta Ppl = \Delta V/C + R\dot{V} + I\ddot{V}$$

Resting animals breathe slowly, flow rates are low, acceleration is minimal, and the primary work of the respiratory muscles is to overcome the elasticity of the lung. When respiratory rate increases as during exercise, flow rates increase, and more energy is used to generate flow against the frictional resistance of the airways. Increases in frequency increase acceleration also and, therefore, inertial forces.

It is useful to consider factors affecting pulmonary elasticity and frictional resistance to breathing in turn. Disease can cause changes

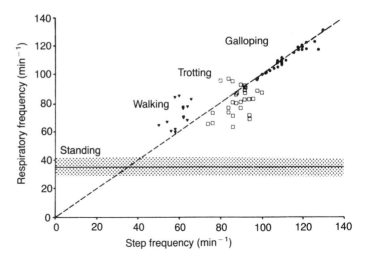

Figure 43–4. The relationship between gait and respiration in the horse. At the walk and trot, step and respiratory frequency are not correlated. At the gallop (and canter), respiratory and step frequency bear a 1:1 relationship. (Hörnicke H, Meixner R, Pollman U: Equine Exercise Physiology. Cambridge, Granta Editions, 1983, p 7.)

in both elasticity and resistance, and increase the work of breathing. Inertial forces are usually negligible and are not discussed further here.

Lung Elasticity Is Due to Tissue and Surface Tension Forces

When the thorax is opened and *pleural pressure* becomes atmospheric, the lung collapses to its *minimal volume*. At minimal volume, some air remains trapped within the alveoli behind closed peripheral airways. This collapse of the lung demonstrates its inherent elasticity, but accurate documentation of the lung's elasticity requires generation of a *pressure-volume curve* by inflating the lung and concurrently measuring the difference between the airway pressure (P_{ao}) and the pressure surrounding the lung. When the lung is excised or the thorax is opened, the pressure around the lung is atmospheric, but in the thorax it is pleural pressure. The pressure difference required for inflation is known as *transpulmonary pressure* (P_L). When the lung is inflated with air from the gas-free state (Fig. 43–6), a large pressure is required to exceed the critical opening pressure of the bronchioles. Once the bronchioles open, the lung inflates more easily until its elastic limits are reached at a P_L of approximately 30 cm H_2O. The volume of air in the lung at this point is the *total lung capacity* (TLC). The lung does not deflate along the same pressure-volume curve; less pressure is required to maintain a given volume than during inflation. This difference in lung elastic properties on inflation and deflation is known as *pressure-volume hysteresis*.

The lung is gas-free only in the fetus and for a few seconds after birth until the first breath is taken. Usually, during life, the lung inflates from functional residual capacity, about 40–45% of TLC. It then exhibits little hysteresis, in part because the bronchioles are already open and their critical opening pressure does not need to be exceeded.

Differences Between Air and Saline Pressure-Volume Curves Are Due to Surface Tension

Inflation of the lung with saline abolishes pressure-volume hysteresis, and the pressure required to maintain a given volume is less than when the lung is inflated with air (see Fig. 43–6). *Surface forces that arise in the fluid film overlying the alveolar epithelium* are present during air inflation but absent when the air liquid interface is abolished by filling the alveoli with saline. Therefore, surface tension forces are responsible for a considerable part of the elastic recoil of the lung and for the lung pressure-volume hysteresis. The elastic recoil of the saline-filled lung is because of connective tissues such as elastin and collagen. *Elastin fibers* form a network around the alveoli and peripheral airways much like the fibers in a nylon stocking. During inflation of the lung, the fibers change their orientation but elongate little.

If the alveoli were lined with water or an ultrafiltrate of plasma, the normal resting transpulmonary pressure of 5 cm H_2O would be insufficient to maintain inflation of such small spheres. Therefore, stability of the alveoli depends on the presence of a *pulmonary*

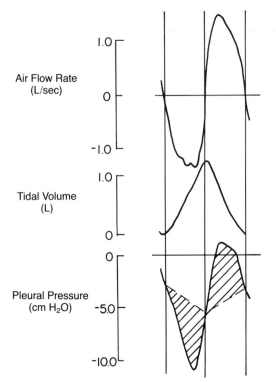

Figure 43–5. Air flow rate, tidal volume, and pleural pressure during inhalation (left) and exhalation (right). During inhalation, pleural pressure decreases as the thorax enlarges, air flow rates increase, and the volume of air in the lung increases. At the end of inhalation, flow rates return to zero, and pleural pressure increases slightly. During exhalation, pleural pressure increases as the thorax decreases in size, flow rates increase to a peak and then decrease again, and the volume of air in the lung decreases. The broken line shows the change in pleural pressure necessary to overcome the elasticity of the lung (proportional to volume). The shaded area represents the change in pleural pressure necessary to overcome the frictional resistance of the airways. The peaks of pleural pressure on both inhalation and exhalation coincide with peaks of flow.

surfactant that reduces surface tension of the alveolar lining. Figure 43–7 shows that the surface tension of the alveolar lining film is not constant: surface tension decreases as lung volume decreases and the alveolar surface area is reduced. Composition of pulmonary surfactant is similar among species. It is a mixture of lipids and proteins, the most common lipid component being *dipalmitoyl phosphatidylcholine.* Surfactant is produced in *type II alveolar cells,* and its hydrophilic and hydrophobic portions cause it to seek the surface of the alveolar lining. As lung volume decreases and the surface area shrinks, surfactant molecules become concentrated on the alveolar surface, reducing surface tension and promoting alveolar stability.

Pulmonary surfactant is released into the alveolar spaces and tracheal fluid late in gestation (0.85 gestation in the sheep), its appearance correlating with the rise in fetal plasma cortisol. *Premature birth* can be followed by respiratory distress because of inadequate surfactant. Surfactant maturation can be induced also by glucocorticoid administration.

The Lung Mechanically Interacts with the Thoracic Cage

Because the visceral and parietal pleurae are maintained in close apposition by a thin layer of pleural fluid, the lung and thoracic cage interact mechanically. Figure 43–8 shows the pressure-volume curves of the lung, thorax, and total respiratory system. At functional residual capacity, the respiratory system is at equilibrium; the inward elastic recoil of the lung is balanced by the outward recoil of the *chest wall.* Below functional residual capacity,

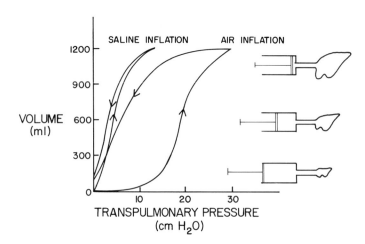

Figure 43–6. Pressure-volume curve of the lung during inflation with saline and with air. The pressure gradient across the lung (transpulmonary pressure) is shown on the abscissa and lung volume on the ordinate. During air inflation, the inflation and deflation curves are separated, i.e., there is pressure-volume hysteresis. Hysteresis is abolished by inflating the lung with saline. The lung inflates more easily (i.e., it takes less pressure for a given volume) with saline than with air.

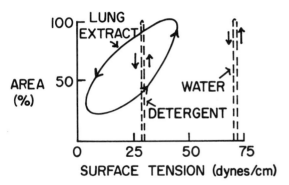

Figure 43–7. The effect of a change in surface area on the surface tension of lung extract, water, and a detergent solution. The surface tension of water is constant at 70 dynes/cm as the area is changed. Although a solution of detergent reduces surface tension, the surface tension does not change with area. The lung extract, by contrast, decreases surface tension as the surface area is reduced, because the surfactant molecules become more tightly packed on the surface of the liquid.

the lung has little elastic recoil, but the thorax increasingly resists deformation, so *residual volume,* the volume of air in the lung at the end of a maximal exhalation, is determined by the limits to which the rib cage can be compressed. Above functional residual capacity, the lung elastic recoil increases. At total lung capacity, the lung approaches its elastic limits, but the chest wall is still compliant.

The slope of the lung-pressure volume curve is called *lung compliance.* Because the pressure-volume curve is alinear, compliance obviously varies with the state of lung inflation. It is usually measured over the tidal volume and, when adjusted for differences in lung size, does not vary greatly between adult mammals.

Consequently, most mammals generate similar pleural pressures during quiet breathing. *Chest wall compliance* is generally less in large than in small animals; the stiff chest wall of the horse and cow contrasts with the very compliant chest wall of small rodents. Neonates have a more compliant chest and a less compliant lung than adults. Species differences in chest wall compliance lead to differences in the equilibrium volume of the respiratory system. In neonatal humans and small rodents, the equilibrium volume is so low that FRC must be maintained by contraction of inspiratory muscles. Species born in a relatively advanced state of maturity, such as foals, may have a sufficiently stiff thorax to maintain FRC passively.

Airflow Is Opposed by Frictional Resistance in the Airways

During ventilation, air flows through the tubes of the *upper airway* and *tracheobronchial tree.* Flow is opposed by the *frictional resistance* between air molecules and the walls of the air passages, and also to a much lesser extent by the *viscous drag* of the tissues. In the resting animal, the nasal cavity, pharynx, and larynx, which warm and humidify the air, provide approximately 50% of the frictional resistance to breathing (Fig. 43–9). Nasal resistance can be decreased, for example, during exercise, by dilating the external nares and vasoconstriction of vascular tissue in the nose. When airflow rates increase during exercise, or when the nasal cavity is obstructed, some species

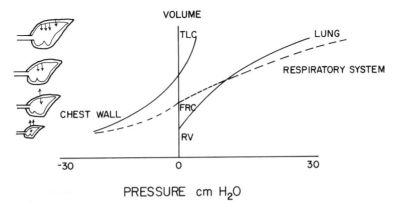

Figure 43–8. The interactions of lung and chest wall pressure volume behavior, which determine lung volumes and the elastic recoil of the respiratory system (shown as a broken line). At functional residual capacity (*FRC*), lung and chest wall elastic recoil are equal and opposite. At residual volume (*RV*), lung recoil is minimal, but the chest wall is resisting compression. At total lung capacity (*TLC*), the lung is approaching its elastic limits and the chest wall is still compliant. Arrows on the diagrams of the lung at the left demonstrate the relative magnitudes and directions of elastic recoil of the lung and chest wall.

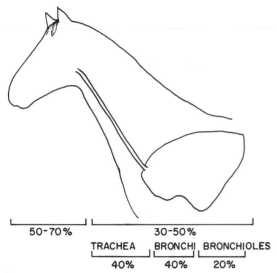

50-70%		30-50%	
	TRACHEA	BRONCHI	BRONCHIOLES
	40%	40%	20%

Figure 43–9. The distribution of airway resistance in a horse.

breathe through the mouth to bypass the high resistance nasal cavity. Other species, such as the horse, are obligate nose breathers and are solely dependent on a decrease in resistance to keep the work of breathing at a reasonable level.

The tracheobronchial tree has up to 24 branches lined by a secretory, ciliated epithelium. The larger airways, *trachea* and *bronchi*, are supported by *cartilage* and supplied with secretory *bronchial glands*. All larger airways, with the exception of the trachea and the first few centimeters of the main stem bronchi, are intrapulmonary and lie within a sheath of loose connective tissue, the *bronchovascular bundle*, which also contains major blood vessels, lymphatics, and nerves. *Bronchioles* lack cartilage and a connective tissue sheath. Alveoli surround the intrapulmonary airways, and the alveolar septa attach to the outer layers of the bronchovascular bundle and to the walls of bronchioles. Except before birth, when the lung contains no air, the alveolar septa are always under tension, which provides radial traction around the airways and maintains their patency.

The lung has six lobes, each supplied by a *lobar bronchus*, which gives rise to daughter bronchi. At each division of the bronchi, the diameters of the daughter airways are not equal. One daughter airway is much narrower than the parent, whereas the diameter of the other is similar to the parent. This *monopodial* system of branching continues through at least the first six generations of bronchi. At the

level of the bronchioles, the diameter of parent and daughter bronchioles is the same. As a result of this branching pattern, the total cross-sectional area of the tracheobronchial tree increases only a little between the trachea and the first four generations of bronchi, but increases dramatically toward the periphery of the lung. Consequently, the *velocity of airflow* diminishes progressively from the trachea toward the bronchioles. The high velocity, *turbulent airflow* in the trachea and bronchi produces the *lung sounds* heard through a stethoscope in a normal animal. *Laminar*, low velocity flow in the bronchioles, produces no sound. As a result of the branching pattern of the tracheobronchial tree, airways greater than 2–5 mm in diameter contribute up to 80% of resistance; bronchioles contribute as little as 20%.

Resistance is determined by the radius and length of the airways. Airway length changes little, but radius can be altered by several passive and active forces. Airways dilate as the lung inflates, because they are mechanically linked to the alveolar septa in which tension increases as the lung volume increases (Fig. 43–10).

A Major Factor Affecting the Diameter of the Tracheobronchial Tree Is Smooth Muscle Contraction

There is *smooth muscle* in the walls of the airways from the trachea to the alveolar ducts. In the trachea, it forms the *trachealis muscle*, which connects the ends of tracheal cartilages. In the bronchi, smooth muscle connects the cartilaginous plates, and in the bronchioles it completely encircles the airways. Smooth muscle actively regulates airway diameter in response to many stimuli. *Parasympathetic* innervation of smooth muscle is through the *vagus nerve* (Fig. 43–11), stimulation of which narrows all airways, but especially the bronchi. In normal animals, there is a small amount of parasympathetically mediated smooth muscle tone that can be abolished by sectioning the vagus nerve or by administering atropine, a *muscarinic receptor* antagonist. When irritant materials such as dusts are inhaled, tracheobronchial *irritant receptors* are stimulated, resulting in reflex bronchoconstriction, the afferent arm of which is through the parasympathetic system. A *noncholinergic excitatory system*, with *substance P* as a transmitter,

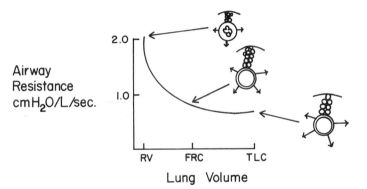

Airway
Resistance
cmH$_2$O/L/sec.

Figure 43–10. The effect of change in lung volume on airway resistance. The airway is represented by the large circle, to which are attached alveoli linking the airway wall to the pleural surface. As the lung volume increases, the alveolar septa become stretched and thus dilate the airway and reduce resistance. *RV,* residual volume; *FRC,* functional residual capacity; *TLC,* total lung capacity.

activated by *axon reflexes* from airway receptors, may cause bronchoconstriction also.

Relaxation of smooth muscle occurs following activation of β$_2$-*adrenergic receptors* by circulating catecholamines released from the ad-

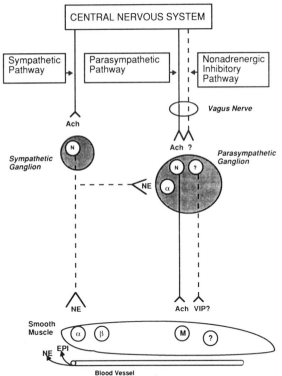

Figure 43–11. Diagrammatic representation of the efferent autonomic innervation of the tracheo-bronchial tree. Smooth muscle has α- and β-adrenergic receptors that are activated by circulating catecholamines or, in a few species, by release of norepinephrine (*NE*) from sympathetic nerves. Muscarinic receptors (*M*) are activated by acetylcholine released from postganglionic parasympathetic nerve terminals. The nonadrenergic inhibitory nervous system that travels in the vagus nerve may release vasoactive intestinal peptide (*VIP*). (Nadel JA, Barnes PJ, Holtzman MJ: Autonomic factors in hyperreactivity of airway smooth muscle. *In* Fishman AP, Macklem PT, Mead J, Geiger SR (eds): Handbook of Physiology, Section 3, Vol 3, Part 2. Bethesda, MD, American Physiology Society, 1986, p 694.)

renal medulla or, in some species, by local release of *norepinephrine* from *sympathetic nerve* endings. Although the lung and airway smooth muscle is richly supplied with adrenergic receptors, particularly β$_2$ receptors, there is considerable species variation in sympathetic innervation to the airways. Sympathetic innervation of muscle seems to be lacking in pigs, sheep, goats, cows, and horses but is present in dogs and cats. Sympathetic innervation of parasympathetic ganglia exists in most species and may modulate parasympathetic activity. Another bronchodilator system, the *nonadrenergic noncholinergic inhibitory nervous system,* exists in some species. The efferent fibers are in the vagus, and the neurotransmitter may be *vasoactive intestinal peptide.*

Airway smooth muscle also contracts in response to many of the *inflammatory mediators,* particularly *histamine* and the *leukotrienes.* Contraction can be modified by an inhibitory factor produced by airway epithelium and accentuated by airway inflammation.

Dynamic Airway Compression Occurs When the Pressure Surrounding the Airway Exceeds the Pressure Within the Airway Lumen

The airway walls are not rigid, and therefore the airways can be compressed or expanded by the pressure gradient across their walls. In the nasal cavity, pharynx, and larynx, *dynamic compression* of the airway tends to occur during inhalation. Pressure within the airways is subatmospheric, and the airways are surrounded by atmospheric pressure. Because of its bony support, the nasal cavity is less prone to compression than less well-supported nares, pharynx, and larynx. Contraction of the abductor muscles of the nares, pharynx, and larynx during inhalation is necessary to prevent collapse of these regions. Failure of the abductor muscles of the larynx to contract during inhalation is responsible for the inspiratory noise and poor performance of horses suffering from laryngeal hemiplegia (roaring).

In the intrathoracic airways, dynamic collapse occurs during *forced exhalation*, when intrapleural pressure exceeds pressures within the intrathoracic airway lumen. Dynamic collapse of the intrathoracic trachea can occur in dogs with collapsing trachea, which puts a mechanical limit on the maximal flow that can be attained during exhalation. *Cough* is a forced exhalation during which dynamic collapse narrows the airways. The high air velocity through the narrowed portion of the airway facilitates removal of foreign material.

The Distribution of Air Depends on the Local Mechanical Properties of the Lung and the Local Changes in Pleural Pressure

Optimal gas exchange requires bringing together air and blood at the alveolus, i.e., matching of ventilation and blood flow. Obviously, gas exchange cannot occur if an alveolus receives blood but no ventilation, or vice versa. Ideally, each region of lung should receive equal amounts of ventilation, but this never occurs in either animals or people. Figure 43–12 illustrates how the mechanical properties of the lungs affect the distribution of ventilation. Region A represents a healthy piece of lung with a normal compliance and a normal airway. Region B has a disease-like interstitial pneumonia in which compliance is decreased, but the airways are normal. Region C has a normal compliance but a narrowed airway, as may occur when airway smooth muscle contracts. When the same decrease in pleural pressure is applied to each region, A and C fill to the same volume, because they have similar compliance, but C fills slowly because of the obstructed airway. Region B fills rapidly, but because of its reduced compliance, achieves a lesser volume than regions A and C. When the model lung is ventilated more rapidly, the volume received by region C decreases, because it has inadequate time to fill. Region C is said to have a long *time constant* (the product of resistance and compliance). This model shows that the distribution of ventilation within the lung is affected by the local lung compliance, regional airway resistance, and the frequency of breathing. Small

degrees of airway obstruction that may cause no signs of respiratory difficulty in the resting animal may result in an uneven distribution of ventilation and hypoxemia when the animal exercises.

Within the thorax, intrapleural pressure is more subatmospheric in the uppermost part of the thorax than in the lowermost parts. Consequently, the lung is more distended and, therefore, less compliant dorsally than ventrally. During inhalation, air preferentially enters the more compliant dependent regions, resulting in a vertical gradient of ventilation (Fig. 43–13). However, the relative distention of different regions of lung is only one of the factors affecting ventilation distribution. Contraction of different muscle groups, increases in flow rate, and local changes in lung and chest wall mechanical properties also affect ventilation distribution. The distribution of ventilation becomes more uneven in the recumbent animal, especially in the supine and laterally recumbent positions because of reductions in lung volume and changes in the pleural pressure gradient.

Collateral Ventilation and Interdependence Tend to Maintain Uniform Ventilation Distribution

Collateral ventilation is the movement of air between adjacent regions of lung through pathways other than the tracheobronchial tree. The collateral movement of air between adjacent regions of lung, most probably through anastomosing respiratory bronchioles, occurs to a small degree in horses and sheep but extensively in the dog. Collateral ventilation is absent in pigs and cattle because of the complete separation of *secondary lung lobules* by *connective tissue septa*. These differences in collateral ventilation mean that gas exchange abnormalities following experimental airway obstruction are more serious in pigs and cattle than in dogs.

Interdependence is the mechanical interaction between adjacent regions of lung and between the lung and chest wall. If one region of lung is lagging in movement behind adjacent regions, the pull of the adjacent lung tissue tends to make it ventilate more synchronously with the remainder of the lung. The dog has good interdependence between adjacent regions of a lobe, but the connective tissue septa between secondary lobules of cow and pig lungs result in limited mechanical interde-

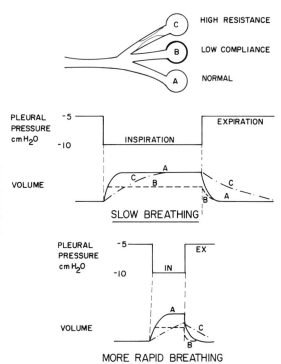

Figure 43–12. The effects of mechanical properties of the lung on airway resistance. Alveolus A is normal, alveolus B has a low compliance, and alveolus C has a high resistance as a result of a partially obstructed airway. Step changes in pleural pressure are applied to these three schematic alveoli, and the changes in volume are shown during slow breathing and during more rapid breathing.

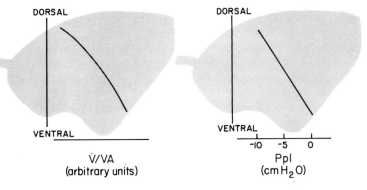

$\dot{V}/VA$
(arbitrary units)

Ppl
(cmH$_2$O)

Figure 43–13. Distribution of ventilation ($\dot{V}/V_A$), perfusion ($\dot{Q}/V_A$), and ventilation/perfusion ratios ($\dot{V}_A/\dot{Q}$) in the standing horse's lung. Ventilation and blood flow per unit lung volume both increase from the dorsal to the ventral part of the lung. As a consequence, there is no vertical gradient of ventilation/perfusion ratios. (Adapted from Amis TC, Pascoe JR, Hornof W: Topographic distribution of pulmonary ventilation and perfusion in the horse. Am J Vet Res 45:1597–1601, 1984.)

pendence between adjacent lobules. In these latter species, the lack of collateral ventilation and limited interdependence frequently result in *atelectasis* (collapse of alveoli) because of complete absorption of gas following airway obstruction.

CLINICAL CORRELATIONS

LUNG FIBROSIS IN THE DOG

HISTORY □ A 3-year-old English setter in respiratory distress is presented at a teaching hospital. The owner first noticed reluctance of the dog to exercise 3 weeks ago. Since that time the animal has had progressive difficulty in breathing. It appears hungry but cannot eat because it gets out of breath.

CLINICAL EXAMINATION □ Inspection reveals a thin dog breathing through its mouth. Respiratory rate is elevated, but the dog seems to be moving little air despite strong inspiratory efforts during which the intercostal spaces sink in. Exhalation presents no difficulty; the ribs collapse rapidly, and there is no accentuated abdominal effort.

Examination reveals slightly blue-colored mucous membranes. Lung sounds are not remarkable. All other systems are normal.

Radiographs of the thorax show diffuse miliary density (whiteness) over the parts of the lung that are normally air-filled. The bronchi are normal. An elevated change in pleural pressure during breathing, normal airway resistance, and decreased static lung compliance are the key findings on lung function testing. Tidal volume is greatly reduced.

COMMENT □ The history and clinical signs point to a respiratory problem. The elevated change in pleural pressure during breathing confirms the increased effort necessary to breathe. This could be due to increased air movement resulting from an increased metabolic rate, airway obstruction, or a decrease in lung compliance (stiffening of the lung). The increased density in the normally air-filled elastic part of the lungs and the normal air passages suggest a decrease in lung compliance rather than airway obstruction. This was confirmed by lung function measurements.

The blue tinge to the mucous membranes indicates desaturation of hemoglobin as a result of impaired oxygen exchange in the diseased lung. The retraction of intercostal spaces during inhalation is a result of the major decrease in pleural pressure as the respiratory muscles work to stretch the stiffened lung. Exhalation is no problem, because the lung has an increased tendency to collapse, and the airways are normal.

This dog has a diffuse disease of the exchange area of the lung, which by decreasing compliance, increases the work of breathing. A biopsy reveals diffuse fibrosis around mineral particles in the walls of the alveoli. The prognosis for the dog is grave.

CHRONIC AIRWAY DISEASE IN THE HORSE

HISTORY □ A 10-year-old horse is presented with a 2-year history of coughing and a progressive loss of exercise tolerance. Recently, the horse's problem has become so severe that it has difficulty breathing while resting in its stall. The cough is frequent. The horse has a normal appetite; however, it is losing weight even though the teeth are normal and the horse is on a parasite control program.

CLINICAL EXAMINATION □ Inspection reveals a thin horse with flared nostrils and an anxious expression. The respiratory rate is elevated, and respiratory movements are accentuated. During inhalation, the intercostal spaces are pulled in between the ribs. The initial part of exhalation is characterized by a rapid relaxation of the rib cage. This is followed by a prolonged contraction of the abdominal muscles, which is terminated immediately before the next inhalation. During the prolonged contraction of the abdominal muscles, wheezes can be heard when you place your ear close to the nostrils.

The horse has an elevated pulse rate. The mucous membranes of the gums have a bluish tint. Auscultation of the thorax reveals increased breath sounds over all the lung fields and musical wheezes audible at end exhalation. Excessive mucus pooled in the airway is viewed through a bronchoscope advanced into the trachea.

Because the horse is being examined at a teaching hospital, there are facilities for measurement of lung function. The change in pleural pressure (ΔPpl) during each breath is 25 cm H_2O (normal = 5 cm H_2O), and airway resistance is 6 cm H_2O/L/second (normal = 1 cm H_2O/L/second). Administration of atropine intravenously decreases ΔPpl to 7 cm H_2O and airway resistance to 3 cm H_2O/L/second. The horse looks less distressed, and wheezes are reduced.

COMMENT □ The respiratory distress, cough, and lack of exercise tolerance point to a respiratory problem. The increased effort of breathing documented by the elevated ΔPpl could be due to airway obstruction, a decrease in lung compliance, or increased breathing due to increased metabolic rate. The latter cause is eliminated, because the horse is resting in the clinic. The mucus in the airway and elevated airway resistance confirm airway obstruction. Musical wheezes at end exhalation typify airway disease and are the result of increased air turbulence or vibration of mucus and the airway walls. Airway obstruction is in part due to bronchospasm resulting from parasympathetic activity, because it is reversed by atropine, a parasympathetic antagonist. Atropine does not return resistance to normal, so there is also considerable obstruction by mucus.

The flared nostrils are an effort to reduce the work of breathing by dilating the upper airway. The blue mucous membranes indicate desaturation of hemoglobin because of impaired oxygen uptake in the diseased lungs.

Retraction of the intercostal muscles during inhalation indicates a major decrease in pleural pressure as the respiratory muscles work against the obstructed airways. The prolonged contraction of abdominal muscles, known as "heaving," represents an effort by the horse to force air out through obstructed airways. Weight loss is probably due to increased work of breathing. Coughing is an effort by the horse to expel the excessive mucus.

This horse has chronic airway disease ("heaves," chronic obstructive lung disease), probably a result of stabling in a dusty barn and eating poorly cured moldy hay. Heaves is the result of an allergic response to antigens in the hay and barn dust. The best treatment for the horse is to keep it out at pasture and supplement its diet with pelleted feed rather than hay.

Bibliography

Goerke J, Clements JA: Alveolar surface tension and lung surfactant. *In* Fishman AP, Macklem PT, Mead J, Geiger SR (eds): Handbook of Physiology, Section 3, The Respiratory System, Vol 3, Mechanics of Breathing, Part 1. Bethesda, MD, American Physiological Society, 1986, pp 247–261.
Leff AR: Endogenous regulation of bronchomotor tone. Am Rev Respir Dis 137:1198–1216, 1988.
Leith DE: Comparative mammalian respiratory mechanics. Physiologist 19:485–510, 1976.
Loring SH, DeTroyer A: Actions of the respiratory muscles. *In* Roussos C, Macklem PT (eds): The Thorax. New York, Marcel Dekker, 1985, pp 327–349.
Murray JF: The Normal Lung. Philadelphia, WB Saunders, 1986, pp 83–119, 121–162.
Robinson NE: Some functional consequences of species differences in lung anatomy. *In* Dungworth DL (ed): Adv Vet Sci Comp Med 26:1–33, 1982.
Slonim NB, Hamilton LH: Respiratory Physiology, 5th ed. St. Louis, CV Mosby, 1987, pp 48–96.

PRACTICE QUESTIONS FOR CHAPTER 43

1. Which of the following lists includes only structures that compose the anatomical dead-space?

   a. Respiratory bronchioles, alveoli, trachea, nasal cavity
   b. Pharynx, bronchi, alveolar ducts, larynx
   c. Capillaries, respiratory bronchioles, trachea, bronchi
   d. Pharynx, nasal cavity, trachea, bronchi
   e. Capillaries, respiratory bronchioles, alveolar ducts, alveoli

2. A horse has a tidal volume of 5 L, respiratory rate of 12 breaths/minute, dead-space/tidal volume ratio of 0.5. Calculate minute ventilation ($\dot{V}_E$) and alveolar ventilation ($\dot{V}_A$).

   a. $\dot{V}_E$ = 60 L/minute; $\dot{V}_A$ = 2.5 L
   b. $\dot{V}_E$ = 30 L/minute; $\dot{V}_A$ = 30 L/minute
   c. $\dot{V}_E$ = 60 L/minute; $\dot{V}_A$ = 30 L/minute
   d. $\dot{V}_E$ = 2.5 L; $\dot{V}_A$ = 1.25 L
   e. $\dot{V}_E$ = 5.0 L/minute; $\dot{V}_A$ = 2.5 L/minute

3. Which of the following occur during inhalation?

   a. Diaphragm contracts, pleural pressure increases, alveolar pressure decreases
   b. Diaphragm relaxes, external intercostal muscles contract, pleural pressure increases
   c. Diaphragm relaxes, pleural pressure decreases, internal intercostal muscles relax

d. External and internal intercostal muscles contract, pleural and alveolar pressure increases
e. Diaphragm and external intercostal muscles contract, pleural and alveolar pressures decrease

4. Lung compliance

a. has the units of pressure/volume (cm H_2O/L).
b. is greater at functional residual capacity (FRC) than at total lung capacity (TLC).
c. is less when the lung is inflated with saline than when the lung is inflated with air.
d. is greater in small mammals than in large mammals, even when adjusted for differences in lung size.
e. is the only determinant of the change in pleural pressure during breathing.

5. Pulmonary surfactant

a. can be deficient in premature newborns.
b. is produced in type II alveolar cells.
c. is in part composed of dipalmitoyl phosphatidyl choline.

d. decreases surface tension of the fluid lining the alveoli.
e. All of the above

6. Which of the following will increase the frictional resistance to breathing?

a. Intravenous administration of a β-adrenergic agonist
b. Contraction of the abductor muscles of the larynx
c. A decrease in lung volume from functional residual capacity (FRC) to residual volume (RV)
d. Relaxation of the trachealis muscle
e. Inhibition of the release of histamine from mast cells

7. The distribution of ventilation within the lung is influenced by

a. gravitational forces.
b. regional variations in airway resistance.
c. regional variations in lung compliance.
d. collateral ventilation and interdependence.
e. All of the above

44

Pulmonary Blood Flow

PULMONARY CIRCULATION

1. The structure of the pulmonary arteries varies among species
2. Functionally, pulmonary blood vessels can be classified into alveolar and extra-alveolar vessels
3. The pulmonary circulation offers a low resistance to flow
4. The distribution of pulmonary blood flow within the lung is influenced by gravity
5. Passive changes in vascular resistance result from changes in lung and vascular volumes, and intravascular pressures
6. Neural and humoral factors cause contraction of the muscular pulmonary arteries
7. Alveolar hypoxia is a potent constrictor of small pulmonary arteries

BRONCHIAL CIRCULATION

1. The bronchial circulation provides nutrient flow to airways, large vessels, and in some species, the visceral pleura

The lung receives blood flow from two circulations. The *pulmonary circulation* receives the total output of the *right ventricle*, perfuses the *alveolar capillaries*, and participates in gas exchange. The *bronchial circulation,* a branch of the systemic circulation, provides nutrient blood flow to airways and other structures within the lung.

PULMONARY CIRCULATION

The pulmonary circulation differs from the systemic circulation in that all the blood passes through only one organ, the lung. When cardiac output increases, as during exercise, the pulmonary circulation must be able to accommodate this increase in blood flow without a large increase in the work of the right ventricle. In addition, control mechanisms must exist to regulate the distribution of blood within the lung so that blood preferentially perfuses the well-oxygenated regions of the lung. The ability to regulate blood flow depends on smooth muscle in the pulmonary arteries.

The Structure of the Pulmonary Arteries Varies Among Species

The main pulmonary arteries that accompany the bronchi are elastic, but the smaller arteries adjacent to the bronchioles and the alveolar ducts are muscular. The adult pig and the cow have a thick *medial muscle layer* in the smaller pulmonary arteries; the horse has less muscle, and the sheep and dog have only a thin muscle layer. The amount of smooth muscle in the media of pulmonary arteries determines the *reactivity* of the vasculature to alveolar hypoxia and other neural and humoral stimuli (see later).

The terminal branches of the pulmonary arteries, the *pulmonary arterioles,* consist of endothelium and an elastic lamina, and lead into the pulmonary capillaries, which form an extensive branching network of vessels within the *alveolar septum* and almost cover the alveolar surface (Fig. 44–1). Not all capillaries are perfused in the resting animal, so vessels can be recruited when pulmonary blood flow increases, for example, during exercise. *Pulmonary veins* with thin walls conduct blood from capillaries to the *left atrium* and also form a reservoir of blood for the *left ventricle.*

Functionally, Pulmonary Blood Vessels Can Be Classified into Alveolar and Extra-alveolar Vessels

Alveolar vessels are the thin-walled capillaries that perfuse the alveolar septum. They are surrounded by a small layer of interstitium and are exposed almost directly to changes in alveolar pressure. *Extra-alveolar vessels,* which include the pulmonary arteries, veins, arterioles, and venules, are surrounded by a layer of loose connective tissue (*the bronchovascular bundle*) bounded by a limiting membrane to which alveolar septa are attached. The behavior of extra-alveolar vessels is determined more by pressure changes within the connective tissue space of the bronchovascular bundle than by changes in alveolar pressure.

The Pulmonary Circulation Offers a Low Resistance to Flow

Pulmonary vascular pressures can be measured by advancing a catheter through the jugular vein into the right ventricle and pulmonary artery. Even though the pulmonary circulation receives the total output of the right ventricle, pulmonary arterial pressures are much less than systemic pressures. Pulmonary arterial systolic, diastolic, and mean pressures average 25, 10, and 15 mmHg in mammals at sea level. This observation shows that the pulmonary circulation offers a low *vascular resistance* to flow. If the catheter is advanced until it

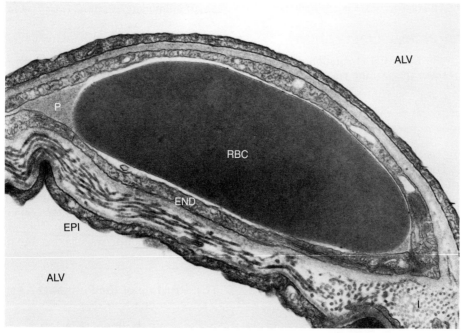

Figure 44–1. Transmission electronmicrograph of a capillary in the alveolar septum of a horse lung. A red blood cell (*RBC*) is shown bathed by plasma (*P*) in a capillary surrounded by endothelium (*END*). Alveoli (*ALV*) are on both sides of the septum and separated from the capillary by the epithelium (*EPI*) and a layer of interstitium (*I*). The interstitium is much thicker on one side of the capillary than on the other. Fluid exchange between the capillary and the interstitium occurs primarily on the thicker side. (Photomicrograph reproduced by courtesy of WS Tyler, Department of Anatomy, University of California, Davis.)

wedges in a pulmonary artery, the occluded vessel becomes an extension of the catheter, allowing estimation of *pulmonary venous pressure (pulmonary wedge pressure)*. Pulmonary wedge pressure (average 5 mmHg) is only slightly greater than *left atrial pressure* (average 3–4 mmHg), which shows that the pulmonary veins provide little resistance to blood flow.

Pulmonary vascular resistance (PVR) is calculated as:

$$PVR = (Ppa - Pla)/\dot{Q}$$

where Ppa is mean pulmonary arterial pressure, Pla is left atrial pressure, and $\dot{Q}$ is *cardiac output.*

Although pulmonary vascular resistance is low in the normal resting animal, it decreases even further when pulmonary blood flow or arterial pressure increases, as occurs during exercise. Recruitment of previously unperfused vessels and distension of other vessels cause the resistance decrease.

Micropuncture studies have shown that approximately half the vascular resistance in the pulmonary circulation is precapillary, and that the capillaries themselves provide a considerable portion of resistance to blood flow (Fig. 44–2). Unlike the systemic circulation, arterioles do not provide a large resistance and, consequently, pulmonary capillary blood flow is *pulsatile*.

The Distribution of Pulmonary Blood Flow Within the Lung Is Influenced by Gravity

Experiments in isolated perfused dog lungs suspended vertically have shown that there is a *vertical gradient of perfusion* that depends on the relative magnitudes of pulmonary arterial, pulmonary venous, and *alveolar pressures* (Fig. 44–3). In zone 1 at the top of the lung, there is no blood flow, because mean pulmonary arterial pressure is insufficient to overcome the hydrostatic pressure imposed by the column of blood connecting the pulmonary artery to the apical blood vessels. Therefore, alveolar pressure exceeds both pulmonary arterial and venous pressure, and the pulmonary capillary, which is a collapsible tube, is closed. In zone 2, pulmonary arterial pressure is greater than alveolar pressure, but exceeds pulmonary venous pressure. The capillary is open for part of its length until the point where alveolar pressure exceeds intravascular pressure. Flow in zone 2 is determined by the difference between pulmonary arterial and alveolar pressure, and is independent of venous pressure. Flow increases down this zone of lung, because pulmonary arterial pressure progressively increases as a result of the hydrostatic gradient. Zone 3 is in the most dependent parts of the lung. Pulmonary arterial and venous pressure both exceed alveolar pressure and increase progressively down the lung. Vessels are perfused throughout their length and are increasingly distended down this zone. As a result, regional blood flow increases progressively down zone 3.

In most quadrupeds, mean pulmonary arterial pressure at rest is sufficient to perfuse the vertical height of the lung, so it is unlikely that a zone 1 exists in normal animals. However, a vertical gradient of perfusion has been demonstrated in standing horses (see Fig. 43–

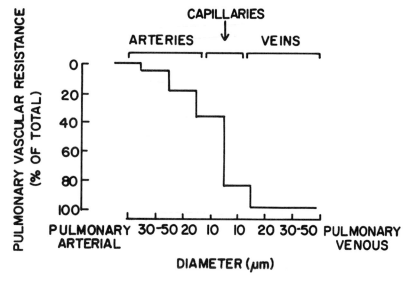

Figure 44–2. The distribution of vascular resistance in the pulmonary circulation, as determined by micropuncture studies. Unlike in the systemic circulation, a major portion of the resistance to blood flow in the pulmonary circulation is in the capillary bed. (From Bhattacharya J, Staub NC: Direct measurement of microvascular pressures in the isolated perfused dog lung. Science 210:327–328, 1980. Copyright 1980 by the AAAS.)

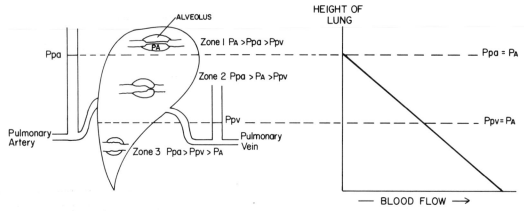

Figure 44–3. Diagrammatic representation of a cross section of a mammalian lung, showing the three zones of vascular perfusion. Mean pulmonary artery pressure (*Ppa*) is represented by the height of the bar on the left and venous pressure (*Ppv*) by the height of the bar on the right. (PA, alveolar pressure.) Within each zone of perfusion, a capillary is shown passing through an alveolus. In zone 1, the capillary is collapsed along its length; in zone 2, the capillary is open along part of its length; and in zone 3, the capillary is distended throughout its length. Graph at the right shows the increase in blood flow occurring from the top of zone 2 to the bottom of the lung.

13). Changes in arterial, venous, and alveolar pressure affect the gradient of blood flow in the lung. During exercise, mean pulmonary arterial pressure increases, thereby increasing the driving pressure for flow in zones 2 and 3, and converting more of the lung from zone 1 to zone 2. *Left heart failure* increases pulmonary venous pressure, which increases pressures upstream in the pulmonary capillaries and even the pulmonary artery. As a result, more of the lung is perfused under zone 3 conditions.

Passive Changes in Vascular Resistance Result from Changes in Lung and Vascular Volumes, and Intravascular Pressures

As the lungs inflate, the bronchovascular bundle is enlarged by the traction of the surrounding alveolar septa. Pressure in the perivascular connective tissue of the bronchovascular bundle decreases and, therefore, extra-alveolar vessels dilate; the degree of dilation depends on the compliance of the vessel.

Alveolar vessels become more elliptical as the alveolar septum stretches during lung inflation. These flattened vessels offer more resistance to flow than the circular cross-section vessels.

The changes in pulmonary vascular resistance during lung inflation reflect the opposing effects on alveolar and extra-alveolar vessels. At residual volume, pulmonary vascular resistance is high, because extra-alveolar vessels are narrowed. As the lung inflates to functional residual capacity (FRC), resistance decreases, primarily because of dilation of extra-alveolar vessels. Further inflation above FRC increases vascular resistance, primarily because of flattening of alveolar capillaries (Fig. 44–4).

Increasing either pulmonary arterial or left atrial pressure or increasing vascular volume decreases pulmonary vascular resistance by distending already perfused vessels and by recruiting previously unperfused vessels.

Neural and Humoral Factors Cause Contraction of the Muscular Pulmonary Arteries

The magnitude of the response of vessels to neural and humoral stimuli is determined to a large degree by the amount of smooth muscle in the small pulmonary arteries. As stated earlier, the amount of smooth muscle varies with species (Fig. 44–5). The increase in pulmonary vascular pressure in response to alveolar hypoxia and other stimuli is greater in calves than in sheep because of the greater amount of muscle in calf pulmonary arteries.

Although pulmonary arteries have both *sympathetic* and *parasympathetic* innervation, the functional role of this *autonomic innervation* is unclear. When vascular tone is elevated, vagal stimulation elicits parasympathetically mediated *vasodilation* through *muscarinic receptors*. This vasodilation is dependent on the presence of a functioning *endothelium*, which produces a factor that relaxes vascular smooth muscle.

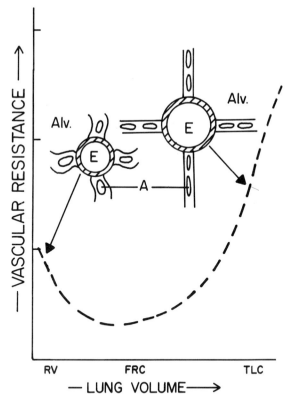

Figure 44–4. The change in vascular resistance occurring with an increase in lung volume. The inset diagrams represent alveolar (*A*) and extra-alveolar (*E*) vessels. At residual volume (*RV*), the extra-alveolar vessels are narrowed, but the alveolar vessels are distended. At total lung capacity (*TLC*), the extra-alveolar vessels are distended, but the alveolar vessels are elliptical because of the tension in the alveolar septum. Minimal vascular resistance occurs close to functional residual capacity (*FRC*). *Alv.*, alveolus.

Depending on the pre-existing level of pulmonary vascular tone, *sympathetic stimulation* can elicit either pulmonary *vasoconstriction* or vasodilation. When vascular tone is low, sympathetic stimulation or infusion of an α-*adrenergic agonist* causes smooth muscle contraction. When vascular tone is elevated, sympathetic stimulation causes vasodilation through β *receptor* stimulation. Although the functional role of the autonomic nervous system and circulating catecholamines in regulation of vascular smooth muscle tone is unclear, sympathetic stimulation at times of stress may stiffen the pulmonary vascular bed, increasing pulsatility and improving perfusion to underperfused regions of lung.

The response of the pulmonary vasculature to a variety of chemical mediators is shown in Table 44–1. Responses may vary with species and with the initial degree of *vascular tone*.

Some mediators, such as catecholamines, bradykinin, and prostaglandins, are taken up or metabolized by the vascular endothelium, so their effects may be modified by endothelial damage. In addition, the *relaxing factor* released by the endothelium modifies the effects of some vasoactive substances.

Alveolar Hypoxia Is a Potent Constrictor of Small Pulmonary Arteries

Alveolar hypoxia occurs in poorly ventilated alveoli, and *hypoxic vasoconstriction* provides a mechanism to redistribute pulmonary blood flow toward better-ventilated regions of lung. Although the vasoconstrictor response to hypoxia is present in all species, the magnitude of the response varies greatly. In domestic mammals, the response is most vigorous in cattle and pigs, less vigorous in horses, and trivial in sheep and dogs (Fig. 44–5). The response to hypoxia is also minimal in the llama, which normally lives under hypoxic conditions at *high altitude*.

In cattle grazing at high altitude, the hypoxia of altitude causes generalized pulmonary hypoxic vasoconstriction (Fig. 44–6). This leads to an increase in pulmonary arterial pressure,

Table 44–1
PULMONARY VASCULAR RESPONSE TO CHEMICAL MEDIATORS

Agent	Action
Angiotensin II	Vasoconstriction.
Histamine	Usually vasoconstriction through H_1 receptors. If vascular tone elevated, vasodilation through H_2 receptors. Acts on both arteries and veins.
Serotonin	Vasoconstriction through S_2 receptors. Action restricted to pulmonary arteries.
Norepinephrine and phenylephrine	Vasoconstriction through α_1 and α_2 receptors.
Epinephrine	Vasoconstriction or vasodilation depending on resting vascular tone and predominance of α or β receptors.
Isoproterenol	Vasodilation through β receptors.
Acetylcholine	Vasodilation when endothelium intact. Vasoconstriction when endothelium removed.
Bradykinin	Variable, usually vasodilation. Acts through vasoactive prostaglandins.
Arachidonic acid	Usually vasoconstriction.
Prostacyclin PGI_2	Vasodilation.
Thromboxane	Vasoconstriction.
Leukotrienes	Usually vasoconstriction.

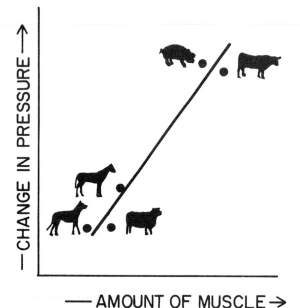

Figure 44–5. The relationship between the amount of muscle in the media of small pulmonary arteries and the change in vascular pressure when animals are exposed to a hypoxic environment. Animals with thicker muscle layers, such as the cow and pig, have a greater vascular response to hypoxia than animals with a small amount of muscle in the small pulmonary arteries, such as the dog and sheep.

which increases the work of the right ventricle and leads to *right heart failure*. The clinical syndrome is known as *brisket disease*, because *edema* fluid accumulates in the brisket. There are genetically determined differences in the response to hypoxia, with Holsteins responding vigorously and thus being highly susceptible to brisket disease. In those species in which the acute hypoxic constrictor response

is most vigorous, chronic hypoxia results in sustained pulmonary hypertension, because the medial muscular layer of the small pulmonary arteries hypertrophies.

The mechanism of hypoxic vasoconstriction is unknown. It can be demonstrated in isolated perfused lungs and, therefore, does not require intact innervation. Various vasoactive agents, such as *histamine, catecholamines, angiotensin,* and *arachidonic acid metabolites,* have been suggested as being involved, but none is clearly the sole mediator. Cellular mechanisms have been invoked also but are not well defined.

The ability of local alveolar hypoxia to cause a local reduction in blood flow has been clearly demonstrated in several species. Under conditions of *atelectasis,* when there is no ventilation to a collapsed region of lung, local blood flow is greatly reduced by a combination of vessel closure as the lung collapses and vasoconstriction in response to the local hypoxia.

BRONCHIAL CIRCULATION

The Bronchial Circulation Provides Nutrient Flow to Airways, Large Vessels, and in Some Species, the Visceral Pleura

The *bronchial circulation,* which receives approximately 2% of the output of the left ventricle, originates from two sources: the *bronchoesphageal artery* and a branch of the bicarotid trunk, the right apical *bronchial artery.* The former supplies the *airways* and the *interlobular*

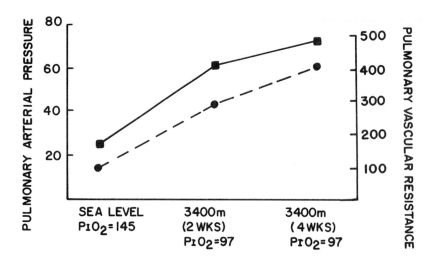

Figure 44–6. The change in mean pulmonary arterial pressure (■—■) and pulmonary vascular resistance (●—●) in calves transported from sea level to 3400 m for a 4-week sojourn. Both vascular resistance and arterial pressure increase when the calves are exposed to the hypoxia of altitude. Pressure and resistance continue to increase while at altitude because of the proliferation of smooth muscle in the small pulmonary arteries. Pressure units are mmHg, resistance units dynes/second/cm^5; PIO$_2$ units are torr. (Compiled from data in Ruiz AV, Bisgard GE, Will JA: Hemodynamic response to hypoxia and hyperoxia in calves at sea level and altitude. Pflugers Arch 344:275–286, 1973.)

septa of most of the lung; the latter supplies the airways of the right apical lobe. Bronchial arteries follow the tracheobronchial tree to the terminal bronchioles, forming a *peribronchial plexus* in the connective tissue along the length of the airways. Branches from this plexus penetrate the smooth muscle layer of the bronchial wall and form a *subepithelial vascular plexus*. Branches are also given off to form the vasa-vasorum of pulmonary vessels. At the level of the terminal bronchiole, bronchial vessels *anastomose* with the pulmonary circulation. There are few anastomoses between bronchial and pulmonary arteries; most anastomoses occur at the capillary or venular level. Species differences occur in the extensiveness of the bronchial blood supply to the pleura. In cattle, sheep, pigs, and horses, the bronchial artery provides blood flow to the *visceral pleura;* in dogs, cats, and monkeys, it does not. The bronchial blood flow to the large extrapulmonary airways drains into the azygos vein; intrapulmonary bronchial blood flow enters the pulmonary circulation at both the pre- and postpulmonary capillary level.

Although the bronchial circulation provides *nutrient blood flow* to many lung structures, the lung does not die if the bronchial circulation is obstructed. The extensive anastomoses between bronchial and pulmonary vessels provide pulmonary blood flow to bronchial vessels. Similarly, when the pulmonary circulation is obstructed, the bronchial circulation proliferates and maintains blood flow to the lung.

Inflow pressure to the bronchial circulation is systemic arterial pressure, but outflow pressure varies, depending on whether venous drainage is through the azygos vein or pulmonary circulation. Changes in pressure in both the systemic and pulmonary vascular beds affect the magnitude of bronchial blood flow. Increasing systemic pressure increases flow, but increasing pulmonary vascular pressures (downstream pressure) reduces and may even reverse flow. Unlike pulmonary arteries, the bronchial arteries dilate in response to hypoxia.

The bronchial circulation proliferates when the pulmonary circulation is obstructed or when there is pulmonary inflammation. Proliferation of the bronchial circulation is extensive in the dorsal regions of the lungs of horses that bleed from the lungs during exercise.

CLINICAL CORRELATION

BRISKET DISEASE IN A HEIFER

HISTORY □ A 2-year-old Hereford heifer was kept during the winter on a farm in the foothills of the Rocky Mountains outside Denver, Colorado. In the late spring, the heifer was transported to Climax, Colorado (altitude 3400 meters) for summer grazing. After 6 weeks, the owners noticed that the animal was having some difficulty breathing, was reluctant to move around the pasture, and had developed an enlarged pendulous brisket and also some swelling between the jaws.

CLINICAL EXAMINATION □ Inspection of the heifer reveals a dejected animal in poor condition. The respiratory and heart rates are elevated, and air seems to be moving well through the nostrils. The most noticeable observation is an enlarged and pendulous brisket. The swelling extends up the neck, and there is also a pendulous area between the jaws. The jugular veins are distended.

Palpation of the swollen brisket reveals that it is heavy; when squeezed, the imprints of the fingers remain for some time. The swelling between the mandibles behaves in a similar fashion when palpated. The mucous membranes of the heifer are a normal color, and the lung sounds are not remarkable.

COMMENT □ The heavy swelling in the brisket and between the mandibles, which pitted upon palpation, is evidence of accumulation of interstitial edema fluid in the dependent areas of the heifer, in which there is loose connective tissue. Accumulation of edema fluid in these regions is an indication of the increase in systemic venous pressure, which is also causing jugular distension. Both are due to right heart failure. The most likely cause of this in a heifer grazing at altitude is diffuse vasoconstriction of the pulmonary circulation as a result of chronic exposure to hypoxia (inspired oxygen tension in Climax is 97 torr, compared with sea level 150 torr). The smooth muscle in the pulmonary arteries contracts in response to hypoxia; if this response is maintained for several weeks, the amount of smooth muscle in the pulmonary arteries increases. Maintenance of cardiac output in the face of the elevated pulmonary vascular resistance leads to right heart failure. If this animal is returned to lowland pasture, it will recover as the vasospasm in the pulmonary circulation diminishes once the hypoxic stimulus is removed. Acutely, this animal could be given oxygen to relieve the hypoxic stimulus. This would cause a reduction in pulmonary arterial pressure, but not to normal levels, because of the increased amount of smooth muscle now present in the pulmonary arteries.

Bibliography

Deffebach ME, Charan NB, Lakshminaryan S, Butler J: State of art. The bronchial circulation: Small, but a vital attribute of the lung. Am Rev Respir Dis 135:463–481, 1987.

Fishman AP: Pulmonary circulation. *In* Fishman AP, Fisher AB, Geiger SR (eds): Handbook of Physiology, Section 3, The Respiratory System, Vol 1, Circulation and Nonrespiratory Functions. Bethesda, MD, American Physiological Society, 1985, pp 93–165.

Murray JF: The Normal Lung. Philadelphia, WB Saunders, 1986, pp 139–162.

Robinson NE: Some functional consequences of species differences in lung anatomy. *In* Dungworth DL (ed): Adv Vet Sci Comp Med 26:1–33, 1982.

Slonim NB, Hamilton LH: Respiratory Physiology, 5th ed. St. Louis, CV Mosby, 1987, pp 109–122.

West JB: Respiratory Physiology: The Essentials, 3rd ed. Baltimore, Williams & Wilkins, 1985, pp 31–46.

PRACTICE QUESTIONS FOR CHAPTER 44

1. Which of the following statements accurately describes the pulmonary circulation?

   a. It receives the total output of the right ventricle except under conditions of alveolar hypoxia, when vasoconstriction reduces pulmonary blood flow.
   b. The medial layer of the main pulmonary arteries is composed of a thick layer of smooth muscle.
   c. The pulmonary veins return blood to the right atrium.
   d. Unlike systemic capillaries, the pulmonary capillaries provide a major resistance to blood flow.
   e. All of the above

2. During exercise, cardiac output can increase fivefold, but pulmonary arterial pressure may not even double. This occurs because

   a. pulmonary vascular resistance decreases during exercise.
   b. unperfused capillaries are recruited during exercise.
   c. previously perfused vessels are distended during exercise.
   d. more of the lung is perfused under zone 2 conditions during exercise.
   e. All of the above

3. Which of the following causes the greatest change in pulmonary vascular pressure?

   a. Exposure of a cow to the hypoxia of high altitude
   b. Administration of a β-adrenergic agonist to a normal dog
   c. Stimulation of the vagus nerve in a sheep
   d. Inhalation of a tidal volume in a horse
   e. An increase in mean pulmonary arterial pressure from 15 to 18 mmHg in a dog

4. The bronchial circulation

   a. receives the total output of the right ventricle.
   b. drains into the pulmonary circulation and azygos vein.
   c. vasoconstricts in response to hypoxia.
   d. supplies nutrient blood flow to bronchi and no other structures.
   e. has a bronchial arterial pressure similar to pulmonary arterial pressure.

5. A radiologist observes that the pulmonary veins in the dorsal region of a horse lung are more distended than normal. This could be indicative of

   a. a major decrease in pulmonary blood flow.
   b. a decrease in pulmonary arterial pressure.
   c. an increase in pulmonary venous pressure.
   d. left heart failure.
   e. All of the above

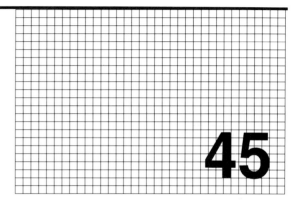

Gas Exchange

45

1. The composition of a gas mixture can be described by the fractional composition or partial pressure
2. Alveolar gas composition is determined by the delivery of fresh gas and the exchange of oxygen and carbon dioxide
3. Exchange of oxygen and carbon dioxide between the alveolus and pulmonary capillary blood occurs by diffusion
4. The exchange of gases between the tissues and blood also occurs by diffusion
5. The amount of alveolar ventilation in relation to pulmonary capillary blood flow, i.e., the $\dot{V}/\dot{Q}$ ratio, determines the adequacy of gas exchange
6. The composition of the mixed arterial blood is determined by the composition of the capillary blood from each of the gas exchange units and the frequency distribution of such units
7. Right-to-left vascular shunts deliver poorly oxygenated venous blood into the oxygenated blood leaving the lung
8. Part of each breath is retained in the anatomical dead-space and does not participate in gas exchange
9. Arterial oxygen (Pa_{O_2}) and carbon dioxide (Pa_{CO_2}) tensions are measured to evaluate gas exchange

The Composition of a Gas Mixture Can Be Described by the Fractional Composition or Partial Pressure

Before beginning a discussion of *gas exchange*, it is necessary to understand how gas composition is measured and the forces causing gas movement within the lungs, blood, and tissues. Air contains 21% oxygen (the *fraction* of oxygen in inspired air, FIO_2, is 0.21). High in the Andes mountains, the air still contains 21% oxygen, yet mammals cannot tolerate the lack of oxygen. Clearly therefore, it is not just the fraction of oxygen that is important for gas exchange. The *hypoxia* of high *altitude* is a result of the low *partial pressure* of oxygen because of the low *barometric pressure*. It is this partial pressure (also called *tension*), and more importantly the partial pressure difference between two parts of the body, that results in gas transfer.

The oxygen tension (P_{O_2}) of a dry gas mixture is determined by barometric pressure (P_B) and the fraction of oxygen (F_{O_2}) in the gas mixture:

$$P_{O_2} = P_B \cdot F_{O_2}$$

In the atmosphere F_{O_2} is 0.21, so P_{O_2} in dry air at sea level is 160 torr:

$$P_{O_2} = 760 \cdot 0.21 = 160 \text{ torr}$$

P_{O_2} decreases at higher altitudes, because barometric pressure decreases.

During inhalation, air is warmed to body temperature and humidified. The concentration of other gases is reduced by the presence of water vapor molecules; therefore, P_{O_2} decreases. The P_{O_2} of humidified gas is calculated as

$$P_{O_2} = (P_B - PH_2O)\ FIO_2$$

where PH_2O equals the partial pressure of water vapor at body temperature, and FIO_2 equals the fraction of oxygen in inspired air. The PH_2O is determined by temperature and percent saturation of the air with water. In a mammal with a body temperature of 38.2°C, PH_2O equals 50 torr; therefore, the P_{O_2} of warmed, completely humidified gas in the conducting airways is

$$P_{O_2} = (760 - 50) \cdot 0.21 = 149\ torr$$

Alveolar Gas Composition Is Determined by the Delivery of Fresh Gas and the Exchange of Oxygen and Carbon Dioxide

In the alveolus, P_{O_2} is less than in inspired air, because oxygen and carbon dioxide exchange occurs continuously. *Alveolar oxygen tension* fluctuates about an average value during breathing, increasing during inhalation and decreasing during exhalation. The average alveolar oxygen tension (PA_{O_2}) of the lung can be calculated from the *alveolar gas equation*, a simplified version of which is shown:

$$PA_{O_2} = (P_B - PH_2O)\ FIO_2 - PA_{CO_2}/R$$

This equation shows that alveolar oxygen tension is determined by the inspired oxygen tension and the exchange of oxygen for carbon dioxide. R is the *respiratory exchange ratio*, CO_2 production/O_2 consumption. Assuming an R of 0.8 and PA_{CO_2} equals 40 torr, PA_{O_2} averages 101 torr.

Because there is only a negligible amount of CO_2 in the inspired air, *alveolar carbon dioxide tension* (PA_{CO_2}) is determined by CO_2 production ($\dot{V}_{CO_2}$) in relation to the amount of *alveolar ventilation* ($\dot{V}_A$):

$$PA_{CO_2} = K \cdot \dot{V}_{CO_2}/\dot{V}_A$$

It is obvious from this equation that if $\dot{V}_{CO_2}$

increases, as occurs during exercise, $\dot{V}_A$ must also increase if PA_{CO_2} is to remain constant. If $\dot{V}_A$ does not increase sufficiently, PA_{CO_2} rises. Similarly, if $\dot{V}_{CO_2}$ remains constant and $\dot{V}_A$ halves, PA_{CO_2} doubles. The alveolar gas equation shows that whenever PA_{CO_2} increases, PA_{O_2} decreases, and vice versa.

Alveolar hypoventilation, a decrease in alveolar ventilation in relation to CO_2 production, elevates PA_{CO_2} and decreases PA_{O_2}. Alveolar hypoventilation occurs to a small extent in cattle exposed to cold. It is observed also when the central nervous system (CNS) is depressed by drugs or injury, when there is severe airway obstruction such as in exercising horses with laryngeal hemiplegia, when there is damage to the thorax and respiratory muscles, or when there is severe lung disease (Fig. 45–1). In *alveolar hyperventilation,* PA_{CO_2} decreases, because ventilation increases in relation to CO_2 production. Concurrently, PA_{O_2} also increases. Hyperventilation occurs when the drive to ventilate is increased by stimuli such as hypoxia, increased production of hydrogen ions, or an increase in body temperature.

A modified form of the alveolar gas equation can be used to determine PA_{O_2} for clinical purposes:

$$PA_{O_2} = (P_B - PH_2O)\ FIO_2 - Pa_{CO_2}/R$$

In this equation, arterial carbon dioxide tension (Pa_{CO_2}) is substituted for PA_{CO_2}.

Exchange of Oxygen and Carbon Dioxide Between the Alveolus and Pulmonary Capillary Blood Occurs by Diffusion

Diffusion is the movement of gases down a concentration (partial pressure) gradient. It occurs passively and does not require energy. The rate of gas movement between the alveolus and the blood is determined by the physical properties of the gas, *surface area* available for *diffusion* (A), the *thickness of the air-blood barrier* (x), and the *driving pressure* gradient of the gas between the alveolus and capillary blood ($PA_{O_2} - Pc_{O_2}$):

$$\dot{V}_{O_2} = D \cdot A \cdot (PA_{O_2} - Pc_{O_2})/x$$

The alveolar surface area available for diffusion is that occupied by perfused pulmonary capillaries. Because of *capillary recruitment,* the surface area increases during *exercise.* Al-

1. Damage to CNS e.g., drugs, trauma

2. Peripheral nerve injury

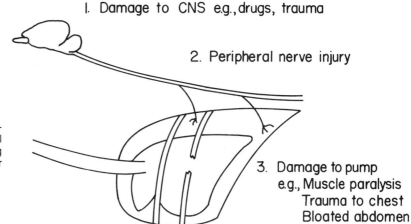

3. Damage to pump
e.g., Muscle paralysis
Trauma to chest
Bloated abdomen

Figure 45–1. Diagrammatic representation of the brain, peripheral nerves, thorax, airways, and lung to show the causes of alveolar hypoventilation.

4. Lung resisting inflation
e.g., Airway obstruction
Decreased lung compliance

though alveolar surface area, capillary volume, and *diffusing capacity* of the lung are generally scaled to body mass ($M^{1.0}$), alveolar surface area is adapted to meet oxygen demands. The horse, by virtue of its smaller alveoli, has a larger alveolar surface area than the cow. This larger surface area is required to supply the higher $\dot{V}_{O_2}$max of the horse.

In the lung, the barrier separating air and blood is less than 1.0 μm thick (Fig. 45–2) but includes a layer of liquid and surfactant lining the alveolar surface, an epithelial layer usually from type 1 epithelial cells, a basement membrane and variable thickness interstitium, and a layer of endothelium. Diffusion also moves gases within the plasma, so oxygen is eventually brought into contact with the erythrocyte and hemoglobin.

The *driving pressure* for gas diffusion varies during inhalation and exhalation and also along the length of the capillary. Cyclic fluctuations in PA_{O_2} occur as fresh air is delivered to the lung. Oxygen tension rises progressively as blood flows along the alveolar capillaries. Alveolar oxygen tension (PA_{O_2}) averages 100 torr and, in the resting animal, mixed venous blood entering the lung has an oxygen tension (Pv_{O_2}) of approximately 40 torr. The driving pressure gradient of 60 torr causes rapid diffusion of oxygen into the capillary, where it combines with *hemoglobin*. Hemoglobin provides a sink for oxygen and helps to maintain a gradient for oxygen diffusion. Normally, equilibration between alveolar and capillary oxygen tensions occurs within 0.25 sec-

ond, approximately one third of the time the blood is in the capillary (Fig. 45–3). During strenuous exercise, mixed venous oxygen tension is low, because muscles extract a lot of oxygen from the blood. In addition, the *velocity of blood flow* through the capillaries is rapid. Because more oxygen must be transferred in

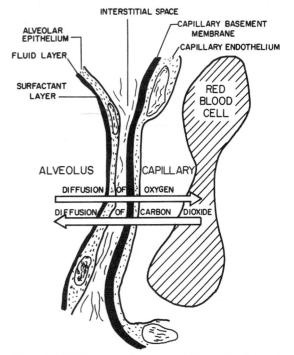

Figure 45–2. Diagrammatic representation of the air blood barrier within the lung, showing the pathway for diffusion of oxygen and carbon dioxide between the alveolus and the erythrocyte within the pulmonary capillary.

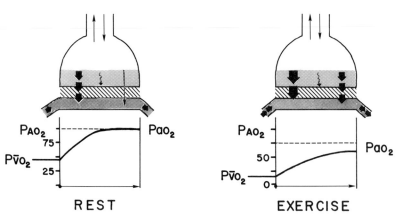

Figure 45–3. Schematic representation of an alveolus and pulmonary capillary, showing the increase in oxygen tension that occurs as blood passes through the capillaries. The shaded area within the alveolus represents mixing of gases by diffusion. The size of the arrows between the alveolus and the capillary represents the magnitude of the oxygen fluxes. In the resting animal, mixed venous oxygen tension (Pv_{O_2}) is approximately 40 mmHg, and blood and air equilibrate rapidly. In the exercising animal, mixed venous oxygen tension is low, and even though oxygen fluxes are high, the blood has not equilibrated with the alveolar oxygen tension before it leaves the alveolus. PA_{O_2}, alveolar oxygen tension; Pa_{O_2}, arterial oxygen tension.

less time than in the resting animal, diffusion equilibrium may not occur, and arterial oxygen tension (Pa_{O_2}) may decrease (Fig. 45–3).

Because of its greater solubility, *carbon dioxide is 20 times more diffusible than oxygen.* Therefore, transfer of carbon dioxide is accomplished with a lesser driving pressure gradient (PA_{CO_2} = 40 torr, Pv_{CO_2} = 46 torr), and failure of diffusion equilibrium for CO_2 is rare.

The Exchange of Gases Between the Tissues and Blood Also Occurs by Diffusion

Arterial blood enters the tissue capillaries with Pa_{O_2} of 85–100 torr and Pa_{CO_2} of 40 torr. As it passes along the capillaries, it is exposed to the tissues that are consuming oxygen and producing carbon dioxide. *Tissue oxygen tension is determined by the rate of delivery of oxygen in relation to its rate of consumption, but* averages 40 torr. Similarly, tissue carbon dioxide tension is determined by the rate of tissue production in relation to the rate of removal by the blood, and averages 46 torr. Therefore, oxygen and carbon dioxide diffuse between the blood and the tissues until the partial pressures of blood and tissue are equal. Tissues with a high oxygen demand have more capillaries per gram of tissue. This provides a larger surface for diffusion and also means that the maximal distance between tissue and capillary is less than in the less well-vascularized tissues (Fig. 45–4). During *exercise,* muscle blood flow increases in part as a result of *recruitment of capillaries* that are not perfused in the resting animal. Capillary recruitment brings blood closer to the metabolizing tissues and slows the rate of blood flow, which allows more time for diffusion equilibrium. Exercise also lowers the tissue P_{O_2} and increases the tissue P_{CO_2} of the muscle and, therefore, increases the driving pressure gradient for diffusion.

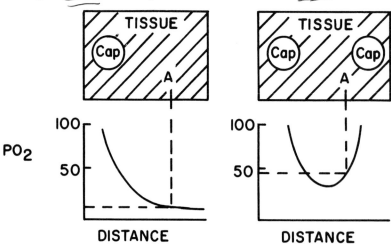

Figure 45–4. Effect of increasing capillary density on tissue oxygen tension (P_{O_2}). Oxygen tension is shown as a function of the distance from the capillary. In the left diagram, point A has an oxygen tension of approximately 10 mmHg, whereas in the right diagram, point A has an oxygen tension of 50 mmHg, because it is now located closer to a second tissue capillary.

The Amount of Alveolar Ventilation in Relation to Pulmonary Capillary Blood Flow, i.e., the V̇/Q̇ Ratio, Determines the Adequacy of Gas Exchange

In the peripheral air spaces of the lung, gas exchange is accomplished by the close approximation of air and blood. In humans, both ventilation (V̇) and blood flow (Q̇) per unit volume of lung increase from the apex of the lung toward the diaphragm. Because the rate of increase of blood flow is greater than the rate of increase of ventilation, the V̇/Q̇ ratio decreases toward the dependent regions of lung. There have been few studies of the *vertical gradient of V̇/Q̇ ratios* in domestic mammals. Even though there is a vertical gradient of ventilation in the horse, it is apparently matched by a similar gradient of blood flow, so there is no vertical gradient of V̇/Q̇ ratios (see Fig. 43–13).

The absence of a vertical gradient of V̇/Q̇ ratios does not preclude differences in V̇/Q̇ matching between peripheral regions of the lung as a result of local variations in vascular and airway resistance or lung compliance. Disease accentuates V̇/Q̇ inequalities and, therefore, impairs gas exchange.

Figure 45–5 shows models (an alveolus adjacent to a capillary) of gas exchange units with a variety of V̇/Q̇ ratios. The unit in Figure 45–5A is ideal. It receives ventilation and blood flow with a V̇/Q̇ ratio of 0.8. Mixed venous blood arrives with oxygen (Pv_{O_2}) and carbon dioxide (Pv_{CO_2}) tensions of 46 torr; it is exposed to alveolar gas tensions and leaves with end *capillary oxygen tension* (Pc_{O_2}) of 100 torr and carbon dioxide tension (Pc_{CO_2}) of 40 torr.

Figures 45–5B and 45–5C show units with low V̇/Q̇ ratios. The gas exchange unit in Figure 45–5B receives a reduced amount of ventilation but continues to receive blood flow. The *oxygen content* of blood leaving this unit is low, and the CO_2 content is high. Low V̇/Q̇ units occur commonly in lung disease because of airway obstruction or localized stiffening of the lung by fibrosis.

Figure 45–5C represents a *right-to-left shunt.* Blood passes through a nonventilated unit, gas exchange does not occur, and the blood leaving the unit has the same composition as mixed venous blood. Right-to-left shunts have a V̇/Q̇ ratio of zero and occur when blood flows past alveoli that are receiving no ventilation. This can happen in acute pneumonia, because the alveoli are flooded with inflam-

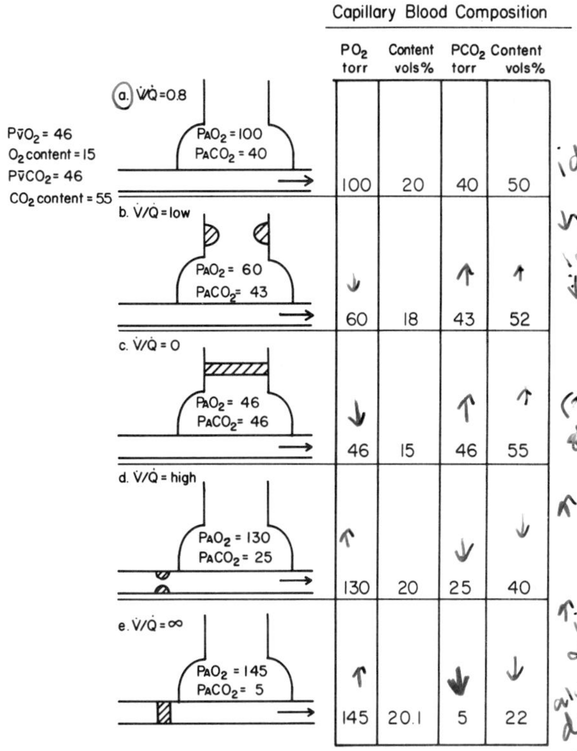

Figure 45–5. Diagrammatic representation of an alveolus and a capillary, showing the effect of differing ventilation:perfusion (V̇/Q̇) ratios on the partial pressure and gas content of blood leaving the alveolus. In the case of (e) V̇/Q̇ = ∞, there is no bulk flow of blood past the alveolus, so capillary blood does not contribute to the arterial blood that leaves the left ventricle. See text for explanation.

matory exudates. Right-to-left shunts can be the result also of complex congenital cardiac defects, such as tetralogy of Fallot, which allow blood to flow from the right to the left side of the heart and, therefore, to bypass the lungs.

Figures 45–5D and 45–5E show high V̇/Q̇ ratio gas exchange units. In Figure 45–5D, ventilation is high in relation to blood flow. This can occur when pulmonary blood flow to part of the lung is reduced by a partial vascular obstruction or by pulmonary hypotension. The blood leaving such a unit has a higher Pc_{O_2} and a lower Pc_{CO_2} than the unit with a V̇/Q̇ unit of 0.8. The CO_2 content of this blood is low, but because of the shape of the *oxyhemoglobin dissociation curve,* the oxygen content of the blood is not increased.

In Figure 45–5E, the gas exchange unit receives ventilation but no blood flow and, therefore, the unit has a V̇/Q̇ ratio of infinity. Such a unit does not contribute to gas exchange and is known as *alveolar dead-space.*

Alveolar dead-space can occur when the pulmonary arterial pressure is so low that many capillaries are unperfused, or when the vessels are obstructed by thrombi.

Extending the concepts demonstrated in Figure 45–5 to the whole lung with its multitude of gas exchange units requires computer simulation and the investigation of the frequency distribution of $\dot{V}/\dot{Q}$ ratios within the lung. In the normal animal, the latter studies have demonstrated a relatively narrow distribution of $\dot{V}/\dot{Q}$ ratios, about $\dot{V}/\dot{Q}$ equals 0.8, symmetrical on a logarithmic scale (Fig. 45–6).

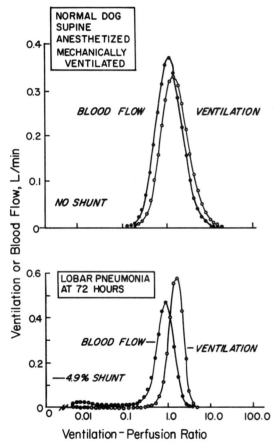

Figure 45–6. The distribution of ventilation and blood flow as a function of the ventilation:perfusion ratio. In the normal dog, shown in the top diagram, most of the blood flow and ventilation is received by gas exchange units with a ventilation:perfusion ratio close to 1.0. No blood flow and ventilation is received by extremely high or extremely low $\dot{V}/\dot{Q}$ units. In the dog with pneumonia, shown on the lower part of the diagram, a considerable portion of the blood flow is received by units with low $\dot{V}/\dot{Q}$ ratios, i.e., units having little ventilation. The amount of blood passing through right-to-left shunts is increased also in pneumonia. (From Wagner PD, Laravuso RB, Goldzimmer E, et al: Distributions of ventilation-perfusion ratios in dogs with normal and abnormal lungs. J Appl Physiol 38: 1099–1109, 1975.)

The Composition of the Mixed Arterial Blood Is Determined by the Composition of the Capillary Blood from Each of the Gas Exchange Units and the Frequency Distribution of Such Units

When blood with differing oxygen or carbon dioxide tensions mixes, the gas tension of the mixed sample is not a simple flow-weighted average of the constituent tensions. Because oxygen and CO_2 are transported in chemical combination as well as in solution, the total gas content must be considered. Consider the effect of mixing two blood samples of equal volume, mixed venous blood (P_{O_2} = 40 torr) and blood from an ideal alveolus (P_{O_2} = 100 torr). If both samples have a hemoglobin content of 15 g/dL, the O_2 content of both samples can be determined from the oxyhemoglobin dissociation curve (see Fig. 46–2). The mixed venous sample has a content of 15 mL/dL, and the ideal alveolar sample a content of 20 mL/dL. Mixing the samples gives an average O_2 content of 17.5 mL/dL, which results in a P_{O_2} equaling 55 torr. This is considerably lower than the 70 torr obtained by averaging the P_{O_2} of the two samples. If the P_{O_2} of the ideal alveolar sample is raised to 500 torr as would occur when breathing oxygen, the oxygen content only increases to 21.2 mL/dL, because hemoglobin was almost saturated with oxygen at P_{O_2} equaling 100 torr. Mixing of the two samples then results in P_{O_2} equaling 60 torr. Similar calculations can be made for CO_2. Because the CO_2 dissociation curve is almost linear over the physiological range, and because mixed venous and ideal alveolar P_{CO_2} differ only by approximately 6 torr, the CO_2 tension of the mixed sample is similar to the average of the P_{CO_2} of the two constituent samples.

Increasing overall $\dot{V}/\dot{Q}$ inequality profoundly depresses Pa_{O_2} and in more extreme forms elevates Pa_{CO_2}. Alveolar dead-space and venous admixture also increase with increasing $\dot{V}/\dot{Q}$ inequality. Venous admixture is the amount of blood with mixed venous composition that must be mixed with blood from ideal alveoli to result in a given Pa_{O_2}.

As the degree of $\dot{V}/\dot{Q}$ inequality increases, the difference between the average alveolar tension and the arterial oxygen tension increases. Normally the *alveolar to arterial oxygen tension difference* (AaD_{O_2}) averages 5 to 10 torr. This occurs because there is a degree of $\dot{V}/\dot{Q}$ inequality even in normal lungs, and because venous blood draining the bronchial and coronary circulations mixes with the oxygenated blood draining the alveoli. The AaD_{O_2} increases when animals are anesthetized or when they have pneumonia, because many poorly ventilated regions of the lung continue to receive blood flow, i.e., the number of low V/Q units increases (see Fig. 45–6). The AaD_{O_2} for carbon dioxide is normally small. It is increased by an increase in alveolar dead-space.

Right-to-Left Vascular Shunts Deliver Poorly Oxygenated Venous Blood into the Oxygenated Blood Leaving the Lung

Normal animals have a shunt fraction of up to 5%, which results from the venous outflow of the bronchial and thebesian veins into the oxygenated blood leaving the lungs. Intrapulmonary right-to-left shunts occur when alveoli are collapsed (*atelectasis*); unventilated because of complete *airway obstruction;* or filled with exudates, as in *acute pneumonia*. The magnitude of right-to-left shunting can be determined by allowing animals to breathe 100% oxygen for 15 minutes. In this situation, all ventilated alveoli receive oxygen, and the blood leaving such alveoli has saturated hemoglobin. The shunt fraction can then be calculated as

$$Qs/Qt = (Cc'O_2 - CaO_2)/(Cc'O_2 - CvO_2)$$

where C equals oxygen content in arterial (a), mixed venous (v), and pulmonary capillary (c') blood. Cc' is derived from PA_{O_2}, assuming 100% saturation of hemoglobin.

Part of Each Breath Is Retained in the Anatomical Dead-Space and Does Not Participate in Gas Exchange

This gas is *wasted ventilation*. In addition, some of the gas ventilating poorly perfused or unperfused, high $\dot{V}/\dot{Q}$ alveoli (alveolar dead-space) is wasted ventilation. The total wasted ventilation (alveolar plus anatomical dead-space) is known as *physiological dead-space*. The ratio of physiological dead-space to tidal volume (VD/VT) can be determined from the partial pressures of CO_2 in mixed expired air (PE_{CO_2}) and arterial blood (Pa_{CO_2}):

$$VD/VT = (Pa_{CO_2} - PE_{CO_2})/Pa_{CO_2}$$

Alveolar ventilation is determined from VD/VT and minute ventilation (VE):

$$\dot{V}A = \dot{V}E\,(1 - VD/VT).$$

Arterial Oxygen (Pa_{O_2}) and Carbon Dioxide (Pa_{CO_2}) Tensions Are Measured Clinically to Evaluate Gas Exchange

Venous gas tensions are inadequate to evaluate gas exchange, because they are largely determined by the blood flow to metabolism ratio of the tissues. *Blood gas tensions* are the end result of the individual processes involved in gas exchange and, thus, are affected by the composition of inspired air, alveolar ventilation, alveolocapillary diffusion, and ventilation-perfusion matching.

Domestic animals normally breathe air containing 20.9% oxygen ($FIO_2 = 0.209$), but in experimental conditions FIO_2 may be changed and result in a change in PIO_2. More commonly, however, PIO_2 varies because of changes in barometric pressure (P_B). The daily fluctuations in P_B caused by atmospheric conditions cause only trivial changes in PIO_2, but the decrease in P_B that occurs at higher altitudes results in a major decrease in PIO_2. As a consequence of the decrease in PIO_2, there is a decrease in PA_{O_2} and, thus, Pa_{O_2} as animals ascend in altitude. Altitude-induced changes in Pa_{O_2} must always be considered when evaluating blood gas tensions.

Adequacy of alveolar ventilation is assessed by examining Pa_{CO_2}. It is elevated above the normal value of around 40 torr when animals hypoventilate, and is decreased during hyperventilation. Hypoventilation also decreases PA_{O_2} and Pa_{O_2}, and hyperventilation increases these tensions. Changes in alveolar ventilation affect Pa_{O_2} but do not change the alveolar-arterial oxygen difference.

Diffusion abnormalities and $\dot{V}/\dot{Q}$ mismatching impair the transfer of oxygen from the alveolus to arterial blood, increase the alveolar-arterial oxygen difference, and reduce Pa_{O_2}. Pa_{CO_2} is rarely elevated by these problems, because the hypoxemia stimulates ventilation, keeping Pa_{CO_2} normal or even reducing it below normal. A decrease in Pv_{O_2} also decreases Pa_{O_2} and increases the alveolar-arterial oxygen difference, even though $\dot{V}/\dot{Q}$ distribution in the lung is unchanged. Strenuous exercise may be accompanied also by hypoxemia, because blood flow through the lung is too rapid for diffusion equilibrium to occur.

In animals with normal lungs, increasing FIO_2 elevates Pa_{O_2}. As $\dot{V}/\dot{Q}$ mismatching becomes more extreme, increasing FIO_2 increases Pa_{O_2} only modestly, especially in the presence of shunts. Concurrently, the alveolar-arterial oxygen difference widens. Because of greater mismatching of ventilation and blood flow, Pa_{O_2} tends to be lower in newborn animals than in adults.

CLINICAL CORRELATIONS

HYPOVENTILATION IN A BULLDOG

HISTORY ☐ A 5-year-old bulldog is presented to you because it refuses to exercise. Previously the dog had been willing to go for short slow walks. Over the past 6 months, the dog has been making an increasing amount of noise when it breathes. When it is awake, it makes a rattling sound during inhalation; when it sleeps, it snores loudly and wakes frequently, standing up, turning around, and then lying down again. On one occasion the owner tried to get the dog to run, but the dog collapsed, making a loud noise in its throat as it struggled to inhale.

CLINICAL EXAMINATION ☐ The bulldog is in good condition, but even as you walk into the room, you notice the loud rattling noises being made by the dog during breathing. You also observe that the mucous membranes of the pendulous lips have a bluish tinge. The dog is standing when you walk in the room, but while you are talking to the owner, the dog lies down and apparently goes to sleep. At this point, the noises of breathing become much louder.

Examination of the dog reveals no abnormalities in the heart or the digestive tract, but examination of the respiratory tract reveals multiple abnormalities. The external nares of the dog are extremely small, and it is difficult to introduce a speculum to examine the nasal cavity. When the dog's mouth is opened, an excessive amount of loosely folded tissue is observed in the pharynx, and it is impossible to move these aside in order to examine the larynx. Listening to the lungs is not helpful, because all the sounds being generated by the loose vibrating tissue in the upper airway are transmitted to the lungs. Radiographs, however, reveal no abnormalities in the lungs, but the trachea is quite narrow. An arterial blood sample is taken for measurement of carbon dioxide

and oxygen tensions. Pa_{O_2} is 50 torr, and Pa_{CO_2} is 75 torr.

OUTCOME ☐ This bulldog represents an extreme form of the brachycephalic syndrome, seen in short-nosed dogs, but particularly in bulldogs. The syndrome usually includes stenosis of the external nares and obstruction of the pharynx by pendulous folds of excessive soft tissue. In some of these dogs, the trachea is also very narrow. These dogs have difficulty breathing, particularly during inhalation, when the subatmospheric pressure within the upper airway sucks the loose folds of tissue into the airway lumen. This can result in total obstruction to ventilation. Generally, these dogs make a lot of noise during inhalation as the loose folds of tissue vibrate. Exhalation presents less difficulty, because the higher-than-atmospheric pressure in the pharynx tends to push back the loose tissue and open the airway. Over a period of time, the chronic, excessively subatmospheric pressure during inhalation can cause deformity of the larynx.

The upper airway obstruction in this bulldog is limiting ventilation so severely that the dog is suffering from alveolar hypoventilation. This is indicated by the elevated Pa_{CO_2}. An elevation in Pa_{CO_2} occurs when alveolar ventilation is not sufficient to remove the carbon dioxide being produced by the body. The accumulating carbon dioxide in the alveolus and the lack of ventilation also depress the alveolar oxygen tension (PA_{O_2}), and this leads to a depression in the arterial oxygen tension, such as is seen in this dog. The hypoxemia then leads to hemoglobin desaturation, which gives the bluish color to the mucous membranes of the dog.

COMMENT ☐ The treatment for this dog is surgical removal of some of the excessive tissues of the upper airway and enlargement of the external nares. This will remove some of the obstruction and may improve ventilation. However, with the narrowing of the trachea observed in this dog, it is unlikely that the dog will ever be able to exercise to a significant degree, although its condition may be improved sufficiently that it can make a suitable pet.

HYPOXEMIA IN AN ANESTHETIZED CLYDESDALE HORSE

HISTORY ☐ A 2-year-old, 750-kg Clydesdale horse is presented for removal of a testicle that has been retained in the abdomen, a procedure that requires anesthesia. You know that anesthesia of heavy draft horses can lead to gas exchange problems, and therefore you have an anesthetic machine available to provide ventilation and to supplement the horse with extra oxygen. The horse is anesthetized with a short-acting intravenously administered barbiturate, an endotracheal tube is inserted, and the horse is connected to the anesthesia machine and allowed to breathe oxygen containing 2–3% halothane for anesthesia. Ventilation is not assisted.

Thirty minutes after the induction of anesthesia, the veterinary technician takes an arterial blood sample to monitor the horse's gas exchange. Arterial oxygen tension (Pa_{O_2}) is 70 torr, and arterial carbon dioxide tension (Pa_{CO_2}) is 65 torr. Are you happy with the results of the blood gas analysis; if not, what can be done to improve gas exchange?

COMMENT □ The elevation of Pa_{CO_2} from the normal value of 40 torr to 65 torr shows that the horse is suffering from alveolar hypoventilation. That is, the ventilation received by the alveoli is insufficient to remove the carbon dioxide being produced by the horse. This is probably a result of depression of the CNS by the anesthetic gases, so ventilatory drive is reduced. In addition, the positioning of the horse on its back for removal of the retained testicle causes the heavy viscera to push on the diaphragm, making it difficult for the horse to ventilate. Alveolar hypoventilation in an anesthetized animal can be corrected by the use of positive pressure ventilation. You have a ventilator as part of the anesthesia machine and choose to ventilate the horse to return the Pa_{CO_2} to acceptable levels.

The Pa_{O_2} of 70 torr shows that the horse has considerable problems in exchanging oxygen. Although a Pa_{O_2} of 70 torr is sufficient to almost saturate hemoglobin and would not be considered particularly low in an animal breathing air, it is very low in an animal breathing 100% oxygen. When animals breathe oxygen, the alveolar oxygen tension is over 600 torr.

$$PA_{O_2} = (P_B - PH_2O) \cdot FIO_2 - Pa_{CO_2}$$
$$= (760 - 50) \cdot 1.0 - 65 = 645 \text{ torr}$$

If the lung is functioning ideally, arterial oxygen should also be close to 600 torr. In this horse, arterial oxygen tension is only 75 torr,

so there is an alveolar-arterial oxygen tension difference of close to 570 torr.

This huge alveolar-arterial oxygen tension difference is not unusual in large anesthetized mammals. The positioning of the horse on its back with the consequent weight of the viscera pushing forward on the diaphragm and compressing the lungs can lead to severe $\dot{V}/\dot{Q}$ inequalities. Parts of the dependent lung are unable to ventilate, although they continue to receive blood flow and, therefore, become right-to-left shunts. These right-to-left shunts result in severe arterial hypoxemia. As long as the Pa_{O_2} is sufficient to saturate hemoglobin, the horse is in no danger. The dangerous point is during recovery from anesthesia. The horse must be supplemented with oxygen until it is sufficiently conscious to be able to rest on its sternum unaided and eventually to stand. Returning to these postures eliminates right-to-left shunts, restores the $\dot{V}/\dot{Q}$ distribution to normal, and improves gas exchange.

Bibliography

Hedenstierna G, Nyman G, Kvart C, Funkquist B: Ventilation-perfusion relationships in the standing horse: An inert gas elimination study. Equine Vet J 19:514–519, 1987.

Murray JF: The Normal Lung. Philadelphia, WB Saunders, 1986, pp 163–172, 183–210.

Slonim NB, Hamilton LH: Respiratory Physiology, 5th ed. St. Louis, CV Mosby, 1987, pp 97–108, 123–134.

Wagner PD, Laravuso RB, Goldzimmer E, et al: Distributions of ventilation-perfusion ratios in dogs with normal and abnormal lungs. J Appl Physiol 38:1099–1109, 1975.

West JB: Respiratory Physiology: The Essentials, 3rd ed. Baltimore, Williams & Wilkins, 1985, pp 21–30, 49–66.

West JB: Ventilation-perfusion inequality and overall gas exchange in computer models of the lung. Respir Physiol 7:88–110, 1969.

West JB: Ventilation-perfusion relationships. Am Rev Respir Dis 116:919–943, 1977.

PRACTICE QUESTIONS FOR CHAPTER 45

1. Calculate the alveolar oxygen tension (PA_{O_2}) of an anesthetized cow when the barometric pressure is 750 torr, PH_2O at body temperature = 50 torr, Pa_{CO_2} = 80 torr. The cow is breathing a mixture of 50% oxygen and 50% nitrogen. Assume the respiratory exchange ratio is 1.0.

a. 270 torr
b. 620 torr
c. 275 torr
d. 195 torr
e. 670 torr

2. Which of the following will decrease the rate of oxygen transfer between the alveolar air and the pulmonary capillary blood?

a. Increasing PA_{O_2} from 100 to 500 torr
b. Perfusing previously unperfused pulmonary capillaries
c. Decreasing the mixed venous oxygen tension from 40 to 10 torr
d. Converting zone 1 of the lung to zone 2
e. None of the above

3. During exercise, recruitment of muscle capillaries that are unperfused in the resting animal results in all of the following except

a. an increase in the velocity of capillary blood flow.
b. an increase in the surface area for gas diffusion between tissues and blood.
c. a decrease in distance between tissue capillaries.
d. maintenance of tissue P_{O_2} in the face of increased demand for oxygen.
e. a shorter distance for gas diffusion.

4. Which of the following could potentially result in more low $\dot{V}/\dot{Q}$ regions within the lung?

a. Atelectasis of one lobe of a dog lung
b. Obstruction of the main pulmonary artery to the right lung
c. Doubling the ventilation to the right cranial lobe while holding blood flow constant
d. Vasoconstriction of the pulmonary arteries of the left lung in a cow
e. None of the above

5. Which of the following statements is correct?

a. Right-to-left shunts represent an extremely high $\dot{V}/\dot{Q}$ ratio.
b. Right-to-left shunts are not a cause of elevated alveolar-arterial oxygen difference.
c. An increase in the VD/VT ratio can result from an increase in the number of high $\dot{V}/\dot{Q}$ units in the lung.
d. The shape of the oxyhemoglobin dissociation curve means that low $\dot{V}/\dot{Q}$ units in the lung are not a cause of hypoxemia (low Pa_{O_2}).
e. Totally occluding the right pulmonary artery increases the right-to-left shunt fraction by 50%.

6. A horse has difficulty inhaling, especially during exercise. Arterial blood gas tensions at rest are Pa_{O_2} = 55, Pa_{CO_2} = 70 torr. After you give the horse oxygen to breathe, Pa_{O_2} increases to 550 torr, and Pa_{CO_2} remains unchanged. The cause of these gas tensions is

a. right-to-left shunt through a complex cardiac defect.
b. atelectasis of 50% of the lung.
c. a 50% decrease in the VD/VT ratio.
d. alveolar hypoventilation.
e. None of the above

Gas Transport in the Blood

OXYGEN TRANSPORT

1. Oxygen is transported in solution in plasma but mainly in combination with hemoglobin
2. A molecule of hemoglobin can reversibly combine with four molecules of oxygen
3. The binding of oxygen and hemoglobin is determined by P_{O_2}
4. The oxyhemoglobin dissociation curve can be displayed with percent saturation of hemoglobin as a function of P_{O_2}
5. The position of the oxyhemoglobin dissociation curve is not fixed but varies with blood temperature, pH, P_{CO_2}, and the intracellular concentration of certain organic phosphates
6. As hemoglobin is depleted of oxygen, its color changes from bright red to bluish red
7. Carbon monoxide, which binds to the same sites on hemoglobin as oxygen, has 200 times the affinity of oxygen for hemoglobin
8. Methemoglobinemia occurs in certain toxicities, notably nitrite poisoning

CARBON DIOXIDE TRANSPORT

1. Like oxygen, carbon dioxide is transported in the blood both in solution in plasma and in chemical combination

GAS TRANSPORT DURING EXERCISE

1. Oxygen demands of exercise are met by increases in blood flow, hemoglobin, and oxygen extraction from blood

OXYGEN TRANSPORT

Oxygen Is Transported in Solution in Plasma but Mainly in Combination with Hemoglobin

When blood in the pulmonary capillaries flows past the alveoli, oxygen diffuses from the alveolus into the blood until the partial pressures equilibrate, i.e., there is no further driving pressure difference. Some of the oxygen dissolves in the plasma, but because oxygen is *poorly soluble,* an oxygen-carrying pigment, *hemoglobin,* is necessary to deliver sufficient oxygen to the tissues. Without hemoglobin, which transports the majority of the oxygen, the cardiac output would have to be inordinately high to maintain the oxygen supply to the tissues.

Even though the amount of oxygen dissolved in plasma is small, it increases directly as partial pressure increases, 0.003 mL dissolving in each 100 mL of plasma at a P_{O_2} of 1 torr (Fig. 46–1). At the alveolar P_{O_2} of 100 torr, therefore, there is 0.3 mL oxygen dissolved in each deciliter of blood. If an animal breathes pure oxygen so that PA_{O_2} is about 600 torr, 1.8 mL of oxygen are dissolved in each deciliter of plasma.

A Molecule of Hemoglobin Can Reversibly Combine with Four Molecules of Oxygen

Mammalian hemoglobin consists of four unit molecules, each containing one *heme* and its associated protein. Heme is a *proto-porphyrin* consisting of four *pyrroles* with a *ferrous* iron at the center. The ferrous iron combines reversibly with oxygen in proportion to P_{O_2}.

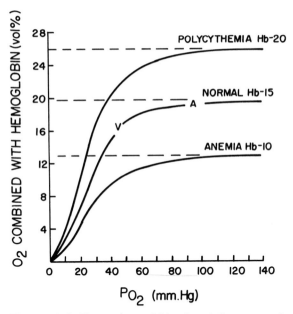

Figure 46–2. The oxyhemoglobin dissociation curve of normal (hemoglobin, Hb = 15 g/dL), anemic (Hb = 10 g/dL), and polycythemic blood (Hb = 20 g/dL). The amount of oxygen combined with hemoglobin is plotted as a function of oxygen tension (P_{O_2}).

The hemoglobin molecule is spheroid, an *amino acid side chain* being attached to each heme. The amino acid composition of the side chains greatly affects the affinity of hemoglobin and defines the different types of mammalian hemoglobin. Adult hemoglobin contains two α and two β *amino acid chains; fetal hemoglobin contains two α and two γ chains.* Closely related species, such as humans and anthropoid apes, have similar amino acid sequences on the side chains, whereas more divergent species have greater numbers of differences in amino acid sequences.

Each hemoglobin molecule can reversibly bind up to four molecules of oxygen. The reversible combination of oxygen with hemoglobin is shown in the *oxyhemoglobin dissociation curve* (Fig. 46–2). Binding is a four-step process, the *oxygen affinity* of a particular heme being influenced by the oxygenation of the others. These *heme-heme interactions* are responsible for the *sigmoid shape* of the oxyhemoglobin dissociation curve.

The Binding of Oxygen and Hemoglobin Is Determined by P_{O_2}

Examination of Figure 46–2 shows that the *oxygen content* of blood, i.e., the oxygen combined with hemoglobin, is determined by P_{O_2}.

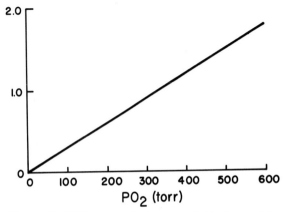

Figure 46–1. The amount of oxygen (mL) dissolved in plasma as a function of P_{O_2}.

Above a P_{O_2} of approximately 70 torr, the oxyhemoglobin dissociation curve is virtually flat. Further increases in P_{O_2} add little oxygen to hemoglobin, and the hemoglobin is said to be saturated with oxygen. This plateau in the oxyhemoglobin dissociation curve above a P_{O_2} of 70 torr allows saturation of hemoglobin with oxygen, even if animals ascend to moderate altitude and PIO_2 decreases.

One gram of saturated hemoglobin can hold 1.36–1.39 mL of oxygen; therefore, average mammalian blood with 10–15 g of hemoglobin per deciliter has an oxygen capacity of 13.9–21 mL of oxygen per deciliter (volumes percent). Anemia, a reduction in the number of circulating erythrocytes with a consequent reduction in the amount of hemoglobin in the blood, decreases oxygen capacity. When the hemoglobin content of blood increases, oxygen capacity increases also. The latter occurs in many mammals, but especially in the horse during exercise; contraction of the spleen forces more erythrocytes into the circulation and increases the oxygen capacity of the blood.

Below P_{O_2} of 60 torr, the oxyhemoglobin dissociation curve has a steep slope. This is in the range of tissue P_{O_2} at which oxygen is unloaded from the blood. Tissue P_{O_2} varies depending on the blood flow/metabolism ratio, but "average" tissue P_{O_2} is 40 torr (Pv_{O_2}). Blood exposed to P_{O_2} equalling 40 torr loses 25% of its oxygen to the tissues. In rapidly metabolizing tissues where P_{O_2} is lower, more oxygen is unloaded from the blood. The oxygen normally remaining in combination with hemoglobin forms a reserve that can be drawn upon in emergencies.

The Oxyhemoglobin Dissociation Curve Can Be Displayed with Percent Saturation of Hemoglobin as a Function of P_{O_2}

Percent saturation of hemoglobin is the ratio of oxygen content to oxygen capacity. Hemoglobin is over 95% saturated with oxygen when it leaves the lungs of an animal at sea level. Percent saturation of mixed venous blood (P_{O_2} = 40 torr) is 75. Although all mammals have similarly shaped oxyhemoglobin dissociation curves, the position of the curve with respect to P_{O_2} varies (Fig. 46–3). This can be described by measurement of P_{50}, the partial pressure at which hemoglobin is 50% saturated with oxygen. The higher P_{50} generally found in small

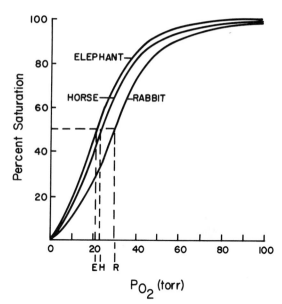

Figure 46–3. The oxyhemoglobin dissociation curve of three species of mammal. Percent saturation of hemoglobin is plotted as a function of oxygen tension. Although the curves have similar shapes in all mammals, they are not superimposed. The differences between the curves can be expressed by the P_{50}, i.e., the partial pressure at which hemoglobin is 50% saturated with oxygen. P_{50} is shown in E, H, and R.

mammals allows unloading of oxygen at a high P_{O_2} to satisfy their higher metabolic demands.

The Position of the Oxyhemoglobin Dissociation Curve Is Not Fixed but Varies with Blood Temperature, pH, P_{CO_2}, and the Intracellular Concentration of Certain Organic Phosphates

An increase in tissue metabolism produces heat, which elevates blood temperature and shifts the oxyhemoglobin dissociation curve to the right (increases P_{50}). Such a shift facilitates dissociation of oxygen from hemoglobin and releases oxygen to the tissues. Conversely, excessive cooling of the blood, as occurs in hypothermia, shifts the dissociation curve to the left so that tissue P_{O_2} must be lower to release oxygen from hemoglobin.

The shift in the oxyhemoglobin dissociation curve resulting from a change in P_{CO_2}, the Bohr shift, results in part from the combination of CO_2 with hemoglobin, but mostly from the production of H^+, which decreases pH. A change in pH alters the oxygen binding by changing the structure of hemoglobin (Fig. 46–4). The Bohr effect is not constant among species; in small mammals, a given change in pH produces a greater shift in the dissociation

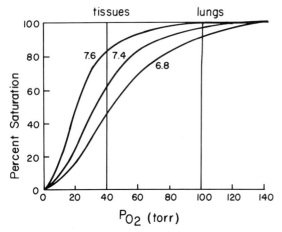

Figure 46–4. The effect of pH on the oxyhemoglobin dissociation curve. A decrease in pH shifts the dissociation curve to the right and therefore assists in unloading oxygen at the tissues. The shift in the dissociation curve has much less effect on percent saturation of hemoglobin when oxygen is being loaded into the blood in the lungs (i.e., above $PO_2 = 90$ torr) than when oxygen is being unloaded at the tissues (below $PO_2 = 65$ torr).

curve than in large mammals, supposedly ensuring the delivery of oxygen during high rates of metabolic activity, when CO_2 production is greatest.

The oxyhemoglobin dissociation curve of mammalian hemoglobin solution generally lies to the left of the curve of whole blood until *organic phosphates,* such as *diphosphoglycerate (DPG)* and *adenosine triphosphate (ATP),* are added to the solution. In erythrocytes, DPG has a molar content equivalent to that of hemoglobin, much higher than in other cells. This DPG regulates the combination of oxygen with hemoglobin. When concentrations of DPG are high, as occurs under anaerobic conditions, the oxyhemoglobin dissociation curve is shifted to the right (P_{50} increases), and the unloading of oxygen is facilitated. In contrast, a reduction in DPG, as can occur in stored blood, shifts the dissociation curve to the left. Not all hemoglobins bind DPG equally. Ruminant hemoglobin in general is unresponsive to DPG, and elephant hemoglobin binds DPG weakly.

As Hemoglobin Is Depleted of Oxygen, Its Color Changes from Bright Red to Bluish Red

This color change, known as *cyanosis,* can be observed in the mucous membranes of animals when the blood in the underlying capillaries is hypoxic. Cyanosis can result from

impaired transfer of oxygen from the alveolus to the blood, but can also result from reduced blood flow to the peripheral tissues. The latter can occur when animals are in cardiovascular failure or are extremely cold.

Carbon Monoxide, Which Binds to the Same Sites on Hemoglobin as Oxygen, Has 200 Times the Affinity of Oxygen for Hemoglobin

Exposure to carbon monoxide levels of less than 1% in air can eventually saturate hemoglobin and displace oxygen. Fortunately, such low levels of CO must be breathed for some time in order to deliver sufficient CO to saturate all the blood hemoglobin, so toxicity is not immediate. Carbon monoxide not only reduces the oxygen content of the blood, it also displaces the oxyhemoglobin dissociation curve to the left, so the release of the remaining oxygen to the tissues occurs at lower than normal tissue P_{O_2}.

Methemoglobinemia Occurs in Certain Toxicities, Notably Nitrite Poisoning

When the normal ferrous iron of hemoglobin is oxidized by *nitrites* and other toxins to ferric iron, brown-colored *methemoglobin* is formed. Methemoglobin does not bind oxygen; thus, the oxygen capacity of the blood is reduced. Nitrite can be ingested directly in spoiled feeds, but ruminants more commonly form nitrite in the rumen following ingestion of nitrate-rich feeds such as Sudan grass or mangel tops.

CARBON DIOXIDE TRANSPORT

Like Oxygen, Carbon Dioxide Is Transported in the Blood Both in Solution in Plasma and in Chemical Combination

Unlike oxygen, which is chemically bound only to hemoglobin, *carbon dioxide* is transported in two chemical combinations (Fig. 46–5). Carbon dioxide is produced in the tissue; therefore, tissue P_{CO_2} is higher than the P_{CO_2} of the blood arriving in the capillaries. Carbon dioxide diffuses down a concentration gradient from the tissues into the blood. When the blood leaves the tissues, P_{CO_2} has risen from 40 to approximately 46 torr, exact values

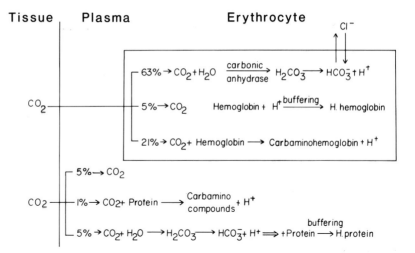

Figure 46–5. The methods of CO_2 transport in the blood. All reactions displayed in this diagram can be reversed when the blood reaches the lung and CO_2 diffuses into the alveolus.

being dependent on the blood flow to metabolism ratio.

Approximately 5% of the CO_2 entering the blood is transported in solution. The majority of CO_2 diffuses into the red cell, where it undergoes one of two chemical reactions. Most of the CO_2 combines with water and forms *carbonic acid,* which then dissociates into *bicarbonate* and *hydrogen ion:*

$$H_2O + CO_2 \longleftrightarrow H_2CO_3 \longleftrightarrow H^+ + HCO_3^-$$

This reaction also occurs in plasma, but in the red cell the presence of *carbonic anhydrase* accelerates the hydration of carbon dioxide several hundredfold. Ionization of carbonic acid occurs rapidly, and H^+ and HCO_3^- accumulate within the erythrocyte. The reversible reaction is kept moving to the right, because H^+ is *buffered* by hemoglobin, displacing K^+, which combines with HCO_3^-. A large part of the HCO_3^- diffuses out of the erythrocyte along a concentration gradient into the plasma. Chloride ion diffuses into the erythrocyte to maintain the *Gibbs-Donnan equilibrium.*

The addition of CO_2 to capillary blood is facilitated by the deoxygenation of hemoglobin occurring in the tissues. Deoxyhemoglobin is a weaker acid than oxyhemoglobin and, therefore, a better buffer. Thus, it combines more readily with H^+ and facilitates the formation of HCO_3^- from CO_2.

The formation of *carbamino compounds* is the second form in which CO_2 is transported in the blood. Carbamino compounds are formed by coupling of CO_2 to the $-NH$ groups of proteins, particularly hemoglobin. Although carbamino compounds account for only 15–

20% of the total CO_2 content of the blood, they are responsible for 20–30% of the CO_2 exchange occurring between the tissues and the lungs.

When venous blood reaches the lungs, carbon dioxide diffuses into the alveoli from plasma and erythrocytes, thus causing the reactions shown in Figure 46–5 to move to the left. Simultaneously, the oxygenation of hemoglobin releases hydrogen ions, which combine with bicarbonate to form carbonic acid and, thus, CO_2.

The blood *content of CO_2* as a function of P_{CO_2} is depicted in the carbon dioxide equilibrium curve shown in Fig. 46–6. Curves are shown for oxygenated blood, for partially deoxygenated blood, and for deoxygenated blood. The curves are almost linear and have no plateau in the physiological range; CO_2 can be added to the blood as long as the buffering capacity is available. The higher CO_2 content

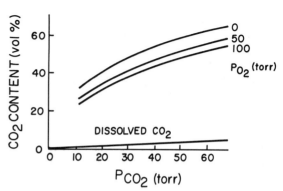

Figure 46–6. Carbon dioxide equilibration curves showing the amount of carbon dioxide contained in the blood as a function of carbon dioxide tension. Curves are shown for dissolved CO_2 and for total CO_2 content at a variety of oxygen tensions (P_{O_2}).

of deoxygenated blood resulting from the higher buffering capacity of deoxyhemoglobin is clearly visible. This effect of oxygenation on CO_2 content is termed the *Haldane effect.*

GAS TRANSPORT DURING EXERCISE

Oxygen Demands of Exercise Are Met by Increases in Blood Flow, Hemoglobin, and Oxygen Extraction from Blood

The demands for gas transport in the blood are not constant but vary with metabolism. Strenuous exercise represents the most extreme demand placed on the gas transport mechanisms. In the galloping horse, oxygen consumption can increase 30-fold. Figure 46–7 shows how this extra demand for oxygen is met. Part of the demand is provided by an increase in *cardiac output,* so the amount of blood flowing through the lungs per minute is increased. This allows an increased uptake of oxygen from the lungs. The cardiac output is redistributed also, with an increased fraction of output going to the exercising muscles. The increase in cardiac output and redistribution serves to increase muscle blood flow by 20-fold.

The horse also meets the increased oxygen demand with an increase in the number of circulating erythrocytes and, therefore, he-

moglobin. Contraction of the spleen can increase the hematocrit from 35 to 50%. This provides almost 50% more binding sites for oxygen. The usefulness of an increase in *hematocrit* is limited, because it increases blood viscosity, which tends to slow the flow of blood through the capillaries and increase the work of the heart. The increase in muscle blood flow and hematocrit together increase the delivery of oxygen to the muscle. Muscle also extracts a bigger percentage of the oxygen from the blood during exercise than at rest. This is accomplished by the decrease in muscle P_{O_2}, which results from the increase in metabolic rate. As a result of the increased extraction of oxygen, the *arteriovenous oxygen content difference* is increased.

Muscle itself contains an oxygen-binding pigment, *myoglobin,* that provides a small store of oxygen. However, myoglobin's main function is the transfer of oxygen within the muscle cell. Myoglobin, like hemoglobin, is an iron-containing pigment, but unlike hemoglobin, it contains only one heme group. As a result, the dissociation curve is not sigmoid but is a rectangular hyperbola. The affinity of myoglobin for oxygen is high, with 75% saturation at a P_{O_2} of 20 torr and the steepest slope of the dissociation curve at P_{O_2} equaling 5 torr. As a result of these dissociation characteristics, myoglobin releases oxygen only when intracellular P_{O_2} is low. Myoglobin is more plentiful in slow-twitch aerobic muscle fibers than in fast-twitch fibers, and the amount of myoglobin is increased by exercise training.

Thus, in exercise the increased demand for oxygen is met by changes in blood flow, hematocrit, and oxygen extraction from blood, and to a small degree, by oxygen release from myoglobin. These mechanisms are available whenever unusual demands for gas exchange arise. In anemia, for example, oxygen capacity is reduced, but oxygen delivery to the tissues can be preserved by an increase in cardiac output and increased extraction of oxygen from the hemoglobin.

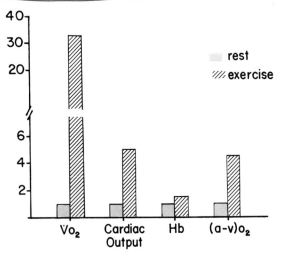

Figure 46–7. Oxygen consumption ($\dot{V}O_2$), cardiac output, hemoglobin (*Hb*), and arteriovenous oxygen difference [(a-v)O_2] in a horse at rest and during a gallop. The 30-fold increase in $\dot{V}O_2$ is accomplished by a fivefold increase in cardiac output, a 50% increase in Hb, and a fourfold increase in (a-v)O_2.

The Respiratory System in Acid-Base Homeostasis

The respiratory system's role in acid-base balance is discussed in Chapter 50.

CLINICAL CORRELATIONS

FLEA INFESTATION IN A CAT

HISTORY □ A cat is presented to you because the owner notices that the cat seems extremely weak and recently has been staggering when it walks around the house. The cat's appetite is good and, apart from the weakness, the owner thinks the cat is normal.

CLINICAL EXAMINATION □ Inspection of the animal shows that it is in reasonable condition and is resting quietly on the examination table. The respiratory rate does not appear to be elevated, and from a distance there are no obvious signs of disease. When you rest your hands on the cat's back, you immediately notice a gritty-feeling material within the fur of the cat. Further examination of the skin shows accumulations of this red-brown material deep within the coat, and you notice many fleas scurrying around when the coat is parted. When you moisten some of the gritty material, it produces a red liquid. The cat's mucous membranes are almost white, and the examination of the mucous membranes produces sufficient struggling that the cat begins to breathe rapidly. The cat's pulse rate is extremely elevated, but the lung sounds are normal. On physical examination, all of the body systems appear to be normal. A blood sample is taken. The packed cell volume (hematocrit) is 10 (normal is 30–45).

COMMENT □ This cat has a severe infestation of fleas. The gritty material in the fur is flea manure, which contains blood products, so when it is wet it produces a reddish liquid. The infestation is further confirmed by the observation of many fleas in the coat. By their blood-sucking method of feeding, fleas can produce anemia when they are present in large numbers, as was the case with this cat. If the flea infestation develops gradually, the anemia is slow in onset, and the host animal may show few clinical signs until the infestation and anemia become extremely severe. The anemia is confirmed in this case by the pale mucous membranes and by the low hematocrit. The rapid heart rate of the cat is a response to the anemia. In order to deliver sufficient oxygen to the tissues, the cardiac output has had to be increased by increasing the heart rate. When the cat is stressed by your examination, it shows signs of respiratory distress, because there is inadequate oxygen delivery to the tissues; this results in production of lactic acid due to anaerobic metabolism. The decrease in pH from the lactic acid stimulates the chemoreceptors, causing the signs of respiratory distress.

TREATMENT □ You can treat the cat in two ways. First, you can administer blood to increase the cat's hematocrit and provide it with sufficient oxygen-carrying capacity until it can generate new erythrocytes. Also you can treat the flea infestation and instruct the owners on how to remove the fleas from the house.

Several weeks later the owner returns with the cat and notes that she has had no further problems. Occasionally, she notes a flea on the cat's coat and treats the cat immediately with flea powder. She is also diligent about regular vacuuming to remove fleas from the house.

ATRIAL FIBRILLATION IN A HORSE

HISTORY □ The owner of a 3-year-old standardbred gelding is concerned because the horse is no longer able to complete its training program. Up until a week ago, the horse had been running well during its daily bouts of training. In the past 2 days, the horse is extremely reluctant to exercise and, if pushed to do so, begins to stagger and appears weak in the rear legs.

CLINICAL EXAMINATION □ Inspection of the horse reveals a normal-appearing standardbred in excellent condition. It is standing in its boxstall, eating, and looks alertly at you and the owner when you enter the stall. Clinical examination reveals normal-colored mucous membranes, no abnormality of lung sounds, and no abnormalities in the gastrointestinal, urinary, or nervous system. When you take the pulse, you note that it is irregular in both amplitude and rate. Several pulses follow one another rapidly, and then there are prolonged pauses. There is no consistent pattern to the irregularity. Auscultation of the heart reveals a similar irregularity in the heart sounds.

You take a blood sample for measurement of the hematocrit, which turns out to be normal. You also perform an electrocardiogram (ECG), which reveals a continuous pattern of multiple

P-waves with occasional and irregularly occurring QRS complexes.

COMMENT ☐ The history, heart sounds, and electrocardiographic findings in this horse are typical of atrial fibrillation. The multiple P-waves observed on the ECG are a result of circuitous depolarization of the atria. In atrial fibrillation the atria do not contract and relax in a coordinated fashion. The atrioventricular (AV) node is activated at intervals that vary considerably from cycle to cycle; hence, there is no constant interval between ventricular contractions. The variable time between ventricular contractions allows for variable degrees of ventricular filling and, therefore, results in uneven stroke volume; consequently, the pulse varies in amplitude as well as frequency.

The irregularity of the ventricular rhythm may be sufficient to maintain cardiac output in the resting animal, but during exercise the cardiac output cannot be maintained. As a result, oxygen delivery to the muscles is inadequate to sustain exercise. This is an example of failure of oxygen delivery due to inadequate blood flow.

TREATMENT ☐ Treatment for atrial fibrillation in the horse is the administration of quinidine sulfate, which has a negative inotropic effect on the myocardium and slows AV conduction time. This allows the re-establishment of normal atrial and ventricular rhythm. The horse's heart rate returns to normal within 5 days and remains so for the following week, at which time training is reinstituted. Several months later the owner reports that the horse is still doing well.

Bibliography

Bartels H: Comparative physiology of oxygen transport in mammals. Lancet 2:599–604, 1964.

Baumann R, Bartels H, Bauer C: Blood oxygen transport. *In* Fishman AP, Farhi LE, Tenney SM, Geiger SR (eds): Handbook of Physiology, Section 3, The Respiratory System, Vol 4, Gas Exchange. Bethesda, MD, American Physiological Society, 1987, pp 147–172.

Dickerson RE, Geis I: Hemoglobin: Structure, Function, Evolution and Pathology. Menlo Park, CA, Benjamin Cummings Publishing, 1983, pp 65–116.

Kitchen H, Brett I: Embryonic and fetal hemoglobin in animals. Ann NY Acad Sci 241:653–671, 1974.

Murray JF: The Normal Lung. Philadelphia, WB Saunders, 1986, pp 172–182.

Prosser CL: Respiratory functions of blood. *In* Prosser CL (ed): Comparative Animal Physiology, 3rd ed. Philadelphia, WB Saunders, 1973, pp 317–361.

Slonim NB, Hamilton LH: Respiratory Physiology, 5th ed. St. Louis, CV Mosby, 1987, pp 135–153.

PRACTICE QUESTIONS FOR CHAPTER 46

1. If 1 g of hemoglobin has an oxygen capacity of 1.36 mL of oxygen, what is the oxygen content of blood containing 10 g of hemoglobin when the blood P_{O_2} is 70 torr?

   a. 13.6 mL/dL (vols %)
   b. 9.5 mL/dL (vols %)
   c. 6.8 mL/dL (vols %)
   d. 21 mL/dL (vols %)
   e. Cannot be calculated from the information provided

2. An increase in pH of blood will

   a. shift the oxyhemoglobin dissociation curve to the right.
   b. decrease P_{50}.
   c. decrease the affinity of hemoglobin for oxygen.
   d. decrease the oxygen capacity of the blood.
   e. All of the above

3. Which of the following decreases oxygen content but does NOT alter Pa_{O_2} or percent saturation of hemoglobin?

   a. Ascent to an altitude of 3,500 meters
   b. Polycythemia
   c. Breathing 50% oxygen
   d. Anemia
   e. Development of a large right-to-left shunt

4. All of the following shift the oxyhemoglobin dissociation curve to the right except

   a. an increase in pH.
   b. an increase in P_{CO_2}.
   c. an increase in 2,3-DPG.
   d. an increase in temperature.

5. Quantitatively, the most important form of CO_2 transport is

   a. HCO_3^- produced in plasma.
   b. CO_2 dissolved in plasma.

c. HCO_3^- produced in the erythrocyte.
d. CO_2 dissolved in the erythrocyte.
e. CO_2 combined with plasma proteins.

6. Oxygenation of hemoglobin in the lungs assists with the release of CO_2 from the blood because

    a. oxygen combines with the NH groups on hemoglobin and displaces CO_2 from carbamino compounds.

    b. oxygen combines with HCO_3^- and produces CO_2.

    c. oxygen facilitates the movement of chloride ions out of the erythrocyte.

    d. oxygen combines with hemoglobin, making it a better buffer, which retains H^+.

    e. None of the above

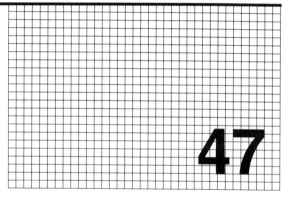

Control of Ventilation

CENTRAL CONTROL OF RESPIRATION

1. Respiratory rhythmicity originates in the medulla and is modified by higher brain centers and inputs from peripheral receptors

PULMONARY AND AIRWAY RECEPTORS

1. Pulmonary stretch receptors, irritant receptors, and juxtacapillary receptors can influence the rhythm of breathing
2. Muscle spindle stretch receptors monitor the effort exerted by respiratory muscles

CHEMORECEPTORS

1. Hypoxia, acidosis, and hypercapnia are all potent stimuli for ventilation
2. Peripheral chemoreceptors are the only receptors monitoring blood oxygen levels
3. The ventilatory response to CO_2 is mediated through a medullary chemoreceptor
4. Ascent to high altitude is accompanied by a decrease in inspired oxygen tension and, consequently, hypoxemia, which leads to an increase in ventilation
5. Because the tissues demand more oxygen and produce more carbon dioxide, ventilation must increase during exercise

Respiratory control mechanisms monitor the chemical composition of the blood, the effort being exerted by the respiratory muscles on the lungs, and the presence of foreign materials in the respiratory tract. This information is integrated with the other nonrespiratory activities, such as thermoregulation, vocalization, parturition, and eructation, to produce a pattern of breathing that maintains gas exchange.

A *feedback control diagram* for the respiratory system is shown in Figure 47–1. The *central controller* regulates the activity of the respiratory muscles, which by contracting give rise to alveolar ventilation. Changes in alveolar ventilation affect blood gas tensions and pH, which are monitored by the *chemoreceptors*, signals being returned to the central controller, and necessary adjustments made in ventilation. *Mechanoreceptors* in the lungs monitor the degree of stretch of the lungs and changes in the airways and vasculature. Stretch receptors (*proprioceptors*) in respiratory muscles monitor the effort of breathing.

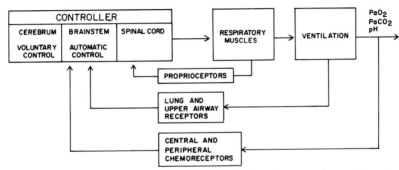

Figure 47–1. Feedback control diagram for the regulation of ventilation. The controller, which includes centers in the cerebrum and brainstem, drives the respiratory muscles that bring about ventilation. Changes in ventilation can cause changes in blood-gas tensions and pH that are monitored by central and peripheral chemoreceptors. Receptors in the lung detect the stretch in the lung tissues and the presence of materials in the lungs and airways. Proprioceptors in the respiratory muscles monitor the amount of effort being applied by the muscles.

CENTRAL CONTROL OF RESPIRATION

Respiratory Rhythmicity Originates in the Medulla and Is Modified by Higher Brain Centers and Inputs from Peripheral Receptors

Brainstem transection experiments have identified the regions of brain essential for maintenance of rhythmic breathing. Figure 47–2 shows the results of such experiments performed with the vagi intact and sectioned. Transection between the *spinal cord* and *medulla* arrests breathing, indicating that the *rhythmicity of breathing* originates in the brain, not in the spinal cord or respiratory muscles. Sectioning between the medulla and *pons* causes a regular gasping respiration unaffected by cutting the vagus *(vagotomy)*. Midpontine sectioning coupled with vagotomy causes prolonged inspiratory efforts *(apneusis)*, but slow deep breathing with vagi intact. Cutting the brain between the pons and midbrain has little effect if the vagi are intact. However, vagal sectioning causes slow deep breathing. These types of experiments have been interpreted as showing that respiratory rhythmicity originates in the medulla but is tuned by afferent information in the vagus and by higher centers in the pons. The pons may be the location of an *off-switch* that terminates inhalation. Apneusis results when medullary centers are deprived of information from both the pontine off-switch and information in the vagus nerve.

Within the medulla, two groups of neurons fire in association with respiration (see Fig. 47–2). The *dorsal respiratory group* (DRG) is located in the ventral lateral portion of the *nucleus tractus solitarius*, and the *ventral respiratory group* (VRG) is located in the *nucleus ambiguus* and *retroambiguus*. The DRG neurons fire primarily during inhalation, and VRG neurons fire during both inhalation and exhalation. The DRG axons project through *bulbospinal pathways* to inspiratory spinal motoneurons (primarily those supplying the diaphragm) and to the VRG. Axons from the VRG project to spinal motoneurons of both expiratory and accessory inspiratory muscles. The source of respiratory rhythmicity within or close to these groups of neurons is unknown, but the loca-

Figure 47–2. Diagrammatic representation of the pons, medulla, and spinal cord, showing centers involved in the regulation of respiration. The effect of sectioning the brain at the levels designated by the horizontal lines is shown on the right side of the diagram.

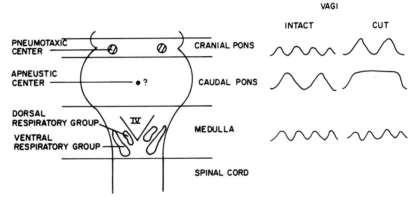

tion of the DRG within the tractus solitarius makes it the recipient of afferent information in the ninth and tenth cranial nerves.

Current ideas suggest that rhythmic respiration results not from reciprocal inhibition of inspiratory and expiratory neurons, but by rhythmic inhibition of inspiratory activity. During inhalation there is an increase in inspiratory neuron activity, the slope of this ramp of activity increasing with increasing chemical respiratory drive, such as hypoxia. Termination of inspiration can be a result of inputs from pulmonary stretch receptors or from a central pontine off-switch. Following vagotomy, the pontine off-switch terminates inhalation after a fixed time for inhalation (TI), which is independent of chemical drive. When *pulmonary stretch receptors* are intact, there is an interaction between TI and tidal volume (Fig. 47–3), such that tidal volume is greater, TI is shorter, and therefore respiratory frequency is greater when there is an increased chemical drive to ventilate.

When inhalation is terminated, inspiratory neurons are inhibited, so exhalation occurs passively as a result of the elastic recoil of the lung and chest wall. There is activity in some inspiratory neurons early in exhalation leading to inspiratory muscle activity, which provides a "brake" on exhalation and regulates the rate of expiratory air flow. Later in exhalation, braking is removed. It is during this latter part of exhalation that expiratory muscles may be

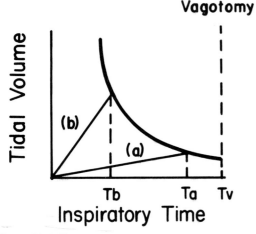

Vagotomy

Figure 47–3. The interactions of tidal volume and inspiratory time. When respiratory drive is low (*a*), the volume of air in the lung increases slowly and inspiratory time is prolonged (*Ta*). When respiratory drive is enhanced (*b*), lung volume increases rapidly and inspiratory time is shortened (*Tb*). The curved dark line defines the possible combinations of tidal volume and inspiratory time. When the vagus is cut, inspiratory time lasts for a fixed period (*Tv*).

activated. When respiratory drive is low, this second phase of exhalation is initiated later than when drive is increased.

The "automatic" breathing described earlier is overridden frequently by demands from higher brain centers. Vocalization, parturition, swallowing, defecation, and many other activities require the active participation of the respiratory system.

PULMONARY AND AIRWAY RECEPTORS

Pulmonary Stretch Receptors, Irritant Receptors, and Juxtacapillary Receptors Can Influence the Rhythm of Breathing

Three types of receptors with vagal afferents have been identified within the lung: *slowly adapting stretch receptors* and *irritant receptors,* both of which have *myelinated afferents,* and *C-fibers* with *unmyelinated axons.* Slowly adapting stretch receptors are nerve endings associated with smooth muscle in the trachea and main bronchi, but to a lesser degree in the intrapulmonary airways. They are stimulated by deformation of the wall of larger airways, for example, when intrathoracic airways are stretched during lung inflation. Because firing rates from these receptors increase progressively as the lung inflates, they are thought to be responsible for the inhibition of breathing caused by lung inflation (Hering-Breuer reflex). Termination of input from these receptors by vagotomy leads to a slowing of respiration and an increase in tidal volume. Slowly adapting stretch receptors may be responsible also for adjustments in the rate and depth of respiration to minimize the work of the respiratory muscles.

Rapidly adapting stretch or irritant receptors are thought to be unmyelinated nerve endings ramifying between epithelial cells in the larynx, trachea, large bronchi, and intrapulmonary airways. They are stimulated by mechanical deformation of the airways such as occurs during lung inflation, bronchoconstriction, and mechanical irritation of the airway surface. Irritant gases, dusts, histamine release, and a variety of other stimuli can cause these receptors to respond also. Stimulation of rapidly adapting irritant receptors leads to *cough, bronchoconstriction, mucus secretion,* and rapid shallow breathing (hyperpnea), i.e., protective responses to clear irritant materials from the respiratory system. These receptors may initiate the *sighs* that are thought to redistribute pulmonary surfactant over the alveolar surface.

Pulmonary C-fibers ramify in the pulmonary interstitium close to pulmonary capillaries (*juxtacapillary receptors*), where they may monitor blood composition or the degree of distention of the interstitium. They may be responsible for the hyperpnea that follows injury of the lung in allergic or infectious diseases.

In addition to intrapulmonary receptors, there are *receptors in the upper airway*. Stimulation of receptors in the nasal cavity causes sniffing and sneezing, whereas stimulation of laryngeal and pharyngeal receptors may cause cough, apnea, or bronchoconstriction.

Muscle Spindle Stretch Receptors Monitor the Effort Exerted by Respiratory Muscles

The density of *muscle spindle stretch receptors* varies greatly in different respiratory muscles, and the effects of stimulating these receptors can vary with the anatomical location of the muscle group. The diaphragm has few muscle receptors, but intercostals are well supplied with *tendon organs* and muscle spindles. Muscle receptors reflexly control the strength of respiratory muscle contraction and adjust the strength of contraction when ventilation is impeded by, for example, airway obstruction.

CHEMORECEPTORS

Hypoxia, Acidosis, and Hypercapnia Are All Potent Stimuli for Ventilation

Chemoreceptors monitor oxygen, carbon dioxide, and hydrogen ion concentration at several sites in the body. In the minute by minute regulation of breathing, carbon dioxide and hydrogen ion are apparently more important than oxygen. Small changes in Pa_{CO_2} and $[H^+]$ produce major changes in ventilation, whereas small changes in Pa_{O_2} in the physiological range have little effect on breathing.

Chemoreceptors are located at several sites in the body. Peripheral chemoreceptors are the *carotid and aortic bodies*, and their removal eliminates the respiratory response to hypoxia. The response to hypercapnia persists, because it is also detected by a *central chemoreceptor*. Changes in blood $[H^+]$ are detected by both the peripheral and central chemoreceptors.

Peripheral Chemoreceptors Are the Only Receptors Monitoring Blood Oxygen Levels

The carotid bodies are located close to the bifurcation of the internal and external carotid arteries, and the aortic bodies around the aortic arch. The latter appear to be most active in the fetus and of little importance in the adult. Carotid bodies are small structures with high blood flow per kilogram. The aortic bodies are supplied by the *vagus nerve*, and a branch of the *glossopharyngeal nerve* supplies the carotid body. Fibers within these nerves are primarily afferent except for a few parasympathetic efferents to blood vessels. Sympathetic efferents from the superior cervical ganglion innervate blood vessels, and preganglionic efferents provide a limited nerve supply to the glomus cells.

Carotid bodies contain two main cell types. *Glomus cells* containing *catecholamines*, especially *dopamine*, may modulate chemosensitivity by releasing a neurotransmitter. *Sustentacular cells* support axons and blood vessels that ramify within the carotid body and may be necessary for the full expression of *chemosensitivity*. Afferent nerve terminals, which are probably the location of chemosensitivity, reciprocally innervate glomus cells.

When the carotid bodies are perfused with blood having a low P_{O_2}, high P_{CO_2}, or low pH, firing rates in the carotid sinus nerve afferents increase. As P_{CO_2} increases and pH decreases, there is an almost linear increase in ventilation. The response to P_{O_2} is alinear. Modest increases in firing rate and ventilation occur as P_{O_2} decreases from unphysiological levels of 500 torr to 70 torr. Further decreases cause a more rapid increase in ventilation, particularly below P_{O_2} equaling 60 torr, i.e., the P_{O_2} at which hemoglobin begins to desaturate (Fig. 47–4). Because neither modest anemia nor carbon monoxide poisoning increases ventilation, it is thought that P_{O_2} is more important than oxygen content as a stimulus to the carotid bodies.

The mechanism of chemosensitivity of the carotid bodies is unknown. Hypoxia, hypercapnia, and changes in blood pH may all alter the local $[H^+]$ in the vicinity of the nerve terminals. Alternatively, the same stimuli, particularly hypoxia, may release messengers from the sustentacular cells by disrupting their metabolism and reducing adenosine triphosphate (ATP) levels. The nonlinearity of the response to hypoxia has been suggested to be

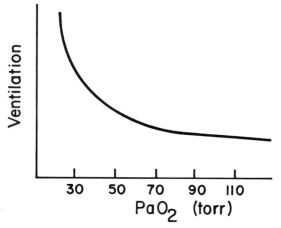

Figure 47–4. The effect of arterial oxygen tension (Pa_{O_2}) on ventilation.

due to the presence of a *cytochrome* or other substance with oxygen-binding characteristics similar to those of hemoglobin.

The Ventilatory Response to CO_2 Is Mediated Through a Medullary Chemoreceptor

Chemosensitive tissue has been localized to the ventrolateral surface of the medulla, lateral to the pyramids, and medial to the roots of the seventh through tenth and the twelfth cranial nerves, but the specific chemosensitive cells have not been identified. These areas are distinct from the DRG and VRG neurons. The central chemoreceptor apparently responds to changes in the pH of the *interstitial tissue fluid* in which it lies. A decrease in pH increases ventilation, and an increase in pH decreases ventilation. Because the central chemoreceptor is bathed by brain interstitial fluid in communication with cerebrospinal fluid (CSF), changes in ventilation can be induced by changes in the composition of arterial blood (Fig. 47–5) and by changes in the [H⁺] of CSF.

The central chemoreceptor is separated from blood by the *blood-brain barrier*, which is freely permeable to CO_2, but less permeable to H⁺ and HCO_3^-. An increase in blood P_{CO_2} causes a rapid increase in P_{CO_2} in the region of the central chemoreceptor. Carbonic acid forms and dissociates into H⁺ and HCO_3^- and, because the interstitial fluid is poorly buffered, pH around the chemoreceptor decreases and stimulates ventilation. Similarly, infusing H⁺ or HCO_3^- into the CSF changes interstitial fluid pH and affects ventilation.

An acute increase in blood [H⁺] is not re-flected immediately by a decrease in interstitial fluid or CSF pH, because the blood-brain barrier is relatively impermeable to H⁺. Therefore, acute increases in [H⁺] are detected by the peripheral chemoreceptors. However, changes in brain interstitial fluid pH may follow those in the blood within 10–40 minutes. Infusion of H⁺ into the blood may initially cause a paradoxical increase in CSF pH, because the increase in blood [H⁺] stimulates peripheral chemoreceptors, thus increasing ventilation and decreasing Pa_{CO_2}. The latter leads to diffusion of CO_2 from the CSF into the blood and, therefore, the paradoxical increase in CSF pH.

The composition of CSF and, hence, brain interstitial fluid has a major effect on the response of the central chemoreceptor. If the [HCO_3^-] of the CSF decreases, as occurs in *metabolic acidosis*, the buffering capacity of the CSF is reduced. An increase in P_{CO_2} then causes a greater decrease in CSF pH than would occur in the presence of a normal buffering capacity, so the ventilatory response to CO_2 is more vigorous than normal (Fig. 47–6). Conversely, in *metabolic alkalosis*, the CSF [HCO_3^-] increases, and the response to CO_2 is depressed. The CSF composition is regulated by active transport of ions at the *choroid plexus*. In metabolic acidosis and alkalosis, CSF [HCO_3^-] tends to follow changes in blood [HCO_3^-], but with a phase lag of several hours.

Ascent to High Altitude Is Accompanied by a Decrease in Inspired Oxygen Tension (PIO_2) and, Consequently, Hypoxemia, Which Leads to an Increase in Ventilation

The ventilatory response to the hypoxia of altitude varies depending on whether it lasts for less than an hour, for several days, or for longer periods. The acute hypoxia experienced on first ascending to high altitude causes hyperventilation mediated through the peripheral chemoreceptors. However, hyperventilation decreases Pa_{CO_2}, which dampens the response to hypoxia. After several hours to days, ventilation increases further and remains somewhat elevated, even after the hypoxic stimulus is removed. This short-term *acclimatization* cannot be explained by changes in CSF pH and may be due to altered excitability of respiratory neurons. Prolonged residence in high altitude leads to a loss of the hyperven-

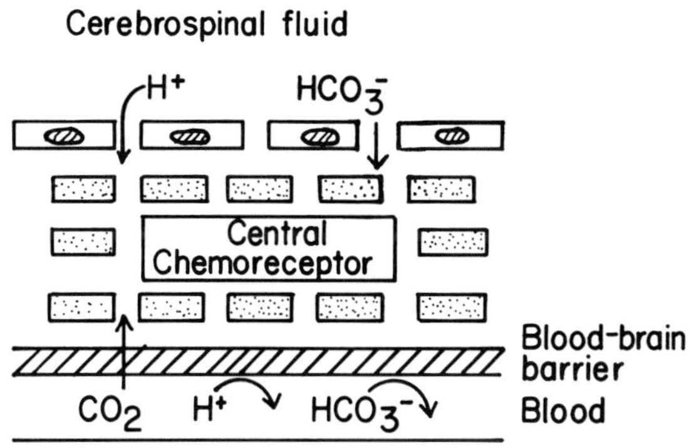

Cerebrospinal fluid

Figure 47–5. Diagrammatic representation of the central chemoreceptor separated from blood by the blood-brain barrier, which allows passage of carbon dioxide but is less permeable to hydrogen ion and bicarbonate. The central chemoreceptor is bathed by brain interstitial fluid, which is in communication with the cerebrospinal fluid.

tilatory response observed during short-term acclimatization.

Because the Tissues Demand More Oxygen and Produce More Carbon Dioxide, Ventilation Must Increase During Exercise

The increase in ventilation following the onset of *exercise* is initially rapid, then occurs more slowly and, provided the work load remains constant, reaches a steady state after about 4 minutes. Although the ventilatory response to exercise has been well described, the reasons for the increase in ventilation are still not well understood.

The primary chemical stimuli for ventilation, i.e., Pa_{O_2}, Pa_{CO_2}, and pH, do not change in most animals during moderate *aerobic exercise*.

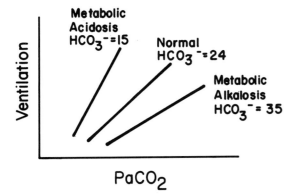

Figure 47–6. The effect of arterial carbon dioxide tension ($PaCO_2$) on ventilation, in a normal animal and in animals with metabolic acidosis and alkalosis. A decrease in the bicarbonate level increases the ventilatory response to carbon dioxide.

This shows that the increase in ventilation is well matched to the needs of the tissues, and also that there must be factors other than chemical drive that increase ventilation during exercise. These other factors may be (1) reflexes originating from motion of the exercising limbs, (2) factors related to the increase in cardiac output, (3) thermoregulatory factors, and (4) psychogenic factors as the animal anticipates exercise.

Once the *anaerobic threshold* is exceeded, the production of *lactic acid* decreases blood pH. The latter stimulates an increase in ventilation, which leads to a decrease in Pa_{CO_2}. In the horse, the increase in ventilation that can occur during exercise may be limited by the fact that respiratory rate is linked, one for one, with stride frequency. During strenuous anaerobic exercise, the horse's arterial pH decreases progressively, although ventilation remains constant. When exercise ceases, there is a further increase in ventilation, presumably because the restrictions imposed by locomotion are removed.

CLINICAL CORRELATIONS

HYPOXEMIA WITH HYPERVENTILATION IN AN 8-MONTH-OLD SAMOYED

HISTORY □ An 8-month-old Samoyed is presented to you because it is reluctant to exercise. Ever since the owner obtained the puppy, she has noticed its behavior is not puppy-like; it tires easily and prefers to sleep rather than to play.

CLINICAL EXAMINATION □ The puppy is not well grown. Even though the owner thinks it has been growing, for a Samoyed of 8 months of age the dog is rather small. When it is standing quietly in the examination room, the dog breathes normally, but when you call it and it runs toward you, its respiratory rate increases, and it begins to pant. At this point, you notice that the dog's tongue and gums have a distinct bluish tinge.

Before examining the dog further, you are already suspicious of a congenital cardiac anomaly. You arrive at this suspicion because of the dog's age, its history, and the fact that it became cyanotic with only a small amount of exercise.

Palpation of the dog shows that even though

it is small, it is not thin. The major abnormality is the cyanosis of the mucous membranes, an extremely elevated heart rate, and loud abnormal cardiac sounds. There is a loud murmur audible over the tricuspid valve area during systole. The murmur is loud enough to produce a palpable vibration on the chest wall. You explain your suspicions of a cardiac defect to the owner, and together you decide to perform some angiographic studies to determine the nature of the defect.

Prior to angiographic studies, an arterial blood gas sample is taken to determine the suitability of the dog for anesthesia. Pa_{O_2} is 61 torr, and Pa_{CO_2} is 23 torr.

Angiography is performed successfully. A catheter is floated into the right atrium of the dog, and dye is injected at this site. Some of the dye passes into the right ventricle, but a large portion passes from the right atrium into the left atrium and out into the systemic circulation. While the dog is under anesthesia, it breathes pure oxygen, and at this time Pa_{O_2} is only 75 torr.

COMMENT □ The blood gas results are fairly typical of an animal with a major oxygen exchange problem, in the case of this dog a right-to-left vascular shunt through a cardiac defect. A large amount of the mixed venous blood returning to the heart is bypassing the lungs, resulting in the low Pa_{O_2}. The Pa_{O_2} is low enough to cause a major increase in ventilation by stimulating the peripheral chemoreceptors. This increase in ventilation causes excessive elimination of carbon dioxide, resulting in the reduced Pa_{CO_2}. Perhaps ventilation could have increased further, but the low Pa_{CO_2} acting on the central chemoreceptor slows down the increase.

In a normal dog, Pa_{O_2} when breathing 100% oxygen is 500 torr or more. The large alveolar arterial oxygen difference when breathing 100% oxygen, coupled with the shunting of blood from the right to the left atrium, suggests that the dog has a large intracardiac defect. You advise the owner that the chances of correcting the defect are slight, and the dog is euthanized.

On postmortem examination, a patent foramen ovale is found. Normally this would not result in right-to-left shunting of blood, because the pressure in the left atrium is normally higher than that in the right atrium. However, this dog also has abnormalities of the tricuspid valve that cause a partial obstruction. This is sufficient to increase the pressure in the right atrium and cause blood to flow from right to left through the foramen ovale.

HYPOVENTILATION IN AN ANESTHETIZED SAINT BERNARD

HISTORY □ A 2-year-old Saint Bernard is presented to you for treatment of a fractured femur. You elect to place an intramedullary pin in the femur, for which procedure the dog will require anesthesia. The dog is anesthetized with a barbiturate, an endotracheal tube is placed, and the dog is allowed to breathe oxygen containing 2% halothane. It is not ventilated but is allowed to breathe the anesthetic mixture spontaneously. The veterinary technician observing the dog notices that the gas reservoir bag on the anesthesia machine is not moving much when the dog breathes. Therefore, she draws an arterial blood gas sample for measurement of blood gases. Measurement reveals Pa_{O_2} equal to 480 torr, and Pa_{CO_2} equal to 90 torr.

COMMENT □ This is an example of alveolar hypoventilation. Carbon dioxide is being eliminated by the lungs less quickly than it is produced by the tissues, so the Pa_{CO_2} is elevated above the normal value of 40 torr. The lung's ability to exchange oxygen is not impaired; the oxygen tension is acceptable in a dog breathing oxygen. Hypoventilation is a common occurrence in anesthetized dogs, particularly those induced with a barbiturate drug. Perhaps the dog was slightly overdosed with barbiturate, resulting in the severe hypoventilation observed in this case. Hypoventilation occurs because the ventilatory response to CO_2 is depressed by anesthesia and, therefore, it takes a larger increase in Pa_{CO_2} than normal to trigger an increase in ventilation.

Bibliography

Berger AJ, Mitchell RA, Severinghaus JW: Regulation of respiration. N Engl J Med 297:92–97, 138–143, 194–201, 1977.

Murray JF: The Normal Lung. Philadelphia, WB Saunders, 1986, pp 233–260, 268–272.

Sant'Ambragio G: Information arising from the tracheobronchial tree of mammals. Physiol Rev 62:531–569, 1982.

Slonim NB, Hamilton LH: Respiratory Physiology, 5th ed. St. Louis, CV Mosby, 1987, pp 172–197.

von Euler C: Brain stem mechanisms for generation and control of breathing patterns. *In* Fishman AP, Cherniak NS, Widdicombe JG, Geiger SR (eds): The Respiratory System, Vol 2, Control of Breathing, Part I. Bethesda, MD, American Physiological Society, 1986, pp 1–67.

PRACTICE QUESTIONS FOR CHAPTER 47

1. The rhythmicity of breathing is thought to originate solely in

   a. the ventral respiratory group of medullary neurons.
   b. the apneustic center.
   c. the pneumotaxic center.
   d. slowly adapting pulmonary stretch receptors.
   e. None of the above

2. Which of the following receptors have afferent nerve fibers in the glossopharyngeal nerve?

   a. Carotid bodies
   b. Slowly adapting pulmonary stretch receptors
   c. Aortic bodies
   d. Intercostal stretch receptors
   e. Rapidly adapting pulmonary stretch receptors

3. Which of the following statements correctly describes the carotid bodies?

   a. Carotid bodies can increase ventilation in response to low Pa_{O_2}, but not in response to an increase in Pa_{CO_2}.
   b. Carotid bodies have a low blood flow to metabolism ratio.
   c. Chemoreception is thought to occur in the glomus cells.

   d. Carotid bodies are located near the bifurcation of the internal and external carotid arteries.
   e. All of the above

4. The duration of inhalation

   a. is independent of chemical drive.
   b. is independent of chemical drive only following vagotomy.
   c. is determined by the ventral respiratory group of neurons.
   d. is shortened by vagotomy.

5. The ventilatory response to a change in Pa_{CO_2}

   a. is mediated through a change in pH of interstitial fluid bathing the central chemoreceptors.
   b. is accentuated in metabolic acidosis, because there is less buffering of the interstitial fluid around the central chemoreceptors.
   c. is modified during exercise, so Pa_{CO_2} remains constant despite a large increase in carbon dioxide production.
   d. can occur in the absence of the peripheral chemoreceptors.
   e. All of the above

6. Which of the following receptors are thought to initiate a cough in response to mechanical deformation of the airway?

   a. Juxtacapillary receptors
   b. Rapidly adapting stretch receptors
   c. Slowly adapting stretch receptors
   d. Intercostal tendon organs
   e. None of the above

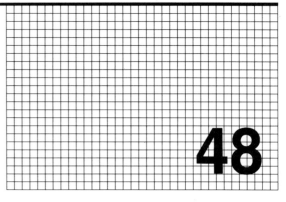

Nonrespiratory Functions of the Lung

DEFENSE MECHANISMS OF THE RESPIRATORY SYSTEM

1. The extensive, delicate gas exchange surface of an animal's lung is protected by a variety of specific and nonspecific defense mechanisms
2. Particle deposition onto the mucociliary system is dependent on particle size and occurs by impaction, sedimentation, and diffusion
3. The respiratory tract is lined by a mucociliary blanket consisting of a ciliated epithelium overlain with a layer of mucus
4. Alveolar macrophages scavenge particles deposited on the alveolar surface

PULMONARY FLUID EXCHANGE

1. The lung continuously produces lymph as a result of the net fluid movement from the pulmonary microvasculature into the pulmonary interstitium
2. The small volume of pleural fluid originates by filtration from capillaries in the visceral and parietal pleura

METABOLIC FUNCTIONS OF THE LUNG

1. The lung removes many hormones and toxins from the blood and inactivates many others

DEFENSE MECHANISMS OF THE RESPIRATORY SYSTEM

The Extensive, Delicate Gas Exchange Surface of an Animal's Lung Is Protected by a Variety of Specific and Nonspecific Defense Mechanisms

When an animal is grazing in a rural environment, the air contains few potentially harmful particles and little in the way of pollutant gases. If, however, the animal is intensively housed or is being transported, the air may be rich with particles such as dust, spores, pollen, bacteria, and viruses and with pollutant gases such as ammonia, diesel fumes, oxides of nitrogen, and ozone. The respiratory system has a variety of defense mechanisms to protect it against potentially injurious substances. Nonspecific defenses protect against many inhaled substances. Specific defenses involve the immune system and are directed against specific injurious agents, such as a bacterium. Respiratory defense mechanisms, which may provide adequate protection to an animal in its pastoral environment, are frequently overwhelmed by the stresses of intensification. The animal is then more susceptible to respiratory disease.

Particle Deposition onto the Mucociliary System Is Dependent on Particle Size and Occurs by Impaction, Sedimentation, and Diffusion

Harmful material is inhaled either suspended in air as *aerosols* or as a gas. Particles and aerosols are removed from the air when they contact the moist epithelial surface of the tracheobronchial tree (Fig. 48–1). The depth of penetration of particles and aerosols depends on particle size. Larger particles greater than 5 μm in diameter contact the airway wall by *inertial impaction*. Inertial impaction occurs at the bends in the large airways, because the large particles traveling at high velocity fail to negotiate the turns. Sites of inertial impaction are provided with *lymphoid tissue, such as tonsils* and *bronchus-associated lymphoid tissue*. As air flow rates diminish deeper in the lung, particles between 0.2 μm and 5.0 μm *sediment* onto the walls of the airways. The smallest particles, less than 0.5 μm in diameter, reach the peripheral airways and alveoli, where by *diffusion* they contact the epithelial surface.

The deposition of particles within the respiratory tract is influenced by the pattern of breathing. Slow deep breathing transports particles deep into the lung, whereas rapid shallow breathing enhances inertial deposition in the larger airways. Bronchoconstriction enhances deposition of particles in more central airways, whereas bronchodilation favors more peripheral distribution.

The deposition of toxic gases depends on their solubility and concentration. Very soluble gases, e.g., SO_2, in low concentrations are removed by the nose, but in higher concentrations penetrate deeper into the lung. Less soluble gases may reach down to the alveoli. Toxic gases stimulate a variety of protective mechanisms, such as *bronchospasm*, mucus hypersecretion, coughing, and sneezing.

The Respiratory Tract Is Lined by a Mucociliary Blanket Consisting of a Ciliated Epithelium Overlain with a Layer of Mucus

Particles deposited on the epithelial surface of the respiratory tract are transported on the *mucociliary escalator* to the pharynx; they are then swallowed or engulfed by *alveolar macrophages* or other cells recruited from the blood. The mucociliary system consists of *sol and gel mucus* layers overlying epithelial cells (Fig. 48–2). The low viscosity sol layer, in which the *cilia* beat, bathes the surface of the epithelial cells. On its forward stroke, the extended cilium catches the overlying viscous gel layer, in which inhaled particles are entrapped, and propels it up the tracheobronchial system or through the nasal cavity. Differential rates of mucus transport are necessary in small and

Particle Deposition

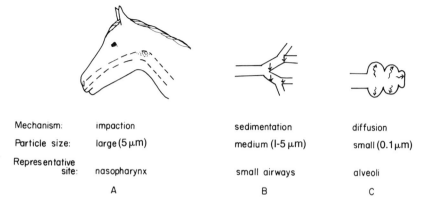

Mechanism:	impaction	sedimentation	diffusion
Particle size:	large (5 μm)	medium (1-5 μm)	small (0.1 μm)
Representative site:	nasopharynx	small airways	alveoli
	A	B	C

Figure 48–1. Mechanisms of particle deposition in the tracheobronchial tree. Large particles are deposited by impaction in the larger bends in the larger airways. Medium-sized particles are deposited in the smaller airways by sedimentation, and small particles move by diffusion and contact the walls of the alveoli.

BRONCHUS   **BRONCHIOLE**

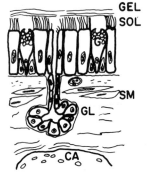
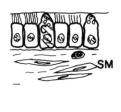

Figure 48–2. Diagram of the epithelium and submucosa of a bronchus and bronchiole. In the bronchus, the epithelium is pseudostratified columnar and includes goblet cells (G), ciliated cells, and basal cells that do not reach the surface of the epithelium. A bronchial gland (GL) is shown in the submucosa with its duct passing between the smooth muscle (SM). Cartilage (CA) underlies the mucosal layer. The cilia beat within a sol layer over which is a layer of gel-type mucus. In the bronchiole, the epithelium is cuboidal and is a mixture of ciliated cells and secretory Clara (C) cells. Smooth muscle is shown in the submucosa. Bronchioles normally do not have submucosal glands or goblet cells, and there is no cartilage in their walls.

larger airways to prevent the "piling up" of mucus in the trachea. Clearance rates and the beating frequency of cilia are slower in bronchioles than in bronchi and trachea.

Respiratory tract mucus originates from several sites (see Fig. 48–2). In *respiratory bronchioles*, the nonciliated Clara cells are a source of the airway lining fluid. In the *terminal bronchioles* and larger airways, goblet cells produce mucous secretions. In the bronchi, submucosal *bronchial glands* produce both serous and mucous secretion. Secretion is under autonomic regulation. Throughout the respiratory tract, transepithelial movement of water and ions can change the composition of the mucus layer. Ion and fluid reabsorption is assisted by *microvilli* on the surface of epithelial cells.

Changes in the composition and viscosity of mucus occur in response to many stimuli and can be the cause or the result of respiratory disease. A change in the depth or viscosity of the sol layer impairs ciliary function, and changes in the viscoelastic properties of gel alter clearance rates.

Coughing is part of the clearance mechanism of the respiratory tract and is initiated by stimulation of subepithelial irritant receptors most numerous in the larger bronchi. Receptors can be stimulated by mechanical deformation resulting from either material on the epithelial surface or bronchoconstriction. The cough reflex becomes hyper-responsive when the respiratory tract epithelium is injured by viral infections, such as equine influenza or bovine viral rhinotracheitis.

Alveolar Macrophages Scavenge Particles Deposited on the Alveolar Surface

Macrophages constitute approximately 85% of cells in the alveolar lining fluids washed from the lung periphery. Some macrophages originate in bone marrow as *monocytes* and differentiate during their passage from the blood into the alveolus, where their turnover time is in the order of days. The remainder are derived from a self-sustaining pool within the alveolus. *Complement, opsonins,* and *lysozyme* in respiratory tract secretions assist macrophages in the killing and removal of viable particulates, such as bacteria. Once phagocytized, particles are destroyed by the macrophage or transported out of the lung. Some macrophages enter the mucociliary system directly from the alveolus; others traverse the alveolar wall and enter the lymphoid tissues associated with the airways. Because macrophages have adapted to the high oxygen levels of the alveolus, phagocytosis is depressed by hypoxia. Suppression of macrophage function by corticosteroids released from the adrenal glands is an important cause of respiratory disease in stressed animals. Virus infections also suppress macrophage function approximately 7 days after virus inoculation (Fig. 48–3).

Alveolar macrophages are a first line of defense. When large numbers of particles are inhaled, the macrophage is assisted by other phagocytes from the blood, particularly *polymorphonuclear leukocytes*. Toxic *oxygen radicals* and *proteolytic enzymes* released by phagocytic cells to break down particulates may damage the lung tissue also. *Protease inhibitors*, such as α_1-antitrypsin, and antioxidants, such as glutathione peroxidase, protect the lung from its own defense mechanisms.

PULMONARY FLUID EXCHANGE

The Lung Continuously Produces Lymph as a Result of the Net Fluid Movement from the Pulmonary Microvasculature into the Pulmonary Interstitium

Figure 48–4 shows a *capillary* in the *alveolar septum*. Fluid filtration normally occurs be-

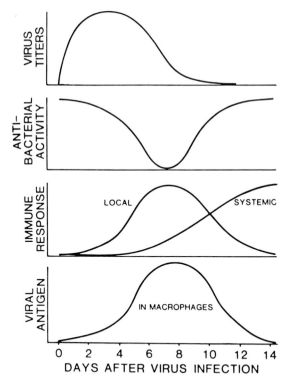

Figure 48–3. The effects of viral infection on antibacterial activity of alveolar macrophages. Antibacterial activity is depressed 7 days after experimental viral infection. At this time, the viral antigen is located in the macrophages, which are damaged by the local immune response to the virus. (From Jakab, GT: Viral-bacterial interactions in respiratory tract infections: A review of the mechanisms of virus-induced suppression of pulmonary antibacterial defenses. In Loan RW (ed): Bovine Respiratory Disease: A Symposium. College Station, TX, Texas A & M University Press, 1984, p 238).

tween the capillary and the *interstitial tissue* on the *thick* side of the alveolar septum, where a layer of interstitium is interposed between the *endothelium* and the epithelial *basement membrane.* On the *thin* side of the septum, the capillary endothelium shares a basement membrane with the *alveolar epithelium,* there being no interstitial tissue. Fluid movement out of the capillary is thought to occur between endothelial cells, but these gaps are too small to allow for passage of *macromolecules.* The latter probably pass through endothelial cells in *vesicles,* which may fuse to form *transendothelial channels.* The alveolar epithelium is less permeable than the capillary endothelium, so fluid does not leak into the alveoli unless the epithelium is damaged, or unless there is considerable fluid accumulation in the interstitium.

The movement of fluid across the endothe-

lium is governed by forces described in *Starling's equation:*

$$\dot{Q}f = Kf\,[(Pmv - Pif) - \sigma(\pi mv - \pi if)]$$

where $\dot{Q}f$ equals the amount of fluid flowing per minute; Kf equals the *capillary filtration coefficient;* Pmv equals *microvascular hydrostatic pressure;* Pif equals *interstitial fluid hydrostatic pressure;* πmv and πif equal *microvascular* and *interstitial colloid osmotic (oncotic) pressures,* respectively; and σ equals the *colloid reflection coefficient* (see also Chapter 22). Figure 48–4 shows average values for vascular and interstitial pressures.

When values shown in Figure 48–4 are inserted into Starling's equation, the net force favors fluid filtration from the capillaries to the interstitium of the lung. The fluid flux between the capillaries and the interstitium varies with changes in vascular permeability, and hydrostatic and oncotic pressures. Capillary hydrostatic pressure increases in left heart failure and during exercise. Because of this, animals that have an increase in fluid filtration across pulmonary capillaries as a result of left heart failure may develop clinically evident *pulmonary edema* during exercise. Increased fluid filtration and pulmonary edema can be a result also of a decrease in plasma oncotic pressure (*hypoproteinemia*), which can be due to starvation or to the overvigorous administration of intravenous (IV) fluids. Increased *vascular permeability* occurs in many inflammatory lung diseases, such as pneumonia, due to the effects of neutrophil products, probably oxygen radicals, on the endothelium. Protein-rich fluid leaks into the interstitium, elevating interstitial fluid oncotic pressure and causing osmotic attraction of water from the vasculature.

Fluid filtered from capillaries moves through the interstitium toward the perivascular and peribronchial tissues, where *lymphatics* are located. Fluid transport along lymphatics is aided by lymphatic vasomotion, valves, and the pumping action of the lungs during breathing. Lymphatics can accommodate quite large increases in fluid flux, and compliant peribronchial and perivascular spaces also provide intrapulmonary "sinks" for fluid accumulation. Fluid does not accumulate in the alveoli and cause clinically evident pulmonary edema unless there is a large increase in the amount of fluid being filtered from the capillaries. Alveolar flooding occurs once the peri-

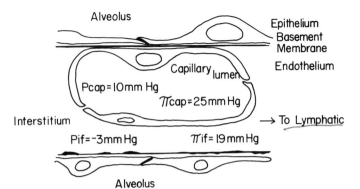

Figure 48–4. Diagrammatic representation of a capillary in the alveolar septum. On the top side of the diagram the capillary endothelium and alveolar epithelium share a basement membrane. On the lower side of the diagram, the endothelium and epithelium are separated by a layer of interstitial tissue. Values for capillary and interstitial hydrostatic pressures (*Pcap* and *Pif*) and capillary and interstitial fluid oncotic pressures (πcap and πif) are shown.

bronchial capacity is exceeded, fluid probably entering the air spaces across alveolar epithelial cells or at the level of the bronchioles. The foaming fluid typical of clinical pulmonary edema probably results from the mixing of air, edema fluid, and surfactant within the airways.

The Small Volume of Pleural Fluid Originates by Filtration from Capillaries in the Visceral and Parietal Pleura

Even though the protein content of pleural fluid is normally low (1.5 g/dL), the net Starling's forces favor filtration of fluid into the pleural space. Fluid is removed by lymphatics that communicate directly with the pleural space through holes (*stomata*) in the surface of the parietal pleura. Fluid accumulates in the pleural cavity when capillary pressures increase, or when vascular permeability is increased by inflammation of the pleura (pleuritis). If fibrin accumulates in the pleura, lymphatics may be obstructed, and drainage of the pleural space may be impaired. As a result, large volumes of fluid can accumulate between the lungs and chest wall.

METABOLIC FUNCTIONS OF THE LUNG

The Lung Removes Many Hormones and Toxins from the Blood and Inactivates Many Others

Because it receives the total cardiac output, the pulmonary capillary bed with its vast endothelial surface is ideally placed to cleanse the blood of substances produced in other parts of the body. The cell surface, which is enlarged by projections and by depressions known as *caveoli*, is the site of many enzymes involved in the uptake and metabolism of vasoactive substances. Serotonin is almost totally removed by uptake into endothelial cells, where it is degraded by monoamine oxidase. Norepinephrine is also removed to some degree, but acetylcholine, epinephrine, and histamine are not removed. The peptides bradykinin and angiotensin are metabolized by angiotensin-converting enzyme located on the endothelial surface. Bradykinin is inactivated, whereas angiotensin I is converted into angiotensin II. The lung degrades the majority of prostaglandin E_2 and prostaglandin $F_{2\alpha}$, but prostacyclin is unaffected. Leukotrienes are broken down by neutrophils, which are numerous in the pulmonary circulation. Many exogenous toxic substances are removed also from the blood by the pulmonary endothelium. This process can at times cause severe lung injury. For example, the toxins from *Crotalaria* species of plants can cause smooth muscle hypertrophy in the pulmonary arterioles and pulmonary hypertension.

CLINICAL CORRELATIONS

PLEURITIS IN A THOROUGHBRED HORSE

HISTORY □ You are asked to examine a 3-year-old thoroughbred, which on the previous day had arrived by truck from a racetrack in New York. On arrival, the horse appeared depressed; this morning it refuses to eat and drink and is breathing rapidly. The owner reports that in New York the horse was at a racetrack where there was much through-traffic of young horses, many of which were coughing.

CLINICAL EXAMINATION □ On arrival at the farm, you meet an anxious owner who leads you to a stall, where the thoroughbred is standing with its elbows slightly abducted, its head lowered, its nostrils flared, and an anxious look in its eye. The grain and hay from the morning's feed are untouched. The horse has a respiratory rate of 65 (normal = 12–20). On further questioning, the owner reports that the horse looked much as it does now when it arrived from New York, but he thought that this was just because it was tired from the truck ride. The trucker reported that the horse drank little when it was offered water on the way across country and had only nibbled at its hay. It was in the truck with four other younger horses. The condition of these horses is unknown.

You examine the horse and find that it is febrile, and its pulse rate and respiratory rate are greatly elevated. The horse becomes anxious when approached and particularly when hands are laid upon the thoracic cage. The horse's mucous membranes are a dull red. Auscultation of the abdomen reveals little in the way of gastrointestinal sounds, and there is no evidence of feces in the stall. You listen to the respiratory system and note louder, harsher sounds than normal in the trachea and in the dorsal part of the lung. However, the ventral part of the lung is notably silent.

You elect to take thoracic radiographs and notice that there is a fluid accumulation in the ventral half of the thorax, obscuring the cardiac shadow and much of the lung. In the dorsal part of the thorax, the lung tissue has a number of radiographic densities that have a fluffy appearance, suggesting they are in the alveolar spaces. A cannula is placed in the pleural cavity to drain the pleural fluid, which is foul-smelling and purulent. Fifteen liters are removed, and radiographs then reveal that the alveolar densities extend into the ventral part of the thorax.

Bacterial cultures of the pleural fluid grow an anaerobic organism (*Bacteroides fragilis*), which is probably responsible for the foul smell of the pleural fluid. A complete blood count reveals a decreased number of circulating neutrophils and a large number of immature forms of neutrophils. This is an indication that the neutrophil resources of the body are being depleted, and the bone marrow is putting out immature forms. Presumably, the neutrophils are being sequestered within the lung and pleural cavity.

COMMENT □ The history and clinical findings in this horse are fairly typical of a case of pleuropneumonia. In New York, the horse was exposed to other animals that were coughing, probably as a result of a viral infection, such as equine influenza or equine rhinopneumonitis. Respiratory viruses generally impair the defense mechanisms of the lung in two ways. First, they denude the tracheobronchial epithelium of cilia and, therefore, reduce mucociliary clearance of the airways. Second, they impair macrophage function. This combination of events results in the deposition of bacteria in the lung and failure of the lung to remove them by either the ciliary system or the macrophages. As a result, the bacteria multiply. The stress of shipping, with limited intake of water, probably resulted in the release of corticosteroids from the adrenal gland, and this further suppressed the defense mechanisms of the lung. As a result of these events, the horse acquired an overwhelming bacterial infection of the lung, which resulted in the migration of large numbers of neutrophils into the alveoli. This resulted in the fluffy densities on the radiograph.

When the infection spread to the pleural cavity, neutrophils migrated to this region also. The release of neutrophil products designed to kill bacteria caused extensive damage to the membranes of the alveolar epithelium, pulmonary capillaries, and pleural capillaries. The protein that leaked into the alveolar spaces, interstitium of the lung, and pleural cavity raised the osmotic pressure within these regions. This resulted in the movement of fluid from the vascular space into the alveolar spaces, interstitium, and pleural cavity. Within the pleural cavity, the fluid accumulates ventrally because of gravity, and it is probably this accumulation of fluid that results in the inability to hear lung sounds in the ventral part of the thorax.

TREATMENT □ The chest tube is left in the pleural cavity so the fluid can be drained repeatedly. The horse is given high levels of antibiotics and a prostaglandin-synthetase inhibitor, flunixin, which should reduce the inflammation and make the horse more comfortable. With the degree of alveolar involvement, the presence of an anaerobic organism, and the large amount of fluid in the pleural cavity, the prognosis for this horse is not good.

MITRAL INSUFFICIENCY IN A DOG

HISTORY □ A 12-year-old cocker spaniel is brought to a veterinary hospital because of a recent deterioration in its condition. The dog has been a faithful pet and has always enjoyed exercising with its owner, but over the past few months, the owner has noticed an increasing reluctance to exercise. The dog has also coughed, especially when it gets up from resting. In the last few days, the dog has refused to leave the house and is eating little. The owner has noticed that the cough is much more frequent and seems to be moist.

CLINICAL EXAMINATION □ You have examined this dog on many occasions, and it has always been friendly, but when you walk in the examination room, the dog greets you with only a modest tail wag. It stands with its head down and its tongue hanging out; it is panting. It walks reluctantly toward you when you call it. The dog was formerly fat, but is now in about normal flesh, so over the past few months it has lost some weight.

You lift the dog onto the examination table and begin by looking at the mucous membranes, which appear normal in color. The dog's temperature is normal. The dog is panting, which makes auscultation of the chest difficult, but on the occasions when the dog breathes without panting, you notice some increased sounds in the trachea and in all the lung fields, which sound like fluid bubbling within the air spaces of the lungs. The heart rate is dramatically increased, and there is a loud murmur audible over the mitral area during systole. You tell the owner that you suspect that the dog has a heart problem, which is leading to the accumulation of fluid in the lungs. You take chest radiographs and an arterial blood sample for measurement of blood gas tensions. The chest radiograph shows an enlarged heart, particularly the left ventricle. The lungs are diffusely more dense than normal, and the densities have a fluffy appearance, suggesting they are in the air spaces of the lungs. There is also increased density along the walls of the major airways.

Arterial oxygen tension (Pa_{O_2}) is 70 torr, and arterial CO_2 tension (Pa_{CO_2}) is 30 torr. The radiographs confirm your suspicions. The left side of the heart is enlarged, suggesting there is left heart failure.

COMMENT □ Left heart failure is accompanied by insufficiency of the mitral valve, so blood leaking back into the left atrium during systole creates a murmur. The elevation in left atrial pressure as a result of mitral regurgitation is leading to an increased pressure in the pulmonary veins and capillaries, causing fluid filtration into the interstitium and now into the alveolar air spaces. It is likely that this condition has been progressing for some time, and only when it became severe enough for fluid to accumulate in the air spaces of the lung did the owner notice the deterioration in the dog's condition.

The hypoxemia is a result of ventilation-perfusion mismatching because of accumulation of fluids within the alveolar spaces. These fluid-filled spaces are still perfused, but the blood passing through this region does not pick up a sufficient amount of oxygen. This results in hypoxemia. The hypoxemia stimulates ventilation, and the increase in total ventilation to the lung is sufficient to eliminate more carbon dioxide than normal, so Pa_{CO_2} is 30 torr, rather than the normal level of 40 torr.

TREATMENT □ The dog is treated with a diuretic and a digitalis glycoside. The diuretic causes fluid elimination by the kidneys, which reduces vascular volume and intravascular pressures and, therefore, reduces the amount of fluid being filtered into the lung. In time, this causes resolution of the edema. The digitalis glycoside increases the contractility of the heart and, therefore, the dog's cardiac output, which improves the ability of the dog to exercise.

Bibliography

Bakhle YS, Ferriera SH: Lung metabolism of eicosanoids: Prostaglandin, prostacyclin, thromboxane, and leukotrienes. *In* Fishman AP, Fisher AB, Geiger SR (eds): Handbook of Physiology, Section 3, The Respiratory System, Vol 1, Circulation and Nonrespiratory Function. Bethesda, MD, American Physiological Society, 1985, pp 365–386.

Becker KL, Gazdar AF: The Endocrine Lung in Health and Disease. Philadelphia, WB Saunders, 1984.

Brain JD: Macrophages in the respiratory tract. *In* Fishman AP, Fisher AB, Geiger SR (eds): Handbook of Physiology, Section 3, The Respiratory System, Vol 1, Circulation and Nonrespiratory Function. Bethesda, MD, American Physiological Society, 1985, pp 447–471.

Brain JD, Valberg PA: State of the art. Deposition of aerosol in the respiratory tract. Am Rev Respir Dis 120:1325–1373, 1979.

Green GM, Jakab GT, Low RB, Davis GS: State of the art. Defense mechanisms of the respiratory membrane. Am Rev Respir Dis 115:479–514, 1977.

Jakab GT: Viral-bacterial interactions in respiratory tract infections: A review of the mechanisms of virus-induced suppression of pulmonary antibacterial defenses. *In* Loan RW (ed): Bovine Respiratory Disease: A Symposium. College Station, TX, Texas A&M University Press, 1984, pp 223–286.

Murray JF: The Normal Lung. Philadelphia, WB Saunders, 1986, pp 283–337.

PRACTICE QUESTIONS FOR CHAPTER 48

1. Particles greater than 2 μm in diameter are deposited in the respiratory tract by

   a. inertial deposition in small airways.
   b. sedimentation in airways.
   c. diffusion in the alveoli.
   d. inertial deposition in large airways.
   e. sedimentation in the alveoli.

2. The mucociliary system

   a. consists of a gel layer in which cilia beat, overlain by a sol layer that entraps particles.
   b. extends from the larynx to the end of the bronchi, but not into the bronchioles.
   c. consists in part of mucus produced by goblet cells in the respiratory bronchioles and by Clara cells in the trachea.
   d. has a more rapid transport rate in the trachea than in the bronchioles.
   e. lacks ciliated cells in the bronchioles, so mucus must be pulled into the larger airways by viscous drag.

3. Phagocytosis of inhaled particles

   a. is generally by type II alveolar cells.

   b. can always be accomplished by alveolar macrophages.
   c. sometimes requires both macrophages and neutrophils.
   d. is accentuated by alveolar hypoxia.
   e. Both c and d

4. The transport of fluid from the capillaries to lung lymphatics

   a. does not occur in a normal animal.
   b. is accentuated by an increase in capillary hydrostatic pressure.
   c. is accentuated by an increase in capillary oncotic pressure.
   d. occurs through the surface of alveolar air spaces.
   e. Both b and d

5. Which of the following occurs as a result of enzymes localized on the pulmonary endothelium?

   a. Conversion of angiotensin I to angiotensin II
   b. Conversion of angiotensinogen to angiotensin I
   c. Release of renin
   d. Conversion of renin to angiotensin II
   e. None of the above

N. EDWARD ROBINSON

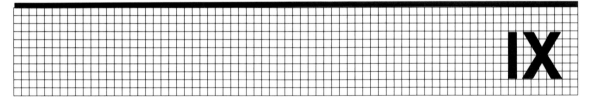

IX

HOMEOSTASIS

49

Fetal and Neonatal Oxygen Transport

1. The fetus depends on the placenta for exchange of gas, nutrients, and metabolic byproducts
2. The efficiency of gas exchange at the placenta depends on the arrangement of fetal and maternal blood vessels, which varies with species
3. The fetal circulation mixes oxygenated and deoxygenated blood at several points, so the fetus exists in a state of hypoxemia
4. Fetal oxygen transport is assisted by fetal hemoglobin, which has a high affinity for oxygen
5. The lung, which is an outgrowth of the foregut, develops in three stages, and surfactant must be present at the time of birth
6. At the time of birth or shortly thereafter, umbilical vessels rupture, pulmonary vascular resistance decreases, and the foramen ovale and ductus arteriosus close

The Fetus Depends on the Placenta for Exchange of Gas, Nutrients, and Metabolic Byproducts

From conception until birth, the *embryo* and *fetus* depend on the mother for a supply of oxygen and nutrients and for removal of carbon dioxide and other metabolic byproducts. Until the *placenta* develops, the embryo exchanges these substances by diffusion through the uterine fluids. As the *conceptus* increases in size, the specialized exchange organ, known as the placenta, becomes essential. The placenta brings maternal and fetal blood into close apposition over a large surface area that is provided by a network of capillaries.

The gross appearance of the placenta of different species varies widely. In horses and

pigs, the placenta is *diffuse* and covers most of the uterine epithelium. In ruminants, the placenta consists of rows of discrete circular to oval *cotyledons* that are attached to highly vascularized *caruncles*, approximately 100 in number, in the uterine epithelium. In dogs, the placenta is *zonary*, forming a circular band around the *allantochorion* of the puppy. A complete listing of types of placentation of different species is provided in Table 49–1.

As well as differing in the amount of uterine surface to which they are attached, placentas also differ in the number of layers of cells that separate the maternal and fetal blood (Table 49–1). In horses, pigs, sheep, and cows, the fetal *chorion* is applied to the maternal *uterine epithelium* (*epitheliochorial* placentation), whereas in carnivores, the chorion is applied

593

Table 49–1
PLACENTATION OF DOMESTIC MAMMALS

Species	Classification	
	Gross	*Histologic*
Horse	Diffuse	Epitheliochorial
Pig	Diffuse	Epitheliochorial
Cow	Cotyledonary	Epitheliochorial
Sheep	Cotyledonary	Epitheliochorial
Goat	Cotyledonary	Epitheliochorial
Dog	Zonary	Endotheliochorial
Cat	Zonary	Endotheliochorial
Rabbit	Discoid	Hemochorial
Guinea pig	Discoid	Hemochorial

to the *endothelium* of maternal vessels (*endotheliochorial* placentation); in rodents and most primates, the chorion invades the uterine mucosa and erodes the maternal capillaries, so it becomes bathed by maternal blood (*hemochorial* placentation).

The Efficiency of Gas Exchange at the Placenta Depends on the Arrangement of Fetal and Maternal Blood Vessels, Which Varies with Species

The exchange of gases and other substances across the placenta is determined by several factors, including the amount of surface apposition between fetal and maternal tissues, and the number of layers of cells separating

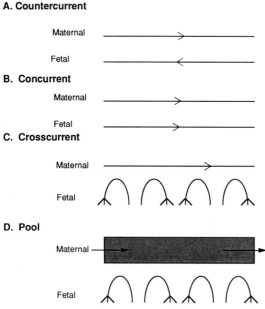

Figure 49–1. Schematic representation of possible arrangements of fetal and maternal blood vessels. (From Dawes GS: Foetal and Neonatal Physiology. Chicago, Year Book Medical Publishers, 1968.)

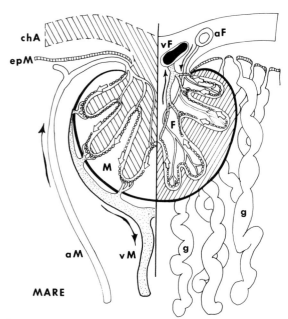

Figure 49–2. Diagram showing the arrangement of maternal and fetal blood vessels in the microcotyledons of the equine placenta. Small open arrows demonstrate the postulated countercurrent directions of maternal and fetal blood flows. *aM*, maternal artery; *vM*, maternal vein; *chA*, chorioallantois; *epM*, uterine epithelium; *g*, endometrial glands; *aF*, fetal artery; *vF*, fetal vein; *F*, fetal; *M*, maternal. (Based on data in Tsutsumi Y: Journal of Agriculture, Hokkaido (imp.) University 52:372–482, 1962; reproduced with permission from Cross GS, Comline KS, Nathanielzs PW (eds): Foetal and Neonatal Physiology: Proceedings. Sir Joseph Barcroft Centenary Symposium. Cambridge, Cambridge University Press, 1973, pp 245–271.)

fetal and maternal blood. However, a major factor determining exchange is the arrangement of fetal and maternal blood vessels within the small interdigitating *villi* of the placenta. Figure 49–1 gives schematic representations of the possible arrangements of vessels. *Countercurrent* flow of maternal and fetal blood provides the most efficient exchange and allows equilibration of fetal and maternal arterial gas tensions. *Concurrent* flow of fetal and maternal blood allows fetal vessels to equilibrate with the maternal venous gas tensions. In *crosscurrent* and *pool* types of *equilibrators*, fetal capillaries loop down to maternal vessels or into a pool of maternal blood. These types of exchangers are not easily described by any simple model. It is likely that several different arrangements of vessels are found in the placentas of all species, but some seem to have more of the characteristics of countercurrent exchangers, and others those of venous equilibrators.

Figure 49–2 shows the arrangement of vessels in the *microcotyledon* of the horse, a species in which fetal and maternal blood flow is primarily countercurrent. The cotyledonary placenta of sheep functions as a venous equilibrator, whereas the labyrinthine hemochorial placenta of the rabbit seems to be a countercurrent exchanger.

Placental gas exchange has been best studied in the sheep and is summarized in Figure 49–3. Maternal blood enters the uterus with a P_{O_2} of 80 torr and leaves with a P_{O_2} of 50 torr. Some of this blood supplies the *myometrium* and *endometrium*, but most participates in gas exchange in the cotyledon. Fetal arterial blood enters the cotyledon with a P_{O_2} of 24 torr, but after gas exchange only has a P_{O_2} of 32 torr. This is because the sheep placenta is a venous equilibrator, so the maximal possible P_{O_2} would be 50 torr. However, this maximum is not reached, because venous blood, which has provided nutrient blood flow to the chorion, dilutes the better oxygenated blood draining from the cotyledon. The countercurrent exchanger of the horse is apparently more efficient, because umbilical venous P_{O_2} averages 48 torr.

The amount of placenta available for exchange in part determines the ultimate size of the fetus. If uterine caruncles are surgically removed from sheep so there are less sites for formation of fetal cotyledons, the full-term weight of lambs is reduced. Similarly, in horses, it is rare to see twins survive to term and be of equal size. The diffuse placenta of the horse apparently can support only one full-size fetus. One foal in a set of twins is usually very small or dies *in utero.*

The Fetal Circulation Mixes Oxygenated and Deoxygenated Blood at Several Points, So the Fetus Exists in a State of Hypoxemia

In the adult, the *cardiac output* of the right and left ventricles is separated and perfuses the pulmonary and systemic circulations, respectively. In the fetus, the output of the two sides of the heart mixes at several points, so it is convenient to use the term cardiac output to refer to the combined output of the right and left ventricles. The combined cardiac output averages 500 mL/minute/kg in fetal sheep, with the output of the right ventricle exceeding that of the left. Figure 49–4 is a diagram of the fetal circulation showing the percentage of the

cardiac output traversing the major vessels and the P_{O_2} within these vessels.

The placenta, which has a low vascular resistance, receives 45% of the cardiac output through the *umbilical arteries.* The *umbilical veins* drain the placenta toward the liver. In species such as the sheep, most of the umbilical venous blood passes through the liver through a low resistance channel known as the *ductus venosus;* in other species, such as the pig and horse, the ductus venosus disappears early in gestation, and umbilical venous blood flows through the liver capillaries. Within the liver, the oxygenated blood from the placenta is mixed with a small amount of less well-oxygenated blood draining the liver sinusoids. The hepatic venous blood enters the posterior vena cava, where it mixes with poorly oxygenated blood, draining the hind end of the fetus, so the blood returning to the right atrium has a P_{O_2} of 25 torr.

A low resistance pathway, the *foramen ovale*, connects the right and left atria, and a structure known as the *crista dividens* directs the better oxygenated blood from the posterior vena cava through the foramen ovale to the left atrium. The poorly oxygenated blood returning to the *right atrium* in the cranial vena cava is directed into the right atrium and *right ventricle.* Most of the output of the right ventricle does not go through the lungs, however, because in the fetus the lungs have a high vascular resistance. Another low resistance channel, the *ductus arteriosus*, connects the *pulmonary artery* with the *aorta* and allows blood to bypass the lungs. It is important to note that the arrangement of the fetal circulation allows the better oxygenated blood to enter the left ventricle, from where it reaches the brachycephalic vessels and the front of the animal. The less well-oxygenated blood from the ductus arteriosus enters the aorta downstream from the brachycephalic vessels. The tissues of the hind end of the animal and the placenta receive blood with a P_{O_2} of approximately 22 torr.

Flow of blood from the right to the left atria through the foramen ovale, and from pulmonary artery to aorta through the ductus arteriosus, requires that the pressure in the right side of the fetal circulation is greater than that in the left side. This occurs because the low resistance placenta receives a large part of the output of the left ventricle, whereas the output of the right ventricle is opposed by the high resistance pulmonary circulation. At term, arterial pressure in the lamb is about 42 mmHg.

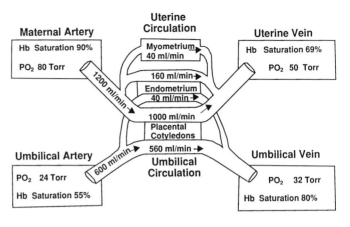

Figure 49–3. Numerical data that demonstrate normal conditions of placental oxygen transfer in sheep. (From Battaglia FC, Meschia G: An Introduction to Fetal Physiology. Orlando, FL, Academic Press, 1986, p 157).

The fetal circulation is not a passive system but is capable of considerable regulation, particularly as the fetus matures. *Fetal hypoxia* can stimulate vasodilation in the heart and brain, and vasoconstriction in the gut, kidneys, and skeletal tissues. The fetal pulmonary circulation constricts vigorously when the fetus is hypoxic. This constriction diverts more blood through the ductus arteriosus to the systemic tissues.

Fetal Oxygen Transport Is Assisted by Fetal Hemoglobin, Which Has a High Affinity for Oxygen

Fetal arterial blood has a low P_{O_2} because the placenta is not a highly efficient gas exchanger, and because oxygenated and venous blood mix at several points in the fetal circulation. The fetus is adapted to this state of chronic hypoxia in two ways. First, it has a high cardiac output that delivers a large volume of blood per minute to the tissues. Secondly, the fetus produces erythrocytes containing hemoglobin with a high *affinity* for oxygen.

The production of erythrocytes initially occurs in the *yolk sac*. These embryonic erythrocytes are nucleated and contain embryonic hemoglobin, the oxygen affinity of which is not clearly defined. At the termination of the embryonic period, erythrocyte production shifts to the liver and spleen. Depending on the species, fetal red cells contain either *fetal* or *adult hemoglobin* (see later). Simultaneously, there are changes in glycolytic enzymes to provide the fetal concentrations of *2,3-diphosphoglycerate* (2,3-DPG). Fetal erythrocytes have a higher affinity for oxygen than maternal erythrocytes, i.e., the fetal blood oxyhemoglobin dissociation curve lies to the left of the adult curve (Fig. 49–5). In some species, such as the cat, the difference in P_{50} between fetus and adult is small, whereas in ruminants the difference is 10–20 torr.

Three different mechanisms account for the position of the fetal oxyhemoglobin dissociation curve. In ruminants, the higher oxygen affinity results from synthesis of fetal hemoglobin with a high intrinsic oxygen affinity. Fetal hemoglobin of these species is unresponsive to 2,3-DPG. After birth there is gradual replacement of fetal by adult hemoglobin. In primates, there is little intrinsic difference in the oxygen affinity of fetal and maternal hemoglobin, but fetal hemoglobin has a decreased interaction with DPG. In horses and pigs, there is no fetal hemoglobin; embryonic hemoglobin is replaced immediately by adult hemoglobin. The fetal erythrocytes of these species have a low concentration of 2,3-DPG. Following birth, there is an increase in the concentration of 2,3-DPG, which gives the hemoglobin its adult dissociation curve.

The high affinity of fetal hemoglobin for oxygen allows the hemoglobin in the umbilical veins with a P_{O_2} of 30 torr to be 80% saturated with oxygen, and the hemoglobin in the aorta with a P_{O_2} of 22 torr to be 56% saturated. Although fetal hemoglobin allows the transport of oxygen at the low P_{O_2} existing in fetal arteries, it also necessitates low oxygen tensions in fetal tissues in order to unload oxygen from fetal hemoglobin. Therefore, the fetus exists in a state of tissue hypoxia when compared to the adult.

The Lung, Which Is an Outgrowth of the Foregut, Develops in Three Stages, and Surfactant Must Be Present at the Time of Birth

By the time of birth, the lung must be ready to assume the gas exchange functions of the

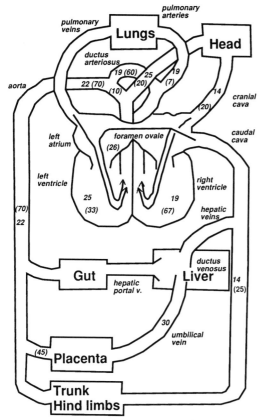

Figure 49–4. Diagrammatic representation of the fetal circulation showing the oxygen tension in torr and percentage of cardiac output *(parentheses)* in different parts of the circulation.

placenta. The lung develops in three stages of equivalent duration. Beginning as an outgrowth of the foregut, the lung bud invades the *mesenchyme* of the thorax and divides into all the major airway branches in the first third of gestation. Because these *primordial airways* are lined with a *cuboidal epithelium* and look like a gland in cross section, this stage of development is known as the *glandular stage.* In the second phase of development, the lung is invaded by blood vessels (the *canalicular stage*). In the final or *alveolar sac stage,* alveolar sacs and, in some species, *alveoli*, develop. The stage of maturity of the lung at birth in general matches the maturity of the fetus. Lambs and piglets have well-developed alveoli, but humans and, more especially, rodents have thicker walled alveolar sacs. In these latter species, alveoli develop as the animal grows postnatally.

Pulmonary surfactant is essential if the lung is to remain inflated after birth (see Chapter 43). Beginning at about mid-gestation, there is

an increase in the synthesis of surfactant components, such as lecithin, within the lung. This increase in *lecithin* synthesis coincides with the appearance of *type II alveolar cells,* the source of surfactant, and with an increase in pulmonary blood flow. Some of this lecithin is secreted into the alveolar lumens and appears in the amniotic fluid, where it can be measured as an indicator of the state of lung maturity. Lung maturity coincides with an increase in *serum cortisol* in the fetus.

Until the time of birth, the *vascular resistance* of the fetal pulmonary circulation is high for several reasons. The fetal lung is not inflated; therefore, the large vessels are not pulled open by the surrounding *alveolar septa.* In addition, the hypoxia of the fetus maintains the pulmonary vascular smooth muscle in a state of contraction that narrows the arteries. Both of these conditions are alleviated by the first few breaths.

The fetal lung continuously secretes fluid until about 2 days before birth. This fluid, which is rich in chloride and low in bicarbonate and protein, travels up the trachea into the *amniotic cavity.* The fluid in the alveolar spaces and airways is in part squeezed out of the lung as the thorax is compressed during birth. The majority is reabsorbed by lymphatics and blood vessels shortly after birth.

In late gestation, the fetus makes *breathing movements,* although it moves little of the viscous fluid to and fro in the airways. These movements apparently prepare the respiratory muscles for their postnatal function.

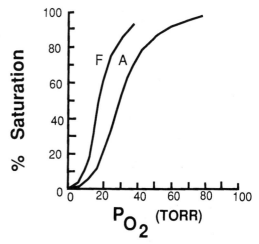

Figure 49–5. Oxyhemoglobin dissociation curves of fetal (*F*) and adult (*A*) sheep.

At the Time of Birth or Shortly Thereafter, Umbilical Vessels Rupture, Pulmonary Vascular Resistance Decreases, and the Foramen Ovale and Ductus Arteriosus Close

At term, the fetus is dependent on the placenta and its dam for exchange with the environment, but the lung and other organs must be ready to assume their postnatal functions. During a normal birth, the newborn emerges from the birth canal at about the time the placenta is detaching from the uterine wall. Placental gas exchange probably continues well into third-stage *labor*. If labor is prolonged, the placenta may detach before the newborn is delivered.

Immediately after delivery, the newborn takes the first breath. The stimuli for this include (1) hypoxia and hypercarbia, which result from the loss of the placental gas exchanger; (2) cooling as the fetal fluids evaporate from the skin; and (3) a generalized increase in sensory input to the fetus as it is licked and nuzzled by its dam. Moving the first air into the lungs requires a considerable effort as viscous fluids must be inhaled down the airways before air can enter the alveoli. The critical opening pressures of the fluid-filled small airways and alveoli must be exceeded also. All alveoli may not inflate during the first breath, but subsequent inhalations will inflate all the lung and distribute surfactant over the alveolar surface. This surfactant makes the alveoli stable and prevents their collapse, so a stable *functional residual capacity* can be established. After the first few breaths, arterial oxygen tension is much higher than in the fetus, yet breathing continues. It appears, therefore, that breathing is inhibited *in utero*, and the chemoreceptors are insensitive to hypoxia. Inhibition is removed after birth.

Inflation and oxygenation of the lung reduce the pulmonary vascular resistance and, therefore, decrease pressure in the pulmonary artery, right ventricle, and right atrium. At about the same time, the umbilical vessels rupture, because the animal struggles. Umbilical blood flow is arrested by local vasoconstriction in the umbilical vessels. The loss of the low resistance placental circulation increases systemic vascular resistance, which increases pressure in the aorta, left ventricle, and left atrium. As a result of these changes, aortic pressure exceeds pulmonary arterial pressure, and left atrial pressure exceeds right atrial pressure. Blood flow through the ductus ar-

teriosus and foramen ovale reverses. Flow reversal in the foramen ovale causes a flap valve to close and occlude the foramen. Over succeeding days to weeks, this valve becomes adherent to the wall of the atrium, thus permanently closing the foramen. Reversal of flow in the ductus arteriosus exposes the ductus wall to well-oxygenated blood. This causes constriction of smooth muscle in the wall of the ductus, thus arresting blood flow.

Ductus closure involves a change in *prostaglandin* levels. Administration of drugs, such as indomethacin, that inhibit prostaglandin synthesis constricts the ductus in fetal sheep, and administration of prostaglandin-E_2 dilates it. Once the ductus has constricted and flow has been arrested, the ductus gradually is converted into a fibrous band of scar tissue.

The changes described in the previous paragraphs convert the fetal circulation into the adult circulation able to support the gas exchange function of the lung. The amazing thing is that these changes happen routinely and without medical assistance in almost all animal births.

CLINICAL CORRELATION

PATENT DUCTUS ARTERIOSUS IN A POMERANIAN

HISTORY ☐ A 7-week-old female Pomeranian puppy is presented to you because it is not growing as fast as its litter mates. The breeder says it is lethargic and prefers to sleep when the other puppies play.

CLINICAL EXAMINATION ☐ Clinical examination reveals a small puppy with a rapid heart rate. The mucous membranes of its gums are pink, and its temperature is normal. While holding the puppy around the thorax, you notice a vibration in the region of the heart. When you listen with a stethoscope, you hear a loud murmur that is almost continuous through systole and diastole, and you recall that this is called a "machinery murmur." It is difficult to listen to the breath sounds because the murmur is audible all over the thorax. A radiograph reveals an enlarged heart, but the lungs appear normal, although a little compressed by the heart.

COMMENT ☐ The clinical and radiographic

findings in a puppy of this age are characteristic of a patent ductus arteriosus. In some animals the ductus fails to close after birth, and blood continues to flow through it, usually from the aorta to the pulmonary artery. This presents the animal with two problems. First, the left ventricle must increase its output to supply the systemic tissues because so much is blood is passing through the ductus. Second, the pulmonary circulation has a volume overload that increases the pressure against which the right ventricle must work. These extra loads result in dilation of the ventricles and sometimes in hypertrophy of the myocardium. This is seen on radiographs as an enlarged heart. The puppy is not growing and is listless because the tissues are not receiving a normal blood flow. The patent ductus must be closed surgically. It would be unwise to breed this animal in the future, because the condition is inherited.

Bibliography

Battaglia FC, Meschia G: An Introduction to Fetal Physiology. Orlando, Academic Press, 1986, pp 1–48, 154–211.

Dawes GS: Foetal and Neonatal Physiology. Chicago, Year Book Medical Publishers, 1968.

Faber JJ, Thornburg KL: Placental Physiology: Structure and Function of Fetomaternal Exchange. New York, Raven Press, 1983, pp 1–32.

Murray JF: The Normal Lung: the Basis for Diagnosis and Treatment of Pulmonary Disease, 2nd ed. Philadelphia, WB Saunders, 1986, pp 1–21.

Silver M, Steven DH, Comline RS: Placental exchange and morphology in ruminants and the mare. *In* Comline KS, Cross KW, Dawes GS, Nathanielzs PW (eds): Foetal and Neonatal Physiology. Proceedings of the Sir Joseph Barcroft Centenary Symposium. Cambridge, Cambridge University Press, 1973, pp 245–271.

PRACTICE QUESTIONS FOR CHAPTER 49

1. The vascular channel that allows fetal blood to pass from the pulmonary artery to the aorta is known as the

   a. foramen ovale.
   b. ductus arteriosus.
   c. ductus venosus.
   d. fetal cotyledon.
   e. allantois.

2. Which of the following fetal blood vessels contains blood with the highest P_{O_2}?

   a. Aorta
   b. Ductus arteriosus
   c. Pulmonary artery
   d. Left ventricle
   e. Umbilical artery

3. Which of the following statements about the fetal circulation is true?

   a. Right atrial pressure is higher than left atrial pressure.
   b. Pulmonary vascular resistance is high.
   c. The placenta receives about 45% of the combined output of both ventricles.
   d. The output of the right is greater than that of the left ventricle.
   e. All of the above

4. Which of the following does NOT correctly describe the lung *in utero*?

   a. Type II cells, which produce surfactant, are present within the first few days of gestation in sheep.
   b. Chloride-rich fluid is secreted into the airways and flows into the amniotic cavity.
   c. Components of surfactant can be detected in the amniotic fluid when the lung approaches maturity.
   d. All the major branches of the tracheobronchial tree are present at birth, but alveoli continue to multiply postpartum.
   e. Breathing movements occur *in utero*, but the volume of fluid moved in and out of the lungs is small.

5. Which of the following lists the events that follow birth in the correct sequence?

   a. Closure of foramen ovale, first breath, rupture of umbilical vessels
   b. Decrease in right atrial pressure, first breath, closure of the ductus arteriosus
   c. First breath, closure of the ductus arteriosus, decrease in pulmonary arterial pressure
   d. First breath, decrease in pulmonary arterial pressure, closure of the foramen ovale
   e. Closure of the foramen ovale, closure of the ductus arteriosus, first breath

6. Fetal oxygen transport is assisted by

    a. fetal hemoglobin, which has a lower oxygen capacity than adult hemoglobin.

    b. fetal hemoglobin, which has a lower P_{50} than adult hemoglobin.

    c. a cardiac output that is less per kilogram of body weight than in the adult.

    d. a cardiac output that preferentially delivers the blood with the highest P_{O_2} to the placenta.

    e. a fetal lung, which is an efficient gas exchanger.

7. Which of the following domestic mammals has a diffuse, epitheliochorial placenta in which fetal and maternal blood flow is countercurrent in the microcotyledons?

    a. Dog

    b. Cow

    c. Horse

    d. Rabbit

    e. Sheep

50

Acid-Base Homeostasis

1. Relative constancy of the body's pH is essential, because metabolism requires enzymes that operate at an optimal pH
2. Hydrogen ion concentration is measured as pH
3. An acid can donate a hydrogen ion, and a base can accept a hydrogen ion
4. Buffers are combinations of salts and weak acids that prevent major changes in pH
5. Hemoglobin and bicarbonate are the most important blood buffers
6. Intracellular buffering is provided by proteins and organic phosphate
7. The first defense against a change in blood pH is provided by the blood buffers, but it is the lungs and the kidneys that must ultimately correct the hydrogen ion load
8. Changes in ventilation can rapidly change P_{CO_2} and, therefore, alter pH
9. Metabolic production of fixed acids requires that the kidneys eliminate hydrogen ions and conserve HCO_3^-

ACID-BASE DISTURBANCES

1. Acid-base abnormalities accompany many diseases, and the restoration of normal blood pH should be a consideration when treating any disease
2. In respiratory acidosis, the accumulation of carbon dioxide in the blood decreases pH
3. In respiratory alkalosis, the loss of carbon dioxide from the blood increases pH
4. In metabolic acidosis, the accumulation of fixed acids or loss of buffer base decreases blood pH
5. Metabolic alkalosis is caused by the excessive elimination of hydrogen ions or by the intake of base, such as HCO_3^-
6. Respiratory compensations occur rapidly; renal compensations occur over several hours
7. Hydrogen and potassium ions are interrelated in acid-base homeostasis
8. The diagnosis of acid-base disturbances depends on interpretation of measurements of arterial blood pH and P_{CO_2} from which $[HCO_3^-]$ and total buffer base are calculated
9. Over the years, a large number of terms have been used to explain acid-base balance

Relative Constancy of the Body's pH Is Essential, Because Metabolism Requires Enzymes That Operate at an Optimal pH

For optimal functioning of the cells constituting the animal, the ionic composition of body fluids is maintained within fairly narrow limits. *Hydrogen* is one of the ions that determines the *acidity* or *pH* of the body fluids. Serious deviations of pH outside the normal range can drastically disrupt cell metabolism and, therefore, body function.

When veterinarians use the term *acidosis* and *alkalosis*, they are comparing the pH of an animal's arterial blood with the normal value of 7.4. A pH below 7.4 is referred to as acidosis, above 7.4 alkalosis. The range of pH compatible with life is 6.85–7.8, but rarely are these extremes approached. The body buffers, lungs, and kidneys all defend the body from onslaught by hydrogen ions from a variety of sources.

The biggest daily load of hydrogen ions (*protons*) arises during the transport of carbon dioxide from the tissues to the lungs. If the lungs eliminate carbon dioxide as fast as it is produced in the tissues, there is no net hydrogen ion gain by the body. However, the balance between carbon dioxide production and elimination may be disturbed during exercise or respiratory disease, thus threatening *acid-base* homeostasis.

Hydrogen ions are also a product of protein metabolism, which produces sulfuric and phosphoric acids, fat metabolism, and the incomplete oxidation of glucose to lactic acid. Hydrogen ions from these sources, although normally small in amount in comparison to that produced in CO_2 transport, must be eliminated continuously by the kidneys. In disease, the hydrogen ion load imposed on the body is frequently increased because of an increase in tissue breakdown (*catabolism*), or because the kidneys fail to eliminate hydrogen ion. In rarer instances, hydrogen ion is lost from the body, e.g., in vomit. To understand how the body regulates pH and how acid-base disorders are diagnosed, it is first necessary to review acids, bases, and buffering.

Hydrogen Ion Concentration Is Measured as pH

Only one in 550 million molecules of water is *ionized*, making the concentration of hydrogen and hydroxyl ions in water 1×10^{-7} mol/L. The *chemical potential* of the hydrogen ions is known as the acidity and is expressed in pH units. pH is the *negative logarithm* of the hydrogen ion concentration. Water with 1×10^{-7} mol/L of hydrogen ion and an equal concentration of hydroxyl ions has a pH of 7.0, i.e., a neutral pH. A decrease in pH indicates increasing acidity; for example, a decrease of 1.0 pH represents a tenfold increase in hydrogen ion concentration. Doubling hydrogen ion concentration decreases pH by only 0.3 unit.

The normal range of blood pH, 6.85–7.80, represents a hydrogen ion concentration of 1.4×10^{-7} to 1.6×10^{-8} Eq/L. Thus, although hydrogen ion concentration is regulated, up to tenfold changes can occur, much greater than the changes observed in the concentration of other ions, such as sodium or potassium.

An Acid Can Donate a Hydrogen Ion, and a Base Can Accept a Hydrogen Ion

Hydrochloric acid (HCl) is a *strong acid*, because it dissociates completely in water into H^+ and Cl^-. Chloride ion is a base, because it has the potential to accept a hydrogen ion, but it is a *weak base*, because HCl is so completely dissociated. Carbonic acid, in contrast, is a *weak acid*, because it is incompletely dissociated in solution to hydrogen and bicarbonate ions. Bicarbonate, however, is a relatively *strong base* that can accept a hydrogen ion and form undissociated carbonic acid. When carbonic acid is formed, hydrogen ions are removed from solution, and the concentration of free hydrogen ions decreases. Bases do not have to be ions. Ammonia, NH_3, is a base, because it can accept a proton and become ammonium ion, NH_4^+. This reaction is of little importance in the blood, but it is important in the distal renal tubule. Proteins act also as buffers by virtue of the terminal amino and carboxyl groups, which can accept and donate protons.

Buffers Are Combinations of Salts and Weak Acids That Prevent Major Changes in pH

Usually buffers are mixtures of weak acids and their salts. Imagine a solution containing sodium bicarbonate and carbonic acid. Sodium bicarbonate dissociates completely into sodium and bicarbonate ions; carbonic acid dissociates incompletely into hydrogen and bicarbonate ions. Thus, in the solution there are sodium, hydrogen, and bicarbonate ions, and undissociated carbonic acid. If a strong acid such as HCl is added to the solution, the added hydrogen ions upset the dissociation equilibrium of carbonic acid. Hydrogen ions combine with bicarbonate ion to form carbonic acid, thus reducing the concentration of hydrogen ions, i.e., preventing a major change in pH.

If, in contrast, sodium hydroxide is added to the solution, the hydroxyl ions, formed by dissociation of sodium hydroxide, combine with hydrogen ion to form water. The decrease in hydrogen ion causes dissociation of more carbonic acid, again preventing a large change in pH.

The dissociation of a weak acid and, therefore, the concentration of hydrogen ion, base, and undissociated acid are determined by the *dissociation constant* (K_A) and can be described by the *law of mass action*. For carbonic acid

$$K_A = \frac{[H^+][HCO_3^-]}{[H_2CO_3]}$$

Taking logarithms of both sides of this equation results in

$$\log K_A = \log \frac{[H^+][HCO_3^-]}{[H_2CO_3]}$$

or

$$\log K_A = \log [H^+] + \log \frac{[HCO_3^-]}{[H_2CO_3]}$$

Rearranging

$$-\log [H^+] = -\log K_A + \log \frac{[HCO_3^-]}{[H_2CO_3]}$$

but $-\log [H^+]$ is pH and $-\log K_A$ is defined as pK. Therefore,

$$pH = pK + \log \frac{[HCO_3^-]}{[H_2CO_3]}$$

This is the *Henderson-Hasselbalch equation* written for the bicarbonate, carbonic acid system. It can be written for any buffering system in the generic form:

$$pH = pK + \log \frac{[base]}{[acid]}$$

This equation shows that the pH of a solution is determined by the ratio of the concentration of base (the hydrogen ion acceptor) and undissociated acid (the hydrogen ion donor), and by the pK of the buffering system.

Figure 50–1 shows the change in pH that results when acid is added to a phosphate buffer with a pK of 6.8. This is a graphical description of the Henderson-Hasselbalch equation. Initially, as acid is added, there is a large decrease in pH. As considerably more acid is added to the solution, pH changes little. Hydrogen ions combine with $HPO_4^=$ and form $H_2PO_4^-$. Finally, pH decreases considerably. The zone over which pH changes little as acid is added, i.e., where buffering capacity is optimal, is within plus or minus one pH unit of pK. Note that when pH equals pK, 50% of the buffer has been consumed. From this buffer curve it is obvious that an effective buffer must have a pK within plus or minus one pH unit of the solution in which it operates. Thus, the optimal blood buffers should have a pK between 6.4 and 8.4. In addition, buffers must be sufficiently plentiful to be effective.

Hemoglobin and Bicarbonate Are the Most Important Blood Buffers

Hemoglobin is an important blood buffer because it is plentiful, and because the *imidazole residues* of globin *histidine* have a pK close to blood pH. In actuality, the pK of hemoglobin

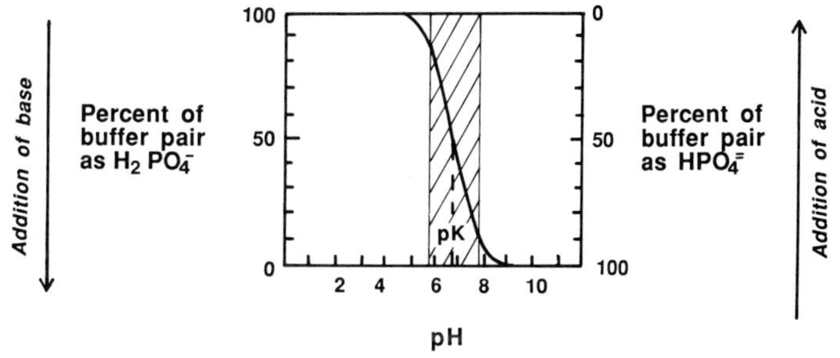

Figure 50–1. Titration curve for the phosphate buffer system. pK is 6.8. The shaded area represents the range of pH over which this buffer is effective.

changes with the degree of oxygenation. Because deoxyhemoglobin has a pK (7.93) closer to blood pH than oxyhemoglobin (pK = 6.68), deoxyhemoglobin provides more buffering capacity. When arterial blood enters the tissue capillaries, oxygen leaves hemoglobin, so the resulting deoxyhemoglobin is an excellent buffer for the hydrogen ions produced when CO_2 is added to the blood.

The other blood buffer with an optimal pK is the $HPO_4^=/H_2PO_4^-$ system with a pK of 6.8 (see Fig. 50–1). The normally low phosphate concentration in the blood makes this buffering system quantitatively unimportant; however, it is important in the renal tubules where phosphate is concentrated. *Plasma proteins* also provide a small amount of blood buffering.

Although a pK of 6.1 would seem to make the HCO_3^-/H_2CO_3 buffer unimportant for blood buffering, this is not so for two reasons. First, there is a large amount of HCO_3^- (24 mEq/L) in blood, and secondly, the concentration of HCO_3^- can be regulated by the kidneys, whereas the concentration of H_2CO_3 can be regulated by the lungs. Because the salt and acid concentration can be regulated, the HCO_3^-/H_2CO_3 system is said to be an open system. Figure 50–2 shows the value of this open system in maintaining body pH.

The HCO_3^-/H_2CO_3 buffering system is also of great value to clinicians, because its components can be readily measured in the clinical laboratory and used to diagnose acid-base disturbances. It is not necessary to measure the components of every buffering system to diagnose acid-base disturbances. If one system is known, changes in other systems can be predicted.

In the Henderson-Hasselbach equation for the HCO_3^-/H_2CO_3 system, it is usual to measure pH and $[H_2CO_3]$, and derive $[HCO_3^-]$. The latter depends on the PCO_2 and a constant α with a value of 0.03. So, the $[H_2CO_3]$ in solution is directly proportional to P_{CO_2}, with one molecule of H_2CO_3 being in equilibrium with 340 CO_2 molecules. The $[H_2CO_3]$ is calculated as $0.03 \cdot P_{CO_2}$; for clinical use, the Henderson-Hasselbach equation for the HCO_3^-/H_2CO_3 system is written:

$$pH = pK + \log \frac{[HCO_3^-]}{[0.03 \, P_{CO_2}]}$$

Under normal conditions, pH of arterial blood is 7.4, $[HCO_3^-]$ is 24 mEq/L, and Pa_{CO_2} is equal to 40 torr.

$$7.4 = 6.1 + \frac{\log 24}{0.03 \cdot 40} = 6.1 + \log \frac{20}{1}$$

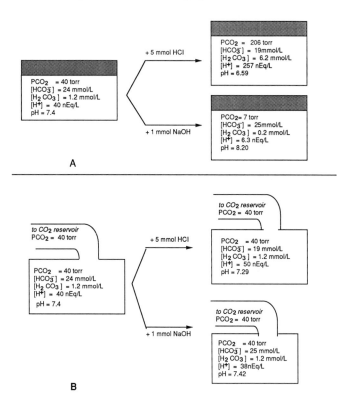

Figure 50–2. Buffer function of the carbonic acid–bicarbonate system under closed (*A*) and open (*B*) conditions. Under closed conditions the *total* quantity of the buffer (acid plus base components) remains constant. Under open conditions the P_{CO_2} of the system, and thus the $[H_2CO_3]$, is maintained at a fixed level by continuous equilibration of the liquid phase with a gas reservoir of constant P_{CO_2}. The term $[H_2CO_3]$ denotes the combined concentration of carbonic acid and dissolved CO_2. (Reprinted with permission from Madias, Nicolaos E, Cohen J: Acid-base chemistry and buffering. *In* Cohen JJ, Kassirer JP (eds): Acid Base. Boston, Little, Brown and Company, 1982.)

This equation demonstrates that a normal blood pH requires a ratio of $[HCO_3^-]/[\alpha P_{CO_2}]$ of 20:1.

Intracellular Buffering Is Provided by Proteins and Organic Phosphate

Whereas the hemoglobin and bicarbonate provide the most immediately available source of buffers to prevent drastic changes in blood pH, *intracellular buffers* within the body tissues provide another large reserve of buffering capacity. In order to enter cells, hydrogen ion must be exchanged with other cations, such as sodium or potassium. Once inside the cell, hydrogen ion is buffered by *amino acids, peptides,* and *proteins,* and by *organic phosphates.* These buffers provide approximately five times the buffering capacity of the extracellular fluid.

The First Defense Against a Change in Blood pH Is Provided by the Blood Buffers, but It Is the Lungs and the Kidneys That Must Ultimately Correct the Hydrogen Ion Load

When body pH is threatened by a change in the production or elimination of hydrogen ions, the first line of defense is provided by buffers within the blood and tissues. However, buffers are only preventing drastic changes in pH; they cannot correct the problem by increasing or decreasing the elimination of hydrogen ions or by replacing lost buffering capacity. Ultimately, pH must be corrected by adjustments in ventilation or by changes in renal function. Because the lungs can alter Pa_{CO_2} and the kidneys can regulate $[HCO_3^-]$, the Henderson-Hasselbalch equation has been written as

$$pH = pK + \log \frac{\text{kidneys}}{\text{lungs}}$$

Changes in Ventilation Can Rapidly Change P_{CO_2} and, Therefore, Alter pH

As blood flows through the tissues, carbon dioxide diffuses into the plasma and the erythrocyte, where carbonic *acid forms* and then *dissociates* into hydrogen and bicarbonate ions:

$$H_2O + CO_2 \rightarrow H_2CO_3 \rightarrow H^+ + HCO_3^-$$

Because the initial concentration of HCO_3^- in

the blood is greater than that of H_2CO_3, the relative increase in $[H_2CO_3]$ is greater than the increase in $[HCO_3^-]$, so the ratio $[HCO_3^-]/[\alpha P_{CO_2}]$ is decreased, and pH decreases. In the lungs, CO_2 leaves the blood, and pH increases again. For these reasons, venous blood is more acidic than arterial blood. Normally, the lungs eliminate carbon dioxide as fast as it is produced by the tissues, so the Pa_{CO_2} and pH of arterial blood remain relatively constant.

The lungs can cause quite rapid changes in blood pH by increasing or decreasing the elimination of CO_2. When ventilation increases in relation to CO_2 production (*hyperventilation*), the ratio $[HCO_3^-]/[\alpha Pa_{CO_2}]$ increases, and pH increases. Conversely, when ventilation decreases in relation to CO_2 production (*hypoventilation*), the ratio $[HCO_3^-]/[\alpha Pa_{CO_2}]$ decreases, and pH decreases. Figure 50–3, a pH/bicarbonate diagram, shows how the $[HCO_3^-]$ and pH change as the Pa_{CO_2} of the blood increases or decreases.

Metabolic Production of Fixed Acids Requires That the Kidneys Eliminate Hydrogen Ions and Conserve HCO_3^- ·

When *fixed acids* are added to the blood, for example, from protein metabolism, the hydrogen ions are buffered in part by HCO_3^-. Buffering results in conversion of HCO_3^- to H_2CO_3

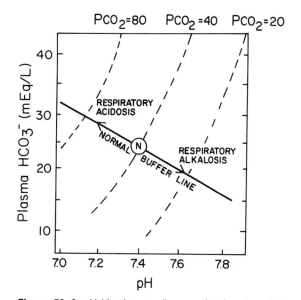

Figure 50–3. pH bicarbonate diagram showing the effect of increasing and decreasing P_{CO_2} on pH and bicarbonate concentration. *N* represents the normal arterial blood composition. As P_{CO_2} increases or decreases, the change in pH and bicarbonate is predicted by the normal buffer line.

and CO_2, which is eliminated from the lungs. Fixed acids are produced continuously and would consume the body's HCO_3^- if the kidneys were not continually regenerating HCO_3^-.

The role of the kidneys in acid-base balance is described in Chapter 42. Large amounts of HCO_3^- are filtered daily through the glomerulus and subsequently reabsorbed in the renal tubule. The amount of HCO_3^- reabsorbed depends on the amount filtered, which is determined by plasma $[HCO_3^-]$ and *glomerular filtration rate*, and the rate of hydrogen ion secretion by renal tubular cells. The latter is controlled in part by the acid-base status of the body.

When P_{CO_2} is high, the reaction

$$H_2O + CO_2 \rightarrow H_2CO_3 \rightarrow H^+ + HCO_3^-$$

within the *renal tubules* is driven to the right, producing more hydrogen ions for secretion into the *tubular lumen* and HCO_3^- for return to the blood. When P_{CO_2} is low, hydrogen ion elimination and, therefore, HCO_3^- reabsorption decrease.

Ammonia, an important buffer in the distal renal tubule, is produced by the action of *glutaminase* on *glutamine*. In acidosis, the activity of glutaminase increases, resulting in increased ammonia production, an increased buffering capacity of the renal tubular fluid and, therefore, increased ability to eliminate hydrogen ions.

ACID-BASE DISTURBANCES

Acid-Base Abnormalities Accompany Many Diseases, and the Restoration of Normal Blood pH Should Be a Consideration When Treating Any Disease

In most diseases, the buffering systems, lungs, and kidneys keep pH within tolerable limits, but in severe disease these homeostatic mechanisms may be inadequate, and life-threatening changes in pH can occur. In diagnosing and treating acid-base abnormalities, it is important to realize that there is a primary abnormality that causes the change in blood pH. Because the body then attempts to correct the abnormality, the clinician must disentangle the data to find the primary cause of the problem. The primary problems are excessive accumulation or elimination of carbon dioxide (respiratory abnormalities), or the excessive accumulation or elimination of fixed acids (metabolic abnormalities).

In Respiratory Acidosis, the Accumulation of Carbon Dioxide in the Blood Decreases pH

Respiratory acidosis is caused by *alveolar hypoventilation*, which can be due to damage to or depression of the respiratory control centers, injury to the respiratory pump (e.g., fractured ribs or bloated abdomen), or severe respiratory disease that either obstructs the airways or excessively stiffens the lungs. Alveolar hypoventilation means that CO_2 produced by the tissues is eliminated incompletely by the lungs, so blood P_{CO_2} increases.

Consider what would happen to blood pH and $[HCO_3^-]$ in the absence of other buffers, such as hemoglobin. The reaction

$$H_2O + CO_2 \rightarrow H_2CO_3 \rightarrow H^+ + HCO_3^-$$

is driven to the right by the accumulating CO_2; H^+ accumulates and pH decreases. Bicarbonate accumulates simultaneously, but the amount is too small to keep the ratio $[HCO_3^-]/[\alpha P_{CO_2}]$ at a normal value of 20/1. If sufficient H^+ (40 nEq/L) is produced to decrease pH from 7.4 to 7.1, the 40 nEq/L of HCO_3^- also produced only increases plasma $[HCO_3^-]$ from 24 mEq/L to 24.00004 mEq/L, an amount insufficient to measure.

In the blood, other nonbicarbonate buffers not only take up H^+ produced by the accumulation of CO_2, but also cause accumulation of HCO_3^- as follows:

$$H_2O + CO_2 \rightarrow H_2CO_3 \rightarrow H^+ + HCO_3^-$$
$$\downarrow$$
$$H^+ + Hb^- \rightarrow HHb$$

By buffering H^+, Hb^- pulls the first reaction to the right, so HCO_3^- accumulates. This accumulation of bicarbonate, shown on the *normal buffer line* in the pH/HCO_3^- diagram (see Fig. 50–3), is still insufficient to maintain a normal $[HCO_3^-]/[\alpha P_{CO_2}]$ ratio, and pH decreases. Therefore, the characteristic findings in acute respiratory acidosis are an elevated arterial Pa_{CO_2}, decreased pH, and a minor increase in $[HCO_3^-]$.

To facilitate the clinical interpretation of acid-base status, investigators use the terms *total buffer base, base excess,* and *base deficit.* Total buffer base is the sum of the concentrations of available blood buffers. Base excess and deficit refer to an increase or decrease, respectively, in total buffer base. In acute respiratory acidosis, total buffer base does not change, because the accumulation of HCO_3^- is accompanied by an equivalent decrease in the concentration of other buffers such as Hb^-. Therefore, there is no base excess or base deficit.

The ideal way to correct respiratory acidosis is to restore alveolar ventilation. Because this option is not open to the animal, other means to correct pH must be used. The elevated P_{CO_2} and decreased pH increase hydrogen ion and NH_3 production in the kidney. This increases elimination of hydrogen ion in the urine and generates new HCO_3^-, so plasma $[HCO_3^-]$ increases; the ratio $[HCO_3^-]/[\alpha P_{CO_2}]$ and pH are restored toward normal. The newly generated HCO_3^- adds to the total buffer base and, therefore, causes a base excess. Figure 50–4 shows how this accumulating HCO_3^- restores pH toward normal, even though P_{CO_2} remains constant.

In Respiratory Alkalosis, the Loss of Carbon Dioxide from the Blood Increases pH

Respiratory alkalosis is caused by *alveolar hyperventilation*, which is due to stimulation of the chemoreceptors by hypoxia or to stimulation of intrapulmonary receptors by lung injury or inflammation. Overly vigorous use of a ventilator can cause hyperventilation in an anesthetized animal. Carbon dioxide is eliminated faster than it is produced by the tissues, so blood P_{CO_2} decreases. The changes in blood chemistry are the inverse of those in respiratory acidosis:

$$H_2O + CO_2 \leftarrow H_2CO_3 \leftarrow H^+ + HCO_3^-$$
$$\uparrow$$
$$H^+ + Hb^- \leftarrow HHb$$

As CO_2 is eliminated, H_2CO_3 is formed from H^+ and HCO_3^-, so pH increases and $[HCO_3^-]$ decreases. Hydrogen ion is supplied by release from nonbicarbonate buffers, such as hemoglobin. The net result of these processes is that Pa_{CO_2} decreases, pH increases, and $[HCO_3^-]$ decreases and is replaced by other buffers. There is no change in total buffer base. The increase in the ratio $[HCO_3^-]/[\alpha P_{CO_2}]$ increases pH.

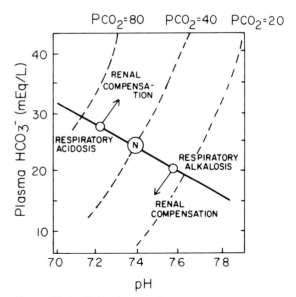

Figure 50–4. pH bicarbonate diagram showing the effects of respiratory acidosis and alkalosis on pH bicarbonate and P_{CO_2} of arterial blood as P_{CO_2} increases. In acute respiratory acidosis, the changes in pH and bicarbonate are predicted by the normal buffer line. Renal compensation leads to an accumulation of bicarbonate, which increases pH, while P_{CO_2} remains constant. In respiratory alkalosis, reverse changes occur.

Figure 50–4 shows the increase in pH and decrease in $[HCO_3^-]$ as P_{CO_2} decreases. In order to restore pH toward normal, hyperventilation must be stopped, or the kidneys must eliminate $[HCO_3^-]$. The latter occurs because the low P_{CO_2} and alkalosis reduce hydrogen ion and NH_3 production by the kidney. When hydrogen ion is not produced in sufficient amounts to capture all the filtered HCO_3^-, the latter spills into the urine.

In Metabolic Acidosis, the Accumulation of Fixed Acids or Loss of Buffer Base Decreases Blood pH

Metabolic acidosis is the most common acid-base abnormality. During metabolism, there is a continuous production of fixed acids. An increase in their production or failure of hydrogen ion elimination by the kidneys are the causes of metabolic acidosis. Increased production of fixed acids occurs as a result of protein catabolism or ketone production in starvation, or as a result of anaerobic metabolism and lactic acidosis. *Diarrhea* can cause metabolic acidosis also, because excessive amounts of HCO_3^- (buffer) are lost in the feces. In ruminants, excessive feeding of carbohydrates can lead to increased H^+ production in the rumen (*rumen acidosis*). The hydrogen ions that are absorbed cause metabolic acidosis.

The accumulation of H^+ in the blood is buffered by HCO_3^- and other buffers. The CO_2 produced by the combination of H^+ and HCO_3^- is lost through the lungs. The loss of buffer base gives rise to a base deficit, and the HCO_3^- depletion decreases the $[HCO_3^-]/[\alpha P_{CO_2}]$ ratio, so pH decreases (Fig. 50–5).

The decrease in pH accompanying metabolic acidosis is a stimulus to ventilation. The increase in alveolar ventilation eliminates carbon dioxide, which decreases P_{CO_2}, restoring the $[HCO_3^-]/[\alpha P_{CO_2}]$ ratio and pH toward normal. This is shown in Figure 50–5. As the P_{CO_2} decreases, pH and HCO_3^- decrease along a line that parallels the normal buffer line. Ultimate restoration of normal acid-base balance requires the restoration of the depleted base by the kidney or by therapy with intravenous fluid containing buffers, such as bicarbonate.

Metabolic Alkalosis Is Caused by the Excessive Elimination of Hydrogen Ions or by the Intake of Base, Such as HCO_3^-

The most common cause of *metabolic alkalosis* is *vomiting*, in which gastric contents rich in

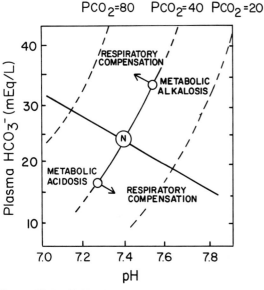

Figure 50–5. pH bicarbonate diagram showing the effect of metabolic acidosis and alkalosis on pH, bicarbonate and P_{CO_2} of arterial blood. In uncompensated metabolic acidosis, there is a decrease in bicarbonate, which leads to a decrease in pH, while P_{CO_2} remains constant. Respiratory compensation results in a decrease in P_{CO_2}, with a subsequent increase in pH and movement of data points parallel to the normal buffer line. In metabolic alkalosis, the reverse changes occur.

hydrogen ion are lost from the body. In ruminants, torsion and dilation of the *abomasum* cause metabolic alkalosis, because hydrogen ions are trapped in the abomasum. Low levels of potassium in the blood (*hypokalemia*) can also cause metabolic alkalosis. When extracellular fluid potassium levels are low, potassium moves from the intracellular to the extracellular fluid and is replaced in part by hydrogen ions that are lost from the plasma, resulting in alkalosis. In addition, hydrogen ion is lost into the urine instead of potassium.

The loss of hydrogen ion from the body frees buffer, so the plasma $[HCO_3^-]$ and total buffer base increase. The ratio $[HCO_3^-]/[\alpha P_{CO_2}]$, pH, and base excess all increase (see Fig. 50–5). The increase in pH reduces the drive to ventilate; alveolar ventilation decreases, so P_{CO_2} increases. This restores the ratio $[HCO_3^-]/[\alpha P_{CO_2}]$ toward normal and, hence, the pH returns toward normal (see Fig. 50–5).

Respiratory Compensations Occur Rapidly; Renal Compensations Occur Over Several Hours

The discussion of acid-base disturbances has shown that the lungs compensate for metabolic problems, and the kidneys compensate for respiratory problems. Because the *chemoreceptors* respond almost immediately to changes in blood pH, and because changes in ventilation rapidly change P_{CO_2}, respiratory compensation for metabolic acid-base problems occurs almost immediately. For this reason, it is rare to observe "pure" metabolic acidosis or alkalosis without a respiratory compensation. The response of the kidneys to a respiratory acid-base disturbance is less rapid. Changes in ammonia and HCO_3^- production occur over about 24 hours.

As compensatory mechanisms restore pH toward normal, there is less "error signal" to drive the compensatory mechanisms, so it is rare for these to return pH to normal. For example, in metabolic acidosis, the low pH drives ventilation to decrease P_{CO_2}. However, as pH returns to normal, the respiratory drive is reduced; therefore, compensation is rarely complete.

Hydrogen and Potassium Ions Are Interrelated in Acid-Base Homeostasis

The interrelationship between potassium and hydrogen ions was pointed out as a cause of metabolic alkalosis. In this situation, a lack of intracellular potassium causes the movement of hydrogen ions into the cells, making the blood more alkaline. In the kidney, the lack of potassium for secretion is made up by hydrogen ions, so the urine is acid when the blood is alkaline. This is, however, not the only example of potassium/hydrogen ion interaction. When there is an excess of hydrogen ion in the blood, such as occurs in metabolic acidosis, hydrogen ion replaces potassium in the cells. The potassium that spills from the cells into the extracellular space would cause life-threatening *hyperkalemia* were it not lost through the kidneys. When the acidosis is subsequently corrected, hydrogen ion leaves the cells and must be replaced by potassium from the extracellular fluid. The intracellular potassium deficit is frequently much greater than can be supplied by the extracellular pool, so it may be necessary to supply potassium to prevent hypokalemia when treating metabolic acidosis.

The Diagnosis of Acid-Base Disturbances Depends on Interpretation of Measurements of Arterial Blood pH and P_{CO_2} from Which [HCO_3^-] and Total Buffer Base Are Calculated

Arterial samples must be used to determine the respiratory component of an acid-base abnormality, and samples must be obtained anaerobically to prevent the loss of CO_2 from the blood. Arterial P_{CO_2} (Pa_{CO_2}) and pH are measured with electrodes in a blood-gas machine. Plasma [HCO_3^-] and total buffer base are determined from normograms or frequently from a built-in program in the blood-gas analyzer.

When analyzing blood-gas data, it is useful to ask the following questions:

1. Is the sample acidotic (pH < 7.4) or alkalotic (pH > 7.4)?
2. What is the respiratory component (is Pa_{CO_2} high, low, or normal) and will it explain the pH?
3. What is the metabolic component (is there a base excess or deficit) and will it explain the pH?
4. How can (1) and (2) be combined to explain the data, bearing in mind that compensations rarely return pH to normal?

Examples are provided in Table 50–1.

Over the Years, a Large Number of Terms Have Been Used to Explain Acid-Base Balance

Some of these terms are defined below:

Anion gap: In the blood, the total cation concentration [$Na^+ + K^+ + Mg^{2+} + Ca^{2+}$] should approximately equal the total anion concentration [$HCO_3^- + Cl^-$]. Usually, the total cations exceed the total anions, so there is an anion gap. This gap is due to unaccounted-for anions from fixed acids, such as lactate. In metabolic acidosis, the anion gap increases because of increased production of fixed acids.

Standard bicarbonate: The plasma [HCO_3^-] when P_{CO_2} is equal to 40 torr is known as standard bicarbonate. Plasma [HCO_3^-] can change as a result of respiratory and metabolic disturbances. If [HCO_3^-] is measured when P_{CO_2} is normal (i.e., 40 torr), the increase or decrease in [HCO_3^-] from normal is due to metabolic disturbances.

Total carbon dioxide (TCO$_2$): Carbon dioxide is present in the blood in solution and as carbamino compounds, but largely as HCO_3^-. Total CO_2 can be measured by adding an acid to the blood and collecting the evolved CO_2,

Table 50–1
EXAMPLES OF BLOOD-GAS ABNORMALITIES

pH	Pa_{CO_2}	HCO_3^-	Base Excess	Base Deficit	Diagnosis
7.4	40	24	0	0	Normal
7.26	60	27	0	0	Uncompensated respiratory acidosis
7.38	60	36	9	0	Partially compensated respiratory acidosis
7.2	40	15	0	12	Uncompensated metabolic acidosis
7.35	22	11	0	12	Partially compensated metabolic acidosis
7.45	20	13	0	11	Partially compensated respiratory alkalosis
7.55	40	34	11	0	Uncompensated metabolic alkalosis
7.2	50	19	0	9	Combined metabolic and respiratory acidosis
7.6	20	20	0	0	Uncompensated respiratory alkalosis
7.3	20	9	0	15	Partially compensated metabolic acidosis

which comes primarily from HCO_3^-. Changes in TCO_2 should be interpreted as changes in $[HCO_3^-]$.

CLINICAL CORRELATIONS

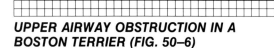

UPPER AIRWAY OBSTRUCTION IN A BOSTON TERRIER (FIG. 50–6)

HISTORY □ A Boston terrier exhibits signs of severe respiratory distress. It has difficulty inhaling and makes a snoring sound during inhalation. The effort of walking magnifies the distress. An arterial blood sample reveals that Pa_{CO_2} equals 80 torr, pH equals 7.3, HCO_3^- equals 39 mEq/L, and base excess equals 10 mEq/L.

CLINICAL EXAMINATION □ Examination reveals excessively narrowed (stenotic) nares and excessive folds of tissue in the soft palate, the latter occluding the glottis. The larynx and trachea appear normal.

Reconstructive surgery is performed on the dog to enlarge the nares and remove the excessive tissues from the palate. Two weeks after surgery, respiratory distress is much less. Blood gas analysis reveals that Pa_{CO_2} equals 45 torr, pH equals 7.39, HCO_3^- equals 27 mEq/L, and base excess equals 2 mEq/L.

COMMENT □ The animal is acidotic with an elevated Pa_{CO_2} and base excess. Only the high Pa_{CO_2} will explain the acidosis; therefore, the dog has respiratory acidosis. The increase in $[HCO_3^-]$ (normal = 24 mEq/L) is due primarily to creation of new HCO_3^- (a base excess) by the kidneys and indicates the condition is of at least several days' duration. Respiratory acidosis is due to alveolar hypoventilation resulting from the upper airway obstruction. Surgery corrects the obstruction and alleviates the hypoventilation. This returns pH to a more normal value. Two weeks after surgery, the base excess has been virtually eliminated.

TORSION OF THE ABOMASUM IN A COW (SEE FIG. 50–6)

HISTORY □ A Holstein cow gave birth 2 weeks ago and became inappetent 2 days ago. Over the last 12 hours she has become depressed, and her right flank is distended. Ex-amination shows she is depressed and dehydrated. Her extremities are cold. Rectal examination reveals a large fluid-filled organ between the rumen and the right abdominal wall. A fluid sample obtained percutaneously from the distended organ is chloride-rich and very acid. An arterial blood sample shows that Pa_{CO_2} equals 50 torr, pH equals 7.6, HCO_3^- equals 50 mEq/L, and base excess equals 24 mEq/L.

COMMENT □ The history and physical findings are typical of a dilatation or torsion of the abomasum. This condition occurs shortly after parturition in dairy cows fed high levels of concentrates and chopped feeds. The abomasum distends and may rotate, so its inlet and outlet are obstructed. Fluid rich in chloride and hydrogen ion continues to be secreted and is trapped in the abomasum. The loss of hydrogen ion from the blood results in a base excess and causes the metabolic alkalosis. The alkalosis depresses ventilation, which elevates Pa_{CO_2}. This is a compensation to restore pH toward normal.

NEONATAL DIARRHEA IN A CALF (SEE FIG. 50–6)

HISTORY □ A 2-week-old calf has profuse diarrhea. It is depressed and cold, its eyes are sunken and dull, and it lies in a pool of feces. The calf's hematocrit is 65, pH equals 7.2, Pa_{CO_2} equals 30 torr, HCO_3^- equals 12 mEq/L, and base deficit equals 15 mEq/L.

COMMENT □ The calf shows typical clinical signs of severe dehydration as a result of excessive fluid loss in the feces. Fluid loss from the intravascular compartment reduces blood volume and cardiac output. To maintain blood pressure, vasoconstriction occurs in the extremities, which therefore have less blood flow and become cold. The loss of fluid from the interstitial space causes the dry eyes and muzzle, the sunken eyes, and inelastic skin. The increased hematocrit of 65 (normal 45) confirms the dehydration.

Feces contain HCO_3^-, and its excessive loss causes a base deficit and a decrease in pH. In addition, poor tissue perfusion results in lactic acidosis. Because the acidosis is not respiratory in origin, it is a metabolic acidosis. The acidosis stimulates ventilation, which reduces Pa_{CO_2} in an attempt to correct pH.

PRIMARY CAUSE	BLOOD CHEMISTRY	COMPENSATIONS	BLOOD CHEMISTRY
Upper Airway Obstruction 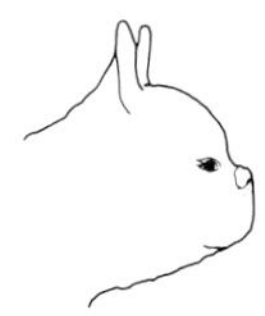 Upper airway obstructed Too little ventilation CO_2 retained	1) Elevated P_{CO_2} 2) Decreased $[HCO_3^-]$ $\quad [\alpha P_{CO_2}]$ 3) Decreased pH	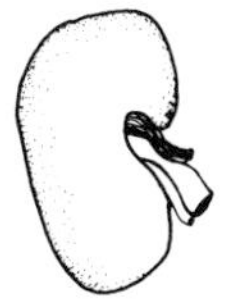 Increased H^+ elimination Increased HCO_3^- retention 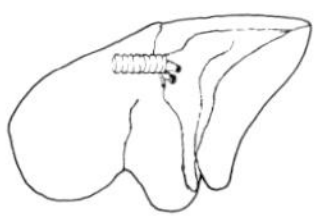 Increased drive to ventilate Animal cannot respond because airway is obstructed	1) Increased $[HCO_3^-]$ 2) Base excess 3) Increased $\dfrac{[HCO_3^-]}{[\alpha P_{CO_2}]}$ 4) pH approaches normal
Abomasal Torsion 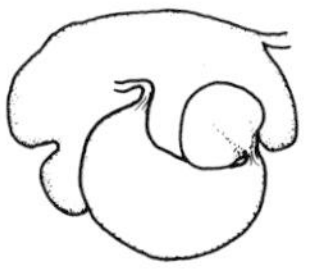 H^+ accumulates in the distended abomasum	1) Increased $[HCO_3^-]$ as less H^+ to buffer 2) Base excess 3) Increased $\dfrac{[HCO_3^-]}{[\alpha P_{CO_2}]}$ 4) Increased pH	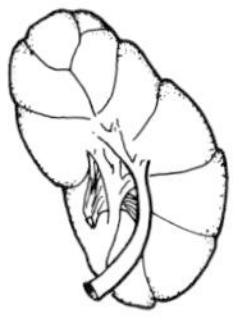 Decreased H^+ production Decreased HCO_3^- retention Increased HCO_3^- elimination 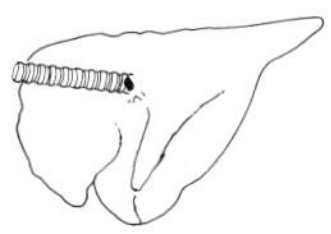 Decreased ventilatory drive Decreased CO_2 elimination	Restoration of $[HCO_3^-]$ 1) Increased P_{CO_2} 2) Decreased $\dfrac{[HCO_3^-]}{[\alpha P_{CO_2}]}$ 3) pH approaches normal

Figure 50–6. Diagrammatic representation of the acid-base changes initiated by upper airway obstruction, abomasal torsion, and neonatal calf diarrhea.

PRIMARY CAUSE	BLOOD CHEMISTRY	COMPENSATIONS	BLOOD CHEMISTRY
<u>Neonatal Diarrhea</u>	1) Decreased $[HCO_3^-]$ 2) Base deficit 3) Decreased $\dfrac{[HCO_3^-]}{[\alpha P_{CO_2}]}$ 4) Decreased pH	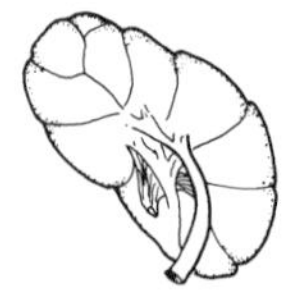	
Fluid and electrolyte, including HCO_3^- loss in feces		Increased H^+ elimination Complete $[HCO_3^-]$ reabsorption Increased $[HCO_3^-]$ production	Restoration of $[HCO_3^-]$
		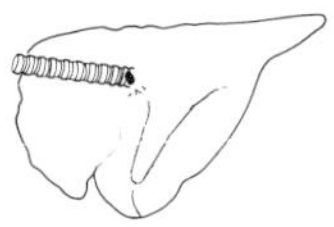	1) Decreased P_{CO_2} 2) Increased $\dfrac{[HCO_3^-]}{[\alpha P_{CO_2}]}$ 3) pH approaches normal
		Increased ventilatory drive Increased CO_2 elimination	

Figure 50–6. Continued

Bibliography

Cohen JJ, Kaiser JP: Acid-base. Boston, Little, Brown and Co, 1982, pp 3–94.

Davenport HW: The ABC of Acid-Base Chemistry, 6th ed. Chicago, University of Chicago Press, 1974.

Gamble JL: Acid-Base Physiology: a Direct Approach. Baltimore, Johns Hopkins University Press, 1982, pp 1–54.

Stubbs DW: The physiology of acid-base balance. *In* Brown AM, Stubbs DW (eds): Medical Physiology. New York, John Wiley & Sons, 1983, pp 567–597.

PRACTICE QUESTIONS FOR CHAPTER 50

1. Elevated Pa_{CO_2}, low pH, and no base excess/deficit are characteristic of

   a. acute respiratory acidosis.
   b. acute respiratory alkalosis.
   c. metabolic acidosis.
   d. metabolic alkalosis.
   e. None of the above

2. Elevated Pa_{CO_2}, alkaline pH, and base excess are characteristic of

   a. chronic respiratory acidosis.
   b. chronic respiratory alkalosis.
   c. metabolic acidosis.
   d. metabolic alkalosis.
   e. None of the above

3. Low Pa_{CO_2}, acid pH, and base deficit are characteristic of

   a. chronic respiratory acidosis.
   b. acute respiratory alkalosis.
   c. metabolic acidosis.
   d. metabolic alkalosis.
   e. None of the above

4. The most likely acid-base disturbance to be found in a dog at the top of Mount McKinley (height = 20,320 ft = 6,353 miles) is

   a. respiratory acidosis.
   b. respiratory alkalosis.
   c. metabolic acidosis.
   d. metabolic alkalosis.
   e. None of the above

5. The distal tubule of the kidney affects acid-base balance by

a. altering the pK of the HCO_3^-/H_2CO_3 buffer.
b. changing $[H_2CO_3]$ in the Henderson-Hasselbalch equation.
c. generating new HCO_3^-.
d. producing ammonia to buffer H^+.
e. Both c and d

6. Which of the following buffers will be most effective in blood (pH = 7.4)?

a. HX/X$^-$, pK = 4.2, plentiful
b. HY/Y$^-$, pK = 7.2, scarce
c. HZ/Z$^-$, pK = 9.6, scarce
d. HW/W$^-$, pK = 7.6, plentiful
e. HA/A$^-$, pK = 10.2, plentiful

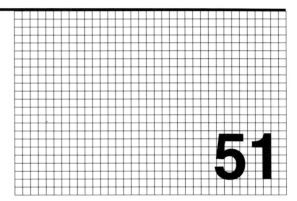

Thermoregulation

INTRODUCTION

1. The temperature of a tissue is one of the major factors affecting its function
2. Depending on the strategies used to regulate body temperature, animals are classified as homeotherms or poikilotherms
3. Body temperature depends on the balance between heat input and output

HEAT EXCHANGE WITH THE ENVIRONMENT

1. Heat loss by convection occurs when a fluid is warmed by the body
2. Heat loss by conduction occurs when the body is in contact with a cooler surface
3. Emission of infrared radiation and its absorption by cooler objects can be a major form of heat loss
4. Evaporative heat loss occurs when the water in sweat, saliva, and respiratory secretions is converted into water vapor

HEAT PRODUCTION

1. Heat is a byproduct of all metabolic processes
2. Shivering produces heat by muscle contraction
3. Nonshivering thermogenesis is an increase in basal metabolic rate, caused especially by the oxidation of fats, to produce heat

HEAT TRANSFER IN THE BODY

1. Because tissues are poor conductors, heat is most effectively transferred in the blood
2. Countercurrent heat exchange along the limbs conserves body heat

TEMPERATURE REGULATION

1. Mammals and birds normally regulate the inputs and outputs of heat to maintain body temperature within a narrow limit
2. Temperature-sensitive receptors are located in the central nervous system, in the skin, and in some internal organs
3. Information from central and peripheral heat-sensitive neurons is integrated in the hypothalamus to regulate heat-losing or conserving mechanisms

INTEGRATED RESPONSES

1. The responses to heat stress are peripheral vasodilation and increased evaporative cooling
2. The responses to cold stress are peripheral vasoconstriction, piloerection, and increased metabolic heat production by shivering and nonshivering thermogenesis
3. Fever is an elevation of body temperature, which results from an increase in the set point brought about by pyrogens

HEAT STROKE, HYPOTHERMIA, AND FROSTBITE

1. Heat stroke occurs when heat production or input exceeds heat output, so body temperature rises to dangerous levels
2. Hypothermia occurs when heat output exceeds heat production, so body temperature decreases to dangerous levels
3. Frostbite occurs when ice crystals form in the tissues of the extremities

INTRODUCTION

The Temperature of a Tissue Is One of the Major Factors Affecting Its Function

Because body function is the result of chemical and physical processes that are sensitive to changes in temperature, animals use a variety of strategies to regulate the temperature of their tissues. If *body temperature* is allowed to decrease too far, metabolic processes are slowed to such an extent that body function ceases. Conversely, an increase in temperature beyond the normal value of about 38°–45°C can denature proteins and also be fatal.

Depending on the Strategies Used to Regulate Body Temperature, Animals Are Classified as Homeotherms or Poikilotherms

Poikilotherms are also called *cold-blooded animals,* because their body temperature varies with the temperature of the environment. However, this does not mean that these animals have no control over their body temperature; rather, they use behavioral methods to prevent major changes in their temperature. The lizard basks on a sun-baked rock to increase its temperature early in the morning and hides beneath the rock later in the day to prevent overheating. Veterinarians are sometimes asked to advise on the management of captive poikilotherms; it is important to remind owners to provide supplemental heat if they want their animals to be active at the cooler times of the year.

Mammals and birds are *homeotherms;* they maintain a constant body temperature in the presence of considerable changes in environmental temperature. Although the maintenance of a constant temperature allows mammals to live in a wide variety of environments and to remain active during the cold times of the year, it is not without cost. Homeotherms must maintain a high metabolic rate just to provide the heat necessary to maintain body temperature. This requires a high energy intake and, therefore, almost constant foraging for food. Poikilotherms require much less energy and are better able to survive times of food shortage. Because most veterinarians are primarily concerned with mammals and birds, this chapter focuses on the maintenance of a normal body temperature by homeotherms.

Body Temperature Depends on the Balance Between Heat Input and Output

Heat inputs to the body are from metabolism and from external sources (Fig. 51–1). Once food energy is ingested, heat is produced at all stages of the metabolic processes, and eventually all food energy is converted into heat, which is dissipated into the environment and radiated into space. Some of this conversion of food energy into heat occurs during metabolism, some when external work is performed. When the running horse pulls a cart, the leg muscles work to overcome the effects of gravity and to oppose the friction in the muscles and joints and in the cart wheels. The heat produced in this process must be dissipated

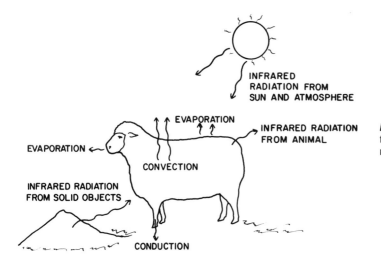

Figure 51-1. Diagrammatic representation of the heat inputs and outputs between a mammal and the environment.

to the environment if body temperature is to remain constant.

Animals gain heat from the environment when ambient temperature exceeds body temperature, and when they are exposed to *radiant heat* sources. The latter occurs when an animal is exposed to sunlight or is placed close to solid objects that are warmer than body temperature.

Heat is lost to the environment by *radiation* from the body surface to a cooler object; by *convection* as the surrounding air or water is warmed by the body; by *evaporation* of respiratory secretions, sweat or saliva; and by *conduction* to cooler surfaces with which the animal is in contact. A small amount of heat is also lost with urine and feces.

Many of the metabolic heat sources, such as the liver, heart, and limb muscles, are remote from the skin, which is the site of heat loss. Therefore, it is necessary to transfer heat between these sites. Body tissues are poor conductors, so heat is mainly transferred by convection in the circulation.

HEAT EXCHANGE WITH THE ENVIRONMENT

Heat Loss by Convection Occurs When a Fluid Is Warmed by the Body

When the air or water in contact with the skin is heated, it flows away, thereby exposing the skin to cooler fluids. Because water has a higher *specific heat* than air, water-dwelling animals lose more heat by convection than terrestrial mammals. The amount of heat lost by convection depends on the *thermal gradient* (temperature difference) between the skin of the animal and the fluid overlying the skin; a bigger thermal gradient results in more heat loss. In *natural convection,* the warmed air or water rises from the surface of the animal, because it is less dense than the cooler fluid. In *forced convection,* cooler fluid is moved over the skin surface by a breeze or current, or simply because the limbs and animal are moving. Forced convection is more effective than natural convection as a mode of heat loss, because the thermal gradient is maintained by the constant renewal of the cooler air or water. Young or small animals left in a cool draft can quickly lose a lot of body heat by convection and should be protected from such situations.

The thermal gradient for heat loss can be altered by changes in skin blood flow and the amount of *insulation* separating the animal from the environment. Increasing blood flow to the skin raises skin temperature and, therefore, heat loss, whereas a reduction in skin blood flow reduces heat loss. Hair traps air and impairs convection. The thickness of the layer of hair can be altered by *piloerection* (making the hair stand up) and by growing a thicker hair coat in winter. The thick layer of blubber in sea mammals also provides a layer of insulation. Reducing body surface area by curling up in a ball or by huddling with other animals also reduces convective heat loss.

Heat Loss by Conduction Occurs When the Body Is in Contact with a Cooler Surface

Because animals usually do not lie on cool surfaces for long periods, conduction is not usually a major form of heat loss. There are, however, some situations in which conductive heat loss can lead to hypothermia. A cold, stainless steel surgery table can form a heat sink for a small anesthetized bird or mammal. Insulation or a heat source should be provided for such animals. Similarly, newborn piglets can lose a lot of heat into a cold concrete floor on which they are lying. Adult pigs cool themselves by conduction when they wallow in cool mud puddles.

Emission of Infrared Radiation and Its Absorption by Cooler Objects Can Be a Major Form of Heat Loss

All solid objects emit invisible *electromagnetic radiation* in the *infrared* range. Warm objects emit on a shorter *wavelength* and more emissions per unit time than cool objects. When these emissions strike another object, some are absorbed and thus transfer heat. Although all objects emit radiant heat, the net heat transfer is from warm to cool objects. It is important to realize that radiant heat loss can occur even when the animal is surrounded by a thermally neutral or warm environment. Heat can be lost from an animal to the uninsulated walls of a building even though the intervening air is warm.

Evaporative Heat Loss Occurs When the Water in Sweat, Saliva, and Respiratory Secretions Is Converted into Water Vapor

The evaporation of 1 L of water into water vapor requires 580 *kilocalories* (kcal), which must be supplied by the body. Evaporative heat loss occurs continuously by the diffusion of water through the skin and by loss of water vapor from the respiratory tract. This water loss is obligatory, but under thermal stress, evaporative cooling can increase greatly, because *sweat glands* are activated or the animal begins to *pant*. Evaporative heat loss becomes increasingly important as the ambient temperature approaches body temperature; it is the only form of heat loss available once ambient temperature exceeds body temperature. The effectiveness of evaporation is reduced as the *relative humidity* increases and the air becomes more saturated with water vapor.

Sweating occurs from two types of coiled, tubular *sweat glands* located in the dermis. *Apocrine* glands found in association with hair

follicles produce a protein-containing secretion, whereas *eccrine* glands produce an aqueous secretion. All placental mammals except rodents and lagomorphs have sweat glands, but in the dog and pig they are poorly developed and of little use in thermoregulation. In hoofed mammals, thermoregulatory sweating is from apocrine glands; eccrine glands are for thermoregulation in primates. Secreted sweat has an ionic composition similar to plasma. As it passes to the surface along the duct, its composition is altered by the reabsorption of ions. If secretion rates are low, almost all the sodium and chloride are absorbed and followed by water. Therefore, the sweat reaching the skin is a concentrated solution of urea, lactic acid, potassium ions, and in the case of hoofed mammals, protein. When secretion rates are high, less sodium and chloride are absorbed, more water is lost, and the other constituents are consequently diluted. In hot environments, acclimatization increases the sweating rates and, because of increased secretion of *aldosterone*, most of the sodium and chloride is reabsorbed before the sweat reaches the skin.

In most species, sweating is under the control of *sympathetic cholinergic* nerve fibers, but in the horse, control seems to be through *sympathetic adrenergic* fibers. Apocrine glands are stimulated to secrete by an increase in circulating *catecholamines*.

Panting is one mode of increasing evaporation from the respiratory tract. Small tidal volumes are moved at rapid frequency (200 breaths per minute) over the respiratory dead-space. Panting occurs close to the resonant frequency of the respiratory system, so the work of breathing is minimized and does not add to the heat load. Vascular engorgement of the respiratory and oral mucosa and increased salivation increase heat loss through evaporation. By ventilating primarily dead-space, severe hyperventilation and respiratory alkalosis are avoided. In birds, *gular flutter* is another method of increasing air flow over the respiratory dead-space. Even in mammals, such as the horse, that do not pant, evaporative heat loss from the respiratory tract probably increases during prolonged exercise, because dead-space ventilation increases.

Mammals vary in the relative importance of different modes of evaporative heat loss. In horses and cattle, sweating is the major form of evaporative heat loss. Sheep sweat, but panting is also of considerable importance. The dog relies almost totally on panting. Even

Table 51–1
HEAT PRODUCTION BY MAJOR FOOD TYPES

	Heat production (kcal)		
Food Types	*Per Gram of Food*	*Per Liter of O_2 Consumed*	*Per Liter of CO_2 Produced*
Carbohydrates	4.1	5.05	5.05
Fat	9.6	4.75	6.67
Proteins (to urea)	4.2	4.46	5.57

in small rodents, which neither pant nor sweat, evaporation is increased by smearing saliva or water on the fur.

HEAT PRODUCTION

Heat Is a Byproduct of All Metabolic Processes

Table 51–1 shows the amount of heat produced by the metabolism of carbohydrates, fats, and proteins. The *basal metabolic rate* is the rate of energy metabolism measured under minimal stress while the animal is fasting. Basal metabolic rate is greater in homeotherms than in poikilotherms, because the former need to generate heat to maintain body temperature. The metabolic rate per kilogram body weight is greater in small than in larger mammals (Fig. 51–2). This is in part necessitated by the greater surface-to-volume ratio of smaller animals. The relatively greater surface area of small animals provides a bigger area for heat loss.

An increase in metabolic rate, as occurs for example during exercise, results in increased heat production and, therefore, necessitates increased heat loss from the animal. An in-

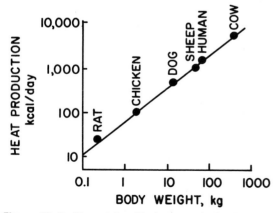

Figure 51–2. The relationship between body size and metabolic rate.

crease in body temperature also increases metabolic rate.

Shivering Produces Heat by Muscle Contraction

Shivering is one method to increase the metabolic production of heat. Antagonistic groups of limb muscles are activated so that they produce no useful work. The chemical energy used in shivering appears as heat. Shivering increases blood flow to the limb muscles, which increases heat loss from the body, but overall there is a net increase in body heat.

Nonshivering Thermogenesis Is an Increase in Basal Metabolic Rate, Caused Especially by the Oxidation of Fats, to Produce Heat

When animals are chronically exposed to cold, they develop the ability to increase metabolic heat production without shivering (nonshivering thermogenesis). The increase in metabolism is mediated through an increase in thyroxine secretion and the calorigenic effects of catecholamines on lipids. Brown fat is a specialized vascular, mitochondria-rich fat found between the scapulae of smaller mammals. Catecholamines increase metabolism in all fats, but particularly in brown fat, and the heat produced is distributed around the body in the blood.

HEAT TRANSFER IN THE BODY

Because Tissues Are Poor Conductors, Heat Is Most Effectively Transferred in the Blood

Because heat is produced primarily in muscles and the liver, and is eliminated at the skin and the respiratory tract, it is necessary to distribute heat around the body. Tissues have a *thermal conductivity* similar to cork; therefore, conduction is not an efficient means of heat redistribution.

The blood perfusing a metabolically active organ collects heat and transfers it to cooler parts of the body. Redistribution of blood flow can deliver heat preferentially to certain body regions or can allow regions to cool when the maintenance of the temperature of the brain and major viscera (*core temperature*) is threatened. When the ambient temperature is high, skin blood flow is increased in two ways. The *arterioles* of skin vascular beds dilate, resulting in increased capillary blood flow. In addition, *arteriovenous anastomoses* open in the limbs, ears, and muzzle. This greatly increases the total blood flow along the limb, and the increased heat delivery warms the limb tissues toward core temperature. Conversely, under cold stress, skin vascular beds vasoconstrict and arteriovenous anastomoses close, so that skin and limb temperatures decrease. This results in reduced heat loss from the skin and in a gradient of temperatures along the limb (Fig. 51–3). Under severe cold stress, the skin temperature of the extremities can approach ambient temperature. Interestingly, the lipids in the limb extremities have a lower melting point than in the core, so fats do not solidify in extreme cold stress.

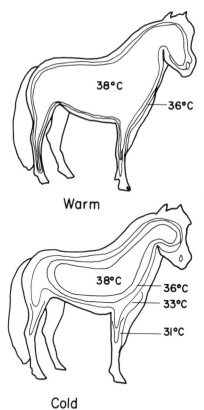

Figure 51–3. Diagrammatic representation of the distribution of temperatures in a pony under warm and cold environmental conditions. Under warm conditions, the core body temperature extends down into the limbs and close to the skin surface of the animal. Under cold conditions, vasoconstriction in the peripheral blood vessels results in a gradient of temperatures between the core and the extremities. The core temperature is maintained only in the abdomen, thorax, and brain of the animal. The more peripheral tissues are allowed to cool considerably.

Countercurrent Heat Exchange Along the Limbs Conserves Body Heat

When environmental temperature is high, the blood perfusing the skin vascular beds returns to the core through superficial veins. Under cold conditions, limb blood flow returns to the core through deep veins that accompany arteries (Fig. 51–4). Heat is transferred by countercurrent exchange from the warm arterial blood to the cooler venous blood and thereby returned to the core of the body.

A similar countercurrent exchange of heat occurs in a *carotid rete* in sheep and some other ungulates. In the latter system, the carotid artery forms a rete bathed in a sinus of venous blood that has drained the nasal cavity. The colder venous blood from the nose cools the arterial blood supplying the brain and protects the temperature of the brain. This mechanism becomes important during exercise, when the increase in ventilation aids in cooling the blood that drains from the nose. As a result, the arterial blood carrying heat from the exercising muscles is cooled before it enters the brain.

TEMPERATURE REGULATION

Mammals and Birds Normally Regulate the Inputs and Outputs of Heat to Maintain Body Temperature Within a Narrow Limit

It has been customary to measure body temperature as a first part of the clinical examination of mammals. This is because body temperature is maintained within fairly narrow limits despite big variations in ambient conditions. In disease the ability to regulate temperature can be impaired by, for example, dehydration. In addition, infectious and other agents produce pyrogens that can increase body temperature. Table 51–2 gives the normal range of *rectal temperature* in some common domestic mammals. Rectal temperature is somewhat lower than the core temperature of the animal, and changes in rectal temperature lag behind changes in core temperature. However, rectal temperature is conveniently measured in domestic mammals and provides a useful indication of core temperature.

In well-hydrated animals living in temperate climates, the range of normal temperature is quite narrow. Mammals living in hot arid climates tolerate a wider range of temperature, allowing body temperature to decrease during

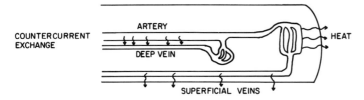

Figure 51–4. Diagrammatic representation of a limb showing the arterial supply and venous drainage by deep veins and superficial veins. Under warm conditions, blood perfuses the more peripheral capillary beds and heat is lost to the environment through the skin. Blood returns from the superficial vascular beds through the superficial veins, which provides an additional source of heat loss. Under cold conditions peripheral vasoconstriction occurs, and the blood flow to the limb is directed to the deeper vascular beds and returns to the trunk through the deep veins. Countercurrent heat exchange between the arteries and veins conserves body heat.

the cool nights, so more heat can be absorbed during the ensuing hot day.

In order to maintain temperature within narrow limits, the animal must regulate its heat inputs and outputs. Clearly, the inputs and outputs cannot be equal at all times. During exercise, for example, heat production exceeds heat loss. Heat is stored in the body and then dissipated when exercise ceases. The specific heat of body tissues is similar to water; therefore, quite large amounts of heat can be stored without a potentially lethal increase in temperature.

Temperature-Sensitive Receptors Are Located in the Central Nervous System, in the Skin, and in Some Internal Organs

To regulate body temperature the animal has a variety of *temperature sensors* at various locations within the body. These sensors relay information to the brain, which then initiates mechanisms to either increase or decrease heat loss or production.

Numerous heat-sensitive neurons are located in the preoptic area of the hypothalamus. These neurons increase their firing rate in response to minor increases in local temperature. In addition, heating of this area immediately initiates heat-losing mechanisms, such as peripheral vasodilation and sweating.

These observations suggest that this region of the brain may be the main center for temperature regulation. Other hypothalamic and mid-brain neurons decrease their firing in response to heat, and yet others increase firing in response to cold. All these temperature-sensitive neurons are monitoring brain or core temperature.

When an animal is exposed to cold, there can be considerable heat loss before a change in core temperature occurs. Therefore, it is advantageous to have temperature-sensitive neurons located in the skin, so environmental temperature changes are detected before they threaten core temperature. The most numerous temperature-sensitive neurons in the skin respond to cold, so chilling of the skin can initiate heat conservation before core temperature decreases. *Skin cold receptors* are particularly sensitive to the rate of decrease of temperature. For this reason, shivering can occur after exercise as the skin is rapidly cooled by sweat evaporation, despite the fact that core temperature may be normal or slightly elevated. Skin receptors sensitive to heat also exist and can initiate heat loss when skin temperature rises.

Temperature-sensitive neurons also exist at various locations in the viscera. Drinking large volumes of cold fluids may stimulate cold receptors in the gastrointestinal (GI) system, so body heat is conserved.

Table 51–2
RECTAL TEMPERATURE OF DOMESTIC MAMMALS IN °C

Species	Average	Range
Cat	38.6	38.1–39.2
Cattle (beef)	38.3	36.7–39.1
Cattle (dairy)	38.6	38.0–39.3
Dog	38.9	37.9–39.9
Donkey	37.4	36.4–38.4
Goat	39.1	38.5–39.7
Horse	37.7	37.2–38.2
Pig	39.2	38.7–39.8
Sheep	39.1	38.5–39.9

Information from Central and Peripheral Heat-Sensitive Neurons Is Integrated in the Hypothalamus to Regulate Heat-Losing or Conserving Mechanisms

Figure 51–5 shows the *feedback control* mechanisms for the regulation of body temperature. Central integration of the information from various receptors occurs in the anterior hypothalamus. The neural circuitry that would bring about such integration is shown in Figure 51–6. Information from central tempera-

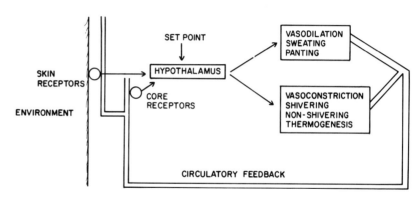

Figure 51–5. Feedback control mechanisms for the regulation of body temperature. Temperature receptors in the skin and the core relay information to the hypothalamus, which adjusts the responses to conserve and produce heat or to lose heat. The results of these responses are relayed to the receptors through the circulation.

ture receptors seems to predominate over information from skin and visceral receptors, so a rise in core temperature of only 0.5°C causes a sevenfold increase in skin blood flow; a modest decrease in core temperature initiates vasoconstriction and shivering. The effect of central receptors is about 20-fold greater than the effect of peripheral receptors.

In the regulation of body temperature, the hypothalamus behaves as if it has a normal *set point*. When core temperature rises above the set point, heat-losing mechanisms are initiated, and when temperature decreases, heat conservation or production begins. Information from peripheral receptors modifies the set point, so shivering begins at a higher core temperature when the skin is cool than when the skin is warm. Similarly, sweating is initiated at a higher core temperature when the skin is cool than when the skin is warm.

INTEGRATED RESPONSES

The Responses to Heat Stress Are Peripheral Vasodilation and Increased Evaporative Cooling

For all mammals and birds, there exists an environmental temperature at which body temperature can be maintained in a normal range primarily by vasomotor mechanisms (Fig. 51–7). This *zone of thermoneutrality* varies with the metabolic rate and the amount of

insulation. Clearly, the pig, which lacks fur, has a higher thermoneutral temperature than the sheep with thick wool. In the thermoneutral zone, body temperature can be regulated by vasomotor mechanisms that increase or decrease skin blood flow and, therefore, change the amount of heat loss by convection and radiation.

When a homeotherm is exposed to heat stress the initial response is vasodilation, which increases skin and limb blood flow. The resulting increase in skin temperature and the extension of core temperature down the limbs increase the temperature gradient between the skin and the environment, resulting in more heat loss by radiation and convection (see Fig. 51–3).

If vasodilation cannot maintain a normal temperature, evaporative cooling is increased by sweating or panting, or both. Evaporative cooling is the only method of heat loss available once environmental temperature exceeds skin temperature and is most effective when relative humidity is low. Figure 51–8 shows that cows at −10°C lose 10% of their heat by evaporation, but as ambient temperature rises to 30°C they lose 80% by evaporation. As relative humidity rises, it becomes increasingly difficult to lose heat; therefore, exercise in hot humid conditions is likely to cause heat exhaustion.

Animals also use behavioral methods to resist heat stress. These methods, which in-

Figure 51–6. Circuitry proposed for neuroregulation of body temperature. Peripheral (*P*), spinal (*Sp*), and hypothalamic (*Hy*) temperature sensors connect with neurons innervating networks that ultimately control heat-dissipating, heat-conserving, or heat-generating mechanisms. Pluses and minuses refer to excitatory and inhibitory inputs. (From Eckert R, Randall D: Animal Physiology: Mechanisms and Adaptations. New York, WH Freeman and Co, 1983, p 734; adapted from Bligh J: Temperature Regulation in Mammals and Other Vertebrates. Amsterdam, North Holland Publishing Co, 1973, p 190.)

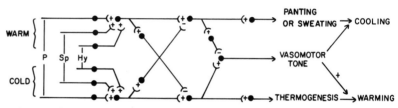

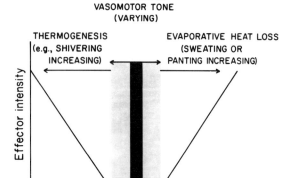

Figure 51–7. Relationship between thermoregulatory responses and core temperature. The set point for temperature regulation is indicated by the black shaded zone. On either side of this set point there exists a zone in which temperature can be maintained by vasomotor responses (gray areas). As the core temperature deviates more dramatically from the set point there is a need to increase thermogenesis or to increase evaporative heat loss. (Modified with permission from Bligh J: Temperature regulation in environmental physiology of animals. *In* Bligh J, Cloudsley-Thompson JL, Macdonald AG (eds): Environmental Physiology of Animals. Oxford, Blackwell Scientific Pub, 1976, p 426.

clude seeking of shade, standing in water, or wallowing in mud, are not available to intensively managed livestock. The producer must assume increased responsibility for the animals' comfort and survival.

The Responses to Cold Stress Are Peripheral Vasoconstriction, Piloerection, and Increased Metabolic Heat Production by Shivering and Nonshivering Thermogenesis

As ambient temperature decreases, homeotherms initially conserve heat by peripheral vasoconstriction. This sets up a temperature gradient along the limbs and reduces skin temperature, so there is little temperature gradient for radiation and convective heat loss (see Fig. 51–3). Piloerection provides insulation and also decreases heat loss. Further cold stress initiates increases in metabolic heat production by shivering or nonshivering thermogenesis. All adult mammals can shiver, and neonates born in an advanced state of development, such as lambs and foals, can also shiver. Puppies and other less-developed neonates cannot shiver and rely on the warmth of mother and the nest to protect them from cooling. *Brown fat* occurs in some of the latter

neonates and in other small mammals, and provides a source of nonshivering thermogenesis.

Chronic exposure of animals to cold results in increased secretion of *thyroxine* and an increase in basal metabolism, which increases basal heat production. When animals are housed where they receive natural light, there is an increased thickness of the hair coat at cold times of the year. Hair growth is the result of decreasing day length as cold weather approaches.

Fever Is an Elevation of Body Temperature, Which Results from an Increase in the Set Point Brought About by Pyrogens

Pyrogens are extremely potent substances that act on the hypothalamus to increase the set point for body temperature. Pyrogens include bacterial products such as *endotoxin* from gram-negative bacteria and proteins produced by body tissues, particularly white blood cells. The exogenous pyrogens, such as endotoxin, can stimulate leukocytes to produce endogenous pyrogen.

When the hypothalamus is exposed to pyrogen, the set point increases, and the animal initiates responses to conserve and produce heat until the body temperature reaches the new set point (Fig. 51–9). Shivering, peripheral vasoconstriction, piloerection, and huddling behavior are all characteristic of the onset of fever. Once the new set point is reached, the animal maintains its body at the new temperature until the pyrogen is metabolized and production ceases. When this occurs, the set point decreases back to normal, and the animal initiates heat-losing mechanisms to decrease body temperature.

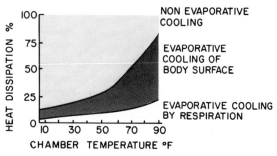

Figure 51–8. Methods of heat loss used by a cow as the environmental temperature increases. At low temperatures, the majority of heat loss is by nonevaporative cooling, but as the environmental temperature increases, the cow becomes increasingly dependent on evaporation.

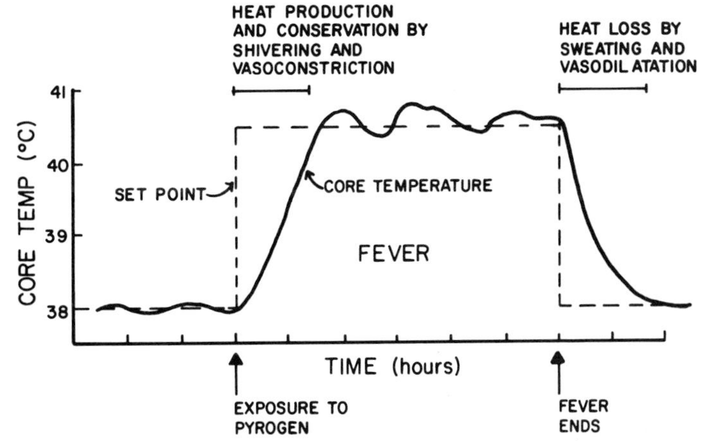

HEAT PRODUCTION AND CONSERVATION BY SHIVERING AND VASOCONSTRICTION

HEAT LOSS BY SWEATING AND VASODILATATION

Figure 51–9. The events involved in fever. Exposure to a pyrogen increases the set point of the temperature-regulating system. This results in heat production and conservation to elevate body temperature, resulting in fever. When the fever ends, the set point decreases, and heat must be lost from the body.

The local production of *prostaglandin-E₁* in the hypothalamus is thought to be involved in increasing the set point. For this reason, cyclo-oxygenase blocking drugs, such as aspirin or phenylbutazone, are used to treat fever.

HEAT STROKE, HYPOTHERMIA, AND FROSTBITE

Heat Stroke Occurs When Heat Production or Input Exceeds Heat Output, so Body Temperature Rises to Dangerous Levels

In hot, humid weather it is difficult for animals to lose heat, because evaporative cooling cannot occur effectively. Strenuous exercise under these conditions can lead to a dangerous increase in body temperature. Similarly, when dogs are closed in cars in the sun, their panting saturates the air with water vapor, so further heat loss is impossible. As body temperature rises, metabolic rate increases, and more heat is produced. In addition, panting or sweating, or both, leads to dehydration and circulatory collapse, so it is more difficult to transfer heat to the skin. Once body temperature exceeds 41.5–42.5°C, cellular function is seriously impaired, and consciousness is lost.

Hypothermia Occurs When Heat Output Exceeds Heat Production, so Body Temperature Decreases to Dangerous Levels

Small or sick animals exposed to a cold environment may lose more heat than they can generate, and body temperature may decrease to a point that the animal can no longer invoke heat-regulating mechanisms. The ability of the hypothalamus to regulate body temperature is greatly impaired below a temperature of 29°C. Cardiac arrest occurs at around 20°C. Neonates seem to be able to withstand cooling more than adults, and apparently comatose lambs, piglets, and puppies can be warmed and revived.

Frostbite Occurs When Ice Crystals Form in the Tissues of the Extremities

In extremely cold conditions, when the extremities are vasoconstricted to conserve heat, the tissues may cool below the freezing point of tissue water. Ice crystals disrupt the tissue integrity, and gangrene can result. Frostbite is normally prevented by the fact that vascular smooth muscle dilates in extreme cold, causing an inflow of warm blood. The latter mechanism apparently works adequately in animals that winter outdoors in northern climates.

CLINICAL CORRELATIONS

INFLUENZA IN PIGS

HISTORY □ You are called to examine a group of 3-month-old pigs in an intensively managed fattening house. The group of 20 pigs is in a pen, and there are multiple similar pens within the barn. In the last 2 days in this particular pen of pigs, the animals have been reluctant to eat and have started huddling together. The owner has observed that the outer pigs in the huddle continually try to burrow toward the center of the pile of pigs, and that the ones on the outside appear to be trembling. At this time the remaining pigs in the barn are not affected. When you enter the barn and the pigs are disturbed, they begin sneezing and coughing, and some are reluctant to move.

CLINICAL EXAMINATION □ Three pigs are caught, and the rectal temperature is found to be 41°C (normal = 38.5°C). There is a nasal discharge, and the conjunctiva and nasal mucosa are congested. You treat the pigs with antibiotics, and over a period of several days the pigs recover; however, the disease spreads progressively through the remaining pens in the fattening house. All pigs show the same clinical signs, and no pigs die from the disease. Blood samples are taken for virus neutralization tests from the acutely affected pigs 2 weeks after they have recovered.

The diagnosis from the viral neutralization test is swine influenza, which has a high morbidity, but low mortality.

COMMENT □ The clinical signs produced by this disease are largely due to the development of fever. The pigs examined had an elevated body temperature, because the infection had adjusted the set point of the thermoregulatory center to a high value. In order to raise body temperature to this new value, the pigs huddled together, and the pigs on the outside shivered in order to generate metabolic body heat. Once the infection is overcome and pyrogen is metabolized, the behavior of the pigs changes; they need to lose heat, so they separate and move around the pens more freely.

HEAT STROKE IN A BOSTON TERRIER

HISTORY □ At 3:00 P.M. on a 95°F day in August, you receive a frantic phone call from a client. The client went to a shopping mall and left her car parked in the lot. She had her Boston terrier with her, but because she thought she would only be a few minutes, she left the dog in the car. While in the mall, she was delayed by an uncooperative clerk at a store. When she came out of the store, her dog was prostrate with its tongue hanging out of its mouth, and it was unresponsive to the owner's attentions. You instruct the owner to bring the dog over to the practice immediately and to drive with the windows open for the one-half-mile trip.

CLINICAL EXAMINATION □ On arrival at the clinic, the dog is laid on the examining table, where it fails to respond to its name. Its mouth is open, its tongue is distended, and its mucous membranes are dry. Body temperature is 42.2°C.

From the history, the animal's body temperature, and its lack of response, you diagnose heat stroke. The dog is placed in a bath of cool water, and fluids are administered intravenously. Within 5–10 minutes, the dog begins to look around, and recognizes its owner. The water bath treatments are continued for 2 hours, at which time the body temperature is close to normal. The dog remains in the hospital overnight and is then discharged to a delighted owner the next day.

COMMENT □ The temperature inside a car parked in the hot sun rises rapidly to above body temperature. At this time, the only mechanism available to lose heat is evaporation of water from the respiratory tract, which the dog attempts by panting and salivating. For a while this is an effective means of losing heat, but water vapor is transferred to the air in the car and progressively saturates the atmosphere with water. As the per cent saturation of the air increases, evaporation and, therefore, heat loss become more and more difficult. Eventually the animal cannot lose heat, and body temperature begins to rise. Once body temperature exceeds 41.5–42.5°C, animals may lose consciousness. In addition, the panting results in dehydration and reduces the ability of the dog to deliver heat from the core of the body to the extremities. Brachycephalic dogs, such as Boston terriers, have an added disadvantage in temperature regulation. The short nose and convolutions in the wall of the pharynx increase the work of breathing, especially when the dogs pant. This increased work is an additional source of body heat, and the anatomy of the upper airway probably makes evaporative cooling less effective.

Therapy for this condition is to reduce body temperature and to restore circulatory function as rapidly as possible. For this reason, the dog is placed in a cool water bath to reduce body temperature, and also receives intravenous fluids to rehydrate it by expanding its circulatory volume and restoring the ability of the circulation to redistribute heat within the body.

Bibliography

Eckert R, Randall D: Animal Physiology. New York, WH Freeman and Co, 1983, pp 689–744.

Hales JRS: The partition of respiratory ventilation of the panting ox. J Physiol 188: 45–68, 1966.

Heller HC, Crawshaw LI, Hammel HT: The thermostat of vertebrate animals. Sci Am 239: 102–113, 1978.

Taylor CR, Schmidt-Nielsen K, Raab JL: Scaling of energetic costs of running to body size in mammals. Am J Physiol 219: 1104–1107, 1970.

PRACTICE QUESTIONS FOR CHAPTER 51

1. Sweating is an effective cooling mechanism because

   a. sweat secretion produces heat, which is carried to the skin surface in the sweat.
   b. conversion of sweat into water vapor requires heat, which is supplied by the skin.
   c. sweat dripping from the body carries away large amounts of heat.
   d. reabsorption of ions from sweat requires heat energy from the skin.

2. In the cold, animals both conserve and produce heat. Which of the following is a method of heat conservation?

   a. Shivering
   b. Brown fat metabolism
   c. Increased thyroxine secretion
   d. Countercurrent heat exchange in the limbs
   e. All of the above

3. Which of the following methods of heat loss can occur in an animal (body temperature = 38°C) standing in a room (temperature = 40°C) with relative humidity of zero? The walls of the room have a temperature of 30°C.

   a. Convection and evaporation
   b. Convection and radiation
   c. Evaporation and radiation
   d. Radiation alone
   e. Convection, evaporation, and radiation

4. Which of the following describes thermoregulation?

   a. Temperature receptors in both the brain and skin can initiate thermoregulatory responses.
   b. The brain temperature receptors have a greater influence on thermoregulation than do skin receptors.
   c. The core temperature at which shivering begins is lower if the skin is cold than if the skin is warm.
   d. Skin cooling can initiate shivering even if core temperature is normal.
   e. All of the above

5. Which of the following correctly describe fever?

   a. It results when the set point for body temperature decreases.
   b. It is accompanied by sweating to lose heat as body temperature rises.
   c. It is accompanied by shivering to gain heat as body temperature decreases once pyrogens are metabolized.
   d. It can be initiated by pyrogens from bacteria or leukocytes
   e. All of the above

PRACTICE ANSWERS

Chapter 1

1. b 2. c 3. d 4. b 5. d

Chapter 3

1. e 2. c 3. a 4. b 5. a

Chapter 4

1. d 2. b 3. b 4. b 5. b

Chapter 5

1. d 2. a 3. d 4. d 5. e

Chapter 6

1. c 2. c 3. a 4. c 5. b

Chapter 7

1. a 2. d 3. e 4. c 5. e

Chapter 8

1. a 2. c 3. b 4. e 5. e

Chapter 9

1. b 2. e 3. c 4. e 5. a

Chapter 10

1. c 2. d 3. a 4. c 5. d

Chapter 11

1. c 2. d 3. b 4. b 5. a

Chapter 12

1. d 2. b 3. a 4. d 5. a

Chapter 13

1. b 2. d 3. b 4. d 5. e

Chapter 14

1. b 2. a 3. a 4. c 5. a

Chapter 15

1. b 2. d 3. d 4. a 5. a

Chapter 16

1. c 2. b 3. b 4. a

Chapter 17

1. c 2. e 3. a 4. e 5. a

Chapter 18

1. e 2. a 3. c 4. b 5. c

Chapter 19

1. b 2. b 3. e 4. d 5. a

Chapter 20

1. b 2. d 3. e 4. e 5. a

Chapter 21

1. b 2. e 3. c 4. a 5. a

Chapter 22

1. d 2. a 3. a 4. b 5. c

Chapter 23

1. d 2. b 3. c 4. a 5. b

Chapter 24

1. e 2. b 3. c 4. a 5. a

Chapter 25

1. b 2. d 3. c 4. e 5. e

Chapter 26

1. d   2. d   3. e   4. b   5. d

Chapter 27

1. d   2. b   3. c   4. e   5. d

Chapter 28

1. d   2. a   3. b   4. a   5. c

Chapter 29

1. b   2. c   3. e   4. b   5. a   6. c

Chapter 30

1. d   2. c   3. a   4. c   5. d

Chapter 31

1. c   2. d   3. e   4. b   5. a

Chapter 32

1. c   2. c   3. c   4. e   5. b

Chapter 33

1. a   2. c   3. b   4. d   5. d

Chapter 34

1. d   2. d   3. d   4. c   5. c

Chapter 35

1. b   2. b   3. a   4. e   5. d

Chapter 36

1. e   2. e   3. c   4. e   5. f   6. f

Chapter 37

1. c, d, e, f   2. b   3. c   4. e   5. f

Chapter 38

1. d   2. d   3. b   4. c   5. c

Chapter 39

1. c   2. d   3. a   4. d   5. e

Chapter 40

1. a   2. d   3. b   4. e   5. b

Chapter 41

1. a   2. e   3. c   4. d   5. e

Chapter 42

1. c   2. a   3. a   4. c   5. b

Chapter 43

1. d   2. c   3. e   4. b   5. e   6. c   7. e

Chapter 44

1. d   2. e   3. a   4. b   5. d

Chapter 45

1. a   2. e   3. a   4. a   5. c   6. d

Chapter 46

1. e   2. b   3. d   4. a   5. c   6. e

Chapter 47

1. e   2. a   3. d   4. b   5. e   6. b

Chapter 48

1. b   2. d   3. c   4. b   5. a

Chapter 49

1. b   2. d   3. e   4. a   5. d   6. b   7. c

Chapter 50

1. a   2. d   3. c   4. b   5. e   6. d

Chapter 51

1. b   2. d   3. c   4. e   5. d

INDEX

Note: Page numbers in *italics* refer to illustrations; page numbers followed by *t* refer to tables.